Ambulatory Surgical Nu

EDITOR

THERESA L. CLIFFORD, DNP, RN, CPAN, CAPA, FASPAN, FAAN

Perioperative Nurse Manager
Surgical Services
Northern Light Mercy Hospital
Portland, Maine
Nurse Liaison for Special Projects
American Society of PeriAnesthesia Nurses
Cherry Hill, New Jersey

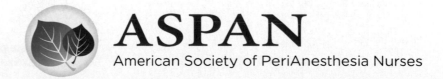

ASPAN
American Society of PeriAnesthesia Nurses

Elsevier
3251 Riverport Lane
St. Louis, Missouri 63043

Senior Content Strategist: Yvonne Alexopoulos
Director, Content Development: Ellen Wurm-Cutter
Senior Content Development Specialist: Kathleen Nahm
Publishing Services Manager: Julie Eddy
Project Manager: Becky Langdon
Design Direction: Bridget Hoette

Printed in India

Last digit is the print number: 9 8 7 6 5 4 3 2 1

Working together
to grow libraries in
developing countries

www.elsevier.com • www.bookaid.org

Contributors

Sylvia J. Baker, MSN, RN, CPAN (retired), FASPAN
Professional Development Specialist (Retired)
Professional Development
Northwestern Medicine, DeKalb, Illinois

Carol Bell, BS, RN
Clinical Nurse Manager
St. Thomas Surgicare, Nashville, Tennessee

Amy Berardinelli, DNP, RN, NE-BC, CPAN, FASPAN
Clinical Nurse Manager
Department of Surgical Services
Akron Children's Hospital, Akron, Ohio
Associate Editor
AORN Journal
AORN, Denver, Colorado

Katrina L. Bickerstaff, BSN, RN, CPAN, CAPA
Staff Nurse
Nursing, Tucson Medical Center Integrative Pain Center, Tucson, Arizona

Brandy Rae Boissoneault, MSN, RN
Clinical Nurse Lead
ACU/PACU
Northern Light Mercy Hospital, Portland, Maine

Elizabeth Card, DNP, APRN, FNP-BC, CPAN, CCRP, FASPAN, FAAN
Research Nurse Practitioner
Medicine and Anesthesiology
Vanderbilt University Medical Center, Nashville, Tennessee

LeighAnn Chadwell, MSN, RN, NE-BC
Manager
Holding Room, PACU, Radiology Recovery
Monroe Carell Jr. Children's Hospital at Vanderbilt, Nashville, Tennessee

Theresa L. Clifford, DNP, RN, CPAN, CAPA, FASPAN, FAAN
Perioperative Nurse Manager
Surgical Services
Northern Light Mercy Hospital, Portland, Maine
Nurse Liaison for Special Projects
American Society of PeriAnesthesia Nurses, Cherry Hill, New Jersey

Jacque Crosson, DNP, RN, CPAN, FASPAN
Perianesthesia (Preop/PACU) Nurse Manager
Surgical Services
Mayo Clinic Hospital, Phoenix, Arizona
Standards & Guidelines SWT Coordinator
American Society of PeriAnesthesia Nurses, Cherry Hill, New Jersey
Member Education Committee
ERAS USA, Beverly, Massachusetts

Denise Faraone Diaz, MSN, BA, RN, CPAN, CAPA
Clinical Nurse
Post-Anesthesia Care Unit
Thomas Jefferson University Hospital, Philadelphia, Pennsylvania

Ronda E. Dyer, MSN, BSPA, RN, CPAN, CAPA, CNE
Staff Registered Nurse
PACU
Adventist Medical Center-Hanford, Hanford, California

Helen C. Fong, DNP, RN, CPAN, PHN, FASPAN
Health Facilities Evaluator Nurse
Center for Health Care Quality
California Department of Public Health, Sacramento, California

Terri A. Gray, MEd, BSN, CPAN
Nursing Professional Development Specialist
PAS/POHA/PACU
Corewell Health Beaumont Hospital, Dearborn, Michigan

Regina Hoefner-Notz, MS, BSN, RN, CPAN, CPN, FASPAN
Clinical Manager
Perioperative Services
Children's Hospital Colorado, Aurora, Colorado

Kristen Lemorie, MSN, RN, AGCNS-BC, CPAN, CAPA
Clinical Nurse Specialist
Ambulatory Procedures
University of Michigan Health, Michigan Medicine, Ann Arbor, Michigan

Myrna Eileen Mamaril, DNP, RN, NEA-BC, CPAN, CAPA, FAAN, FASPAN
Clinical Nurse Specialist
Perioperative Services
Johns Hopkins Hospital, Baltimore, Maryland

Deborah Moengen, BSN, RN, CPAN
Director of Perioperative Clinical Practice
Surgical Services
CentraCare, South Haven, Minnesota
Region 3 ASPAN Board of Directors 2019-2023
American Society of PeriAnesthesia Nurses, Cherry Hill, New Jersey

Rachel Moses, MSN, RN, CPAN
Manager Innovation and Research
Institute of Nursing Excellence
Peace Health Sacred Heart Medical Center, Springfield, Oregon

Denise O'Brien, DNP, RN, ACNS-BC, CPAN (retired), CAPA (retired), FASPAN, FCNS, FAAN
Perianesthesia Clinical Nurse Specialist
Consultant
Self-Employed, Ypsilanti, Michigan

Valerie A. Pfander, DNP, APRN, ACCNS-AG, CPAN, FASPAN
Clinical Nurse Specialist
Perianesthesia
Munson Medical Center, Traverse City, Michigan
Assistant Professor
College of Nursing
Michigan State University, Lansing, Michigan

Carre Smith, MSN, RN
Supervisor of Surgical Services
Porter Medical Center
University of Vermont Health Network, Middlebury, Vermont

Daphne Stannard, PhD, RN, CNS, NPD-BC, FCCM
Emerita Associate Professor
School of Nursing
San Francisco State University, San Francisco, California

Angelique Weathersby, MSN, MBA, RN
Assistant Unit Manager
PACU
Arrowhead Regional Medical Center,
    Colton, California

**Hazel Marie Barmore Wiegert, MAN,
BSN, RN, CPAN, CAPA**
Staff Registered Nurse
PACU
Hennepin Healthcare, Minneapolis,
    Minnesota

**Antoinette A. Zito, MSN, CPAN,
FASPAN**
Perioperative Education Program
    Coordinator
Surgical Services
Cleveland Clinic, Cleveland, Ohio

Reviewers

Aliah Anderson, BSN, RN
El Paso Children's Hospital
El Paso, Texas

Linda J. Beagley, MS, RN, CPAN, FASPAN
Manager Nursing Education
Swedish Hospital, NorthShore
  University HealthSystem
Chicago, Illinois

Joni M. Brady, DNP, RN, PMGT-BC, CAPA
International Collaboration of
  PeriAnaesthesia Nurses Chair, Board
  of Directors
Nurse Consultant
Alexandria, Virginia

Rebekah Hill, MS, AGACNP-BC
Certified Registered Nurse Practitioner
UPMC Pinnacle
Harrisburg, Pennsylvania

Beverly J. Jackson, BSN, RN
Neuromodulation VNS Therapy Case
  Manager
Texas A&M University Corpus Christi
Corpus Christi, Texas

Ilana Jesse, BSN, RN
Colorado Springs, Colorado

Wesla DeShun Johnson-Brown, BSN
OR Services, Preoperative Services
Cedars Sinai Medical Center
Los Angeles, California

Minhas Moon, APRN FNP-C, MSN, RN, BSN
University of Miami Health System
Miami, Florida

Natalie Mae Peters, BN, RN, AHPRA
Registered Nurse
La Trobe University
Wodonga, Victoria, Australia

Carrie Quinn, MSN, RN, ACCNS-AG, CPAN, CNL-BC
Clinical Nurse Specialist, Perioperative
  Services
Penn Medicine Lancaster General
  Health
Lancaster, Pennsylvania

Lisa Paula Rudd, BSN, MSN, CNE, PCCN, RN-BC (Cardiac-Vascular/ Medical Surgical Nursing)
Registered Nurse
Cone Health
Greensboro, North Carolina

Don Sim, MSN, RN, PHN, CCRN, CHFN
Stanford Hospital
Palo Alto, California

Alyssa J. Straight, BSN, RN
Preoperative/PACU Registered Nurse
Texas Orthopedics Surgery Center
Austin, Texas

Acknowledgments

I am grateful to every individual contributor, each a friend and colleague, who willingly participated in the development of this book. All have helped to shape this book into a contemporary text, and it is hoped that this book, with their contributions, will inform and guide perianesthesia nurses as their roles expand in the setting of ambulatory surgery.

It is impossible to produce a quality nursing reference book without expert partners in the publishing industry. I would like to particularly thank Kathleen Nahm, senior content development specialist, and Yvonne Alexopoulos, senior content strategist, who patiently and generously kept me focused on the task at hand in spite of the challenges that the pandemic imposed on the team of writers and the process. Thank you both for your guidance and support.

Theresa L. Clifford, DNP, RN, CPAN, CAPA, FASPAN, FAAN

Preface

The first nursing textbook that focused on the ambulatory setting for perianesthesia nurses, *Ambulatory Surgical Nursing*, was published in 1993 and updated in 2000.[1] It was written by perianesthesia nursing expert Nancy Burden and her associates and provided a foundation for the specialty of outpatient surgery. The text delivered guidance to nurses on patient care and surgical procedures that were being introduced in the ambulatory surgery setting. The exciting option of providing clinical care and defining the standards of practice in this setting was emerging at the time for perianesthesia nurses. The first outpatient surgery center had opened in 1970, and by the 1990s, care options in the outpatient setting were expanding at incredible rates.[2] Now, several decades later, the medical sciences and related technologies continue to evolve in and change the outpatient surgical landscape.

In 1998 there were 2634 freestanding surgery centers,[1] but in 2023, there were an estimated 8469 ambulatory surgery centers in the United States, representing an increase of more than 200%.[3] As mentioned, the first ambulatory surgery practice was introduced in 1970 in Sioux City, Iowa. Dr. Ralph Waters realized that the movement of certain procedures to the outpatient setting would help reduce costs, improve efficiencies, and enhance patient satisfaction.[2] These goals continue to drive the movement of procedures into the outpatient setting. The differences in the past several decades have included the opportunity to provide safe and high-quality care to higher-acuity patients having more complex surgeries in the outpatient setting.

Today's perianesthesia nurse, whether working in the clinical setting of a hospital-based surgical practice, an office-based surgery practice, or an outpatient ambulatory surgery center, faces a myriad of challenges previously not imagined. The science of anesthesia has advanced clinical practice. Both propofol and sevoflurane have emerged as top choices for short-acting anesthetics with a rapid onset, which are perfect for the outpatient setting.[4] The discovery and utilization of readily metabolized agents along with technological advances have supported the development and introduction of clinical guidelines for reducing common postanesthesia complications such as unwanted sedation, minimizing postoperative nausea and vomiting, and improving pain and comfort management. Multimodal techniques improve the quality of clinical care while providing services to patients with multiple co-morbidities, resulting in enhanced safety and optimal outcomes for higher-risk patients (e.g., obese patients, extremely young or old patients). Robotic surgical programs are moving into outpatient practices, providing surgeons and patients with a wider array of options for surgical care.

Readers of this book will find seven primary sections exploring topics ranging from leadership theories to clinical inquiry to challenges in pain management. Each chapter includes learning objectives related to the content, a case study to stimulate critical thinking, and chapter highlights to summarize key points. In addition, evidence-based practice boxes identify a brief but relevant topic. As the twenty-first century has unfolded, emerging issues have presented a variety of learning opportunities, as well as challenges, for the perianesthesia nurse. Today's perianesthesia nurse should be familiar with the principles of enhanced recovery protocols and theories related to preoperative optimization. The perianesthesia nurse now encounters patients with substance use disorders with greater frequency than ever before. Embracing diversity, equality, and inclusion has become crucial for establishing a healthy relationship with a patient and family during the short time in which the nurse provides care. Lastly, nurses need information on the different types of surgical specialties now being offered in the in the outpatient setting, as well as the procedural and interventional practices, such as cardiovascular and endoscopic procedures, being provided.

REFERENCES

1. Burden N. *Ambulatory Surgical Nursing*. 2nd ed. WB Saunders, 2000.
2. Merrill DG. Practice management/role of the medical director. *Anesthesiol Clin*. 2014;32(2):529-540. https://doi.org/10.1016/j.anclin.2014.02.021
3. IBISWorld. Ambulatory Surgery Centers in the US: Number of Businesses 2005-2029. September 6, 2023. https://www.ibisworld.com/industry-statistics/number-of-businesses/ambulatory-surgery-centers-united-states/.
4. Smith I, Skues MA, Philip BK. Ambulatory (outpatient) anesthesia. In Gropper MA, ed. *Miller's Anesthesia*. 9th ed. Elsevier, 2019.

Dedication

This book, *Ambulatory Surgical Nursing*, is dedicated to perianesthesia nurses who work in all phases of perianesthesia care for the patient having outpatient and ambulatory surgery. I also want to thank my friends and colleagues at the American Society of PeriAnesthesia Nurses and the staff I manage at Northern Light Mercy Hospital for their ongoing support and encouragement of my professional journey.

Special thanks to my best friend and "sister from another mother," Julie, who spent countless hours wondering if I would ever emerge from my office. I appreciate your support and patience throughout this important time. Lastly, I dedicate this work to the memory of my mother, Lorraine, who taught me both the joys and heartaches that come with being "just a nurse."

Theresa L. Clifford

Contents

Introduction

1 The History of Ambulatory Surgery and the Nurse's Role

Denise O'Brien, DNP, RN, ACNS-BC, CPAN (retired), CAPA (retired), FASPAN, FCNS, FAAN

EVOLUTION OF AMBULATORY SURGERY

In the early 1970s, the evolution of ambulatory surgery began. The first step was the acceptance of the concept of providing surgical care for elective procedures for young, healthy patients and allowing them to return home on the same day that the procedures were performed. Over the intervening years, ambulatory surgery has expanded to encompass a wider variety of procedures, patients, and structures. Procedures with greater complexity and patients with multiple co-morbidities have become the norm rather than the exception. Health care insurance, managed care companies, and Medicare initiatives drive these changes to reduce costs and improve financial performance. Technologic advances in surgery and anesthesia have improved the safety of performing more complex procedures, and effective short-acting medications with minimal side effects, as well as improved anesthetic and pain management techniques, have encouraged a more rapid and trouble-free recovery from anesthesia.

The Beginnings

Ambulatory surgery is an ancient art; evidence of surgery has been recorded in drawings dated as far back as 3500 BC. Trephining of the skull and amputations were illustrated. Documented references can also be found in ancient Babylonian, Egyptian, Eastern Indian, Greek, and Roman civilizations.[1] It was not until early Christian times that churches began to develop hospitals where patients were cared for in designated places besides their homes after surgery.

Between 1899 and 1908, a series of ambulatory surgeries were performed with great success on 8988 children at the Glasgow Royal Hospital for Sick Children in Scotland.[2] The procedures addressed orthopedic problems, cleft lip and cleft palate, spina bifida, depressed skull fractures related to birth, hernias, congenital pyloric stenosis, and others. No children required admission following their procedures. Contemporary accounts describe similar results from that era.

In 1916, Dr. Ralph D. Waters opened the Down-Town Anesthesia Clinic in Sioux City, Iowa, and administered the first reported general anesthesia used in the western hemisphere for an ambulatory surgery patient.[3]

"His second publication (Waters, 1919) describes the original way in which he met a pressing need in many communities. Dentists and aural surgeons, as well as general practitioners, are frequently compelled to perform operations which, though of a minor nature, demand anaesthesia for a short period of time. The patients are usually in good health and need not lie in bed when once they are fully recovered from anaesthesia.

Waters, therefore, provided a small operating suite for the purpose. In addition to the operating room itself, there were small adjacent 'recovery wards' in which a patient could lie on a cot under the supervision of a trained nurse, until sufficiently recovered to go home. This establishment, which he called 'The Down-town Anesthesia Clinic', was at the disposal of his colleagues at such times as he was not occupied in the operating rooms of the local hospitals."[4]

The medical community was apparently not ready for this innovation, and his idea was not successfully adopted in other areas. Neither were many physicians ready to accept the concept of early postoperative ambulation suggested by Dr. Emil Ries of Chicago in 1899.[5] Suggesting that patients walk and eat within hours of surgery was a radical departure from tradition, and, although we now know it to be beneficial, it was not until the 1940s and 1950s that early ambulation came into widespread use.

By the 1960s, physicians began testing and stretching established traditions. Taking a cue from emergency rooms that historically have discharged patients soon after minor surgical procedures, physicians began to provide surgery without hospitalization. Economic advantages began to emerge that contributed to the trend toward outpatient surgery. Hospital beds became scarce, physicians began to undertake private surgical enterprises for profit, the public began to accept newer methods, and anesthesiologists responded with more appropriate techniques.

The Butterworth Hospital in Grand Rapids, Michigan, became the first hospital in the country to offer outpatient surgery and opened what is considered to be the country's first established ambulatory surgery program in 1961. Between 1963 and 1964, the staff performed 879 ambulatory procedures.[6] Other hospitals developed similar programs. In 1970, the first successful freestanding ambulatory surgery facility, Surgicenter, was opened in Phoenix, Arizona. Drs. Wallace Reed and John Ford were assisted in the development and opening of this facility by a registered nurse, Sharon Schafer. This center moved into a new facility and is part of the Banner Health System. The freestanding facility market continues to compete with hospitals, each driving the others to develop better products and services that address community needs for ambulatory surgery.

As managed care companies, the U.S. government, and private insurers continue to control the amounts of payments for procedures, the most cost-effective settings will flourish. All types of facilities are striving to meet that goal. Third-party payers require many surgeries to be performed in an ambulatory setting to avoid costly hospitalizations and are even requiring that certain procedures be performed in physicians' offices to further reduce costs. It is expected that competition will continue, and that new concepts and services will be developed.

Nursing Practice Changes Associated with Ambulatory Surgery

As ambulatory surgery procedures and requirements have evolved, nursing practice has developed ways to address varying patient needs. Specific nursing standards of practice have been developed and continue to evolve specifically for ambulatory surgery populations.

Various nursing processes applicable to the ambulatory surgery setting have been refined over the past 50 years. These include preadmission telephone calls, virtual visits or interviews, postdischarge telephone contacts to evaluate the effectiveness of nursing interventions, postoperative smart phone applications for ongoing patient follow-up, preoperative facility tours, the development and application of discharge standards, and the development and refinement of wellness approaches to encourage patients to participate in self-care. In many facilities, structured preadmission testing clinics have been developed to meet the assessment, educational, emotional, and physical preparatory needs of patients.

Ambulatory Surgery Today

Ambulatory surgery continues to evolve, earlier discharge occurs, and more complex procedures are performed. Now, ambulatory surgery includes concepts of care other than the immediate discharge of patients after their initial recovery from anesthesia and minor surgery. Short-stay admissions, up to 23 hours, have become more common as procedures have become more complex and patients with more complex disorders have undergone ambulatory surgery. The concept of short-stay admissions addresses the needs of patients who require a longer period of recuperation while still meeting acceptable criteria for ambulatory surgery, primarily to ensure third-party payment. In addition to same-day discharge, most people having major operative or interventional procedures enter the hospital on the morning of surgery rather than the night before. These patients may be admitted and cared for before surgery in hospital-based ambulatory surgery units, although some larger institutions may have separate units strictly for this category of patients, sometimes referred to as "AM admissions (AMA, AM Admit)." Special units for these morning admission patients have many names, such as "To Come In Unit (TCI)," "Admission Day Surgery Program (ADP), or "Same Day Admission (SDA)."

A multitude of names have been given to individual ambulatory surgery departments in hospitals and freestanding centers throughout the country, but regardless of the name attached to a department, patients in these units share similar needs and similar challenges. Sociologic, economic, and technologic influences have expanded the trend toward surgery performed on an ambulatory rather than an inpatient basis.

The high acuity and volume of critically ill patients in some hospitals may result in competition for hospital beds, and these beds are becoming scarce. Bed shortages are sometimes caused by bed closings at the hands of licensing agencies, by economic forces in the facility, and sometimes by nursing staff shortages. Additionally, the increasing demand for hospital beds due to the coronavirus SARS-CoV2 disease (COVID-19) pandemic and other emerging infectious diseases has limited the numbers and types of procedures that may be performed in the hospital setting. This situation forced lower-acuity patients to rely on such out-of-hospital services as home care and ambulatory surgery programs.

In addition, the current financial state of the healthcare industry and pressures from the government and third-party payers to contain and lower associated costs make ambulatory surgery programs economically attractive to providers and consumers. Not only does a third-party payer benefit from patients being cared for in the lower-cost setting of ambulatory care but the patient can derive a benefit as well. If patients are responsible for a deductible (e.g., the amount of money that they must pay before their insurance plan pays for health benefits), they may have to pay it regardless of the setting in which care is given. However, the co-payment amount is often defined in terms of a percentage of the total cost of care. Thus, the lower the overall charges from the healthcare institution, the less the co-payment.

The U.S. Balanced Budget Act of 1997 affected reimbursement plans for the Medicare segment with the development of a prospective payment system, much like the hospital diagnosis-related group payment plan. Plans to implement this system in freestanding ambulatory surgery centers (ASCs) were delayed until after the year 2000 for several reasons. First, year 2000 computer compatibility needed to be ensured throughout federal systems. Also, the freestanding market, led by its professional organizations, demanded and was granted a delay in earlier implementation to allow more time for industry responses and the Health Care Financing Administration's study of the proposed rule. The new payment system was enacted along with a similar plan for hospital-based outpatient surgery reimbursement (Outpatient Prospective Patient System). In 2010, under the Patient Protection and Affordable Care Act and as amended by the Health Care and Education Reconciliation Act (collectively known as the Affordable Care Act), the Secretary of Health and Human Services was required to develop a plan to implement a value-based purchasing program for payments under the Medicare program for ASCs. Revisions to these programs are ongoing.

Technologic advances in surgery provide alternatives to more invasive major procedures, thus allowing the rapid return of normal functions and earlier patient discharges. The variety of equipment available to the surgeon has expanded significantly, and newer techniques allow surgeons to accomplish procedures with less trauma to surrounding tissues. Use of lasers, laparoscopes, endoscopes, fiberoptic light sources, robotics, and other complex computerized equipment has increased the volume and types of ambulatory surgery procedures. Advancements in anesthetic techniques, pain management, and pharmaceuticals have also impacted ambulatory surgery. The use of newer anesthetic approaches, highly specific anesthetic agents and sedatives with short half-lives, and new analgesics and antiemetic drugs has helped reduce the complications of postanesthesia recovery, promote early discharge, and improve patient outcomes.

Access to technology has altered both the assessment and learning modalities for patients. Widespread Internet connectivity now provides patients with access to innumerable health-related sites. Preadmission education may include videos accessed through websites, smartphone-based applications, and virtual online classes or sessions. Postdischarge follow-up can be accomplished via telephone, virtual real-time video conversations, or phone or computer applications so that symptoms can be surveyed and care recommendations offered.

The Internet, a worldwide interconnected network of computers and digital technology, has opened a universe of information to the masses, including medical information that was previously not readily available to the lay public. Multiple sites of varying quality and content exist. Patients should be instructed as to which websites and virtual resources are acceptable and recommended. Nurses caring for patients today must remain professionally current so that they are prepared to interpret, explain, and correct information patients and families may learn from the Internet or other sources.

Critical pathways (e.g., clinical pathways, care paths, care maps, clinical maps, clinical trajectories, integrated plans of care) delineate the expected progress of a patient from the beginning to the end of the process related to a specific procedure or type of procedure. These pathways outline the plan for the provision of clinical services with expected time frames and resources targeted to specific diagnoses or procedures. These pathways prospectively link clinical care activities and associated costs with predetermined time points and outcomes, thus allowing the analysis of both clinical and economic effectiveness.

Care paths are developed by an interdisciplinary team and are based on historical data as well as on expected and desired outcomes. Care paths or maps are highly individualized to the facility or program and are dependent on collaboration among medical, nursing, and other practices, as well as on patient demographics and acuity. By setting "normal" or "average" parameters expected along the patient's continuum of care, they provide a standard against which an individual patient's progress can be compared and allow for interventions to improve progress and outcomes of care.

Care maps do not replace physicians' orders, but they do provide a suggested best treatment plan. Given to a patient in a format the patient can understand, a care map can help the patient anticipate the timing of various stages or activities. Care maps have been developed to address progress during a hospital stay and generally are expressed in terms of day of surgery, postoperative day one, day two, and so on. For the ambulatory surgery setting, the time frame is compressed and typically includes preadmission, day of procedure, immediate postoperative care, and discharge.

More recently, enhanced recovery pathways (ERPs) or enhanced recovery after surgery (ERAS) protocols, incorporating evidence-based practice guidelines and best practices, have been developed and shown to reduce complications and improve patient outcomes for ambulatory surgery patients.[7] The purpose of these pathways or protocols is to reduce postoperative complications and shorten the patient length of stay. Additionally, these pathways standardize care, reducing variations in perioperative care and improving patient outcomes. Included in the ERPs are preoperative considerations (e.g., procedure and patient selection, patient/family education, hydration and carbohydrate loading recommendations, prehabilitation), interoperative considerations (e.g., use of fast-track anesthesia techniques, fluid management, multimodal anesthesia/antiemetic techniques, glycemic control), and postoperative considerations (e.g., emphasis on patient-related outcomes, pain management, antiemetic therapy, surgical care). ERPs ideally are developed by the interdisciplinary care team and incorporate evidence-based guidelines and best practices.

STATISTICS OF OUTPATIENT SURGERY

Surgery, with its accompanying period of recuperation, has transitioned into the outpatient arena on a grand scale. Procedures may be performed in hospital outpatient departments, in co-located hospital or freestanding settings, or in privately owned ASCs. According to the Leapfrog group,[8] in 1982, outpatient surgeries represented just 4.7% of Medicare surgical billings. Today, 53% of all surgeries are done in an outpatient setting.[8]

There are multiple reasons that ambulatory surgery, either in freestanding surgery centers or hospital-associated outpatient facilities, is a thriving activity. These reasons include convenient locations, high patient satisfaction, and overall cost savings for patients. For physicians, the benefits include efficient scheduling and good accessibility, as well as cost savings. Other benefits include fewer bureaucratic issues, and this "lack" allows ASCs to provide innovative technologies and promotions of quality care because of greater physician investment in quality outcomes.[9]

Data related to the volume of ambulatory surgery procedures since 2019 have been skewed by the COVID-19 pandemic and its impact on access and care for non-COVID–related surgical needs. Data related to types of procedures between 2014 and 2019 identified the procedures shown in Table 1.1 as the most common procedures performed in the ASC setting. Cataract surgery remained the most frequently provided ASC service in those years, according to a recently released report by the Medicare Payment Advisory Commission.[10]

ASC surgeons perform an estimated 22.5 million procedures each year. On average, Medicare saves more than $4.2 billion annually when surgical procedures are performed at ASCs instead of hospital outpatient departments.[11] Likewise, Medicaid and other insurers benefit from lower prices for services performed in the ASC setting.

All surgical specialties are represented in ambulatory surgery. In a report from the Agency for Healthcare Research and Quality, 2019 data from hospital-owned ambulatory surgery facilities identified lens and cataract procedures as the most common, accounting for 8% of all major ambulatory procedures.[12] Highlights of this report are shown in Table 1.2. Table 1.3 shows the top 20 major ambulatory surgeries performed in hospital-owned facilities in 2019.

The fact that a surgery is completed in an ambulatory care facility makes it no less important or serious. Safe execution of surgery requires total attention to all the details of preparation, execution, and aftercare during the perioperative period. Hospitals that offer ambulatory surgery programs must provide care that is of the same quality as that provided for hospitalized counterparts.[13] Similarly, freestanding centers must provide a standard of medical, anesthesia, and nursing care equal to that provided in a hospital setting. In fact, freestanding units are sometimes obliged to show that they provide even more vigilance, patient attention, and emergency preparedness than nearby hospitals. This is in order to compensate for the concerns of some people in the public or healthcare community about the safety (or possible lesser safety) of self-contained centers in comparison with hospital-based settings.

The past 50 years have seen the proliferation of freestanding outpatient surgery centers in the United States. As of

TABLE 1.1 Top 10 Procedures in Ambulatory Surgery Centers in 2019

1	Cataract with intraocular lens insert	18.5%
2	Upper GI endoscopy, biopsy	7.8%
3	Colonoscopy and biopsy	6.8%
4	Lesion removal colonoscopy	6.5%
5	Inject foramen epidural; lumbar, sacral	4.6%
6	After-cataract laser surgery	4.1%
7	Inject paravertebral; lumbar, sacral	3.4%
8	Injection spine; lumbar, sacral (caudal)	2.5%
9	Colorectal screen, high-risk individual	2.1%
10	Destroy lumbar/sacral facet joint	1.7%

Source: Newitt P. 10 most common procedures in ASCs. *Becker's ASC Review.* 2021. https://www.beckersasc.com/benchmarking/10-most-common-procedures-in-ascs.html?oly_enc_id=2548E9889712G3W

TABLE 1.2 Highlights from the Agency for Healthcare Research and Quality: Major Ambulatory Surgeries Performed in Hospital-Owned Facilities in 2019

The number of encounters for major ambulatory surgeries was 11.9 million

Females, adults aged 65 years and older, White individuals, and people living in rural communities had the highest rates of encounters for major ambulatory surgeries

Most encounters involving major ambulatory surgeries took place at facilities owned by private, not-for-profit hospitals, teaching hospitals, and hospitals located in urban areas

Lens and cataract procedures accounted for 8% of all major ambulatory surgeries and represented the most common surgery overall, for those aged 65+ years, for all races and ethnicities except Hispanic, and for patients with Medicare as the expected payer

Seven of the top 20 ambulatory surgery categories were related to the musculoskeletal system and accounted for 22% of all major ambulatory surgeries

Tonsillectomy and/or adenoidectomy, as well as myringotomy, were the most common major ambulatory surgeries among children

Hernia repair was among the top major ambulatory surgeries for all adult male age groups, whereas obstetric/gynecologic surgeries were among the most common major ambulatory surgeries for younger adult females

Source: McDermott KW (IBM Watson Health), Liang L (AHRQ). Overview of Major Ambulatory Surgeries Performed in Hospital-Owned Facilities, 2019. HCUP Statistical Brief #287. December 2021. Agency for Healthcare Research and Quality, Rockville, MD. http://www.hcup-us.ahrq.gov/reports/statbriefs/sb287-Ambulatory-Surgery-Overview-2019.pdf

August 2022, there were over 11,800 ASCs in the nation.[14] Of these, more than 5900 were Medicare-certified.[11] To be eligible for Medicare, reimbursement centers must meet federal standards. Today, 43 states require state licensure.

AMBULATORY SURGERY VERSUS TRADITIONAL IN-HOSPITAL SURGERY: SIMILARITIES AND DIFFERENCES

Similarities and differences can be identified in comparisons of the ambulatory setting with the traditional in-hospital surgical setting (Table 1.4).[14] While these comparisons were first identified 30 years ago, they remain pertinent today. Some relate to patients' physical and emotional needs, others to broader facility-related issues. Obvious in both settings is the patient's basic need for surgical intervention. In both types of units, the patient is highly dependent on surgeons, anesthesia providers, and perianesthesia nurses. The ambulatory setting further extends that net of responsibility to families.

Patients face many of the same fears in all surgical settings, whether ambulatory or inpatient. They fear pain, the unknown, anatomic loss or alterations, the outcome of the procedure, possible embarrassment or loss of dignity, and financial problems. They also fear appearing ignorant when asking or answering questions. Patients may be worried about a potential change in ability to function within the family unit, an impending unfavorable diagnosis, or even the possibility of death.

Although published in 1991, a study of 76 adults undergoing ambulatory surgery for the first time remains pertinent today. In it, the patients were asked what concerned them the

TABLE 1.3 Top 20 Major Ambulatory Surgeries Performed in Hospital-Owned Facilities in 2019

	Procedure	Number	Percentage
1	Lens and cataract procedures	1,235,400	7.9
2	Other (select) therapeutic procedures on muscles and tendons	1,158,600	7.4
3	Cholecystectomy and common duct exploration	643,200	4.1
4	Other (select) operating room therapeutic procedures on joints	594,500	3.8
5	Other (select) operating room therapeutic procedures on nose, mouth, and pharynx	537,800	3.4
6	Other (select) operating room therapeutic procedures on skin and breast	537.700	3.4
7	Inguinal and femoral hernia repair	494,900	3.2
8	Hernia repair other than inguinal and femoral	470,500	3.0
9	Tonsillectomy and/or adenoidectomy	460,400	2.9
10	Decompression of the peripheral nerve	449,200	2.9
11	Excision of semilunar cartilage (meniscus) of knee	433,500	2.8
12	Hysterectomy, abdominal and vaginal	419,000	2.7
13	Myringotomy	371,900	2.4
14	Lumpectomy, quadrantectomy of breast	347,500	2.2
15	Other (select) operating room therapeutic procedures on bone	334,500	2.1
16	Arthroplasty knee	317,800	2.0
17	Insertion, revision, replacement, removal of cardiac pacemaker or cardioverter/defibrillator	310,200	2.0
18	Appendectomy	308,500	2.0
19	Partial excision bone	307,100	2.0
20	Laminectomy, excision intervertebral disc	296,200	1.9
		10,028,500	64

Source: McDermott KW (IBM Watson Health), Liang L (AHRQ). Overview of Major Ambulatory Surgeries Performed in Hospital-Owned Facilities, 2019. HCUP Statistical Brief #287. December 2021. Agency for Healthcare Research and Quality, Rockville, MD. www.hcup-us.ahrq.gov/reports/statbriefs/sb287-Ambulatory-Surgery-Overview-2019.pdf

TABLE 1.4 Ambulatory Versus Inpatient Surgery

SIMILARITIES BETWEEN AMBULATORY AND INPATIENT SURGERY PROGRAMS
Basic pathology that requires surgical intervention
Surgical techniques/technology
Skill and knowledge required of personnel
Patient's need for anesthetics
Patient's fears/emotional impact
Information/teaching needs
Strict aseptic technique required
Technologic support/instrumentation
Potential for emergencies to occur
Patient's dependence on staff during surgery and anesthesia

DIFFERENCES FOUND IN THE AMBULATORY SETTING
Emphasis on the concept of wellness
Control of patient's compliance with preoperative preparations at home
Generally healthier patients
Alterations in anesthesia (shorter-acting agents, regional techniques)
Use of premedicants
Local infiltration of operative site
Generally shorter surgical times
Family involvement in care
Patient and family responsibility
Impact on home environment
Compressed time for assessment and interventions
Usually elective procedures

Source: Burden N. The specialty of ambulatory surgery. In: Burden N, Quinn DMD, O'Brien D, Dawes BSG. *Ambulatory Surgical Nursing.* 2nd Ed. WB Saunders, 2000. P. 15.

most about having their surgery on an outpatient basis.[15] Six areas of concern were identified:

1. The availability of professional care following discharge
2. The need for information (this need varied considerably, with some people wanting complete information and others not wanting to know any details ahead of time)
3. Concern about the process of surgery, for instance, waiting before surgery or being discharged too soon
4. The outcome in relation to health
5. The recovery process, including complications, pain, and integration back into home responsibilities
6. Personal vulnerability.[15]

Similarities between the two types of settings include the need for maintaining appropriate levels of asepsis in the operating and procedural rooms, and the proper and safe use of technology and instrumentation. Each setting identifies quality improvement and infection control procedures that must be addressed. Staff preparation for emergencies is essential in both the ambulatory surgery and hospital settings.

Differences exist between the ambulatory and inpatient surgery settings. Generally, a healthier patient population is found in ambulatory surgical settings than in hospital surgical settings. Although many ambulatory units serve large numbers of elderly and systemically sick people, these patients usually present with relatively well-controlled diseases. Personnel in freestanding ASCs most often perform elective surgical procedures, but units associated with large hospitals and

medical centers may accommodate patients with minor emergencies in their daily schedules.

Rapid patient turnover, shorter surgical times, reduced overall patient stays, and increased family involvement in care are all typical of an ambulatory setting. Nurses have significantly less time for preoperative and postoperative assessment, intervention, patient teaching, and evaluation. Nursing staff must encourage patient and family responsibility for care. Nurses support a medication protocol that relies on a combination of minimal sedation and appropriate multimodal pain management to support the patients' rapid return to self-care.

Ambulatory surgery creates unique problems for perianesthesia nurses. For instance, nurses often cannot monitor, much less verify, a patient's compliance with preoperative home preparations, such as bathing and complying with fasting (NPO [nothing by mouth]) status. Same-day discharge requires discharge planning and attention to the physical setup of the patient's home, transportation needs, home support requirements, emergency resources, and the occasional need for unexpected hospitalization. Fear about being at home after surgery without nursing or medical supervision may affect some patients and should be considered in an overall nursing care plan.

An open, flexible mind and an innovative and creative spirit are trademarks of the ambulatory surgery staff. These characteristics can result in certain advantages for an ambulatory surgery setting over traditional hospitalization. For instance, ambulatory surgery departments often provide a more home-like and inviting atmosphere, an emphasis on wellness, and a greater inclusion of family or friends in patient care and instructions.

A freestanding ambulatory surgery center is well suited to offer new ways of addressing patient needs without bureaucratic restrictions. For instance, recliners may be used to replace stretchers, patients may retain dentures and sensory aids during surgery, patients may walk to and from the operating room when appropriate, and families may wait in the immediate postoperative area. Some of these practices are possible because of the layout of the units or centers. Others may be associated with attitude changes and the freedom from hospital traditions.

Many hospital-based outpatient surgery units offer these and other innovative services. However, some hospital-based units find it difficult to break away from the rules requiring more traditional policies and procedures. Whenever possible, restrictive policies should be updated to support a more progressive view toward individualized patient care.

PATIENT RIGHTS AND RESPONSIBILITIES

Given the climate of consumerism in today's healthcare industry, patients are generally better informed about what to expect, and even what to demand, from healthcare providers. High-quality care is expected. The patient is faced with the frightening experience of giving up control of both body and life. Patients should be able to trust that the people providing care are not only medically capable but also sensitive to patients' potential fears and emotional needs. It is expected that the patient's dignity will be preserved and that any details of care will be held in confidence.

In all surgical settings, patients assume that clear, accurate instructions will be provided, along with an opportunity for questions in a setting that is not intimidating. That expectation has special significance for the ambulatory surgical patient who must assume a certain amount of responsibility for self-care at home after surgery. Clear discharge instructions and explanations are essential components of nursing care, as is support of the patient's sense of self-confidence, which nurses can help to nurture. In addition, ambulatory surgery patients need assurance that they will not knowingly be sent home prematurely.

Inherent in the process of providing high-quality care is a recognition that every patient cared for in an ambulatory surgery facility has both responsibilities and rights. Established policies should define and identify patients' rights and responsibilities and the facility's overall goals of care. By establishing such a philosophy, the ASC helps its staff members to focus collectively and individually on clearly defined goals that promote staff unity and purpose. There are different approaches to facility goals and to patient rights and responsibilities. Patient rights may be addressed in terms of expected outcomes or in terms of process and expectation (Table 1.5).[14] The goals of an ambulatory surgery program are often designed from the viewpoint of the facility staff rather than the patient. Typical goals include providing comprehensive preoperative assessment and education, ensuring that appropriate candidates are selected, and verifying the home support for patients before giving preoperative sedation. The ASC should ensure that every employee is knowledgeable and supportive of its philosophy and policies. All healthcare facilities should ensure that patients' rights are communicated to patients, families, and employees. This information may be posted in public view and on the facilities website. A written copy may also be provided to each patient and caregiver.

Patients also have responsibilities, such as reporting accurately on their medical histories, following the treatment protocol, and paying their bills. Ambulatory surgery demands that patients assume additional responsibilities, for example, the need to have a responsible adult companion to accompany the patient home from the surgery facility and an adult to be responsible for the patient after surgery. These are frequently abused or misapplied responsibilities that deserve serious attention. Patients who refuse to accept these or other responsibilities inherent in having surgery on an ambulatory basis may find their surgeries cancelled if other arrangements cannot be made to ensure their safe postoperative course.

PERIANESTHESIA NURSE'S ROLE IN AMBULATORY SURGERY

Whether patients and families accept the concept of same-day discharge because they are well instructed and well prepared or whether they tolerate it because they have no other alternative is unclear. Regardless, the ambulatory surgical nurse is a primary resource for care, instruction, and support.[16] This adage remains to this day even as ambulatory surgery nursing has evolved over the subsequent years. The nurse addresses diverse and ever-changing questions and problems. Ambulatory surgery patients challenge nurses to

TABLE 1.5 Patient Rights and Responsibilities

AS A PATIENT, YOU HAVE THE RIGHT TO:

Considerate, respectful care at all times and under all circumstances with recognition of your personal dignity.

Personal and informational privacy.

Confidentiality of records and disclosures. Except when required by law, you have the right to approve or refuse the release of records.

Information concerning your diagnosis, treatment, and prognosis, to the degree known.

The opportunity to participate in decisions involving your healthcare.

Competent, caring healthcare providers who act as your advocates.

Know the identity and professional status of individuals providing a service.

Adequate education regarding self-care at home written in language you can understand.

Make decisions about medical care, including the right to accept or refuse medical or surgical treatment and the right to initiate advance directives such as a living will or durable power of attorney. If you already have a living will or other directive or you wish to initiate one, please speak with a nurse.

Information concerning implementation of any advance care directive.

Impartial access to treatment regardless of race, color, sex, national origin, religion, handicap, or disability.

Receive an itemized bill for all services.

Report any comments concerning the quality of services provided to you during the time spent at the facility and receive fair follow-up on your comments.

Know about any business relationships among the facility, healthcare providers, and others that might influence your care or treatment.

AS A PATIENT, YOU ARE RESPONSIBLE FOR:

Providing, to the best of your knowledge, accurate and complete information about your present health status and past medical history and reporting any unexpected changes to the appropriate practitioner(s).

Following the treatment plan recommended by the primary practitioner involved in your case.

Providing an adult to transport you home after surgery and an adult to be responsible for you at home for the first 24 hours after surgery.

Indicating whether you clearly understand a contemplated course of action and what is expected of you and asking questions when you need further information.

Your actions if you refuse treatment, leave the facility against the advice of the practitioner, and/or do not follow the practitioner's instructions relating to your care.

Ensuring that the financial obligations of your healthcare are fulfilled as expediently as possible.

Providing information about and/or copies of any living will, power of attorney, or other directive that you desire us to know about.

Source: Burden N. The specialty of ambulatory surgery. In: Burden N, Quinn DMD, O'Brien D, Dawes BSG. *Ambulatory Surgical Nursing*. 2nd Ed. WB Saunders, 2000. P. 17.

assess, plan, implement, and evaluate care on many levels. The patient's clinical, emotional, social, and educational needs must be considered concurrently.

The nurse shares the responsibility for evaluating and addressing patient needs with the healthcare team. In fact, a team approach-interaction among physicians, certified registered nurse anesthetists, nurses, families, and patients is vital to the success of the ambulatory surgery process. Mutual trust and overlapping responsibilities exist among team members in successful programs.

ELEMENTS OF A SUCCESSFUL PROGRAM

Many elements contribute to the ultimate success of any ambulatory surgery program. Especially important are patient and procedure selection, patient and family education, adequate home support, appropriate anesthesia technique, careful staff selection, and constant reinforcement of the wellness philosophy in a climate of caring concern. Nurses play a central role in each of these elements and are fundamental to the program's quality and success.

Patient and Procedure Selection

Patient and procedure selection begins in the surgeon's office. The surgeon, the anesthesiologist, and sometimes other physician consultants evaluate the patient's physical condition and tolerance for surgery and anesthesia. The patient's medical status must allow for adequate protection against the impact of surgery and anesthesia, and the care provided must support the patient's physical condition.

Medically compromised and older patients are cared for in the ambulatory surgery setting in increasing numbers. Often, medically compromised patients receive more intensive medical care after surgery because they see their own primary physicians frequently.

Contraindications to being considered for an ambulatory setting may include an inadequate home support system or an educational or intelligence level that precludes the understanding of proper self-care. Emotional or mental conditions that may cause undue fear or panic for the patient (or frighten other patients in an ambulatory surgery unit) might make hospital admission advisable, especially if the security or safety of patients or others is a factor. A person who has a high probability of requiring more extensive surgery than is typically undertaken in the ambulatory setting should be screened well before the decision is made for ambulatory care. Nurses are in an ideal position to assess and communicate many of these and other patient characteristics.

The procedure must lend itself to early patient discharge. With current economic pressures, improved technology, and an increasing demand for hospital beds, more complex and invasive procedures are being performed on an ambulatory basis. Examples include vaginal hysterectomy, thyroidectomy, simple mastectomy, spine procedures (e.g., minimally invasive lumbar decompression, lumbar fusions), and total joint replacements (e.g., hips, knees, shoulders). For a particular procedure to be appropriate for an individual, however, the patient's emotional and intellectual status must be considered, as well as the physical status. Also, each surgeon's technical and supportive skills should be considered, as well as both the physician's and the patient's histories of postoperative complications.

Although selection is the physician's responsibility, the ambulatory perianesthesia nurse also has a mechanism for input on issues regarding both procedure and patient selection. The nurse often provides surgeons and anesthesiologists with information that is important to selection. An in-depth preoperative nursing interview, best accomplished before the day of surgery, provides an opportunity for social, emotional, and physical assessments.

The nurse often elicits more detail and encourages patients and families to share information that they may have not shared with the surgeon or anesthesia provider. The ambulatory surgical nurse who discovers data that may influence the decision to proceed with or cancel a particular surgery is responsible for communicating that information to physicians responsible for that patient.

Although all these factors affect the selection process, third-party payers, namely the U.S. government and private insurers, affect the selection process more than any other force. This requires healthcare providers to respond to the needs of many patients who may, in fact, be poor candidates for early discharge but who are placed in that situation by the reimbursement process that limits the patient's care to the ambulatory surgery setting.

Patient and Family Education

Patient and family education plays a key role in the patient's successful, uncomplicated recuperation. Without proper instruction, the family and the patient may be uninformed about the physical needs and restrictions involved both before and after a particular surgical procedure. Furthermore, they may not even realize their need for more information. They may feel uneasy asking what they consider simple or inconsequential questions, so it is the nurse's role not only to educate but also to objectively assess their learning needs. While offering preoperative and aftercare instructions and explaining the patient's and family's responsibilities, the nurse assesses each learner's level of understanding and alters the teaching plan accordingly. The nurse provides a nonjudgmental atmosphere to help the patient and family feel comfortable asking any questions. Nurses need to be receptive to any information needs that are expressed and offer explanations that meet the patient's and family's learning needs.

The need for written instructions to accompany verbal information is paramount both before and after surgery. By supplying written directions, the nurse provides the patient with a reliable reference for later use. These instructions may be available on paper or via a patient portal dependent on the needs of the patient and family. Before surgery, patients' anxiety levels may be competing with their attention to instructions and their ability to comprehend and retain the information being provided. After surgery, the insightful postanesthesia nurse understands that patients may seem wide awake and alert during postoperative teaching sessions, although the effects of anesthetics, sedatives, and analgesics often erase that period from patients' memories. The need to provide written instructions and to include family or support persons in the instruction process in that setting is obvious. When possible, reviewing postoperative instructions preoperatively may benefit both the patient and family and allow for questions while the patient is not sedated.

Ensuring an Adequate Home Support System

Reliable home support should be available during the patient's postoperative course, particularly for intervention in the event of complications after discharge. This support system may be an adult family member, a friend, or a healthcare professional who is engaged by the patient for a specific period to provide care. The patient and family member should feel confident to handle the recuperation period at home.

They must all understand that a person recuperating from anesthesia should not be left unattended after returning home on the day of surgery.

Through the provision of personalized preoperative counseling before the day of surgery, the nurse contributes to the patient's and family's confidence, helps decrease anxiety, and helps eliminate unfounded fears and false expectations. Certainly, the adult patient has the ultimate responsibility for establishing the necessary support for home and transportation needs. However, the entire team—physician, patient, family, friends, and nurse—must work together to ensure the availability of an appropriate support system.

Preparation of the physical home environment also helps ensure a smooth preoperative and postoperative course. This involves having the right equipment, supplies, and medications available; providing a safe, comfortable, and clean environment; and making sure that appropriate foods and beverages are available. Sometimes the home may not be well suited to the patient's immediate postoperative needs, and modifications or an alternate plan should be instituted. Predicting and addressing these types of issues are vital to an uncomplicated recovery. After surgery, some people may need a level of supervised medical attention in the time between hospitalization and discharge to home. Reasons for this may include an inadequate support system, a complex or lengthy surgical procedure, actual or high potential for complications, prior poor physical and emotional health, prior untoward experience with surgery, or the preferences of the family, physician, or patient.

Medical hotels, home health nursing care, overnight stays at the physician's office, 23-hour admission programs, and surgical recovery centers are examples of systems that offer an intermediate level of care. Some facilities have established the concept of a phase III recovery area or short-stay unit for patients who likely will be discharged within a few more hours but who require an extended period of observation after surgery. If a person comes to an ambulatory surgery facility on the day of surgery without having established any responsible adult as a support system, surgery is often postponed if an adequate alternative cannot be established or until postoperative hospitalization can be approved.

Influencing Anesthesia Technique

Anesthesia technique is a variable that is usually beyond the nurse's direct control but is rarely beyond the nurse's influence. The nurse's documentation, suggestions, and attention to the postanesthesia patient's responses enable the anesthesia department to obtain clear information on which decisions about techniques and medications used for ambulatory surgical procedures are based.

When minimal or no preoperative medication is given, the nurse provides reassurance and emotional support to patients and reduces patient anxiety by use of relaxation techniques and other nursing interventions. The anesthesia and surgical team attempt to provide a postoperative course with a low incidence of pain, somnolence, nausea, and vomiting. Nursing measures in the perianesthesia period should complement the anesthetic approach and focus on promoting readiness for discharge without complications.

SELECTION OF NURSING STAFF MEMBERS

Selection of nursing staff members is another avenue that significantly affects the quality of the ambulatory surgical process. Choosing nurses with appropriate knowledge, skills, and experience is essential, but with those qualities being equal among all candidates for a position, it makes sense for the manager to select the nurse who can quickly establish rapport with patients and others. This is especially true because time for personal interactions and making a good impression is at a premium in the ambulatory surgery setting.

A warm, outgoing, caring, and cheerful demeanor is often what clinical leadership seeks. The patient and family sense the attitudes of nurses as quickly as they observe the nurses' skills and abilities. A positive attitude on the part of patients, which is so important to the ambulatory surgery process, is enhanced when patients meet and interact with nursing and medical staff members who genuinely care about the patient, the family, and the success of the surgery.

The way nurses care for a patient's dignity, emotions, and feelings is the subject of many more compliments on or complaints about postdischarge evaluations than is the patient's perception of the physical care that was received. Not only does it make ethical and moral sense to hire the nurse who shows a true concern and respect for patients and the facility, it also makes financial and business sense. Kind, caring nurses are the ambulatory unit's best marketing tools.

As in other busy departments, nurses in the ASC also should be able to interact pleasantly with other nurses, physicians, business and administrative personnel, and other health professionals. Well-developed time management skills are essential in ASCs, which are usually very busy departments with greatly fluctuating caseloads. Especially during times of peak volume, nurses should work well together toward a common goal of safe and efficient patient care.

To promote the maximum efficiency of the department, each nurse should be willing to work in any area of need if that nurse is competent and has been appropriately oriented in that department. Nurses in freestanding centers have the added challenge of having no other nursing or ancillary departments to call on during emergencies. Each nurse must have complete confidence in the dependability and the assistance of other nurses in the center. Like most nursing settings, the ambulatory surgery unit requires nurses who are concerned with details: nurses who assess, plan, act, and reassess with vigilance. Innumerable details must be coordinated both within the facility and in the patient's home setting. Anything less than total attention to such details could lead to incomplete patient preparation before surgery, the delay or cancellation of surgery, and the lack of a proper support system for the postoperative period. Nurses who care about, and take action to correct, deficiencies in the patient's care plan may find themselves addressing many issues, such as missing diagnostic reports, the patient's incomplete understanding of the surgical procedure, special positioning needs for arthritic or poorly mobile patients, and special emotional support for a person suffering with depression.

Because postoperative and postanesthetic complications can have much more serious effects when they occur in the home setting, the nurse must meticulously assess, direct, and evaluate every parameter of the nursing care provided within the ASC. What the nurse does or does not notice, teach, act on, report, or intervene about greatly affects patient outcomes. Caring about every aspect of the process is intrinsic to the ambulatory surgical nursing concept.

CHAPTER HIGHLIGHTS

- Changes in healthcare over the past several decades have led to the expansion of procedures and services in the outpatient setting.
- In addition to socioeconomic factors impacting the need for acute care beds and lower cost care, scientific advances in technology and anesthesia support safer ambulatory-based care

- Successful outpatient surgery programs include appropriate patient selection, education, staff training, and quality monitoring to ensure safe provision of care

Special thanks and credit to Nancy Burden, MS, RN, CPAN, CAPA, who is the author of the original text this chapter is based on in *Ambulatory Surgical Nursing*, 2nd Edition.

REFERENCES

1. Davis J. History of major ambulatory surgery. In: Davis J, ed. *Major Ambulatory Surgery*. Williams & Wilkins; 1986:3-31.
2. Nicoll JH. The surgery of infancy. Proceedings of the 77th Annual Meeting of the British Medical Association. *BMJ*. 1909;2:753-754. Available at: https://drcesarramirez.com/files/te_interesa/Nicoll_THE_SURGERY_OF_INFANCY.pdf.
3. Epstein BS. Exploring the world of ambulatory surgery. *Ambul Surg*. 2005;12(1):1-5. Available at: https://doi.org/10.1016/j.ambsur.2005.01.001.
4. Gillespie NA. Ralph Milton Waters: a brief biography. *Br J Anaesth*. 1949;21(4):197-214. Available at: https://doi.org/10.1093/bja/21.4.197.
5. Ries E. Some radical changes in the after-treatment of celiotomy cases. *JAMA*. 1899;XXXIII(8):454-456. Available at: https://doi.org/10.1001/jama.1899.92450600020001g.
6. Aquavella J. Ambulatory surgery in the l990s. *J Ambul Care Manage*. 1990;13(1):21-24. Available at: https://doi.org/10.1097/00004479-199002000-00005.
7. Joshi GP. Enhanced recovery pathways for ambulatory surgery. *Curr Opin Anaesthesiol*. 2020;33(6):711-717. Available at: https://doi.org/10.1097/ACO.0000000000000923.
8. Leapfrog. *ASC Survey*. Factsheet: Same Day Surgery, 2022. 2022. ASC Outpatient Surgery Fact Sheet_0.pdf. Available at: leapfroggroup.org.
9. Newitt P. *10 Most Common Procedures in ASCs*. Becker's ASC Review; 2021. Available at: https://www.beckersasc.com/benchmarking/10-most-common-procedures-in-ascs.html?oly_enc_id=2548E9889712G3W.
10. Ambulatory Surgery Center Association. *Medicare Cost Savings*. (no date). Available at: https://www.ascassociation.org/advancingsurgicalcare/reducinghealthcarecosts/costsavings.
11. McDermott KW, Liang L. *Overview of Major Ambulatory Surgeries Performed in Hospital-Owned Facilities*. 2019. HCUP Statistical Brief #287. Agency for Healthcare Research and Quality; 2021. Available at: https://www.ncbi.nlm.nih.gov/books/NBK577044/.
12. The Joint Commission. *Comprehensive Accreditation Manual for Hospitals: The Official Handbook: CAMH*. The Joint Commission; 2022.
13. Definitive Healthcare. *How Many Ambulatory Surgery Centers are in the U.S.?* 2022. Available at: https://www.definitivehc.com/blog/how-many-ascs-are-in-the-us.
14. Burden N. The specialty of ambulatory surgery. In: Burden N, Quinn DMD, O'Brien D, Dawes BSG, eds. *Ambulatory Surgical Nursing*. 2nd ed. WB Saunders; 2000:15.
15. Caldwell LM. Surgical outpatient concerns: what every perioperative nurse should know. *AORN J*. 1991;53(3):761-767. Available at: https://doi.org/10.1016/s0001-2092(07)68951-0.
16. Burden N. The keys to success: the ambulatory approach. *Breathline. The Newsletter of the American Society of PeriAnesthesia Nurses*. 1987;7:11-s12.

2 Leadership in Ambulatory Surgery

Regina Hoefner-Notz, MS, BSN, RN, CPAN, CPN, FASPAN

LEARNING OBJECTIVES

A review of the content of this chapter will help the reader to:

1. Understand the concepts and components of leadership.
2. Identify various leadership styles.
3. Recognize personal traits and actions associated with leadership.
4. Acknowledge barriers to leadership and opportunities for change process

INTRODUCTION

The concepts associated with leadership are well known; however, the ability to describe leadership's impact on nursing is elusive. Multiple theories on leadership exist, as well as specific information regarding the similarities and differences of various leadership styles. This chapter is not an attempt to describe management principles of nurse leaders but, rather, to provide a reflection of various leadership theories supporting each nurse's ability to lead.

The willingness to examine the various attributes of sound leadership as well as the barriers to good management can offer encouragement to all nurses interested in developing their own style of leadership. This foray into leadership supports the union of a robust, clinically excellent professional practice with a personal life-long learning style that integrates components of leadership. Tim Size describes leadership as "the capacity to help transform the future into reality. Individuals who can and will exercise leadership are like a river's current—a part past, where we stand, a part yet to come. We have an ongoing need to remember and to look toward the next generation."[1]

As nurse leaders we respect our roots, but we all must seek ways to assist our own leadership development, as well as support those seeking to lead. Leadership today will be different tomorrow. How do we get ready for the future?

What Is Leadership?

Although there are various theories about leadership, Peter Northouse proposes the definition of and the action required for this phenomenon to occur.[2] A communications professor, Northouse explains how leadership is a process during which a person influences a group of individuals to achieve a common goal. By using the term *process*, Northouse puts forward the idea that leadership is not a trait, confined to one person, but is more a transaction that occurs between the leader and a follower. He describes leadership as an interactive event, thereby leaving it open to everyone. Leaders and followers are closely linked because without followers, there are no leaders.[2]

The components necessary for leadership to occur are process, influence, groups, and goals.[2]

1. Process. Leadership is a process not limited to individuals of power or authority, and defining it as an action provides opportunities for anyone to become a leader.
2. Influence. Leadership involves influence. The person defined as the leader impacts the actions of followers, thereby exerting a significant influence over the group. Influence is a requirement of leadership; without it leadership does not exist.
3. Groups. Leadership must occur in a group. The group influenced by a leader can be any type or size. In nursing, the leader does not necessarily need to be the formal manager or charge nurse. Informally, a leader can be an individual who has influence over the group.
4. Goals. Leadership must also involve the attainment of a goal or goals. The leader directs the energy of the group to a certain goal or end result.[2]

Elaine Maxwell is an associate professor of leadership in the School of Health and Social Care, London South Bank University. She writes about nursing leadership and how complex this topic is to study and describe. There is overwhelming interest in nursing leadership, but there is little concrete evidence about what actually works in this profession. Because leadership is such a complex process to study and for which specific results are difficult to define, she suspects there is no "one size fits all" answer to what makes good leadership in nursing.[3]

Leadership Styles

Multiple models of leadership have been identified in the literature. At times, situations require specific strategies for effective management and resolution. These same challenges may also require a combination of approaches. This section provides a brief overview of a variety of leadership style examples.

Transformational Leadership

Transformational leadership is the approach to leadership that is the current focus of the nursing Magnet model of the American Nurses Credentialing Center. The model characterizes transformational leaders as "translating vision to action and helping others reach their highest potential."[4] This model was developed in the late 1980s and early 1990s. The primary focus of transformational leadership is to tap into the internal values and ideals of individuals to motivate them to support the greater good.[2] Transformational leadership centers around the four *Is*, or domains.

1. Individualized consideration: identifying the needs of individual members of the staff
2. Intellectual stimulation: questioning the status quo and presenting new ideas
3. Inspirational motivation: presenting a vision in which people can achieve their personal goals through meeting the organization's goals
4. Idealized influence: role-modeling the desired behaviors[3]

This model encourages the leader to provide an environment that is safe and supportive and tailored to the followers' needs. It also encourages others to develop innovative ideas and clinical inquiry, as well as to articulate the need for the highest standards of care. The leader is asked to be inspirational while supporting engagement and open communication.[4] The leader has a vision that might transform people while encouraging them to do their best professional work. Transformational leadership is concerned with emotions, values, ethics, standards, and long-term goals.[5]

Transactional Leadership

Transactional leadership is a behavioral model. In this model, leaders ensure that work is completed through either reward or sanction.[3] The transactional leader does not individualize the needs of the staff nor does the leader focus on personal development.[2] This method is not necessarily negative or in opposition to transformational leadership, and it actually may be used in tandem with transformational leadership to address a specific task. For example, when a unit is short-staffed and a leader offers an incentive to improve staffing, this is considered transactional leadership. The reward enables safe staffing and allows other staff members to be their best selves and deliver safe care in the presence of sufficient staffing numbers.

Servant Leadership

Robert Greenleaf developed the idea of servant leadership almost 44 years ago after observing his company's managers.[6] He noted how some were extremely successful and others were not quite as successful. The successful managers notably put others first, whether employees, customers, or community members. He called them servant leaders.[5] The basic underlying tenet of servant leadership was described by Greenleaf as "the feeling that one wants to serve. Being servant first. Do those served grow as persons? Do they...become healthier, wiser, freer, more autonomous, more likely themselves to become servants?"[6]

The components that make up this leadership model include listening, empathy, healing, awareness, persuasion, conceptualization, foresight, stewardship, commitment to others' growth, and community building.[7] It is interesting to note that there has been a resurgence in servant leadership among some younger individuals who want to make a positive impact on our world and support others who are doing so. Millennials are increasingly seeking solutions to their own concerns. This younger generation is seeking to make a difference through their professional lives. The focus on purchase decisions based on ethical and social values has been identified as an offshoot of both this model and the goals of the younger generation.[6]

Authentic Leadership Empowerment

This newer nursing theory of leadership development combines the theories of authentic leadership and structural empowerment. The theory of authentic leadership empowerment (TALE) is a middle-range theory that has the aim of guiding the professional development of nurses as they take on leadership roles.[8] This theory looks at the value of the authentic leadership model that first appeared in the literature in the 1990s and combines it with Kanter's structural empowerment theory, which evaluates how organizations empower, or do not empower, employees to provide input into their work environments.[8] Kanter's theory has been extensively studied to evaluate nursing workforce issues, leading to the ideas that nurses feel empowered when there is support, information, and an opportunity to influence. The TALE model hopes to empower nurses to cultivate their authentic leadership behaviors.[8] This empowerment process becomes more complex when leaders continue to develop their genuine selves as resilient, confident leaders who are creating their personal leadership styles but find themselves in an organization that continues to place barriers to practice, standards of care, or staffing. Employing this model of nursing leadership aims at the continued growth and development of nurse leaders.[8]

Autocratic/Authoritarian Leadership

When following the principles of the autocratic or authoritarian leadership style, the person in power makes all decisions for the group. People are directed through commands, and there is little input about decision making from the group. All communication flow is downward as questions and suggestions are mostly discouraged. Autocratic leaders have low tolerance for those making mistakes.[5,9,10] This type of leadership can work in specific situations such as the need to enforce policy compliance or when there are legal implications of practice. In general, however, little trust is developed among group participants and many experience missed growth opportunities.[9]

Democratic Leadership

Democratic leaders often consider the various viewpoints of the individual members of a group. Communication is open and feedback is both desired and accepted from the group members. This style of leadership can promote growth opportunities for engaged members of the group, as well as encourage cooperation and collaborative work for the completion of various tasks. While the democratic leader can build trust among group members, the ultimate decision will still be made by the leader. This method may be frustrating to those anxious for quick decisions. Since the opinions of multiple people are solicited, moving ideas forward in a timely manner can sometimes be a struggle.[9,10]

Laissez-faire Leadership

As a laissez-faire leader, the person in charge provides no specific direction for the group. The leader adopts a "hands off" mentality and provides little direction or support unless asked to do so. On the one hand, small, highly functional, experienced teams continue to work well together. However, newer members of the group requiring more specific direction to feel secure in their roles will find this style of leadership disturbing. As a result of the changes in healthcare due to new trends and directions in this fast-shifting environment, laissez-faire leadership can be especially challenging.[9,10]

Why Is Nurse Leadership Important?

Over the next 10 years, one million nurses are expected to retire. In 2015 alone, healthcare lost an estimated 1.7 million years of accumulated nursing experience as a result of retirement from the profession.[11] These numbers suggest that now, more than ever, it is time to support nurses to develop leadership skills.

A study in 2019 indicated that 50% of nurses were interested in securing leadership opportunities. However, the majority of this group with a mean age of 43 years only had 1 to 5 years of nursing experience.[11] This study also indicated that conversely, nurses with over 20 years of nursing experience had less interest in leadership.[11]

It takes time to develop new leaders and leadership skills. Many nurses are unsure how to go about it or how to seek out mentorship opportunities to develop the skill sets required to lead effectively. Nurse leaders with practiced leadership skills can empower others to have a voice in their patient care that impacts changes and outcomes. These already identified leaders serve as role models for the next generation of nurse leaders.

It is important to mention here that healthcare is not the only venue for developing leaders. Professional organizations provide multiple opportunities for involvement in committees and strategic work teams impacting practice at various levels. These organizational means also offer networking opportunities to connect with like-minded professional nurses. Being proactive and self-directed about one's own professional development, using an active voice to articulate the value and contribution of one's role, and advocating on behalf of the profession is essential to the future of nursing.[12]

Nurses must seriously consider their personal accountability to the best practice when defining what that practice entails. Evidenced-based practice changes can become part of an organizational practice when a nurse leader at the local or national level is well-informed about them. Not every nurse will be a chief nursing officer, but every nurse can be part of a professional organization and impact change with the right tools.

Barriers to Leadership

There are many times in a nurse leader's career that a nurse turns to the nurse leader and says, "I wouldn't want your job." This sentiment reflects the perception that some nurses perceive leadership as a negative thing. Skepticism about leadership can occur when actions are taken or decisions made that appear to be lacking in a moral or ethical way.[8] An ongoing lack of transparency frequently leads to distrust and decreased confidence in an organization.

To remove negative thoughts about nursing leadership, it is essential to identify the barriers preventing nurses from securing leadership opportunities. Once that occurs, nurses with potential can be recognized and asked to lead through some of the various activities with which they are already involved, such as shared governance, committee work, or being a charge nurse. This becomes essential, particularly since the National Center for Healthcare Leadership has determined that "gaps in leadership create opportunities for poor results in patient care, staff satisfaction, and business outcomes."[13]

Some of the barriers to leadership identified by nurses include, but are not limited to:

1. Inadequate support from the organization
2. Unreasonable workload
3. Too much responsibility associated with the role
4. Loss of job security
5. Inadequate compensation
6. Loss of patient contact
7. Conflict with personal obligations
8. Too many meetings
9. Labor management issues[13]

Some of the organizational actions identified by nurses as providing support for interest in leadership roles include, but are not limited to:

1. Formal mentoring

2. Leadership development activities and projects
3. Educational opportunities[13]

The biggest concerns that were identified with regard to management issues included, but were not limited to:

1. Managing conflict
2. Dealing with difficult people
3. Engaging in disciplinary actions[13]

Despite challenges for obtaining adequate resources, the best investment healthcare facilities can make is creating a process to identify potential candidates for nursing leadership as well as enabling significant investments in leadership and mentoring programs.

Cultivating Leadership

There is a time and a place for considering whether a nurse should step up into a specific leadership role. However, there are multiple leaders in every workplace, whether formal or informal.

Craig Johnson, in his 2021 published work about leadership, examined the concepts of leaders that cast light or shadow.[14] As would be expected, those that cast light are the moral and ethical ones. "Ethical leadership is a two-part process involving personal moral behavior and moral influence."[14] Leaders who practice in a moral way have self-developed a manner that incorporates traits such as justice, humility, optimism, and courage. They also accept their responsibility to those they lead to promote ethical behaviors in others.[14] Their leadership supports those around them and lifts them up to the next level.

Johnson also describes leaders that cast shadows.[14] These leaders have the potential to do more harm than good and project shadows from a place of inner darkness. There are feelings of internal threats, whether they are due to the leader's intrinsic insecurity, fear, selfishness, or narcissism. As a leader, understanding these differences is important because this knowledge encourages leaders to reflect upon their actions and determine the undercurrent of why they do certain things. This reflection can be very complex or very simple, but what becomes exceedingly important is the ability to scrupulously review actions and behaviors that could be improved upon.

Leaders who seek to understand their dark or shadow side can continue to develop good, ethical leadership skills. Leaders will always have ethical burdens to work through as they receive new tasks and meet new job requirements.[14] One example of evaluating the shadow side might include reflection about communication as one speaks or deals with others. Does the leader allow others to present new ideas or processes, or does the leader shut them down? Doing the latter may be a result of the shadow side. If the leader is reflective, can the leader identify feelings of being threatened by better ideas or someone else gaining power? For a leader, this process presents opportunities for ongoing personal growth.

Leadership Traits and Actions

Several authors have identified various traits co-workers want and expect from nurse leaders. The leadership traits to which younger nurses respond and for which coaching may be needed include[15]:

1. Sincere enthusiasm
   Leaders presenting with sincere enthusiasm and passion about what they do can create a contagiously energetic atmosphere in which to work. This cannot be faked, and people who associate with the leader can discern the sincerity of the leader's actions.
2. Integrity
   As with reflections on light versus shadow in leadership, integrity is essential to gaining trust. Integrity shows up

in multiple ways, such as the quality of a person's work or the ability of a person to give credit to other workers for their ideas or achievements. When one acts with integrity, one does the right thing every time, even when no one else is watching. The primary goal should always be to focus on the patient and family and to do the right thing for them.

3. Great communication skills

Great communication involves being able to motivate, instruct, and discuss difficult issues thoughtfully and empathetically with others. It is about understanding that listening is as important as speaking and is an integral part of the communication process. A leader must stop to listen, must not be distracted by phones or other people, and must communicate in a timely manner.

4. Loyalty

Loyalty is a reciprocal theme for team members and leaders. Loyalty might entail ensuring fairness and consistency for all members of a group. This might mean defining rules that position everyone on the same playing field or ensuring that all team members have the training and resources needed to do their jobs. Loyalty is standing up for team members in crisis and conflict.

5. Decisiveness

Leaders are willing to make decisions in a timely manner. Leaders understand that if their decisions do not result in workable solutions, they will accept personal accountability for them. Although team members may like the democratic process when it is applicable, they often appreciate a leader who can make decisions that resolve the problem at hand.

6. Competence

Many organizations choose nurse leaders who have demonstrated clinical excellence. Although this is an important component of understanding the requirements of the staff, having clinical knowledge and excellence does not necessarily guarantee that one has the ability to lead a group, motivate a team, or competently run a meeting, committee, or unit. These are skill sets that a nurse leader needs to acquire, much like all the others listed.

7. Empowerment

A good leader understands the strengths, as well as the weaknesses, of the team with which they work. Leaders train and develop team members and therefore feel comfortable empowering them to act autonomously within the scope of their job. This action acknowledges that leaders trust in the capacities of the team members, and it also assists the team in making decisions. This trust provides empowerment, allowing the members of the team to create the best situations in the moment.

8. Charisma

Good or bad, some leaders are just more likeable than others. Team members appreciate leaders who are approachable, friendly, and willing to be transparent about their care and concern for the team. These leaders can relate to various people throughout the organization to accomplish the jobs they need to get done.

These traits and behaviors are crucial to developing solid and trustworthy leadership. As leaders continue to advance, they encourage others to join them to reach their own potential. Smart organizations create processes for continuing the development of existing leaders, as well as for identifying and coaching emerging leaders.

Succession Planning

As nurse leaders proceed, it is important that they have, and constantly review, their visions for the future and their plans for fulfilling them. Strategic action is important because it facilitates the creation of a process for transitions. Successful succession planning requires that leaders be cultivated and form partnerships.[16] In best-case scenarios, there is time to identify talent in the people on a team and determine their interest and willingness to manage change.

In recent years, the generation known as baby boomers, born between 1946 and 1964, has formed a large part of the workforce (currently 32% of the nursing workforce).[17] These workers are now beginning to retire, and as they continue to retire the makeup of the nursing population will change significantly. Generation X and millennial nurses will need to be prepared for leadership roles. It is a time to teach, coach, and "equip this workforce with the skills and knowledge and behaviors to lead with ... vision and teamwork."[18] Various journal articles suggest that key roles be identified within an organization and various competencies be categorized that will lead to success in key positions. Describing the roles and required competencies can foster a belief that an organization is willing to invest in personal and professional education and development.[13,18]

Generation X nurses were born between 1965 and 1980. They have learned to manage independently at a young age owing to the influence of various factors. The defining historic moments for them included the AIDS epidemic, the *Roe vs. Wade* decision, the space shuttle *Challenger* explosion, the Watergate investigation, and the historic fall of the Berlin Wall. They are frequently described as latchkey kids because both of their parents worked and they unlocked the door of an empty house after school The professional advancement of this generation has been slowed down by the large number of baby boomers remaining in leadership positions. Gen X individuals tend to be cautious, self-reliant, independent, and extremely comfortable with technology. Directions provided for them should be straightforward and succinct. This group often express a desire to demonstrate their expertise.[17]

Millennial nurses were born between 1981 and 1997. They are achievement-oriented and motivated but desire flexible work schedules to help with their work–life balance. The defining historic moments for this age group were events of violence and terrorism, including the attacks of September 11, 2001, and the Columbine High School shootings. These nurses were born to older mothers, and 60% came from families where both parents worked. During their lifetimes, the world was experiencing a new, unprecedented multicultural and multiethnic awareness. Accordingly, millennial nurses demonstrate more ethical diversity than other generations, have acquired more education, and are extremely comfortable with technology. They are group oriented and network well. From a learning perspective, they want frequent coaching and personal feedback.[17]

Exploring the differences and similarities of the generations of working nurses is not intended to stereotype or categorize nursing colleagues but, rather, to inspire today's nurse leaders to seek better understanding of their learning and communication styles. This insight can prepare nurses to become more engaged and enjoy greater success as nurse leaders. The nursing experiences of younger nurses are very different from those of more senior nurses. Healthcare continues to involve increasingly complex patient conditions and treatments for them. Nurses today are dealing with advancing technology, escalating acuities, rising burnout among staff, and unstable financial grounding.

The notion of self-leadership is a single process that can be used to support all nurses dealing with the frenzy of change and complexity in healthcare. This theory encourages nurses to create and maintain constructive thought patterns. The author describing self-leadership identifies contrasting patterns of thinking related to opportunities and obstacles.[19] Persons engaging in opportunity-focused thinking seek constructive ways to deal with challenges, whereas persons engaging in obstacle-focused thinking dwell on withdrawing and retreating from problems. To disengage from dysfunctional obstacle-focused thinking, the author suggests practicing positive self-talk, visualization, and a thorough exploration of personal beliefs and assumptions.[19]

Nurse leaders can evaluate situations in various ways. They might ask "What can I control?" and "What do I have no control over?" By incorporating this type of self-talk, the nurse leader can shift energy toward situations that can be positively influenced as opposed to those that cannot be. This has the potential to decrease some stress and anxiety. Utilizing visualization, nurse leaders can picture themselves as having positive and meaningful discussions with other nurses, truly listening to their concerns, and acknowledging issues. By looking at beliefs and assumptions the nurse leader can ask questions and clarify a situation to reframe it and make it manageable.[19]

Six questions associated with this clarification and reframing process are particularly powerful for new nurse leaders as they start to deal with multifaceted situations.[19]

1. What do you know, or think you know, about the situation?
2. What do you not know about the situation but would like to know?
3. Why is this situation a problem for you?
4. If this problem were solved, what would you have that you do not have now?
5. What have you already thought of or tried to address regarding this problem?
6. What might you be assuming about this situation that may or may not be true?

These practices, thoughts, and theories should be encouraged through conventional education and formal mentoring programs. The identification of potential leaders allows nurse leaders to share information and set up one-to-one discussions about potential leadership pathways and how to navigate them. As mentors, nurse leaders can share tips regarding what worked well and what did not work as well. Process change for development involves coaching and frequent feedback to validate and celebrate practice.

Reflecting on Maxwell's work specific to nurse leadership, it is apparent that there is no singular style of leadership that will solve all problems and unravel all complications.[3] Various styles should be incorporated to deal with the multitude of situations nurse leaders deal with on a daily, sometimes hourly, basis. Maxwell summarizes leadership development through the acquisition of four skills[3]:

1. Capacity to calibrate and monitor the workload of a team
2. Ability to create a work environment in which all staff feel safe to contribute in a way that is fulfilling
3. Power to create relationships that build resilience
4. Competence to ensure the team delivers safe care and good experiences (for patients, families, and staff) with the most efficient use of available resources[3]

In the end Maxwell writes, "work environment—including leadership—affected nurses' work commitment and their intention to stay. In particular, they found that nurses who felt they had good relationships in their workplace were more committed to the ward than those who felt they were only there to earn a living."[3]

Believing that all nurses are leaders, whether formal or informal, requires an ongoing commitment to educate, inform, and mentor each other to share collective experiences, knowledge, and power. Remaining positive about the profession and making formal leadership attractive to nurses via the correct tools and support are crucial. It is important to remember that leadership is a process, that all nurses serve a role, and that the creation of positive and attractive work environments is needed to continue the important work nurses do each day.

CHAPTER HIGHLIGHTS

- Leadership is described as a transaction that occurs between a leader and followers rather than a character trait.
- There are a number of leadership styles described in the literature, including, but not limited to, the transformational, transactional, servant, authentic empowerment, autocratic/authoritarian, democratic, and laissez-faire styles.
- At times, leadership requires a blend of styles to enhance the effectiveness of a leader.
- Identifying potential nursing leaders is one of the best investments healthcare facilities can make.
- All nurses are leaders whether they are formally or informally identified as such.

CASE STUDY

Janice has been recently promoted to the position of nursing manager of the perianesthesia department. Although she has 25 years of clinical nursing experience, she has never taken formal courses in management. Having worked with many managers along her clinical journey, she can identify the behaviors that she does NOT want to demonstrate. She decides to explore nursing theories on management and leadership to expand her understanding of effective leader behaviors, strategies she is interested in learning and adopting. She learns that a leader who provides little direction or support for the team is effective when the team is small and highly functional. Which style of management does this describe?

REFERENCES

1. Size T. Leadership development for rural health. *N C Med J.* 2006;67(1):71-76.
2. Northouse PG. *Leadership Theory and Practice.* 7th ed. Sage Publications; 2015.
3. Maxwell E. Good leadership in nursing: what is the most effective approach? *Nurs Times.* 2017;113(8):18-21. Available at: https://www.nursingtimes.net/clinical-archive/leadership/good-leadership-in-nursing-what-is-the-most-effective-approach-17-07-2017/.
4. Pearson MM. Transformational leadership principles and tactics for the nurse executive to shift nursing culture. *J Nurse Adm.* 2020;50(3):142-151. Available at: https://doi.org/10.1097/nna.0000000000000858.
5. Marquis BL, Huston CJ. *Leadership Roles and Management Functions in Nursing.* 10th ed. Philadelphia: Lippincott, Williams & Wilkins; 2020.
6. Linuesa-Langreo J, Ruiz-Palomino P, Elche-Hortelano D. New strategies in the new millennium: servant leadership as enhancer of service climate and customer service performance. *Front Psych.* 2017;8:786. Available at: https://doi.org/10.3389/fpsyg.2017.00786.
7. Fahlberg B, Toomey R. Servant leadership: a model for emerging nurse leaders. *Nursing.* 2016;46(10):49-52. Available at: https://doi.org/10.1097/01.nurse.0000494644.77680.2a.
8. Doherty DP, Revell SMH. Developing nurse leaders: toward a theory of authentic leadership empowerment. *Nurs Forum.* 2020;55(3):416-424. Available at: https://doi.org/10.1111/nuf.12446.
9. Posnick S. *5 Nursing Leadership Styles You'll Come to Learn as a Nurse.* The Job Network; 2022. Available at: https://www.thejob-network.com/5-nursing-leadership-styles-utilize-122016. Accessed June 2, 2022.
10. Cornell A. *5 Leadership Styles in Nursing.* Relias; 2020. Available at: https://www.relias.com/blog/5-leadership-styles-in-nursing. Accessed June 2, 2022.
11. Bove LA, Scott M. Advice for aspiring nurse leaders. *Nursing.* 2021;51(3):44-47. Available at: https://doi.org/10.1097/01.nurse.0000733952.19882.55.

12. Martin E, Waxman KT. Generational differences and professional membership. *Nurse Lead*. 2017;151(2):127-130. Available at: http://dx.doi.org/10.1016/j.mnl.2016.11.014.

13. Morris M, Wood F, Dang D. Development and evaluation of a nurse leadership succession planning strategy in an academic medical center. *J Nurs Admin*. 2020;50(7-8):378-384. Available at: https://doi.org/10.1097/nna.0000000000000904.

14. Johnson CE. *Meeting the Ethical Challenges of Leadership*: Casting Light or Shadow. 7th ed. Sage Publishing; 2021.

15. Fries K. *8 Essential Qualities that Define Great Leadership*. Forbes; 2018. Available at: https://www.forbes.com/sites/kimberlyfries/2018/02/08/8-essential-qualities-that-define-great-leadership/.

16. Burke D, Erickson JI. Passing the chief nursing officer baton: the importance of succession planning and transformational leadership. *J Nurs Admin*. 2020;50(7-8):369-371. Available at: https://doi.org/10.1097/nna.0000000000000901.

17. Stutzer K. Generational differences and multigenerational teamwork. *Crit Care Nurse*. 2019;39(1):78-81. Available at: https://doi.org/10.4037/ccn2019163.

18. Martin A. Talent management: preparing a "ready" agile workforce. *Int J Pediatr Adolesc Med*. 2015;2(3-4):112-116. Available at: https://doi.org/10.1016/j.ijpam.2015.10.002.

19. Goldsby EA, Goldsby MG, Neck CP. Self-leadership strategies for nurse managers. *Nurs Manage*. 2020;51(3):34-40. Available at: https://doi.org/10.1097/01.numa.0000654848.10513.11.

2

3 Perianesthesia Nursing Standards

Theresa L. Clifford, DNP, RN, CPAN, CAPA, FASPAN, FAAN

LEARNING OBJECTIVES

A review of the content of this chapter will help the reader to:

1. Define the core principles of nursing standards and scope of practice.
2. Identify perianesthesia practice standards.
3. Describe the purpose and value of perianesthesia nursing standards and practice recommendations.
4. Differentiate principles, standards, practice recommendations, and position statements.

OVERVIEW

In the 1970s, the American Nurses Association (ANA) House of Delegates created action plans to enable the profession to determine the scope of practice for nursing and to define the requirements for the education of assistive personnel.[1] Contemporary specialty nursing organizations continue the work of defining and refining the scope of practice for each associated specialty. Standards provide direction, define accountability, identify outcomes, provide a framework for the evaluation of practice, and define a competent level of nursing practice.[2] The first guidelines for perianesthesia nurses, *Guidelines for Standards of Care*, were published in 1983.[3,4] Since 1983, these standards have evolved with changing practice, emerging new trends in healthcare, and advances in the fields of anesthesia and surgery impacting patient care. Today the term *guidelines* should not be confused with *standards*. Guidelines are narrower in scope and describe specific recommendations for the care of a particular clinical condition or diagnosis. Guidelines are developed systematically and are based on scientific evidence and expert opinion.

The American Society of PeriAnesthesia Nurses (ASPAN) engages a robust process for reviewing and publishing updated practice standards every 2 years, and as needed. This does include the integration of evidence-based practice when identified. The clear intent of the select expert members of the standards and guidelines strategic works teams has been to address the clinical practice needs of all nurses within the perianesthesia setting, regardless of role, caring for all patients of all ages in any clinical setting, including the ambulatory surgery center (ASC). Each rendition of the practice standards as they are published builds upon the previous edition and incorporates current changes in the field of perianesthesia. The purpose of this chapter is to identify the role of standards of practice within perianesthesia nursing as a specialty.

Evidence-Based Practice: Why do standards change?
Given the swift changes in healthcare pathways, frequent reviews and updates to established standards of care are required in order to promote the best possible evidence. Although contemporary advances in healthcare knowledge and experience occur rapidly, standards and guidelines upon which clinical care decisions are based must be grounded in evidence as research and new knowledge emerge.

Adapted from HealthManagement. Raising care standards to enhance patient outcomes. 2017. https://healthmanagement.org/c/hospital/whitepaper/raising-care-standards-to-enhance-patient-outcomes

---

ASPAN Standards

ASPAN standards are divided into several unique sections. Each section serves to provide the perianesthesia nurse with guidance and support upon which clinical excellence in perianesthesia practice can be built. Each section of the standards will be described in detail.

Scope of Practice

The scope of practice is presented to help identify and define perianesthesia nurses and perianesthesia nursing practice. This includes who, what, where, when, and why perianesthesia practice exists (Table 3.1). The practice is complex and yet must remain flexible in order to meet the needs of a constantly changing, if not chaotic, healthcare environment. The core of practice standards is intended to apply to all phases of patient care involving the anesthesia event. This implies that the standards are relevant in any unit where anesthetics, whether for procedural sedation or local infiltration or for general anesthesia, are administered. Given this definition, the standards also apply regardless of the location of the event, including, but not limited to, in hospitals, ambulatory or outpatient surgery centers, and surgical office-based practices. Also, in terms of scope of practice, these standards of

TABLE 3.1 Scope of Perianesthesia Nursing Practice

Who	All perianesthesia registered nurses with an active license to practice
What	Perianesthesia nursing, provision of clinically excellent nursing care and leadership, evidence-based education, and focused research surrounding the perianesthesia experience
Where	All environments where perianesthesia care is provided regardless of phase of care (all phases) or population served (all ages)
When	Anytime, anywhere there is a need for perianesthesia nursing expertise, caring, leadership, practice, or education
Why	The needs of procedural/surgical patients continually change, and the perianesthesia registered nurse's response adapts accordingly

Source: Adapted from American Society of PeriAnesthesia Nurses (ASPAN). *2023-2024 Perianesthesia Nursing Standards, Practice Recommendations and Interpretive Statements.* ASPAN; 2022.

perianesthesia practice are important regardless of the role of the perianesthesia registered nurse. This includes clinical bedside nurses, nurse researchers, nurse educators, nurse leaders, and advanced practice nurses, to name a few.[5]

The scope of practice also provides definitions for the range of clinical care, or the phases of care, provided to patients having perianesthesia experiences. The preanesthesia phase of care is focused on preparation of the patient for the perianesthesia event through a history, an assessment, and patient teaching. This also includes the immediate requirements for surgical and procedural safety through a final assessment and determination of validated preparation. Phase I is the period of time when the nursing roles focus on providing immediate postoperative care during the patient's transition from a totally anesthetized state to one requiring less acute interventions. Phase II is the period of time when the postoperative nursing roles focus on preparing the patient for self- or family-care or for care in an extended-care environment. Extended care, formerly called Phase III, is the period of time when the postoperative nursing roles focus on providing the ongoing care for a patient requiring extended observation and/or additional interventions after transfer from Phase I or II.

Principles

There are currently three main principles related to perianesthesia practice upon which the standards are built. The first principle belongs to the domain of ethical practice. According to the ANA's *Guide to the Code of Ethics for Nurses with Interpretive Statements* revised in 2015, nurses, and in this case perianesthesia nurses, have an obligation to consider the health of the population as well as the safety of patients when providing care.[6] Basic ethical principles are most commonly defined using primary legal terminology (Box 3.1). Given that there is some variation in scope of practice between states, ASPAN adheres to several core domains related to ethical practice. These include competency, responsibility to patients, professional responsibility, collegiality, clinical inquiry, and advocacy. Each domain addresses the very center of the foundation for strong, high-quality, clinically excellent practice (Table 3.2).

The second core principle for perianesthesia nursing is the principle of safety in practice. As a core principle, safety serves as another foundational building block for expert clinical practice. The principle highlights several key elements required to construct a safe model of perianesthesia care. The following elements are defined in the Principles of Safe Perianesthesia Practice[7]:

- Culture, leadership, and governance
- Patient and family engagement
- Workplace safety
- Psychological safety
- Accountability and responsibility
- Teamwork and effective communication
- Negotiation and conflict management

BOX 3.1 Ethical Principles

- *Autonomy*: Patient's right to self-determination
- *Beneficence*: An obligation or responsibility to help the patient; "to do good"
- *Nonmaleficence*: To not intentionally harm the patient; "do no harm"
- *Justice*: To treat the patient fairly

Source: Bordi SK. Geriatrics and anesthesia practice. In: Nagelhout JJ, Elisha S. *Nurse Anesthesia*. 6th ed. Elsevier; 2018.

TABLE 3.2 Definition of the Core Domains of Ethical Perianesthesia Nursing Practice

Competency	Integrates knowledge, attitudes, skills, and behaviors to maintain consistent standards of care
Responsibility to patients	Provides care to each patient while preserving human dignity, autonomy, and confidentiality; protecting patient rights; striving to eliminate health disparities; and supporting the health, well-being, health equity, and health literacy of the patient
Professional responsibility	Responsible and accountable for the care provided and for maintaining compliance with regulatory and professional agencies
Collegiality	Performs as a member of an interprofessional healthcare team providing care to patients
Clinical inquiry	Participates in and/or conducts clinical inquiry projects to improve practice, education, and/or add to the science of nursing
Advocacy	Perianesthesia registered nurses, individually and collectively, serve as advocates for the nursing profession, perianesthesia nursing practice, patients, and their families

Source: Adapted from American Society of PeriAnesthesia Nurses (ASPAN). *2023-2024 Perianesthesia Nursing Standards, Practice Recommendations and Interpretive Statements*. ASPAN; 2022.

- Improvement and measurement
- Continuous learning and competency

Each of the elements listed is crucial to a culture of safety. This concept of a culture of safety is widely different than a historical culture of blame where errors in practice were assumed to be the responsibility of individuals involved. Furthermore, once identified, the individuals involved were expected to assume "blame" for the event when, in fact, organizations as well as individuals must be committed to address unsafe conditions and strive for consistent safety in the workplace. The paradigm of a culture of safety leans toward an integration of system issues (e.g., policies, supplies, manpower), individual responsibilities (e.g., willingness to report unsafe situations, active participation in problem solving), as well as patient compliance as a partner in healthcare.[8]

The final principle is the systematic application of the nursing process during the provision of perianesthesia nursing care. Perianesthesia nurses practice within a wide scope of roles, a wide scope of patient ages, and a wide scope of phases of care in a wide variety of locations. Application of the fundamental nursing process, including the assessment phase, the diagnosis phase, the planning phase, and the implementation phase, followed by the re-evaluation phase, is expected throughout the care continuum. Given the episodic nature of care and the pressure for workflow efficiencies in support of smooth patient throughput, perianesthesia nurses work through this traditional nursing process in rapid progression. Each step requires the comportment of care with critical thinking, clinical judgment, and rapid implementation of action. In the end, perianesthesia nurses provide care that is "patient- and family-centered, holistic, outcome-oriented, and nimble."[6]

Standards

Standards of care are patient- and family-focused, as well as outcome-oriented. Throughout the years, the environment has expanded to include preadmission testing services, day of surgery/procedure ambulatory care settings, postanesthesia care units (PACU phase I and phase II), extended recovery facilities,

TABLE 3.3 Standards

Standard	Key Performance Outcomes	Criteria Example
Standard I: Patient rights and responsibilities	Patient autonomy, confidentiality, privacy, dignity, and worth are maintained throughout the perianesthesia continuum.	Adherence to ANA's Code of Ethics for Nurses with Interpretive Statements
Standard II: Family-centered care	Caring for patients includes caring for families and family-centered care and is incorporated into the professional perianesthesia registered nurse's clinical practice.	Mechanism exists within the facility to encourage and promote family-centered care
Standard III: Environment of care	Healthcare organizations will prioritize safety in the workplace environment to ensure a safe, supportive environment for healthcare personnel, patients, and families or visitors.	Unit/departmental-specific policies and procedures exist for fire, safety, infection prevention/control, internal/external disasters, and hazardous materials
Standard IV: Staffing and personnel management	Staffing patterns reflect an appropriate number of perianesthesia registered nurses with suitable knowledge and skills to provide safe, quality nursing care.	Staff function within written job performance descriptions
Standard V: Clinical inquiry	Research, quality improvement, and evidence-based practice findings guide decision-making in the professional perianesthesia registered nurse's clinical, educational, and leadership roles.	Perianesthesia registered nurses lead or participate in research, quality improvement, and evidence-based practice activities

Source: Adapted from American Society of PeriAnesthesia Nurses (ASPAN). *2023-2024 Perianesthesia Nursing Standards, Practice Recommendations and Interpretive Statements.* ASPAN; 2022.

pain management services, and special procedural areas such as cardiology, radiology, gastroenterology, and oncology, and procedures in physician and dental offices and labor and delivery suites. As a result, the standards have also expanded in their scope and definition. There are five primary standards of clinical practice defined by the ASPAN standards.[6] These include patient rights and responsibilities, family-centered care, environment of care, staffing and personnel management, and clinical inquiry. Refer to Table 3.3 for a brief overview of each standard. Because nursing staff have varied experiences and different educational backgrounds, meaningful standards can provide the framework of reference to ensure that all nursing staff members are providing a high quality of nursing care. Three examples of standards sources include professional nursing associations (e.g., ASPAN, ANA), institution-specific agencies, and regulatory agencies. Nurses are held accountable by law to common nursing standards, as well as community standards for care (e.g., what a prudent nurse would do in the same situation), regardless of membership in any organization.

Practice Recommendations

Practice recommendations mirror slightly the principles of practice guidelines. They have been developed over time as a result of emerging nursing and practice sciences that provide evidence in support of the best and most desirable level of performance expected of perianesthesia nurses. Throughout the continuous process of monitoring clinical activities across the nation and in partnering countries, trends in practice and clinical inquiry are monitored and assessed for practice solutions that both support the safety and outcomes of patients as well as of the healthcare team, particularly the perianesthesia team. Box 3.2 provides a current list of practice recommendations endorsed by practice experts who represent the wide range of clinical roles and settings within this nursing specialty.

Position Statements: Traditional and Collaborative

In general, the purpose of position statements issued by organizations is to highlight current issues, gaps, or concerns related to patient care and practice. The majority of position statements emerge from within the perianesthesia nursing community, while collaborative position statements have

---

BOX 3.2 Practice Recommendations

Patient Classification/Staffing Recommendations
Components of Assessment and Management for the Perianesthesia Patient
Practice Recommendation A: Preanesthesia Phases of Care
Practice Recommendation B: Postanesthesia Phases of Care
Equipment for Preanesthesia/Day of Surgery Phase, PACU Phase I, Phase II, and Extended Care
Competencies, Knowledge, and Skills for the Perianesthesia Registered Nurse
Competencies of Perianesthesia Unlicensed Assistive Personnel/Support Staff
Safe Transfer of Care: Handoff and Transportation
The Role of the Registered Nurse in the Management of Patients Undergoing Procedural Sedation
Perianesthesia Throughput
Family Presence in the Perianesthesia Setting
Obstructive Sleep Apnea in the Adult Patient
The Prevention of Unwanted Sedation in the Adult Patient
Promotion of Normothermia in the Adult Patient
Alarm Management
Safe Medication Administration

Source: American Society of PeriAnesthesia Nurses (ASPAN). *2023-2024 Perianesthesia Nursing Standards, Practice Recommendations and Interpretive Statements.* ASPAN; 2022.

---

their genesis with partnering organizations with a shared vision or common goal. The standards and guidelines team routinely evaluates the necessity of position statements. When enough clinical evidence is found in support of actionable items related to the issue or gap, a position statement may be moved to the higher level of a practice recommendation with leveled evidence to support the action items. In some circumstances, the original issue that generated the statement may have been resolved across the practice and the team recommends retiring the statement. For historical purposes, all retired position statements are retained by ASPAN. Box 3.3 lists the current position statements.

BOX 3.3 Position Statements

A Position Statement on the Perianesthesia Patient with a Do-Not-Attempt-Resuscitation Advance Directive

A Position Statement on Clinician Well-Being in the Perianesthesia Setting

A Position Statement on Digital Professionalism in Perianesthesia Practice

A Position Statement on Acuity-Based Staffing for Phase I

A Position Statement on Air Quality and Occupational Hazards

A Position Statement on Emergency Preparedness

A Position Statement on Contemporary Social Issues

Source: American Society of PeriAnesthesia Nurses (ASPAN). *2023-2024 Perianesthesia Nursing Standards, Practice Recommendations and Interpretive Statements*. ASPAN; 2022.

Resources

The final section of ASPAN standards allows for direct links and material for resources that are commonly referenced. For example, the American Society of Anesthesiologists (ASA) has numerous practice standards that have a direct influence on perianesthesia practice. As partners in the realm of perianesthesia, references by the ASA are vital as perianesthesia nurses advocate for best practice across any unit providing perianesthesia nursing care. Other resources include a recommended timeline for orientation of new staff to the perianesthesia environment.

CHAPTER HIGHLIGHTS

- ASPAN standards are reviewed and revised every 2 years.
- There are several key components of the published standards: scope of practice, principles, standards, practice recommendations, position statements, and resources.
- Continued research is essential to ensure that new practices are in line with established standards.

CASE STUDY

A perianesthesia nurse (RN) submits a query to the clinical practice committee. She was recently hired in an outpatient surgery center and now questions the practices she has observed at the end of the day. While the last patients are recovering and still requiring vigilant care in Phase I recovery, the surgical team in the operating room has completed their tasks of terminal cleaning. The anesthesia provider walks into the unit with his leather jacket and bike helmet in hand, obviously preparing to leave the building. The RN is concerned because in her previous job in a hospital-based outpatient surgery center, the anesthesia providers were "not allowed" to leave the building until all patients were cleared from the Phase I level of care.

Should the RN be concerned? Why? Why not?

What action can the RN take to address her concerns?

What could possibly go wrong if the provider leaves the building?

Special posthumous thanks and credit to my friend and colleague Lois Schick, MN, MBA, RN, CPAN, CAPA, FASPAN, author of the original text this chapter is based on in the *Ambulatory Surgical Nursing*, 2nd edition.[2]

REFERENCES

1. American Nurses Association. *Expanded Historical Review of Nursing and the ANA*. 2019. Available at: https://www.nursingworld.org/~48de6f/globalassets/docs/ana/ana-expandedhistoricalreview.pdf.
2. Schick L. Nursing standards. In: Burden N, Quinn DMD, O'Brien D, Dawes BSG, eds. *Ambulatory Surgical Nursing*. 2nd ed. WB Saunders; 2000:131-135.
3. Odom-Forren J, Clifford TL. Evolution of perianesthesia care. In: Schick L, Windle PE, eds. *PeriAnesthesia Nursing Core Curriculum: Preprocedure, Phase I and Phase II PACU Nursing*. 4th ed. Elsevier; 2021:1-9.
4. American Society of Post Anesthesia Nurses. *Fifty Years of Progress in Post Anesthesia Nursing 1940-1990*. ASPAN; 1990.
5. Ashton KC. Standards of Care and Standards of Practice. *J Leg Nurse Consult*. 2019;30(4):10-13. Available at: https://member.aanlcp.org/wp-content/uploads/2021/03/AALNCJLNCWinter2019.pdf.
6. American Nurses Association. *Guide to the Code of Ethics for Nurses with Interpretive Statements*. American Nurses Association; 2015.
7. American Society of PeriAnesthesia Nurses. *2023-2024 Perianesthesia Nursing Standards, Practice Recommendations and Interpretive Statements*. ASPAN; 2022.
8. Oberfrank SM, Rall M, Dieckmann P, Michaela K, Gaba DM. Avoiding patient harm in anesthesia: human performance and patient safety. In: Gropper MA, ed. *Miller's Anesthesia*. 9th ed. Elsevier; 2020:105-178.

4 Clinical Inquiry: Quality Improvement and Evidence-Based Practice in Ambulatory Surgery

Daphne Stannard, PhD, RN, CNS, NPD-BC, FCCM

LEARNING OBJECTIVES

A review of the content of this chapter will help the reader to:

1. Define clinical inquiry.
2. Differentiate between evidence-based practice, primary research, secondary research, and quality improvement.
3. Describe how clinical inquiry is a vital and required component of ambulatory surgical nursing practice.

OVERVIEW

The *Perianesthesia Nursing Standards, Practice Recommendations and Interpretive Statements*[1] published by the American Society of PeriAnesthesia Nurses (ASPAN) have a dedicated standard for quality improvement, evidence-based practice (EBP), and research. These activities are a constellation of research and scholarly activities that fall under the umbrella term *clinical inquiry*. Clinical inquiry can be defined as the act of deliberate questioning about a practice issue(s), ranging from a structured and systematic investigation to clinical observation, resulting in patient- and family-centered solutions, findings, or recommendations. On a daily basis, nurses working in ambulatory surgical settings engage in clinical inquiry activities, and the purpose of this chapter is to describe and differentiate these different activities and apply them to ambulatory nursing practice.

FACTS AND FIGURES

Healthcare is highly regulated, but many seldom consider the requirements for professional nurses to engage in clinical inquiry. The *Scope and Standards of Nursing Practice*, set forth by the American Nurses Association, has two standards that apply to clinical inquiry. Standard 14 (Scholarly Inquiry) states that a registered nurse will integrate "scholarship, evidence, and research findings into practice."[2] Additionally, Standard 15 (Quality of Practice) states that a registered nurse will contribute to quality nursing practice and specifies that incorporating evidence into nursing practice to improve outcomes is one of the competencies that fulfills that standard.[3] Other competencies under Standard 15 that are germane to clinical inquiry include collecting data to monitor the quality of nursing practice; providing critical review and evaluation of policies, procedures, and guidelines to improve the quality of health care; participating in quality improvement activities; collaborating with the interprofessional team to implement quality improvement plans and interventions; and documenting nursing practice to support quality and performance improvement initiatives.[2]

Regulatory and accrediting bodies, such as the Centers for Medicare and Medicaid Services[3] and The Joint Commission,[4] have standards for hospitals and surgical centers requiring periodic reporting of quality assurance and performance improvement data to ensure that care delivery is safe and provides high-quality outcomes. Some of the required and reportable quality data are considered nursing-sensitive indicators, which demonstrate the specific contributions nursing as a profession makes to the overall health and well-being of a patient.[5] The excellent provision of healthcare services requires an excellent healthcare team—in terms of both structure and process—yet the actions of individual team members, such as nurses, can have a great impact on specific patient outcomes. Finally, teamwork and collaboration must be demonstrated in order to achieve Magnet designation by the American Nurses Credentialing Center (ANCC),[6] in addition to creating new knowledge and applying existing evidence to show contributions to nursing science.

EVIDENCE-BASED PRACTICE

Evidence-based practice (EBP) is a more inclusive offshoot of evidence-based medicine, which was a movement that started in the early 1990s.[7] There are many definitions of EBP, including the oft-cited Sackett et al. definition that states, "Evidence-based medicine is the integration of best research evidence with clinical expertise and patient values."[8] Yet, this definition is more aligned with the discipline of medicine and associated provider-related activities, such as prescribing therapeutic remedies and ordering diagnostic tests based on a differential diagnosis. A more nursing-centered definition is as follows: EBP for nursing is a way of entering the situation with curiosity and engagement and follows the nursing process by responding to the issue or problem at hand using the best available evidence.[7] This definition is general enough to accommodate the variety of nursing roles and settings but is also specific enough to name the practice that provides a questioning stance in response to an emerging issue or problem.

In 1995, Sackett and Rosenberg described what are now considered to be the iconic five steps of EBP: identifying the problem, accessing the best available evidence, critically appraising the evidence, applying the change to practice, and evaluating the change in practice.[9] While these steps are helpful for a small test of change in a clinical setting, every step may not be needed to solve every clinical problem or issue. In fact, most clinicians trying to solve a clinical issue that is limited in complexity and scope can usually answer the question using the first three steps. These three steps can be thought of as EBP at the point of care (Figure 4.1).The fourth and fifth steps of EBP overlap with primary research and quality improvement and typically require additional resources and work conducted away from the point of care to plan, implement, analyze, and disseminate the findings. The fourth and fifth steps will be discussed under primary research.

For example, if a piece of equipment fails in practice, the first step is always to identify the problem. Taking this example

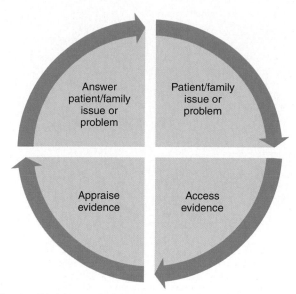

Fig. 4.1 Workflow of evidence-based practice at the point of care.

further, the perianesthesia nurse may recognize that the pulse oximeter waveform is dampened, thus potentially reporting a falsely diminished value. In troubleshooting the low oxygen saturation value, the perianesthesia nurse draws upon education and clinical judgment. Recognizing the dampened waveform and responding to the low saturation alarm is the first step of EBP, namely, problem identification. By moving the pulse oximeter probe to a different digit and moving the hand under the blanket away from competing light sources, the nurse is using the best available evidence to fix the problem. The nurse may need to switch to an ear probe after recognizing that the patient's dark nail polish could be interfering with the signal.

In this example, the third step of EBP at the point of care is not necessary to solve the clinical issue at hand. The perianesthesia nurse had attended workshops and training sessions and read articles providing the best available evidence and internalized this knowledge. Critically appraising the literature was not necessary for the perianesthesia nurse in this example. That is one of the reasons that a flexible definition of EBP is needed for nursing, as nurses confront clinical issues that range in complexity and demand different responses.

If a review of the literature is needed to evaluate what other ambulatory surgical centers (ASCs) have done when confronting a problem, such as an increased incidence in surgical site infections, it is customary to sketch out the issue using a PICO question, whereby the letters of the acronym stand for:

- P for population (patient, problem)
- I for intervention
- C for comparison
- O for outcome

The PICO format is a convention used in EBP to enable the clinician to deconstruct the problem into searchable elements for the second step of EBP, namely, accessing the best available evidence.[7,10] While accessing the literature at face value is fairly straightforward due to the explosion of information that is readily available on frequently used databases, it is helpful to have a plan in terms of which database will be used and what information, in particular, one is seeking. A well-written PICO question helps to guide the clinician in accessing and selecting specific literature that is relevant to the problem at hand. Collaboration with a librarian at this stage is recommended if the PICO question is complex or if the literature is more difficult to access.[11]

The third step of EBP is to critically evaluate the literature that was retrieved for the PICO question. If there are no articles found on the topic, this suggests a flawed PICO question or a search strategy that needs revision (especially if a librarian was used to help locate the evidence). It is possible, of course, that the PICO question points to a truly innovative practice issue and there is no guidance on this topic. In this case, the nurse needs to conduct primary research (discussed below), often with the help of a research team. If multiple research studies have been retrieved using the PICO question, implementing a quality improvement project in the local setting or synthesizing the literature as a systematic review might be most appropriate (see Figure 4.2, Clinical Inquiry Algorithm).[11]

It is usually the case, however, that multiple forms of evidence are found for any given PICO question: perhaps a few primary research articles, a systematic review (described further), several quality improvement projects (described further), some clinical articles, and some gray literature. Critically appraising the literature is the third step of EBP and is the process one uses to carefully evaluate the evidence that has been retrieved. ASPAN has created critical appraisal tools to use when evaluating systematic reviews, quantitative primary research studies, and qualitative or mixed method primary research studies. These tools help to answer whether the retrieved evidence should be considered high-quality evidence and helps the clinician to level or rank the evidence. The ASPAN Hierarchy of Evidence[7] is presented in Figure 4.3.

While it is beyond the scope of this chapter to describe all research methodologies and designs, it should be noted that the highest level of evidence—systematic reviews—is found at the top of the pyramid. As one goes down the pyramid, there is less control over the research, and this can lead to bias. Primary research can employ several different research methodologies and designs, and the research paradigm and level of control exerted by the researchers to avoid systematic bias help to determine the level on the hierarchy of evidence. Clinical articles or what are sometimes referred to as a review of the literature or a narrative review are not considered research studies and thus fall on the lowest level of evidence (expert opinion).

Gray literature is a body of evidence that is often research-based (although not always) and produced by governmental agencies, nonprofit research institutes, and professional organizations that distribute the information outside of customary academic or commercial publications. For this reason, it is often considered unpublished literature, but it may still be a valid source of evidence. Gray literature would be ranked on the hierarchy of evidence in the same fashion as research that was published using traditional publishing channels, such as peer-reviewed journals.[12]

There are also more articles at level 4 than there are at the higher levels. Thus, the hierarchy of evidence pyramid is both a graphic representation of the amount of literature likely to be found on a given topic, as well as a depiction of the rigor associated with each level. It is critical to understand, however, that critical appraisal and the evidence hierarchy must be evaluated together, as one can review a poorly conducted systematic review and a very rigorous observational study.

PRIMARY RESEARCH

Primary research can take many forms depending on the discipline and the research question. In nursing, research is divided into two categories: primary research and secondary research. Primary research is defined as the discovery-oriented systematic investigation to develop or contribute to generalizable knowledge.[13] Most primary research in nursing involves living beings (e.g., animals or humans) and, as such, requires

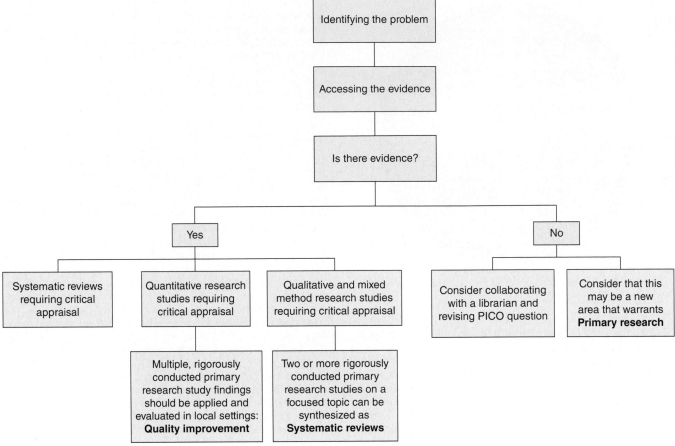

Fig. 4.2 Clinical inquiry algorithm.

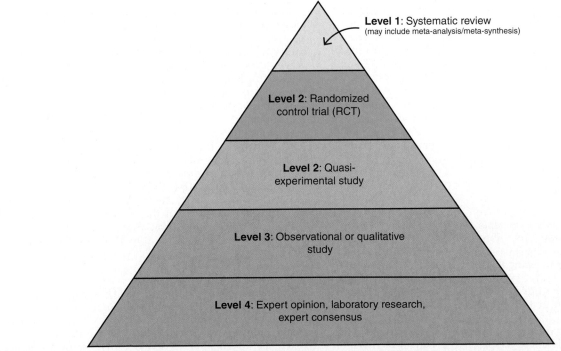

Fig. 4.3 ASPAN hierarchy of evidence. From Stannard D. A practical definition of evidence-based practice for nursing. *J Perianesth Nurs.* 2019;34(5):1080-1084.

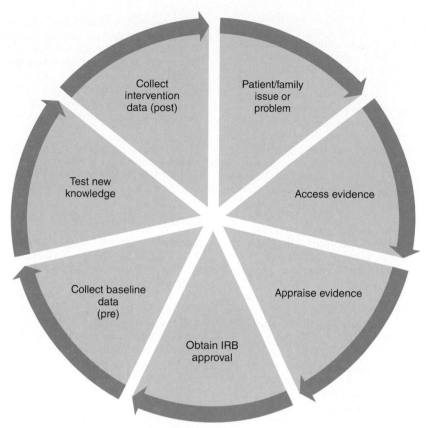

Fig. 4.4 Primary research workflow. From Stannard D. Embracing all types of clinical inquiry. *J Perianesth Nurs.* 2014;29(4):334-337.

approval from an institutional review board (IRB) to ensure protection of animal and human research subjects.[14] In the example of SSIs, if an off-label medication is tested to reduce the incidence of SSIs in an ambulatory surgical facility, the project would have to be approved by an IRB to ensure the safety of the human research subjects. Off-label use refers to unapproved use of an approved drug.[15] The team researching the off-label medication to reduce the incidence of SSI would follow the primary research workflow (see Figure 4.4), but one will notice that the first three steps are identical to the first three steps of EBP at the point of care. The workflow deviates, however, once IRB approval is sought and baseline data are collected to serve as a point of comparison once the intervention has been applied. There are many research designs one can employ to answer a primary research question besides a pre-post design,[16] but for the sake of simplicity, this design was used to illustrate the differences between the different workflows.

SECONDARY RESEARCH

Secondary research involves the investigation of a clinically focused topic using already collected data (see Figure 4.5) and can be divided into two major categories: secondary analysis and systematic reviews. A secondary analysis involves the summary and analysis of an existing data set by posing a new question. For example, a primary researcher may have collected data to answer a research question about medication errors in an ambulatory surgical setting. A secondary analysis could be conducted by the same researcher or someone else and might look for patterns of medication errors in that same data set, for example, but focus instead on errors concerning oral medications occurring in phase II recovery.

This differs from a systematic review, which involves the identification, selection, critical appraisal, and synthesis of the

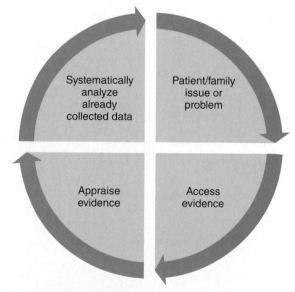

Fig. 4.5 Secondary research workflow.

existing primary research studies on a specific topic.[17] Systematic reviews can only be conducted if at least two or more primary research studies have been conducted on a particular topic. If only one study or no primary research studies exist on a given topic, it is not appropriate to conduct a systematic review until additional primary research has been conducted.

Finally, there is always confusion about systematic reviews and meta-analyses. A meta-analysis is a series of statistical tests one can run on similar data for a quantitative systematic review. These statistical tests can only be used when certain conditions are met, and researchers must often resort to describing their findings with words (often referred to as a narrative write-up), as opposed to using numbers from a meta-analysis. A quantitative systematic review is still a systematic review if it lacks a meta-analysis; the difference is simply that certain statistical conditions regarding the similarity of data were not met. Because a secondary analysis and a systematic review rely on data that have already been collected, IRB approval is not necessary.[13]

Primary research methodologies can support quantitative and/or qualitative data. Examples of primary quantitative data collection methods include surveys and questionnaires that result in the compilation of numerical data (e.g., numbers) that can be analyzed using a variety of statistical methods. Primary qualitative data collection methods include observations, journal entries, structured or unstructured interviews, and other forms of textual evidence that support the gathering of narrative (e.g., words) data. In some research plans, the data can be collected using a mixed-methods approach, often combining both quantitative and qualitative data collection and data analysis methods. Secondary research can also use quantitative and/or qualitative data. A common form of secondary research is a systematic review. The purpose of a systematic review is to conduct a secondary analysis of data that have already been collected from other primary research studies.[18]

Evidence-Based Practice: Qualitative Research

According to de Lima et al., comprehension of the science of nursing has been supported by research studies, essentially quantitative studies, providing a foundation of objective and evidence-based knowledge for clinical practices. Qualitative research, on the other hand, explores a question with the goal of understanding phenomena based on experiences, concepts, themes, and human interactions. Qualitative research in nursing attempts to understand how nurses and patients experience the events surrounding health and nursing care. There are a variety of qualitative research methods, including grounded theory, ethnography, and phenomenological research. Data collection is often performed using surveys, focus groups, interviews, and observations. Once qualitative data is collected it is analyzed following organization of data elements into coding and recurring themes.

Source: de Lima JJ, Miranda KCL, Cestari VRF, de Paula Pessoa VLM. Art in evidence-based nursing practice from the perspective of Florence Nightingale. *Rev Bras Enferm.* 2022;75(4):e20210664.

QUALITY IMPROVEMENT

Quality improvement is defined as the application of previously discovered knowledge in local settings (Figure 4.6). Although primary research is essential for exploring, identifying, and systematically discovering and testing new knowledge, the application of these findings in local settings is necessary to evaluate whether the study results are, in fact, effective in improving care at the site where the quality improvement project is occurring. Local context makes a large impact—what works in one unit, surgical service, or ambulatory surgical center may not work for all.[19] It is vitally important for clinicians and administrators alike to conduct small tests of change in local settings before adopting a large-scale change that might have demonstrated effectiveness at another institution. If a proven intervention does not improve care or outcomes at the local setting, the organizational culture, specific patient population, and a host of other factors may make the proven intervention less effective and may even have a deleterious effect on local outcomes.

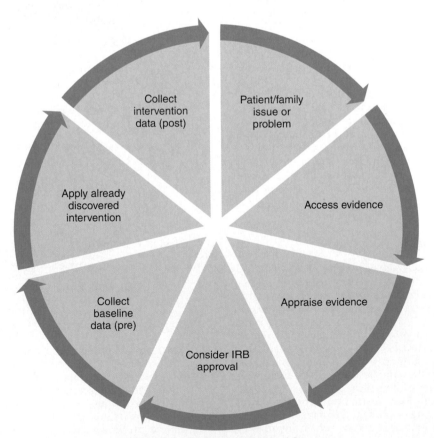

Fig. 4.6 Quality improvement workflow.

This is a growing area in healthcare, and the application of already discovered knowledge in a local setting is classified using many names, such as performance improvement, quality assurance, quality improvement, and implementation.[20] As with the plethora of research methodologies and designs, there are a variety of quality improvement models, approaches, and tools one can use to apply and evaluate a small test of change in a local setting.[21] It should also be noted that data collection (both for presurgical events and postsurgical events) and the application of already discovered knowledge constitute the fourth and fifth steps of EBP, namely, applying the change to practice and evaluating the change in practice.

CHAPTER HIGHLIGHTS

- Clinical inquiry can be defined as the act of deliberate questioning about a practice issue(s), ranging from a structured and systematic investigation to clinical observation, resulting in patient- and family-centered solutions, findings, or recommendations.
- Healthcare is highly regulated, and there are many requirements for professional nurses to engage in clinical inquiry.
- EBP for nursing is a way of entering the situation with curiosity and engagement and follows the nursing process by responding to the issue or problem at hand using the best available evidence.
- Primary research is defined as the discovery-oriented systematic investigation to develop or contribute to generalizable knowledge.
- Secondary research involves the investigation of a clinically focused topic using already collected data.
- Quality improvement is defined as the application of previously discovered knowledge in local settings.

CASE STUDY

Leticia Smith is a 56-year-old woman who has been scheduled for a rhinoplasty procedure in your ambulatory surgical center. She has a significant past medical and surgical history and has an extensive list of medications and supplements that she takes to manage her conditions. She lives with a partner, and they have two grown children who, along with her partner, are with her in the preoperative area to offer emotional support and assistance. As the perianesthesia care nurse you meet the patient and family and begin the preoperative day of surgery screening.

During this process, she mentions several herbal supplements that you know might be contraindicated with her surgical procedure. As an educated and informed professional nurse, you have gone to conferences and read articles that have covered this topic; however, you are not certain that the herbals she has mentioned are inadvisable. You open a web browser and do a quick Internet search for "herbal supplements that are contraindicated for surgery." You search for reputable sources and find a webpage that lists many of the herbal supplements she has taken in the past 24 hours.[22] You bring the medication list to the attention of the anesthesia provider and surgeon, who question the patient further regarding doses and when the supplements were last taken. It is jointly decided to postpone her surgery due to the increased risk of postoperative bleeding secondary to the herbal supplements. You provide the patient and her family with thorough discharge education concerning when to stop these supplements in advance of her newly rescheduled surgery.

In this case, the perianesthesia nurse engaged in clinical inquiry by questioning the herbal supplements the patient was taking. This is an example of EBP at the point of care, as no research or quality improvement was implicated, but, rather, the nurse entered the preoperative setting with curiosity and engagement and followed the nursing process by responding to the patient's medication history by identifying the problem, accessing the evidence, and critically appraising the evidence before bringing it to the attention of the healthcare team. By rescheduling the patient's procedure for a later date, the nurse advocated for patient safety by using EBP at the point of care.

REFERENCES

1. American Society of PeriAnesthesia Nurses. *2021-2022 Perianesthesia Nursing Standards, Practice Recommendations and Interpretive Statements.* ASPAN; 2020.
2. American Nurses Association. *Nursing: Scope and Standards of Practice.* 4th ed. ANA; 2021.
3. *CMS Issues Final Quality Assessment and Performance Improvement Conditions of Participation for Hospitals.* Available at: https://www.cms.gov/newsroom/press-releases/cms-issues-final-quality-assessment-and-performance-improvement-conditions-participation-hospitals. Accessed September 25, 2021.
4. *ORYX Performance Measurement Reporting.* Available at: https://www.jointcommission.org/measurement/reporting/accreditation-oryx/. Accessed September 25, 2021.
5. *Ambulatory Care Nurse-Sensitive Indicator Industry Report.* Available at: https://www.aaacn.org/practice-resources/ambulatory-care/nurse-sensitive-indicators. Accessed September 25, 2021.
6. *Magnet Model: Creating a Magnet Culture.* Available at: https://www.nursingworld.org/organizational-programs/magnet/magnet-model/. Accessed September 25, 2021.
7. Stannard D. A practical definition of evidence-based practice for nursing. *J Perianesth Nurs.* 2019;34(5):1080-1084.
8. Sackett DL, Straus SE, Richardson WS, Rosenberg W, Haynes RB. *Evidence-Based Medicine: How to Practice and Teach EBM.* 2nd ed. Churchill Livingstone; 2000:1.
9. Sackett DL, Rosenberg WMC. The need for evidence-based medicine. *J R Soc Med.* 1995;88:620-624.
10. Fetzer S. Research and evidence-based practice. In: Schick L, Windle P, eds. *ASPAN's Perianesthesia Nursing Core Curriculum: Preprocedure, Phase I and Phase II PACU Nursing.* 4th ed. Elsevier;2021:40-50.
11. Stannard D, Jacobs W. Accessing and selecting the literature: The second step in evidence-based practice. *AORN J.* 2021;114(4):336-338.
12. Bonato S. *Searching the Grey Literature: A Handbook for Searching Reports, Working Papers, and Other Unpublished Research.* Rowman & Littlefield; 2018.
13. Stannard D. Embracing all types of clinical inquiry. *J Perianesth Nurs.* 2014;29(4):334-337.
14. Bankert EA, Gordon BG, Hurley EA, Shriver SP. *Institutional Review Board: Management and Function.* 3rd ed. Jones & Bartlett.
15. *Understanding Unapproved Use of Approved Drugs "Off Label."* Available at: https://www.fda.gov/patients/learn-about-expanded-access-and-other-treatment-options/understanding-unapproved-use-approved-drugs-label. Accessed September 25, 2021.
16. Grove SK, Gray JR. *Understanding Nursing Research: Building an Evidence-Based Practice.* 7th ed. Elsevier; 2019.
17. Holly C, Salmond S, Saimbert M. *Comprehensive Systematic Review for Advanced Practice Nursing.* 2nd ed. Springer; 2017.
18. Stannard D. A systematic approach to systematic reviews. *AORN J.* 2022;115(2):124-127. Available at: https://doi.org/10.1002/aorn.13610.
19. Stannard D. Learning from lessons for change. *AORN J.* 2020;112(5):502-504.
20. Harrison MB, Graham ID. *Knowledge Translation in Nursing and Healthcare: A Roadmap to Evidence-Informed Practice.* Wiley Blackwell; 2021.
21. Rycroft-Malone J, Bucknall T. *Models and Frameworks for Implementing Evidence-Based Practice: Linking Evidence to Action.* Wiley Blackwell; 2010.
22. *Medications and Herbs that Affect Bleeding.* Available at: https://med.stanford.edu/content/dam/sm/ohns/documents/Sinus%20Center/Stanford_Medication_and_Herbs.pdf. Accessed September 25, 2021.

5 Risk Management and Legal Issues

Helen C. Fong, DNP, RN, CPAN, PHN, FASPAN

LEARNING OBJECTIVES

A review of the content of this chapter will help the reader to:

1. Identify terms, definitions, and general information associated with risk management.
2. Acknowledge regulatory requirements in ambulatory surgery centers for patient safety.
3. Describe measures to minimize risks and challenges.

OVERVIEW

Risk management is an essential component of quality management.[1,2] Quality management is important for practice viability (Box 5.1).[2] The goals for risk management include the determination, investigation, and assessment of the risks in healthcare and the designing of plans for the reduction or prevention of the incidence and severity of missed opportunities and errors.[1,3]

The adoption of a comprehensive risk management plan ensures patient safety and quality care and minimizes the financial and legal exposure in ambulatory surgery centers (ASCs).[2,4] The risk management plan must include systems that determine potential hazards and incorporate processes capable of managing events and incidents.[2] This plan must also consider required resources for external benchmarking and education.[2] Data from quality indicators and outcome measures must be utilized for event trending.[2]

Risk management in the outpatient surgery setting is a responsibility of the ASC leadership, including the director and/or manager.[2] The ASC director must ensure that every staff member is educated in detection, prevention, and intervention measures related to potential and actual accidents and injuries.[1] The risk plan also identifies safety risks, aims to reduce both errors and injuries, and tells how to intervene if these risk events occur.[1,2] The possible adverse events in an ASC may include operating on the wrong surgical site, errors in identifying patients, the retention of foreign objects, medication errors,

device-related issues, gas injuries or deaths, anesthetic-related fires or injuries, and infections. Documentation and management of these issues should be done according to facility policies and approved by a governing body. Such policies should also be evaluated on an annual basis in order to maintain their effectiveness and applicability for contemporary needs.[2,4]

Anesthesia providers are playing a key role in patient outcomes as the demand for increased outpatient centers, efficiencies, and ambulatory surgeries has proliferated.[5] Anesthesia providers are the gatekeepers in an ASC.[2,6] These providers are accountable for the criteria for patient selection and suitability to the outpatient ambulatory setting.[6] Patient selection and presurgical assessments are the key elements for ensuring patient safety and optimal health outcomes.[7] Most patients selected for ambulatory surgeries are in good health, and the majority of procedures done are simple and routine.[2,6] The opioid crisis and the need to provide adequate pain management serve as examples of the need to have risk management plans in the outpatient setting. Most recently, anesthesia providers have been using a variety of nerve block techniques for postoperative pain management.[5] Patients have better pain management outcomes and experience earlier discharge when nerve blocks are used.[5] These techniques are effective and safe in controlling postoperative pain. Operational quality metrics and risk management tools are also important for helping to manage adverse events in the ASC.[2,5,6] Difficult outcomes are rare, but they do happen.[2,6]

FACTS AND FIGURES

The first ASC was opened in 1970. The number of ASCs certified by the Centers for Medicare and Medicaid Services (CMS) continued to grow; there were 239 in 1983 and 5316 in 2015.[8] Today, in 2023, there are almost six thousand ASCs certified by Medicare performing more than 30 million surgeries per year.[4] There are four primary organizations recognized by the CMS that are privileged to assess outpatient surgery programs and determine their compliance with CMS requirements. An ASC must be compliant with CMS regulations in order to receive payment for care rendered (Box 5.2).

Over the past several decades, the number of ambulatory surgeries has increased owing to medical and technological advances, as well as demand.[8] The advances in healthcare delivery include improvements in anesthesia and analgesics for pain management.[8] The development of minimally invasive

---

> **BOX 5.1** Definitions of Risk Management and Quality Management
>
> **Risk Management:** A program directed toward identifying, evaluating, and taking corrective action against potential risks that could lead to injury.
> **Quality Management:** A preventive approach designed to address problems efficiently and quickly.
>
> Source: Sullivan EJ. *Effective Leadership and Management in Nursing.* (9th Ed.) Pearson; 2017.

> **BOX 5.2** CMS-Approved Accrediting Organizations
>
> AAAHC: Accreditation Association for Ambulatory Health Care
>
> TJC: The Joint Commission
>
> AAAASF: American Association for Accreditation of Ambulatory Surgery Facilities, Inc.
>
> ACHC: Accreditation Commission for Health Care, Inc.

and noninvasive procedures such as laser surgeries, laparoscopy, and endoscopy has also contributed to this rise.[8] The adoption of enhanced recovery after surgery (ERAS) protocols for an expanding array of surgeries has increased a trend for reducing outpatient admissions to hospitals. Such medical and technological advances are now safely performed outside of hospital settings. In addition, Medicare programs have spurred a growth in ambulatory surgery by expanding their coverage in ASCs both for hospital-based and free-standing facilities.[8] This expansion of Medicare coverage created a strong economic incentive for hospitals to move some surgeries out of the hospital.[8] In January 2020, the CMS removed a number of surgical procedures from the inpatient list. For example, the CMS approved primary total knee arthroplasty and multiple cardiac procedures as billable outpatient procedures in the ASC.[1,4]

RISK MANAGEMENT PLAN

The risk management plan covers every aspect of the prevention of, detection of, and intervention in accidents and injuries.[1,4] Principles of risk management include identification of the potential risks and a regular review of monitoring systems such as "incident reports, audits, committee minutes, oral complaints, and patient satisfaction questionnaires."[1,4] Incident reports or adverse event reports are used to help identify the root causes of actual or near-miss events and further analyze the occurrences to assess their severity and frequency.[1] Data collection must be complete and detailed in order to make certain that an accurate analysis of risks can be conducted.[1,4]

This root cause analysis process related to events and outcomes must include intervention strategies to reduce and eliminate further occurrences and future adverse outcomes.[1,4,9] The collection of data is important in identifying the risk in terms of future events.[9] The process involves careful documentation per institutional policy. The tools used for documentation allow for the complete audit reports of events, identification of probable causes, and ability to predict liabilities and losses.[9] This is done in collaboration with committees such as infection prevention, medical affairs, safety, security, pharmaceutical services, environmental services, and nursing committees.[1] In addition, reviews must include the appraisal of safety and risks associated with specific patient care procedures, physician credentialing policies and procedures, and periodic reviews of physician files. Risk management plans also consider the adherence to federal and state regulations related to patient safety, informed consent, and care.[1,4] These reviews must be communicated to the governing body periodically, which evaluates the outcomes associated with risk management plans.[1,4]

WAYS TO MINIMIZE RISKS
Adherence to Professional Standards and Applicable Standards of Care

Compliance with professional standards is crucial in providing high-quality, safe care.[4,6] Nursing staff and medical personnel working in the ASC must adhere to professional standards set forth by the American Society of PeriAnesthesia Nurses (ASPAN), the Association of periOperative Registered Nurses (AORN), the American Society of Anesthesiologists (ASA), and the Society for Ambulatory Anesthesia (SAA), to name a few.[4,6] ASCs must develop and implement comprehensive credentialing policies and processes for physicians working in the facilities.[4] In addition, following the recommendations from professional organizations mentioned earlier, the framework of the operations of the ASC must provide a safe pathway to quality care. The adoption and utilization of a surgical safety checklist is one example (Figure 5.1). Staff

who adhere to the surgical checklist and timeout procedures before surgery commences safeguard the reduction of adverse events.[10,11] Proper procedures for surgical site marking in the preoperative phase while the patient is awake form yet another safe practice.[10,11]

Compliance with Federal and State Regulatory Standards and Accreditation Requirements

Federal and state regulations, as well as accreditation standards, are designed to ensure that patients receive safe and quality care. Adherence to these regulations as incorporated into the ASC policies promotes quality patient care.

The ASCs must be certified by the CMS to participate in the Medicare program. Thus, ASCs must comply with the federal regulations. The federal regulations for ASCs are found in 42 Code for Regulations (CFR) part 416.[12] Subpart B comprises the general conditions and requirements for participation in Medicare, and Subpart C specifies the various conditions for coverage (Box 5.3). Compliance with the regulations must be on an ongoing basis. Compliance ensures patients receive safe and quality nursing care.

The majority of states regulate ASCs.[6] Every ASC in these states must be licensed to operate and require initial and ongoing inspection and monitoring. out of the states which do require licenses, nearly half require accreditation by a third party. The accreditation organizations include the Accreditation Association for Ambulatory Health Care (AAAHC), American Association for Accreditation of Ambulatory Surgery Facilities (AAAASF), the Accreditation Commission for Health Care (ACHC), and The Joint Commission (see Box 5.2). Although accreditation in some states is voluntary, the ASC with accreditation has the better advantage and is well positioned for third-party payer consideration. The ASCs that are accredited with recognized organizations have deemed status, or, in other words, exceed the clinical expectations for performance, service, and outcomes[13] (Box 5.4).

Robust Implementation of Risk Management Plans

The initial step in a robust implementation of a risk management plan is the identification of risk factors in an ASC.[4] Legal, environmental, regulatory, and safety risks are among the factors to be identified.

It is important that all personnel be educated about the risk management systems put in place to prevent accidental injuries.[4] Implementation of quality measures will be successful if each person in the facility participates and is trained in all procedures and systems designed for promoting and preserving safe practices.[4] Staff also need to be educated on their ethical and legal responsibilities to detect, prevent, and report risks.[4]

Several organizations and tools are available that give leaders of the ASC the opportunity to participate in the ongoing monitoring of and compliance with regulations.[4] ASCs reporting quality indicators provide an opportunity for the public to know the ASCs' commitment to quality care. Data reported can be used for continuous monitoring for improvement.[4] There should be plans in place for responding to sentinel events, as well as processes in place for tracking errors.[4] These include performing a root cause analysis, notifying the patient, and informing the state department, regulatory bodies, and associated boards as appropriate.[4]

Risk management activities include the creation of a safe environment in which to report incidents. Several software tools exist that can detect trends in incidents, as well as allow staff to report incidents without fear of retribution.[1,4] Data from these tools can be used to identify safety trends and

Surgical Safety Checklist

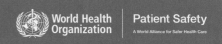

Before induction of anaesthesia	Before skin incision	Before patient leaves operating room
(with at least nurse and anaesthetist)	(with nurse, anaesthetist and surgeon)	(with nurse, anaesthetist and surgeon)
Has the patient confirmed his/her identity, site, procedure, and consent? ☐ Yes	☐ **Confirm all team members have introduced themselves by name and role.**	**Nurse verbally confirms:** ☐ The name of the procedure ☐ Completion of instrument, sponge and needle counts ☐ Specimen labelling (read specimen labels aloud, including patient name) ☐ Whether there are any equipment problems to be addressed
Is the site marked? ☐ Yes ☐ Not applicable	☐ **Confirm the patient's name, procedure, and where the incision will be made.**	
Is the anaesthesia machine and medication check complete? ☐ Yes	**Has antibiotic prophylaxis been given within the last 60 minutes?** ☐ Yes ☐ Not applicable	**To surgeon, anaesthetist and nurse:** ☐ What are the key concerns for recovery and management of this patient?
Is the pulse oximeter on the patient and functioning? ☐ Yes	**Anticipated critical events**	
Does the patient have a:	**To surgeon:** ☐ What are the critical or non-routine steps? ☐ How long will the case take? ☐ What is the anticipated blood loss?	
Known allergy? ☐ No ☐ Yes	**To anaesthetist:** ☐ Are there any patient-specific concerns?	
Difficult airway or aspiration risk? ☐ No ☐ Yes, and equipment/assistance available	**To nursing team:** ☐ Has sterility (including indicator results) been confirmed? ☐ Are there equipment issues or any concerns?	
Risk of >500 ml blood loss (7 ml/kg in children)? ☐ No ☐ Yes, and two IVs/central access and fluids planned	**Is essential imaging displayed?** ☐ Yes ☐ Not applicable	

This checklist is not intended to be comprehensive. Additions and modifications to fit local practice are encouraged.   Revised 1 / 2009   © WHO, 2009

Fig. 5.1 Surgical safety checklist. Source: World Health Organization. https://www.who.int/teams/integrated-health-services/patient-safety/research/safe-surgery/tool-and-resources

---

BOX 5.3 Conditions for Coverage: Medicare Health and Safety Required Standards for ASCs

Compliance with state laws
Governing body management
Surgical services
Quality assessment and performance improvement
Environment
Medical staff
Nursing services
Medical records
Pharmaceutical services
Laboratory and radiologic services
Patient rights
Infection control and prevention
Patient admission, assessment, discharge
Emergency preparedness

Source: Code of Federal Regulations. Title 42, Chapter IV, Subchapter B, Part 416: Ambulatory Surgical Services. 2022.

BOX 5.4 Deemed and Nondeemed ASCs

ASC has "deemed status" when the organization has:

Applied for and been accredited by a CMS-approved accreditation organization (AO)
Been recommended by the AO for Medicare participation
Met all the requirements for certification deemed by the CMS
Complied with the applicable conditions for participation for the purpose of CMS

Nondeemed status applies when the organization:

Operates without accreditation

Source: Code of Federal Regulations. Title 42, Chapter IV, Subchapter B, Part 416 Ambulatory Surgical Services. 2022.

---

processes that need to be changed or developed.[4] Affiliated staff, including the compliance officer, must investigate promptly any sentinel events using methods such as a root cause analysis.[4] ASCs can use technology to track data and focus on corrective actions. This ensures compliance and assists in the reduction of identified problem areas.[4]

There are five high-risk areas in healthcare[1] (Table 5.1): medication errors, complications from diagnostic or treatment procedures, falls, patient or family dissatisfaction with care, and refusal of treatment or refusal to sign consent for treatment.[1] It is crucial to have policies in place to manage these high-risk areas and to safeguard patients from adverse events in these areas.

CREATING A JUST CULTURE

The American Nurses Association (ANA) has provided a position statement regarding a "just culture"[14] (Box 5.5). When an

TABLE 5.1 High-Risk Categories of Adverse Events in ASCs

Medication Errors	Diagnostic Procedures	Falls*	Medical-Legal Incidents	Patient or Family Dissatisfaction with Care
A reportable event when a medication or fluid is omitted, administered to the wrong patient, at the wrong time, at the wrong dosage, or by the wrong route	Any harmful incident occurring before, during, or after any procedures such as blood sampling, x-ray imaging, lumbar puncture, or other invasive procedures	An unplanned event during which a patient comes to rest on ground, floor, or lower level with or without injury to the patient *WHO definition at https://www.who.int/news-room/fact-sheets/detail/falls.	A refusal of a patient or family to receive treatment or sign a consent form	When any dissatisfaction expressed by a patient or family has not been resolved, the event is considered a risk and an incident report has to be filed

Source: Sullivan, EJ. *Effective Leadership and Management in Nursing.* (9th ed.) Pearson; 2017.

BOX 5.5 American Nurses Association Position Statement on Just Culture

Endorsement of the just culture concept to reduce errors and promote patient safety in healthcare

Promotion and dissemination of information on just culture in publications and affiliate organizations

Promotion and collaboration of state governments, boards of nursing, healthcare professional associations, and hospital and long-term care facilities in developing and implementing just culture initiatives

Promotion of continued research related to the effectiveness of the just culture concept in improving patient safety and employee performance outcomes

Commitment of administrators and leaders as stewards of just culture to promote safe systems for safe patient outcomes and protect employees from failure

Encouragement of nurses to advocate for just culture in the practice setting

Incorporation of just culture by nursing educators in nursing curricula at all academic levels

Collaboration of healthcare professional organizations to develop just culture statements

Encouragement for all health care organizations to implement zero tolerance policy of disruptive behavior

Source: Just Culture: Position Statements. 2010. American Nurses Association.

BOX 5.6 Is This a Just Culture or a Culture of Blame?

A patient was brought to the recovery room after undergoing thyroidectomy. The patient started having difficulty breathing, and swelling in the neck area was observed. The nurse caring for the patient attempted to let the surgeon know what was happening but could not find him. She discovered that he had already left the ASC. The nurse made phone calls to the surgeon until he was reached. The surgeon was informed that the patient needed to go back to the operating room, as per the assessment of the anesthesiologist. The surgeon found that a surgical packing had been left in the patient's neck, and this had resulted in swelling and difficulty in breathing. The patient had an unremarkable recovery after the surgical packing was removed.

Did the PACU nurse perform due diligence in this scenario? Would it be a just culture if the perianesthesia nurse was fired in this scenario? What would a just culture look like? Is there a need to look at the processes in place in the operating room? How was the surgical packing missed? If you are the manager of this ASC, how would you handle the situation?

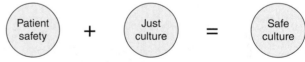

Fig. 5.2 Creating a safety culture.

---

organization adopts a just culture that examines the circumstances surrounding errors, it provides an opportunity for staff to report errors without fear of retribution.[1,14,15] This is in contrast to a toxic culture of blame, in which the fault for errors is often attributed to individuals rather than to issues within a system. Blame cultures promote secrecy because individuals fear that they will receive punitive actions. Lack of reporting can lead to the inability to track errors, thereby increasing the likelihood of other errors and near misses.[15] Approaches to punitive actions will deliberately shut off information needed to identify the faulty system and create a safer one.[14] The case scenario in Box 5.6 is an example. Promoting a blame culture minimizes the ability to learn from mistakes and fix system issues.[14,15] On the other hand, working within a just culture opens avenues for staff to question policies and practices, express concerns, and admit mistakes.[1] A just culture creates an environment where the individual is not held accountable for mistakes of the system over which the individual has no control.[14] This culture of safety helps to identify the predictable relationship between human operators and the systems in which they work.[14] It does not tolerate reckless behaviors that may place the patient at a higher risk of danger.[14] Leaders in a just culture advocate for trust in and rewards and encouragement for staff. Staff in this atmosphere are provided the essential information they need to deliver safe, high-quality care[14] (Figure 5.2). This requires an ongoing collaboration and accountability among leaders, managers, and employees to each other and the system.[1]

A just culture provides opportunities for staff to better understand the risks inherent in the system, as well as the behaviors that might lead to or prevent adverse events.[14] Staff are encouraged to look for risks in the environment and report hazards and errors.[14] They are encouraged and enabled to contribute to the designing of safer systems.[14] Managers have a role to play in executing the environment of a just culture.[14] Managers must determine whether events are the result of human error, at-risk behaviors, or reckless behaviors[14] (Table 5.2). Managers can console the individual if the cause of the event was human error, console and coach if it was at-risk behavior, and manage remedial action if it was reckless behavior.[14] The adoption of a just culture provides opportunities for the improvement of care delivery systems and the forming of healthier workplace environments for those employed in a facility.[14]

TABLE 5.2 Management of Just Culture

Definition	Examples	Management Role
Human error: "Inevitable, unpredictable, unintentional failure" in action, thought, and perception	Mental slip in transposing numbers in a medication dose	Console the individual and redesign the system
At-risk behavior: Behavior an individual chooses when perceiving a risk to be insignificant	Removing medication using the override feature from the automated dispensing machine	Create incentives for healthy behaviors; increase situational awareness
Reckless behavior: Action taken with a conscious disregard for substantial or justifiable risks	Performing duties while intoxicated; falsifying patient records	Taking remedial or punitive action, including following plan for progressive discipline

Source: Just Culture: Position Statement. ANA; 2010.

The Perianesthesia Nurse's Role in Risk Management

The perianesthesia registered nurse has a critical role in risk management.[1] The clinical perianesthesia registered nurse spends the most time providing direct bedside care and is therefore a crucial person in implementing the risk management plan. The responsibilities of ASC perianesthesia nurses cover involvement in various high-risk areas of healthcare.[1]

Accurate documentation in the patient's chart and reporting of incidents are important factors in protecting the organization and the personnel in litigations.[1]

Evidence-Based Practice: The perianesthesia nurse and quality care

The perianesthesia registered nurse symbolizes the culture of the ASC. You are at the bedside and represent the organization while caring for your patient. You are charged to maintain safe and efficient care for your patient. When faced with adverse events, you are the voice to advocate for that patient. As a patient advocate, you can learn how to handle and report adverse events.

Source: Sullivan EJ. *Effective Leadership and Management in Nursing*. 9th ed. Pearson; 2017.

The ASC Manager's Role in Risk Management

The success of the risk management program depends on how the ASC manager adopts and administers the plan.[1] It is important for leaders to help personnel view health and wellness from the patient's standpoint.[1] It is equally important to view the ASC experience from the patient's perspective. This calls for individualized patient care that results in both trust and respect, thereby reducing risk.

LEGAL ISSUES

The Affordable Care Act (ACA) has altered the payment system that reimburses healthcare organizations.[1] Before the ACA, healthcare organizations were paid in *volumes of care* despite outcomes.[1] The greater the number of surgeries and procedures performed, the more the organization got reimbursed.[1] Currently, the ACA has helped shift the focus away from volume-based care to the notion of *value-based care* provided to healthcare consumers.[1] Outcomes associated with value-based care have been measured by an instrument titled the Hospital Consumer Assessment of Healthcare Providers and Systems (HCAHPS).[1] The HCAHPS was instituted by the CMS, Agency for Healthcare Research and Quality (AHRQ), and Department of Health and Human Services (DHHS).[1]

Hospital scores are made public. This public reporting provides initiatives for the leaders of each healthcare organization to strategize ways to maintain high scores.[1]

The Health Information Technology for Economic and Clinical Health Act (HITECH, 2009) is a piece of legislation that has had a profound effect on healthcare services.[1] This law, commonly referred to as "meaningful use," stimulated the use of technology in healthcare to improve the interoperability of the electronic medical record. One form of improvement was the reduction of medication errors through improved communication and enhancement so that medication administration could become safer.[1] The computerized prescriber order entry application, electronic medication administration records, remote pharmacy order reviews, automated bedside dispensing devices, bar code administration tools, smart pumps, and single-unit doses are all technology-assisted strategies that can reduce medication errors.[1]

GENERAL CONSIDERATIONS

Nursing and anesthesia assessments and reviews are crucial strategies for the patients undergoing surgeries in the ASC. Best practice includes an evaluation of the assessment data elements by a medical partner to determine the appropriateness of the patient for the outpatient ASC environment. Medical stratification and adherence to clinical criteria are important to consider in choosing the right candidates for ASC surgeries.[10,16] Appropriate patient selection for ASCs is a great contributory factor in reducing risks in ASCs.[10,16] Patients with minimal co-morbidities will have lower incidences of complications or adverse events.[10,16]

Identifying vulnerabilities in medication administration and patient and staff safety, issues with legal requirements, inefficient practices in diagnostic procedures, and patient dissatisfaction are key in the creation and implementation of risk management plans. A risk management plan supports the accurate tracking of adverse events, as well as the development and implementation of strategic interventions to prevent those adverse events from occurring again. The training and collaboration of all staff in the ASC are important tactics for the successful achievement of risk reduction strategies.

CHAPTER HIGHLIGHTS

Adoption of the following practices ensures patient safety and quality of care:

- Comprehensive diagnostic testing is done to clear the patient for surgery.[3]
- Surgeons assess the patient immediately prior to surgery to discuss the procedures to be performed, risks and benefits of the procedures, and marking of the site and to ensure

that the history has been taken and the physical examination done within 30 days prior to surgery.[3,6,12]

- The informed consent form is signed by the patient and discussed with the surgeon; the discussion includes the risks and benefits of the operation, expectations for the recovery period, and how pain will be managed.[3,12]
- Marking of the site is visible after draping the patient.[3,12]
- Anesthesia providers conduct a preassessment of the patient to evaluate the risks of anesthesia.[3,6,12]
  - Comprehensive diagnostic testing is done to clear the patient for surgery.[3]
  - The informed consent form is signed by the patient and discussed with the anesthesiologist; the discussion includes the risks and benefits of the anesthesia, expectations for the recovery period, and how pain will be managed.[3,12]
- Anesthesia providers conduct a postanesthesia assessment.[6,12]
  - Anesthesia providers assess the patient for discharge readiness and evaluate possible adverse reactions.[3,6,12]
  - State laws are followed on who may perform anesthesia.[6,12]
- Regulations are followed on who is an appropriate candidate for the ASC patient population.[3,6,7,12]
- Evidence-based protocols are adopted for nursing care management in the ASC that encompass preoperative, intraoperative, and postoperative care, and staff training on those protocols is provided.[3]
- Emergency equipment and medications that would be needed in case of complications are available, and staff have been trained in their use.[3,12]
  - A postoperative phone call is made per institutional policy to determine the patient's postoperative status and stability and to answer questions[3,17]
- Patient satisfaction data are gathered to improve the performance on patient outcomes. [3,7]
- Reported complications and medical errors are tracked and trends are noted, and action plans are developed for specific incidents.[3,13]
- The risk management plan must be current and reviewed annually.[2,4]

CASE STUDY

Eve Garden is a 21-year-old patient who was admitted to Eden Surgery Center for a simple **right** ureteroscopy and lithotripsy. During the procedure, Dr. Adam started inserting the scope into the patient's **left** ureter and found that it was blocked, so Dr. Adam placed a stent but did not perform the lithotripsy. At the end of the case, Eve was emerging from anesthesia and brought to the recovery room. While in the recovery room, Dr. Adam realized that the procedure was performed on the wrong side! Dr. Adam went to see the friend of the patient who had accompanied her for the procedure that day. Dr. Adam informed Eve's friend of the error and told her that Eve had to go back to the operating room. After receiving consent from the friend, Eve was brought back to the operating room and the **right** ureteroscopy was performed. The surgeon found the same blockage and placed a stent on the right ureter. The lithotripsy was not performed, and Eve was brought back to the recovery room. The patient had to reschedule another surgical appointment for the lithotripsy.

Was there a system in place for the surgeon to assess the patient before the procedure was performed? Does the system include marking the patient in the preoperative area so the patient can confirm the correct side of the procedure? Was there a "timeout" performed before the procedure started? Did the anesthesiologist and the operating room nurse agree on the correct procedure to be performed on the correct side before the start of the procedure? Was the friend of the patient authorized to consent for the second procedure? Was the patient informed of the error before the second admission to the operating room? Did the ASC conduct a thorough investigation of this wrong-site surgery? Was the error reported voluntarily to the state reporting system? Did the ASC change its preoperative processes in a manner that would reduce the likelihood of a wrong-site surgery? Was peer review done for Dr. Adam? Was he duly credentialed and his license current during the time of the surgery? What corrective actions were done to mitigate the error? Has this happened in the past? Is there a pattern of this error happening in this ASC? Was there a physician assistant assisting Dr. Adam during the surgery? Was this physician assistant allowed to insert the stent? Was the physician assistant performing within the scope of practice?

Examples of resources available to support risk management plans in the ASC

1. Accreditation Association for Ambulatory Health Care (https://www.aaahc.org)
2. Accreditation Commission for Health Care, Inc. (https://www.achc.org)
3. Agency for Healthcare Research and Quality (https://www.ahrq.gov)
4. Ambulatory Surgery Center Association (https://www.ascassociation.org)
5. American Association for Accreditation of Ambulatory Surgery Facilities (https://aaaasf.org)
6. Institute for Safe Medication Practices (https://www.ismp.org)
7. National Committee for Quality Assurance (https://www.ncqa.org)
8. Institute for Healthcare Improvement (https://www.ihi.org)
9. National Quality Forum (https://www.qualityforum.org)
10. The Joint Commission (https://www.jointcommission.org)

REFERENCES

1. Sullivan EJ. *Effective Leadership and Management in Nursing*. 9th ed. Pearson; 2017.
2. Dutton RP. Quality Management and Registries. *Anesthesiol Clin*. 2014;32(2):577-586. Available at: https://doi.org/10.1016/j.anclin.2014.02.014.
3. Coverys Insights Blog. *The ASC Risk Management Best Practices Checklist*. Coverys; 2018. Available at: https://www.coverys.com/knowledge-center/The-ASC-Risk-Management-Best-Practices-Checklist.
4. Stinchcom D. Risk Management for ASCs. *AE*. 2010:68-69. Available at: https://progressivesurgicalsolutions.com/wp-content/uploads/2020/06/Risk-Assessments-for-ASCs_AE_MayJune-2020_DS.pdf.
5. Chelly JE, Ben-David B, Williams BA, Kentor ML. Anesthesia and postoperative analgesia: outcomes following orthopedic surgery. *Orthopedics*. 2003;26(Suppl 8):s865-s871. Available at: https://doi.org/10.3928/0147-7447-20030802-08.
6. Semo JJ. Legal Aspects of Ambulatory Anesthesia. *Anesthesiol Clin*. 2014;32(2):541-549. Available at: http://doi.org/10.1016/j.anclin.2014.02.009.
7. Centers for Medicare and Medicaid Services (CMS). *Regulations and Guidance*. Available at: https://www.cms.gov/Regulations-and-Guidance/Legislation/CFCsAndCoPs/ASC.
8. Hall MJ, Schwartzman A, Zhang J, Liu X. *National Health Statistics Report*. Number 102. Feb 28, 2017. Available at: https://www.cdc.gov/nchs/data/nhsr/nhsr102.pdf.
9. Krenzischek DA. Chapter 8: Safety. In: Schick L, Windle PE, eds. *PeriAnesthesia Nursing Core Curriculum: Preprocedure, Phase I and Phase II PACU Nursing*. 2nd ed. Elsevier; 2010:82-89.
10. Thompson NB, Calandruccio JH. Hand surgery in the ambulatory surgery center. *Orthop Clin North Am*. 2018;49(1):69-72. Available at: http://dx.doi.org/10.1016/j.ocl.2017.08.009.
11. World Health Organization. *Surgical Safety Checklist*. 2009. Available at: https://apps.who.int/iris/bitstream/handle/10665/44186/9789241598590_eng_Checklist.pdf?sequence=2&isAllowed=y.

12. Code of Federal Regulations. Part 416 – Ambulatory Surgical Services. Title 42. Chapter IV. Subchapter B. Part 416. Available at: https://www.ecfr.gov/cgi-bin/text-idx?node=pt42.3.416&rgn=div5.

13. The Joint Commission. *Federal Deemed Status and State Recognition*. The Joint Commission. Available at: https://www.jointcommission.org/resources/news-and-multimedia/fact-sheets/facts-about-federal-deemed-status/.

14. American Nurses Association. *Just Culture: Position Statement*. 2010. Available at: https://www.nursingworld.org/~4afe07/globalassets/practiceandpolicy/health-and-safety/just_culture.pdf.

15. Barnsteiner J, Disch J. A just culture for nurses and nursing students. *Nurs Clin North Am.* 2012;47(3):407-416. Available at: http://dx.doi.org/10.1016/j.cnur.2012.05.005.

16. Marois AJ, Jones CA, Throckmorton TW, Bernholt DL, Azar FM, Brolin TJ. Candidacy for ambulatory outpatient shoulder arthroplasty: a retrospective review. *Semin Arthroplasty.* 2021;31(4):848-855. Available at: https://doi.org/10.1053/j.sart.2021.05.016.

17. Centers for Medicare and Medicaid Services (CMS). *Ambulatory Surgery Centers*. 2021. Available at: https://www.cms.gov/Medicare/Provider-Enrollment-and-Certification/Certificationand Complianc/ASCs.

6 Safety Standards

Deborah Moengen, BSN, RN, CPAN

LEARNING OBJECTIVES

A review of the content of this chapter will help the reader to:

1. Describe safety standards for the ambulatory surgery center.
2. Identify key components of a safe patient care environment in the ambulatory setting.
3. Discuss regulatory sources impacting care delivery and design.

OVERVIEW

Nurses working in an ambulatory surgery center (ASC) need to be aware of and compliant with safety standards. Patient safety is the highest priority in any clinical setting in the ASC. There are many regulatory agencies that address safety, but in this chapter, the primary focus is on the federal agency Centers for Medicare and Medicaid Services (CMS). The chapter outlines topics such as the design of the building housing an ASC, the service workflow, and the standards according to which care must be delivered. This chapter is not completely inclusive but is intended to provide an overview of common, basic safety concepts.

More than 60% of surgical procedures can now be performed in an ASC.[1] Regulatory standards are in place to guide perianesthesia nurses during the provision of safe patient care. The focus of this chapter is primarily on the standards impacting the perianesthesia nurse working in the ASC setting. The content here will only skim the surface of the standards and regulations available and should not be used as the sole reference for safe patient care. Safety standards and requirements may vary from state to state and between various facilities and associated policies. The perianesthesia nurse is encouraged to research specific state and local laws and to use this chapter as a point of reference. Nurses caring for patients in the ambulatory setting must be knowledgeable about the nature of safety standards and their sources.

The CMS is a federal program designed to oversee major healthcare programs.[2] Private insurance companies use CMS-recommended regulations and policies as a baseline for safety requirements. Most of the requirements discussed in this chapter are based on CMS regulations, which serve as a foundation for safety guidance in healthcare. Healthcare consumers can shop for their medical care and can consult many resources, including online databases, to find where the best, most cost efficient, and safest care is being provided. Therefore, in this competitive market, following safety standards is more important today than ever. ASCs have lower overhead and require fewer resources than hospitals, and therefore, ASC leaders can invest in building designs that attract patients, families, and staff.

GENERAL REGULATIONS FOR AMBULATORY SURGERY CENTERS

Building Design Regulations

An ASC is a convenient alternative to a hospital for outpatient procedures. The design of the building in which ambulatory surgery is performed is one factor in the provision of ASC services. This building is unique and distinguishable from other healthcare facilities or office-based physician practices. This does not necessarily suggest that the ASC must be a physically separate building. According to the National Fire Protection Association Life Safety Code, surgery centers must have walls constructed to provide at least a 1-hour separation from a fire source.[3] The physical space may be shared with other services, but not during the same concurrent or overlapping operating hours. The entrances and lobbies are maintained and must be free of obstruction during patient care hours. The location and building designs are typically attractive and offer a pleasant patient experience.

State Regulations

Each state has its own set of regulations. States vary considerably in their licensure requirements for entities that meet the Medicare definition of an ASC. These regulations may also vary from regulations generated at the federal level. Leaders of each ASC should conduct a comparison of the two sources of regulations, and the narrower set of regulations should be followed. Some states may not require separate federal and state licensure of an ASC, although all states require licensure of healthcare professionals providing services within the ASC.

Staff Licensure and Credentialing

Registered nurses are required to be licensed in every state. It is the ASC's responsibility to verify that licenses are current and have not been suspended or revoked.[4]

Board certification is the premier designation clinicians can earn to demonstrate they are experts in their chosen specialty areas.[1] Physicians who perform surgery and anesthesia personnel are not required to be board certified, although patients may prefer it. All advanced providers and physicians practicing in the ASC must be duly credentialed according to the governing body of a facility and must also be compliant with the medical bylaws and administration of the facility. The requirements for these privileges are to be specifically listed in the approved policies and procedures of each facility.[4]

Nursing certifications validate a nurse's knowledge in a specialty much like a board certification for a physician. Certifications require specific education, experience, and demonstration of skills. The perianesthesia nursing standards state the nurse administering sedation and caring for patients in phase I recovery will have advanced life support skills and current certificates such as those required for advanced cardiac life support (ACLS).[5] Nurses who administer sedation to or care for pediatric patients must have certification in pediatric advanced life support (PALS) or pediatric emergency assessment recognition and stabilization (PEARS).[5]

Training Requirements

One of the biggest differences in the ambulatory setting is the reduction of clinical resources for training and education. Support systems and experts are not as readily available as they are in a larger acute care hospital or academic institution. Staff may be required to perform many different tasks and cross train for different areas, especially late in the day and through the evening. ASCs are well advised to ensure that the protocols are in place for emergent situations whenever patients are in the building. This may include scheduling perianesthesia registered nurses who can provide emergency treatment or who have training in ACLS throughout the course of the day.

Staff are required to show competence in many areas, and proof of competence should always be documented. Training for emergency responses can include pathways for managing a malignant hyperthermia crisis and protocols for responding to a massive hemorrhage or cardiac or respiratory arrest. Fire safety precautions should be up to date, and evacuation procedures should be known to all staff. Most facilities conduct practice drills or mock codes to validate that staff can respond when a real crisis occurs. Documentation of these types of drills can serve as validation for a regulatory surveyor.

New employee onboarding should be standardized and comprehensive.[6] Training in preventing and controlling healthcare-associated infections, such as methods to prevent exposure to and transmission of infections and communicable diseases, is recommended as part of annual educational offerings. Some topics may include, but are not limited to, proper hand hygiene, correct donning and doffing of personal protective equipment, thorough methods of surface disinfection, and safe handling of laboratory specimens and blood products.

Evidence-Based Practice: Onboarding of new staff
The creation of a positive onboarding program can lead to higher retention and job satisfaction for new hires. In order to best provide each staff member with relevant new information, mentors and educators must first conduct an assessment to determine what level of knowledge and experience the new nurse is bringing to the experience. Focusing solely on clinical skills, policies, and procedures alone can lead to disengagement if the orientee actually needs to develop critical thinking skills. Personalizing orientation by way of learner-driven strategies helps to address actual gaps in knowledge and skill application.

Adapted from: Valdes EG, Sembar MC, Sadler F. Onboarding new graduate nurses using assessment-driven personalized learning to improve knowledge, critical thinking, and nurse satisfaction. *J Nurses Prof Dev.* 2023;39(1):18-23. https://doi.org/10.1097/nnd.0000000000000805

Licensure and Accreditation

The CMS requires that healthcare services follow the federal regulations outlined in the Medicare Conditions for Coverage in order to receive Medicare and Medicaid payments and reimbursements. CMS provides a *State Operations Manual* that addresses survey and certification activities and policies.[7] This manual describes the preparation and design of program surveys to determine the extent to which an ASC is compliant with guidelines for safety and optimal care.

Forty-six states require licensure of ASCs. Additionally, accreditation often raises the performance criteria for a facility above and beyond the minimal requirements required by CMS for operating as an ASC. In this case, the facility leadership hires supplementary services to conduct additional surveys. Generally, these supplementary standards are more rigid than those of the CMS. The Accreditation Association for Ambulatory Health Care (AAAHC) and The Joint Commission (TJC) are examples of private accreditation agencies that Medicare recognizes and will certify as having "deemed status." This means that Medicare recognizes the certification efforts of the AAAHC and The Joint Commission. As a result, the CMS does not require an ASC survey of an otherwise accredited program, although the CMS still may survey at any time.

Environmental Regulations

The byproduct of anesthesia gases is called waste anesthetic gases (WAGs). After a patient is removed from a closed-circuit anesthesia ventilator, the patient will begin to exhale residual anesthesia gases into the environment. These gases are potentially harmful to those caring for the patient and to other patients through cross contamination. In the post-anesthesia care unit (PACU), the ventilation system should exchange the air over a minimum of a total of six air exchanges per hour with a minimum of two air exchanges of outdoor air per hour.[5] The National Institute for Occupational Safety and Health (NIOSH), Centers for Disease Control and Prevention (CDC), and Occupational Safety and Health Administration (OSHA) publish recommendations for engineering and administrative controls to manage anesthetic agents.[8]

Medical waste such as blood-borne pathogens must be handled with special attention. Disposal is regulated by the Environmental Protection Agency (EPA) and local authorities. Exposure to blood often happens during the care of a patient while handling sharps. The CDC has published guidelines for handling sharps, including how to prevent needlestick injuries and injuries from contaminated sharps.[9]

Under the Occupational Safety and Health Act of 1970, employers are responsible for providing a safe and healthy workplace. Thousands of employers across the United States already manage safety using injury and illness prevention programs, and OSHA maintains that all employers can, and should, do the same. Thirty-four states have requirements or voluntary guidelines for workplace injury and illness prevention programs.[10] Facilities such as eyewash stations are required for staff who may be exposed to injurious substances and need to have immediate care. Personal protective equipment and other devices can protect staff from respiratory hazards. Hearing protection should be provided if noise is an issue. Ergonomically designed workstations and equipment can prevent fatigue and injuries.

Providing clean air to breathe during procedures is important to the surgical team and patients. Surgical smoke containing hazardous chemicals is a byproduct of procedures in which electrosurgical devices or lasers are used for the thermal destruction of tissue.[11] Oregon joined Rhode Island, Colorado, and Kentucky in providing smoke-free operating rooms for all hospitals and ASCs in these states. The Association of periOperative Registered Nurses (AORN) is advocating for the adoption of similar legislation in other states. Removal of this smoke or wearing a mask that can filter a minimum of 0.1 microns protects those in the presence of the smoke.

Procedures for maintaining the temperature and humidity in the operating room and for the sterile storage of supplies are outlined in the accepted standards of practice. Measures for monitoring these issues and providing guidance for restoring compliance with the procedures when errors occur need to be included in the policies for and training of personnel. Corrective action plans should be in place to manage aberrancies in the clinical environment that have the potential to impact staff and patient safety.

Governing Body and Management

The ASC must have a governing body that assumes full legal responsibility for determining, implementing, and monitoring policies governing the ASC's total operations. The governing body has the oversight of and accountability for the quality assessment and performance improvement program, ensures that the facility policies and programs are administered to provide quality healthcare in a safe environment, and develops and maintains a disaster preparedness plan.[2]

Emergency Care Resources

Emergency preparedness is a critical focus for staff and physicians working in an ASC, as they typically do not have rapid response or code teams on site. Staff may be expected to serve in many roles and have multiple functions. Plans for dealing with fires, evacuations, and violent active shooters are required. Discussions of the emergency response provide an ideal opportunity for intraprofessional teams to work on the creation and dissemination of emergency protocols. Input from the various members of the support staff and ancillary services staff can add rich macroscopic information in situations where resources may be limited.

Emergency Equipment

Staff are trained to use the emergency equipment available. The CMS environmental requirements as a condition for coverage state that emergency equipment must be either in or immediately available to the operating room.[2] When a patient experiences an unplanned critical event, the equipment needed may be minimal in an ASC (e.g., arterial line for monitoring, ventilators). Efforts to stabilize the patient at this critical time require personnel trained in cardiopulmonary resuscitation.[2] In addition, the emergency equipment in an ASC must be age- and size- appropriate for the population of patients being served. This equipment must always be well maintained and functional.

Sterile Processing

Surgical instruments are available in a quantity that is proportionate to the ASC's expected daily procedural volume. Scheduling should allow for appropriate cleaning and sterilization of equipment between surgical cases, if necessary. All operating room equipment must be inspected, tested, and maintained appropriately by the ASC, per federal and state laws and regulations.[2] Additionally, staff must adhere to the manufacturers' recommendations for the cleaning and storage of supplies. The ASC does not have to have all the equipment and supplies needed for sterilization on-site, so long as they are provided to the ASC as a service using contractual agreements. If equipment is transported off-site, many local and state regulations are in place for hazardous waste items.

Laboratory Services

Typically, the ASC does not have full laboratory services. However, any form of laboratory service must meet the requirements of the CMS. If the ASC does not have on-site laboratory services, there must be an appropriately certified laboratory available to provide testing.[2] The results of these tests must be readily accessible for staff. Point-of-care testing, such as fingerstick blood glucose evaluations and pregnancy urine tests, require training and waivers in order for the appropriate staff to conduct the tests at the bedside.

Radiologic Services

Proper safety precautions must be maintained against radiation hazards. This includes adequate shielding of patients, personnel, and facilities, as well as appropriate storage, use, and disposal of radioactive materials.[2] Lead aprons are to be maintained and stored properly, with documentation of this process. There must be an identified employee qualified per state law and ASC policy who is responsible for ensuring that all radiologic services are provided per the requirements.[2] Exposure is a risk when working with radiation, and the exposure meters must be checked periodically for those who are working near radiation sources. When a provider or staff person operates radiologic equipment, documentation of competencies and the ability to perform these duties must be included in policies governing radiologic care in the ASC.

Pharmaceutical Services

Resources for a full formulary of medications are usually not available in the ambulatory setting. A designated individual with appropriate training and education in pharmacy and therapeutics provides oversight of the process of providing drugs and biologicals. The designee will provide direction for the pharmaceutical services and is on-site routinely.[2] If a patient requires specialized medication(s) unavailable in the ASC, a transfer to an increased level of care may be required. In addition, the staff providing direct care will need knowledge of how to stabilize the patient with potentially limited resources. Attention to policies on how drugs are handled according to infection control practices should be in place. Controlled substances are closely monitored with excellent documentation to prevent drug diversion in the facility. Medical records and policies on these practices are reviewed. When an adverse drug reaction occurs, the situation is reported to the physician responsible for the patient and the event is documented in the record.[2] In the medical record a written order is documented as soon as possible when a verbal order is given to a nurse.[2] It is good practice when receiving a verbal order to repeat the order using a read-back method to ensure accuracy of the order and to prevent errors.

Patient Criteria and Planning

Not every patient is a candidate for an ASC. ASCs have limited resources, and patients must be able to be discharged home within 24 hours. Each ASC must develop and maintain a protocol to identify inclusion and exclusion criteria. This includes identifying those patients who may be at higher risk for surgery in the outpatient setting by evaluating the history and physical examination. The history and physical examination address, but are not limited to:

1. Patient age
2. Diagnosis
3. Procedure(s) planned

4. Co-morbidities
5. Plan for anesthesia level

The best method for selecting patients safely is usually to use established criteria. Policies address the criteria used to perform risk assessments and ensure consistency among assessments. Nursing and anesthesia providers work together to review patients to evaluate their appropriateness for care in an ASC. Nursing assessment skills are used while interviewing patients and reviewing the documentation to identify any potential unresolved issues prior to surgical and anesthesia care. A physician examines the patient immediately before surgery to evaluate the risk of anesthesia and the procedure to be performed.[2] Physician documentation of this examination is required, as well as notation of the time and date the examination occurred. This information is often reviewed by surveyors to assess compliance. The medical record includes documentation of an immediate postsurgical assessment by the physician, as well as a discharge order. The anesthesia provider must also document an assessment following recovery from anesthesia after surgery. The patient is provided with written discharge instructions and overnight supplies as needed.[2] Every patient must be discharged with a responsible individual (e.g., someone who can call for help if help is needed), except those patients exempted by the attending physician or anesthesia provider. Each facility's policies clearly define these exemptions.

Patient rights are posted in writing in one or more places visible to patients in a language and manner that ensures that patients can understand them.[2] Patients with an advanced directive may present for surgery in an ASC. It is a patient's right to determine the care that is provided in the event of cardiopulmonary arrest.[2] Discussion with anesthesia providers regarding a plan of care needs to occur before surgery to ensure that there is a consensus between the patient, family, and surgical team in light of a desired do-not-resuscitate condition.

Safe Care of the Patient

For patient safety, standards of care are followed and used when developing policies. The CMS includes the following as a standard of practice:

- Proper patient identification and surgical site marking when indicated
  - Preprocedure verification process using relevant documents (including the patient's signed informed consent)
  - Marking of the procedure site by the physician or another member of the surgical team
  - A timeout is performed before starting the procedure to confirm the correct patient, procedure, and site

Surgical fires in the operating room are a concern in every procedure using a fuel and ignition source and an oxidizer. These procedures include electrosurgery or the use of a cautery instrument or laser. Alcohol-based skin preparations may be a hazard, as well, in the environment. Staff training includes measures to minimize the risk of fires and procedures for responding in the event they occur. One measure to include in this training is the appropriate application of skin preparations to ensure that there is no pooling of solutions. It is also important to allow the amount of drying time recommended by the manufacturer prior to making an incision. These measures are documented in the patient's record. The expectations for these procedures need to be outlined in policies.[2]

Staffing

According to the CMS, the nursing services of the ASC must be directed and staffed to ensure that the nursing needs of all patients are met. The perianesthesia nursing standards state there must be perianesthesia registered nurses providing and directing nursing care in the recovery room. Patient needs are the highest priority and necessitate the presence of perianesthesia registered nurses to care for and assess the patients. There must also be a perianesthesia registered nurse available for emergency treatment whenever there is a patient in the ASC.

The American Society of PeriAnesthesia Nurses provides the standards of care for all patients of all ages having anesthesia for procedural or surgical events. The *2021–2022 Perianesthesia Nursing Standards, Practice Recommendations and Interpretive Statements* include a practice recommendation for nurse-to-patient staffing ratios.[6] Staffing must be based on acuity, census, patient flow processes, availability of support resources, and the physical facility. During phase I (e.g., immediately postoperatively), there must be two registered nurses, one of whom is a perianesthesia nurse competent in phase I postanesthesia nursing, in the same room or unit where the patient is receiving phase I care. The phase I perianesthesia nurse must have immediate access and a direct line of sight when providing patient care. The second nurse should be able to directly hear a call for assistance and be immediately available to assist. The need for additional nurses and support staff is dependent on the patient acuity, age, complexity of patient care needed, family support, patient census, and features of the physical facility. These staffing recommendations should also be maintained during "on-call" situations.[6]

Length of Stay and Patient Transfers

By definition, patients cannot plan to stay more than 24 hours in an ASC. Every patient reacts differently to anesthesia and surgery. Before a patient is discharged to the patient's own home, pain and nausea must be controlled. In the event that a patient needs additional care, a transfer to an acute setting is necessary. It is required that the physician or anesthetist evaluate the patient before discharge to a higher level of care.[2] Staff and physicians need to be competent in this transfer of care and complete appropriate documentation. Each ASC has a transfer agreement with a nearby hospital that can accept these patients when needed. The ASC must have an effective procedure for the immediate transfer, to a hospital, of patients requiring emergency medical care beyond the capabilities of the ASC.[2] Upon survey by the CMS, a review of all cases of patients transferred from the ASC to a hospital is conducted.[2]

Quality Monitoring

The CMS requires the provision of quality data as a measurement of the provision of high-quality, appropriate care.[2] Exploring opportunities to improve patient outcomes (e.g., by preventing infections and other adverse events) must be part of every program. Reviewing events for system failures or opportunities for improvement is a healthy way of developing a robust, high-quality program. Implementing ways to prevent errors in the future can improve future patient outcomes. Patients expect and trust that their healthcare providers are providing the best care and that they will have the best outcomes from their procedures. Reviewing data and quality indicators while setting clinical priorities is required for a quality program. A number of resources are available to generate ideas for quality indicators, including the National Quality Forum, Agency for Healthcare Research and Quality, American College of Surgeons, and CDC (Table 6.1). Improving care and the patient experience needs to be part of every program to ensure the best outcomes for patients.

A culture of safety within the healthcare setting has been determined to support the best outcomes for patients. When

TABLE 6.1 Examples of Quality Indicators

Agency	Recommendations
National Quality Forum	Correct site for surgery Retention of foreign object Assault Death Significant patient injury
Agency for Healthcare Research and Quality	Consumer Assessment of Healthcare Providers and Systems (CAHPS) Patient return to emergency department Adverse drug events
American College of Surgeons	Disruptive provider management Adherence to protocols Reporting of adverse events
Centers for Disease Control and Prevention	Monitoring of air quality Tracking of postoperative infections Same-day discharge failures

an error occurs, healthcare personnel need to speak up and report events without fear of retaliation. Bullying in the workplace occurs, and measures need to be in place for reporting and addressing the behavior by every member of the healthcare team. Dealing with dysfunctional communication can take its toll on those who may be targeted, and this may lead to high turnover in staff and unfortunate errors in the administration of care. Sustained attention to ensure positive healthy communication is needed to prevent incivility.

Patient perception indicators can measure a patient's experience of the care received. The Consumer Assessment of Healthcare Providers and Systems Outpatient and Ambulatory Surgery Survey (OAS CAHPS) was the first nationally standardized, publicly reported patient satisfaction survey. This survey collects information about patients' experiences of care in hospital outpatient departments and ASCs. These data are collected and posted publicly so that consumers can evaluate the care provided. Surgical teams can review this data to generate strategies to improve the overall patient experience.

Infection Prevention

Preventing infections for patients in the ASC is a healthcare priority. The ASC needs to have an infection control program that is directed by an individual trained in infection control.[2] Preventing surgical site infections is a goal for all. The CMS provides strategies known to reduce the incidence of infection. Preventing infections begins with how the patient is prepared for surgery and how instruments are sterilized, and it even includes what personnel wear in the operating room. The operating room attire is generally applied according to AORN guidelines. A policy needs to be in place to describe the acceptable attire and traffic flows. Cleaning the operating room between cases, including terminal cleaning at the end of the day, needs to be part of the ASC's training and policies. The skills for and adherence to aseptic techniques by all individuals in the operating room must be carefully monitored to ensure the best patient outcomes. The techniques for handling, sterilizing, packaging, and storing equipment should follow the Association for the Advancement of Medical Instrumentation (AAMI) standards. These activities must be conducted per professionally recognized standards of infection control practice. Examples of national organizations that promulgate nationally recognized infection and communicable disease control guidelines and/or recommendations include the CDC, Association for Professionals in Infection Control and Epidemiology (APIC), Society for Healthcare Epidemiology of America (SHEA), and AORN.[2] The

ASC is responsible for following up on each patient after discharge to identify and track infections associated with the patient's stay in the ASC.[2]

Reportable Events

The U.S. Food and Drug Administration regulates the use of many drugs and medical devices. If a medical device fails, the failure must be reported for tracking and follow-up. Recalls are necessary at times, and each facility should have a process in place for notifying the proper personnel of a problem in the facility and handling the recall. The National Quality Forum and the state hospital associations have a means by which a facility can report adverse events. A process for reviewing the events needs to be based on a safe culture without blame. Learning from an event and investigating the reasons why it occurred help to improve the future care of patients.

CHAPTER HIGHLIGHTS

- Caring for patients in an ASC is a unique experience for nurses.
- Care is taken to be sure a review of the safety standards is in place and observed.
- The safety standards are intended to protect both the patients and the staff who work in the ASC.
- Choosing an ASC is a wonderful option for properly selected patients.
- The safety standards highlighted here provide an overview, but additional safety standards exist and should be reviewed. Local, state, and federal manuals on safety regulations for ASCs should be consulted for complete and up-to-date requirements.

CASE STUDY

Serena has been promoted to a clinical nursing leadership position within a hospital-based outpatient surgery center. Her primary role will include the onboarding and annual competency development of the clinical staff within the service. What general topics should be included in the orientation of new staff to the outpatient surgery environment? Which annual competencies should be included in the education plan for all clinical nursing staff? Which professional organizations can Serena access for support and guidance in terms of standards of care within the outpatient surgery practice?

REFERENCES

1. Leapfrog Group. *ASC Survey Measures.* 2022. Available at: https://ratings.leapfroggroup.org/measure/asc/asc-survey-measures.
2. Centers for Medicare & Medicaid Services. *Ambulatory Surgical Centers (ASC) Center.* 2021. Available at: https://www.cms.gov/Center/Provider-Type/Ambulatory-Surgical-Centers-ASC-Center. Accessed September 11, 2022.
3. National Fire Protection Association (NFPA). *NFPA 101® Life Safety Code.* NFPA; 2021.
4. Electronic Code of Federal Regulations. *Part 416 – Ambulatory Surgical Services.* 2022. Available at: https://www.ecfr.gov/current/title-42/chapter-IV/subchapter-B/part-416.
5. American Society of PeriAnesthesia Nurses. *2021-2022 Perianesthesia Nursing Standards, Practice Recommendations and Interpretive Statements.* ASPAN; 2020.
6. American Society of PeriAnesthesia Nurses. *A Competency-Based Orientation Program for the Registered Nurse in the Perianesthesia Setting.* ASPAN; 2019.
7. Centers for Medicare & Medicaid Services. *State Operations Manual. Appendix L – Guidance for Surveyors: Ambulatory Surgical Centers.*

2022. Available at: https://www.cms.gov/Regulations-and-Guidance/Guidance/Manuals/Downloads/som107ap_l_ambulatory.pdf.

8. Occupational Safety and Health Administration. *Anesthetic Gases: Guidelines for Workplace Exposures*. 2000. Available at: https://www.osha.gov/waste-anesthetic-gases/workplace-exposures-guidelines.

9. Centers for Disease Control and Prevention (CDC). Sharps safety for healthcare settings. 2015. https://www.cdc.gov/sharpssafety/index.html Accessed August 8, 2023.

10. Occupational Safety and Health Administration. *Safety and Health Programs in the States*. White Paper. 2016. Available at: https://www.osha.gov/sites/default/files/Safety_and_Health_Programs_in_the_States_White_Paper.pdf.

11. Linchantra IV, Fong Y, Melstrom KA. Surgical smoke exposure in operating room personnel: a review. *JAMA Surg*. 2019;154(10);960-967. Available at: https://doi.org/10.1001/jamasurg.2019.2515.

7   The Environment of Care

Elizabeth Card, DNP, APRN, FNP-BC, CPAN, CCRP, FASPAN, FAAN;
LeighAnn Chadwell, MSN, RN, NE-BC;
Carol Bell, BSN, RN

LEARNING OBJECTIVES

A review of the content of this chapter will help the reader to:

1. Describe key components of a safe healthcare environment.
2. Identify factors that adversely impact the quality and safety of the perianesthesia healthcare environment.
3. Describe key performances and behaviors of perianesthesia nurses that will positively influence the health of the workplace.

OVERVIEW

Healthcare organizations are charged with attaining a high reliability of their systems. Complex organizations that deliver high-quality, safe, and consistent services or products while reducing and minimizing risks or adverse outcomes in a rapidly changing environment demonstrate high reliability.[1] Airlines and other organizations that use aeronautic devices are leading examples of organizations that have developed highly reliable systems, and other organizations can study them to obtain similar results. Efforts to obtain equally safe, high-quality, efficient environments of healthcare must be guided by collaborative interdisciplinary leaders with a shared vision.[2] Leaders have the responsibility for the creation and maintenance of a safe and efficient environment of healthcare.

There are guiding principles that can assist leaders in accomplishing this task. Regulatory bodies such as The Joint Commission (TJC) or Centers for Medicare and Medicaid Services (CMS) define some of the requirements that must be met by healthcare units and institutions. These are verified through in-person site visits. The identification and implementation of the elements needed for creating a highly reliable environment can become an additional strategy that leaders can utilize.

Perianesthesia nurses provide care in several areas of an ambulatory surgery center (ASC). They may provide preoperative testing that can enhance patients' postoperative outcomes by maximizing their health status. These nurses are also found in preoperative holding areas in which patients are prepared immediately before a procedure takes place, postanesthesia care units (PACUs) in which patients are recovering from anesthesia, and extended postanesthesia care units in which a continuum of care is provided until a patient is discharged and sent home. The success of these units and environments of care needs to be ensured before the first brick is placed for a new building or work gets underway for refurbishing a unit by having nurse leaders on the planning teams of these spaces. Healthcare spaces must be designed to serve the diverse needs of specific populations. In hospitals, for instance, neonatal intensive care units require different types of equipment and space allocations for newborn patients, and these needs differ substantially from the needs of adults in a general emergency room. This chapter focuses on the specific needs of patients in perianesthesia settings in ASCs.

CODES AND REGULATIONS

In a number of states, a Certificate of Need (CON) must be granted before a new healthcare facility, institution, or service can be built or an existing one modified at a specific designated location. Recent laws have placed a new emphasis on the quality of healthcare provided by the institution applying for the CON. The oversight of the granting of CONs has been strengthened, and the funding structures of agencies applying for CONs have been reviewed. In many states, the CON program is one way to monitor and deliver high-quality or improved access to healthcare, as well as cost savings for citizens and governments; it does this through its planned oversight and growth management of the state's healthcare systems. The criteria and standards for granting CONs are set by the state body involved in health planning, which also serves as the body that makes decisions about the implementation of criteria and standards.

The Joint Commission

The Joint Commission (TJC) has been a global leader of quality improvement and patient safety in healthcare for over 70 years. The Joint Commission establishes standards focused on guiding healthcare organizations to deliver safe, high-quality care. In 2002, The Joint Commission established the National Patient Safety Goals (NPSGs) to assist accredited organizations in addressing patient safety concerns. The universal protocol for preventing wrong site, wrong procedure, wrong patient surgery was developed from The Joint Commission's NPSGs.[3]

Accreditation Association for Ambulatory Health Care

The Accreditation Association for Ambulatory Health Care (AAAHC), founded in 1979, is an organization that accredits ambulatory healthcare centers. It reviews primary care practice centers, office-based surgery centers, occupational health centers, and even large dental and medical group practices located in over 25 states. The AAAHC specializes in providing accreditation surveys on-site for all types of outpatient care centers. The organization also advocates for the standardizing and ensuring of high-quality healthcare and safety for patients. This is done by a broad range of ambulatory healthcare experts who create, review, and update standards, evaluate institutions' compliance with standards and governing policies and procedures, and develop resources and tools to achieve continuous quality improvement. The standards are revised annually to align with emerging technologies and current trends in healthcare. Institutions and organizations that meet or exceed these standards can receive a certification from the AAAHC.[4]

There may be additional local and state building codes to which healthcare facilities must adhere, but a discussion of them is beyond the scope of this chapter. Readers should be aware that they exist and consult them when appropriate.

PROVISION OF SAFETY IN HEALTHCARE ENVIRONMENTS

A safe healthcare environment is crucial for the well-being of all who are cared for or provide care within it. Strategic leaders can utilize policies, regulations, and experience as a roadmap for designing such environments. There are two broad populations to be considered in establishing safety: patients and their families and staff.

Safety for Perianesthesia Patients

The National Academy of Medicine, formerly known as the Institute of Medicine, mandated that 90% of healthcare decisions be evidence-based by 2020.[5] However, many of the practice changes that might have achieved this goal were challenging to institute. For example, in 1999 the American Society of Anesthesiologists (ASA) released an evidence-based recommendation for allowing patients to consume clear liquids up to 2 hours before receiving anesthesia, and yet the practice is still nothing by mouth (NPO) after midnight in many institutions 20 years later.[6] There is ample evidence that maintaining a well-hydrated status and consuming a carbohydrate-rich drink 2 hours before a procedure stabilizes blood glucose levels and reduces post procedure adverse events.[6] The adoption of evidence-based recommendations and adherence to standards and guidelines will optimize the safety and therapeutic nature of the environment.[7] Additionally, there is ample evidence that patients who are cared for by nurses who are certified in an appropriate area of specialty are safer, experiencing fewer failures to rescue and having improved patient outcomes.[8-10] Managers and leaders who encourage nurses to obtain specialty certification are also cultivating patient safety and high-quality care.

Safety for Nurses and Other Staff

Appropriate staffing ratios are crucial for delivering safe, high-quality care. One of the responsibilities of the American Society of PeriAnesthesia Nurses (ASPAN) is to define standards of safe staffing practice in the perianesthesia setting. Practice recommendations regarding patient classification and staffing recommendations can be found in ASPAN's *2023–2024 Perianesthesia Nursing Standards, Practice Recommendations and Interpretive Statements*. It is ASPAN's position that "an appropriate number of perianesthesia registered nurses with demonstrated competence [be] available to meet the individual needs of patients and families in each phase of perianesthesia care based on patient acuity, census, patient throughput, and physical facility." Ross points out that since the start of the 2020 pandemic and the related exodus of healthcare workers, the ability to comply with infection control protocols has been compromised, resulting in significant increases in infection rates.[11]

WORKPLACE VIOLENCE AND BULLYING

The American Nurses Association 2016 survey of 18,537 nurses revealed that approximately half of the respondents reported experiencing workplace incivility. This number has undoubtedly increased with the additional stress of the Covid-19 pandemic. Recent predictions of the nursing shortage estimate 4.3 million unfilled positions by 2026.[12,13] Reasons cited for this include the retirement of nurses in the baby boomer generation coupled with 30% to 60% of new nurses voluntarily leaving their first job within 12 months. The top reason cited

for this exodus is workplace bullying and incivility.[12,13] Sadly, 64% of those leaving identified other nurses as the source of these behaviors.[14] These numbers jump to 90% when surveys are expanded to the initial 3 years of nurses' careers.[15] Older generations of nurses have experienced higher amounts of incivility and distress than other generations, indicating that this negative workplace stress impacts all nurses.[16] Left unchecked, incivility contributes to poor health outcomes, nurse suicides, and increased healthcare costs.[14,17] Perhaps the most profound result of incivility is the uptake of these behaviors by former victims.[13] Incivility is associated with job burnout, as well as a decreased quality and performance of work.[18,19] The reported financial impact of these behaviors is 4 billion U.S. dollars.[13] Additionally, there is ample evidence that work environments accepting these behaviors will experience much more of them.[13,17,19] Nurse incivility is a problem that nursing leaders can address by implementing interventions that improve the well-being of the perianesthesia workplace environment. Encouraging civility and eliminating workplace violence and bullying are everyone's responsibilities. There are evidence-based interventions that can be translated easily to the perianesthesia work environment to increase the well-being of the workplace and safety of the patients.

Workplace violence is not isolated to behaviors amongst colleagues within the healthcare environment. The current socioeconomic and political climate within communities has had an adverse impact on the psychological health of many disadvantaged individuals who struggle with poverty, healthcare disparities, and mental health issues, to name a few. Today, more than ever, healthcare organizations must have security plans and measures in place to avert unsafe events from occurring within the system. The ASPAN Standard for Environment of Care urges perianesthesia nurses to be aware of their employer's security recommendations and adhere to safety practices.[7] Examples of these safety recommendations include training to manage aggressive behaviors; using badge identification tags to access locked doors and restricted areas; increasing video surveillance devices, personal security tags, and lighting; and providing easy access to system alarms.

CREATING AN ENVIRONMENT FOR FLOURISHING

The culture of the workplace is created by leaders and reflected in those who function within the environment. Adherence to a code of conduct and zero tolerance has been associated with improvements in workplace violence. However, there is much more that can be done to encourage growth and nurture a place for flourishing. The next generation of nurses and future workforce hope to find a work–life balance as one benefit of the workplace, and organizations that do not address issues and try to provide this balance will be challenged to attract new nurses. Support and an opportunity to contribute to decisions, as well as having access to information about a unit's successes or challenges, are low-hanging fruit that leaders can address and embrace.

SAFETY CONSIDERATIONS FOR PATIENTS, EMPLOYEES, AND VISITORS
Waste Anesthetic Gases

Waste anesthetic gases (WAGs) are invisible, but exposure to them affects living organisms in ways that are visible and measurable. Recognition of the hazards related to the occupational exposure to WAGs was first reported in the late 1960s.[20] In the following 5 decades, researchers uncovered the relationship between the exposure to WAGs in high concentrations for even very short periods of time and the development of headaches;

irritability; fatigue; nausea;, difficulties with concentration, judgment, audiovisual processing, and coordination; the development of liver and kidney disease and malignancies of the lymph and immune systems; and alterations in the metabolization of vitamin B_{12}, or pernicious anemia.[7] The National Institute of Occupational Safety and Health (NIOSH) and the Occupational Safety and Health Administration (OSHA), both U.S. federal agencies, have recognized this hazardous occupational exposure for those working in operating rooms where anesthetic gases are administered. OSHA has created strict regulatory engineering controls and surveillance structures and systems to protect surgical teams from inhaling WAGs. It has also put into place legal obligations to which healthcare facilities must adhere in order to meet these standards. It is recognized that anesthetic gases are not metabolized by patients but rather are exhaled by patients as gases that are 95% unmetabolized.[21,22] Findings from Krenzischek et al.[23] revealed that PACU nurses have measurable metabolites in their breath from exposure to WAGs up to 3 days after their last shift worked. Additionally, metabolites were measured in patients who did not receive general anesthesia but were in the PACU, indicating that cross contamination can occur through WAGs in the ambient air of the PACU.[23]

Solutions can be put into place by unit and hospital leaders to reduce this occupational hazard and reduce exposure to visitors and other patients. Increased fresh air exchanges of heat and air systems, as well as the use of a mask that scavenges WAGs, can alleviate this problem. ASPAN recently created a Position Statement on Waste Anesthetic Gases Outside of the Operating Room, which is supported by the American Industrial Hygiene Association.[7] This position statement gives additional guidance, recommendations, and resources for unit and hospital leaders within the perianesthesia space to improve the health and well-being of the perianesthesia workspace and those contained within it.

Nurses are advocates for healthy work environments, as well as the health of the individuals for whom they care. A specialty nursing organization gives voice to many nurses, advocating for issues that impact the organization's members and those for whom they care. In addition, ASPAN's Position Statement on Air Quality and Occupational Hazards and Position Statement on Waste Anesthetic Gases Outside of the Operating Room set the foundation for advocating for and implementing measures to improve the health of the work environment by mitigating occupational exposure to WAGs.[7]

Infection Control

Preparedness for and awareness of infectious diseases are ongoing challenges that leaders and nurses must face. Knowing the most recent evidence and having up-to-date information on infectious threats is vital. Adhering to universal precautions, coupled with having appropriate personal protective equipment available for all levels of isolation precautions, is essential for ensuring the safety of the perianesthesia work environment. Additionally, general training and annual updates are required to keep staff informed, educated, and safe. Surgical care improvement initiatives for reducing surgical site infections should be incorporated into practice protocols, including but not limited to, appropriate patient screening, measures to prevent skin sepsis, the careful selection of antibiotics, and the provision of patient warming measures.

Maintaining the Physical Safety of Units

Perianesthesia units in the ambulatory setting should be maintained with the same level of cleanliness, disinfection, sterilization, and organization of supplies as hospital-based units. The physical conditions of a unit are not limited to appearance but also include noise, temperature, and lighting levels. Personnel, in addition to adhering to protocols for infection prevention, engage in measures for maintaining hand hygiene practices to reduce the transmission of microbes.[24] Other key components of a safe environment of care are facility-based resources, including emergency backup systems such as generators; fire alarm systems; and comprehensive life-safety plans, such as evacuation plans, blood-borne pathogen exposure protocols, and emergency operations plans.[25] Documentation of these plans, downtime options for power failures, and staff education regarding these tools for safety are crucial in the ambulatory setting, where resources tend to be limited (Table 7.1).

TABLE 7.1 Sample Utilities Failure Plan

Utility System	Failure	Action
Electricity	Loss of power to normal power outlets	Plug all critical patient support devices into red outlets NO new procedures should be initiated while generator power is being used Check warmers and coolers to ensure supplies and medications are safe
Electricity	Loss of power to all outlets	Manually support all critical patient devices Use any equipment that runs on batteries in the meantime Maintain battery supply Use flashlights Check warmers and coolers to ensure supplies and medications are safe
Water	Loss of water pressure	Reduce use to minimum Notify maintenance department
Water	Loss of all water	Do not attempt to use water Turn off faucets Notify maintenance department
Oxygen	Loss of oxygen from wall outlets	Provide tank oxygen for patients in need
Vacuum	Loss of vacuum from wall outlets	Use portable suction devices
Medical air	Loss of medical air pressure	Manually support patients on medical air devices
Air conditioning (HVAC)	Loss of air conditioning	Use fans if needed Ensure operating rooms have adequate temperature and humidity ranges Postpone starting new cases until integrity of supplies is determined Notify maintenance department

Continued

TABLE 7.1 Sample Utilities Failure Plan—cont'd

Utility System	Failure	Action
Heating	Loss of heat	Use extra blankets if necessary Postpone starting new cases Notify maintenance department
Communications	Phones not working	Adhere to communication failure plan Use cell phones Designate a runner if necessary
Communications	Loss of data system	Revert to downtime procedures for documentation
Elevators	Elevators not working	Use stairs Notify maintenance department
Elevators	Stuck in elevator	Use emergency phone to notify operator Stay calm Do not try to climb out of elevator

Source: Adapted from Burden N, DeFazio DMD. The environment of care. In: Burden N, Quinn DMD, O'Brien D, Dawes BSG. *Ambulatory Surgical Nursing.* 2nd ed. WB Saunders, 2000.

Evidence-Based Practice: Hand hygiene

Mouajau et al., provided an overview of hand hygiene compliance (HHC) studies. The relationship between hospital-acquired infections and the practice of hand hygiene has been well established. Based on this overview, HHC is reportedly between 60 and 70%. The Ambulatory Surgery Center should consider the implementation of an HHC monitoring program, ideally incorporating direct observers. In settings where compliance was below 60%, healthcare acquired infection rates were higher. Environmental cleaning, in addition to HHC, serves a critical role in prevention of healthcare acquired infections.

Source: Mouajou V, Adams K, DeLisle G, Quach C. Hand hygiene compliance in the prevention of hospital-acquired infections: a systematic review. *J Hosp Inf.* 2022;119:33-48. https://doi.org/10.1016/j.jhin.2021.09.016

LESSONS FROM PAST PATHOGENIC EVENTS

Often a historical event has a profound impact that is not recognized until well after the event has resolved. For example, the 1918 Spanish influenza pandemic was later named by historians as the deadliest global acute infectious disease outbreak in modern history. The Spanish Flu pandemic was triggered by the H1N1 influenza virus and resulted in an estimated 20 to 50 million deaths around the globe. The highest mortality rates were in young adults between 20 and 40 years of age, an unusual population to be impacted. The population in the years immediately following World War I was decimated by this pathogen in addition to the war, and a huge amount of the workforce was lost. In the late twentieth century, the human immunodeficiency virus (HIV) and the acquired immunodeficiency syndrome (AIDS) that it caused resulted in the deaths of an estimated 35 million people.

The Covid-19 pandemic, caused by the SARS-CoV-2 virus, which emerged in 2020 is sadly not likely to be the last pandemic that the world will experience. The virus was felt to have originated in animals and was then transmitted from animals to humans and humans to humans.[26] HIV, the Ebola virus, the Middle East respiratory syndrome coronavirus (MERS-CoV), and SARS-CoV-2 are the most recent major examples of pathogens that have successfully jumped from animals to humans.[27] The expansion of human populations has resulted in increased human-to-wildlife exposures, and changes in weather patterns have impacted the complexity of food systems. These changes have set the stage for the future development of zoonotic infectious diseases; nearly 75% of the new emerging pathogens infecting humans are zoonotic in nature.[28] This underlines the importance of bio surveillance at the animal-to-human interface. Health systems, policy makers, researchers, and leaders should establish bio surveillance to anticipate and recognize the next potential pathogenic threat and establish policies for reducing its impact.[29]

One Health, a division of the Centers for Disease Control (CDC), is based on the recognition that the environment, planet, and plant, animal, and human health are all intertwined.[30] One Health is a unique collaborative framework of research, educational, industrial, and health systems and governmental agencies from the global to local levels. The goal is to work together to share information and discoveries and to identify zoonotic infections and mitigate their impacts before they become pandemics.[29] So far, health systems and decision-makers have failed to establish bio surveillance at the human-to-animal interface that would allow actions to be taken to thwart pandemics. They have, however, learned from past experiences and identified the barriers to sharing information, funding research, and sharing goals, tools, priorities, and processes that contributed to the failure to predict, prevent, and respond to the Covid-19 pandemic. Interdisciplinary and interagency collaborations and data sharing using a robust One Health framework will allow the world not only to be better prepared for the next crisis but perhaps to prevent it from happening at all.[29]

CHAPTER HIGHLIGHTS

- High-reliability organizations deliver safe, high-quality care.
- The ability to provide safe, high-quality care relies on the multidisciplinary collaboration that can develop and implement safety protocols and procedures within the ambulatory setting.
- Perianesthesia nursing practice promotes and maintains a safe, comfortable, and therapeutic environment for patients, families, and healthcare personnel.

CASE STUDY

It is a typical busy Monday morning in the outpatient surgery center. A new service line has been introduced to the clinical staff however, the provider's office staff have not yet established an efficient routine. Patients arrive randomly, not in sync with the surgical schedule. At one point there are six patients waiting to be admitted, six patients in the preop holding area, four operating rooms running, and five patients in the phase I area of care. The resource nurse for the unit is feeling nervous that the number of staff is not adequate for the number of patients and their current phase of care. What is the appropriate number of perianesthesia registered nurses for this volume of patients? How is this number determined? Which organization is the best resource for staffing recommendations? What factors should be considered when creating a safe staffing plan?

REFERENCES

1. Alavosius MP, Houmanfar RA, Anbro SJ, Burleigh K, Hebein C. Leadership and crew resource management in high-reliability organizations: a competency framework for measuring behaviors. In: Ludwig TD, ed. *Sources of Behavioral Variance in Process Safety.* 1st ed. Routledge; 2019:113-141.
2. Wells N, Card EB. Identifying significant evidence-based practice problems within complex health environments. In: Christenbery TL, ed. *Evidence-Based Practice in Nursing: Foundations, Skills, and Roles.* Springer Publishing Company; 2017.
3. The Joint Commission. *National Patient Safety Goals.* 2022. Available at: https://www.jointcommission.org/standards/national-patient-safety-goals/.
4. Accreditation Association for Ambulatory Health Care. *Certification for Surgery Centers.* 2022. Available at: https://www.aaahc.org/certification/surgical/.
5. Ohio State University. *Evidence-Based Health Care: The Care You Want, But Might Not Be Getting: New Study Reveals One Reason Many Hospitals Struggle with Quality, Safety, and Costs.* ScienceDaily. 2016. Available at: https://www.sciencedaily.com/releases/2016/02/160201215950.htm.
6. Denton TD. Southern hospitality: how we changed the NPO practice in the emergency department. *J Emerg Nurs.* 2015;41(4):317-322. Available at: https://doi.org/10.1016/j.jen.2014.12.001.
7. American Society of PeriAnesthesia Nurses. *2023-2024 Perianesthesia Nursing Standards, Practice Recommendations and Interpretive Statements.* ASPAN, 2022.
8. Cary AH. Certified registered nurses: results of the study of the certified workforce. *Am J Nurs.* 2001;101(1):44-52. Available at: https://doi.org/10.1097/00000446-200101000-00048.
9. Curley MA. Patient-nurse synergy: optimizing patients' outcomes. *Am J Crit Care.* 1998;7(1):64-72.
10. Fukuda T, Sakurai H, Kashiwagi M. Impact of having a certified nurse specialist in critical care nursing as head nurse on ICU patient outcomes. *PloS One.* 2020;15(2):e0228458. Available at: https://doi.org/10.1371/journal.pone.0228458.
11. Ross J. Nursing shortage creating patient safety concerns. *J Perianesth Nurs.* 2022;37(4):565-567. Available at: https://doi.org/10.1016/j.jopan.2022.05.078.
12. American Nurses Association. *Violence, Incivility, and Bullying.* N.D. Available at: https://www.nursingworld.org/practice-policy/work-environment/violence-incivility-bullying/.
13. Gilbert RT, Hudson JS, Strider D. Addressing the elephant in the room: nurse manager recognition of and response to nurse-to-nurse bullying. *Nurs Adm Q.* 2016;40(3):E1-E11. Available at: https://doi.org/10.1097/naq.0000000000000175.
14. Hartin P, Birks M, Lindsay D. Bullying in nursing: how has it changed over 4 decades? *J Nurs Manag.* 2020;28(7):1619-1626. Available at: https://doi.org/10.1111/jonm.13117.
15. Smith LM, Andrusyszyn MA, Laschinger HKS. Effects of workplace incivility and empowerment on newly-graduated nurses' organizational commitment. *J Nurs Manag.* 2010;18(8):1004-1015. Available at: https://doi.org/10.1111/j.1365-2834.2010.01165.x.
16. Leiter MP, Price SL, Laschinger HKS. Generational differences in distress, attitudes and incivility among nurses. *J Nurs Manag.* 2010;18(8):970-980. Available at: https://doi.org/10.1111/j.1365-2834.2010.01168.x.
17. Davidson JE, Accardi R, Sanchez C, Zisook S, Hoffman LA. Sustainability and outcomes of a suicide prevention program for nurses. *Worldviews Evid Based Nurs.* 2020;17(1):24-31. Available at: https://doi.org/10.1111/wvn.12418.
18. Card E, Hyman S. Prevalence and risk factors for burnout in the perianesthesia setting. *J Perianesth Nurs.* 2015;30(4):E40-E41. Available at: https://doi.org/10.1016/j.jopan.2015.05.107.
19. Card E, Tabet CH, Krenzischek D. An introduction to the AANA, AORN, and ASPAN Joint Civility Position Statement. *J Perianesth Nurs.* 2022;37(3):294-295. Available at: https://doi.org/10.1016/j.jopan.2022.02.007.
20. Vaĭsman AI. Working conditions in surgery and their effect on the health of anesthesiologists. *Eksp Khir Anesteziol.* 1967;12(3):44-49.
21. Kharasch ED. Biotransformation of sevoflurane. *Anesth Analg.* 1995;81(6 suppl):S27-38. Available at: https://doi.org/10.1097/00000539-199512001-00005.
22. Sherman J, Le C, Lamers V, Eckelman M. Life cycle greenhouse gas emissions of anesthetic drugs. *Anesth Analg.* 2012;114(5):1086-1090. Available at: https://doi.org/10.1213/ANE.0b013e31824f6940.
23. Krenzischek DA, Schaefer J, Nolan M, et al. Phase I collaborative pilot study: waste anesthetic gas levels in the PACU. *J Perianesth Nurs.* 2002;17(4):227-239. Available at: https://doi.org/10.1053/jpan.2002.34166.
24. Akyüz N, Özbas A, Çavdar I. Safety of personnel working in endoscopy units. *AORN J.* 2007;85(1):181-187. Available at: https://doi.org/10.1016/s0001-2092(07)60024-6.
25. Blackwell LA. A successful life safety survey in an ambulatory surgery center. *AORN J.* 2014;99(3):431-434. Available at: https://doi.org/10.1016/j.aorn.2014.01.001.
26. Ahmad T, Khan M, Haroon, et al. COVID-19: zoonotic aspects. *Travel Med Infect Dis.* 2020;36:101607. Available at: https://doi.org/10.1016/j.tmaid.2020.101607.
27. Sabin NS, Calliope AS, Simpson SV, et al. Implications of human activities for (re)emerging infectious diseases, including COVID-19. *J Physiol Anthropol.* 2020;39(1):29. Available at: https://doi.org/10.1186/s40101-020-00239-5.
28. Karesh WB, Dobson A, Lloyd-Smith JO, et al. Ecology of zoonoses: natural and unnatural histories. *Lancet.* 2012;380(9857):1936-1945. Available at: https://doi.org/10.1016/s0140-6736(12)61678-x.
29. Mackenzie JS, Jeggo M. The one health approach-why is it so important? *Trop Med Infect Dis.* 2019;4(2):88. Available at: https://doi.org/10.3390/tropicalmed4020088.
30. Centers for Disease Control and Prevention. *One Health.* 2023. Available at: https://www.cdc.gov/onehealth/index.html.

Clinical Emergencies and Preparedness in the Ambulatory Setting

Terri A. Gray, MEd, BSN, CPAN

LEARNING OBJECTIVES

A review of the content of this chapter will help the reader to:

1. Describe preventive measures utilized when preparing patients for safe surgery.
2. Describe the most common respiratory complications encountered in the PACU and the appropriate management for them.
3. State two preprocedural actions used to prevent postoperative nausea and vomiting.
4. List three signs and symptoms of local anesthesia system toxicity (LAST).
5. Identify the medications used in the treatment of malignant hyperthermia to stop the crisis.
6. Demonstrate knowledge of the nursing responsibility in the management of postoperative complications.

OVERVIEW

All surgical and anesthesia events have the potential for risks and complications. The ability to predict which patients could develop a surgical complication would enable the team to change the surgical or anesthesia plan or delay or cancel surgery. Many processes are in place to ensure that the ambulatory environment is the appropriate location for the patient. Individualized patient assessments are completed to determine the risk of complications given the nature of the surgery, the anesthesia method planned, the patient's co-morbidities, the American Society of Anesthesiologists (ASA) patient classification, the preoperative medical assessment, and the success of any optimization efforts. The volume of ambulatory surgical procedures has increased significantly owing to advances in the areas of surgical techniques, perioperative processes, and patient selection. The emergence of office-based anesthesia as a subspecialty of ambulatory anesthesia is a result of economic and social factors, as well as of the development of improved and innovative surgical techniques and anesthetic drugs.[1] The outpatient movement has also included an increase in the pediatric patient population. Outpatient anesthesia offers an option for children to undergo minor surgical procedures when conditions can be optimized for safety.

The qualifications and overall competence of the institution and staff members, in addition to the experience of the anesthesiologist, are crucial for high-quality, safe results, particularly for specialty populations (e.g., pediatric patients, obese patients, or patients with chronic respiratory disease). In the ambulatory setting, there is an expectation of a speedy recovery and discharge of patients. This critical objective requires the selection of the appropriate patient population. The movement of more complex procedures into the ambulatory environment raises the potential for staff members to see a wider variety of procedural complications. Complication rates in the postanesthesia care unit (PACU) are hard to compare because studies often measure a variety of complications differently and the sources of these complications have a wide variety of factors. Complications may occur in patients with little or no coexisting disease, and in some cases this can lead to serious sequelae, including cardiac arrest.[2] Complications can be costly to both the patient and the organization, with delayed discharges, additional treatments, decreased patient satisfaction, or transfers to a higher level of care. A patient with complications could have a lengthy recovery time and possible further complications, causing additional financial burdens, physical and emotional burdens, and a change in the quality of life.

FACTS AND FIGURES

There are reasons to be concerned when looking at the number of adverse everts in the PACU. However, a majority of them are minor in nature, caught by observation, and easily managed. Berg and Braehler reported a prospective study involving over 18,000 patients receiving care in the phase I PACU.[3] The findings suggested that the complication rate was nearly one in every four patients, or 24%.[3] According to this study, the most common issues encountered were postoperative nausea and vomiting (PONV) (9.8%), airway management requirements (6.8%), and hypotension (2.7%).[3] Further problems observed included hypoxia, hypothermia, shivering, and cardiovascular instability.[3] Previous studies showed that the overall adverse events in the PACU ranged between 5% and 30%.[4-6] In earlier studies, minor complications appeared to present much more frequently, at 22.1%, than major events, at 0.2% (Figure 8.1).[5]

Specific surgical procedures have particular risks, and many of these procedures are being done in the ambulatory setting. Aside from cardiac surgery, vascular surgery is associated with some of the highest rates of surgical and anesthesia risks.[7] Lower-risk procedures include procedures involving the breast, skin, urologic system, and orthopedic system.[7] Anesthesia techniques and the effects of anesthetic pharmacology can also have an adverse effect on patients. In the early 1990s, a higher incidence of PACU complications was seen in those patients who received a general anesthetic than in those who were given either a regional anesthetic or monitored anesthesia. Moderate sedation, deep sedation, regional anesthesia, total intravenous anesthesia, and general anesthesia are all utilized in the ambulatory setting. Figure 8.2 shows a schematic of the number of factors impacting outcomes.

Postoperative complications make up one focus of quality in ambulatory surgery centers (ASCs), and despite the provision of timely and appropriate perioperative care, complications still can and do occur.[8] Successful surgical outcomes are the result of a coordinated team effort.[9] Major adverse events in the PACU are reduced as a result of preventive processes. These processes involve a robust preadmission pathway, including patient optimization, patient and family education,

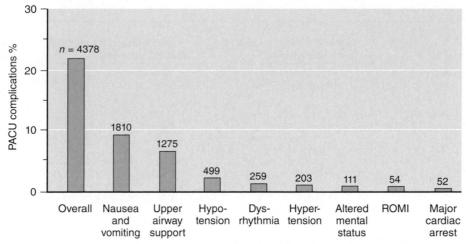

Fig. 8.1 Overall complication rates. Source: Berg SM, Braehler MR. The postanesthesia care unit. In: Gropper MA, ed. *Miller's Anesthesia.* 9th ed. Elsevier; 2020; Figure 80.1.

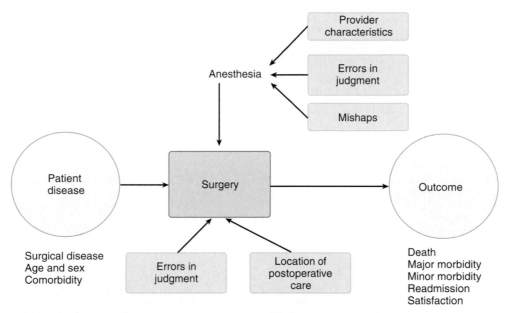

Fig. 8.2 Factors impacting poor outcomes. Source: Hadler RA, Neuman MD, Fleisher LA. Risk of anesthesia. In: Gropper MA, ed. *Miller's Anesthesia.* 9th ed. Elsevier; 2020; Figure 30.1.

standardization, enhanced staff skills, and preparedness. ASCs do not usually have an abundance of resources available for responding to a crisis, and as a result, staff orientation and training are imperative.

PREVENTION OF COMPLICATIONS

Whenever complications occur, it is important to explore the factors that influenced them. Kluger and Bullock reported in a small study in the early 2000s that factors contributing to complications included errors of judgment, communication failures, and inadequate preoperative preparation.[5] In this same study, factors shown to minimize these incidents included having clinical staff with previous experience, detection by monitoring, and the availability of skilled assistance.[5] The standardization of care of perianesthesia patients, including select premedication protocols, multimodal pain therapy options, PONV prophylaxis, and vigilant postoperative monitoring, helped to eliminate variations in outcomes, ensure safety, and improve the quality of care.

Patient Selection

The preanesthesia assessment and evaluation are critical elements for screening patients. However, concern about patient safety remains, as the outpatient surgical population has increased not only in volume but also in age and complexity, necessitating improved preoperative screening.[10] Often, the presurgical assessment identifies patients early in the process who present with risks too concerning to be candidates in an ambulatory environment. For ambulatory-based outpatient surgery, identifying the appropriate patient and proper procedure is one of the key components of safety. One major criterion used to determine a patient's risk during anesthesia is the American Society of Anesthesiologists physical status (ASA PS) classification (Table 8.1).

The ASA PS classification is a simple anesthesia risk stratification tool for surgeries in the inpatient and outpatient settings. Foley's study found that the ASA PS classification system was accurate in identifying the risk level for patients.[11] Patients with higher ASA PS scores subsequently developed medical complications or died at a greater frequency than patients with lower

TABLE 8.1 ASA Physical Status Classification

ASA Physical Status Classification	Definition	Adult Examples (including but not limited to)	Pediatric Examples (including but not limited to)	Obstetric Examples (including but not limited to)
ASA I	A normal healthy patient	Healthy, nonsmoking, no or minimal alcohol use	Healthy (no acute or chronic disease), normal body mass index (BMI) percentile for age	
ASA II	A patient with mild systemic disease	Mild diseases only without substantive functional limitations. Current smoker, social alcohol drinker, pregnancy, obesity (30 < BMI < 40), well-controlled diabetes mellitus (DM)/hypertension (HTN), mild lung disease	Asymptomatic congenital cardiac disease, well-controlled dysrhythmias, asthma without exacerbation, well-controlled epilepsy, non–insulin-dependent DM, abnormal BMI percentile for age, mild/moderate obstructive sleep apnea (OSA), oncologic state in remission, autism with mild limitations	Normal pregnancy, well-controlled gestational HTN, controlled preeclampsia without severe features, diet-controlled gestational DM
ASA III	A patient with severe systemic disease	Substantive functional limitations; one or more moderate to severe diseases. Poorly controlled DM or HTN, chronic obstructive pulmonary disease (COPD), morbid obesity (BMI ≥40), active hepatitis, alcohol dependence or abuse, implanted pacemaker, moderate reduction of ejection fraction, end-stage renal disease (ESRD) undergoing regularly scheduled dialysis, history (>3 mo) of myocardial infarction (MI), cerebrovascular accident (CVA), transient ischemic attack (TIA), or coronary artery disease (CAD)/stents	Uncorrected stable congenital cardiac abnormality, asthma with exacerbation, poorly controlled epilepsy, insulin-dependent DM, morbid obesity, malnutrition, severe OSA, oncologic state, renal failure, muscular dystrophy, cystic fibrosis, history of organ transplantation, brain/spinal cord malformation, symptomatic hydrocephalus, premature infant postconceptual age (PCA) < 60 weeks, autism with severe limitations, metabolic disease, difficult airway, long-term parenteral nutrition, full-term infants < 6 weeks of age	Preeclampsia with severe features, gestational DM with complications or high insulin requirements, a thrombophilic disease requiring anticoagulation
ASA IV	A patient with severe systemic disease that is a constant threat to life	Recent (<3 mo) MI, CVA, TIA, or CAD/stents, ongoing cardiac ischemia or severe valve dysfunction, severe reduction of ejection fraction, shock, sepsis, disseminated intravascular coagulation (DIC), acute respiratory distress syndrome (ARDS), or ESRD not undergoing regularly scheduled dialysis	Symptomatic congenital cardiac abnormality, congestive heart failure, active sequelae of prematurity, acute hypoxic-ischemic encephalopathy, shock, sepsis, DIC, automatic implantable cardioverter-defibrillator, ventilator dependence, endocrinopathy, severe trauma, severe respiratory distress, advanced oncologic state	Preeclampsia with severe features complicated by HELLP syndrome or other adverse event, peripartum cardiomyopathy with ejection fraction < 40, uncorrected/decompensated heart disease, acquired or congenital
ASA V	A moribund patient who is not expected to survive without the operation	Ruptured abdominal/thoracic aneurysm, massive trauma, intracranial bleed with mass effect, ischemic bowel in the face of significant cardiac pathology or multiple organ/system dysfunction	Massive trauma, intracranial hemorrhage with mass effect, patient requiring extracorporeal membrane oxygenation (ECMO), respiratory failure or arrest, malignant hypertension, decompensated congestive heart failure, hepatic encephalopathy, ischemic bowel or multiple organ/system dysfunction	Uterine rupture
ASA VI	A declared brain-dead patient whose organs are being removed for donor purposes			

Source: Pardo MC. Preoperative evaluation. In: Pardo MC, ed. *Miller's Basics of Anesthesia*. 8th ed. Elsevier; 2023; Table 13.16.

ASA PS scores after outpatient surgery. These results confirmed the theory that the ambulatory setting may not be able to meet the needs of high-risk patients.[11] Generally, patients with an ASA PS score of 1 or 2 are eligible for ambulatory surgery, and occasionally a patient with an ASA PS score of 3 meets approval. Currently, some ambulatory settings accept patients with an ASA PS score of 3 or 4, particularly in the office-based environment. Although the ideal patient for an office-based procedure has an ASA PS score of 1 or 2, nearly one third of patients served in this setting in 2014 had an ASA PS score of 3.[11]

Foley's study reported a total of 34,000 patients classified as ASA PS 4 who had undergone ambulatory surgery. After adjusting for potential confounding factors, ASA PS 4 patients had an 89 times greater chance of dying after ambulatory surgery than ASA PS 1 (healthy) patients.[11]

Coordination of care, including patient optimization, is a critical factor for successful outpatient care. Both the anesthesia team and the surgeon or proceduralist should collaborate on optimization goals prior to surgery. The anesthesia provider will have the responsibility of reviewing the history and physical status to determine if the patient is a candidate for the ambulatory setting. Additionally, postprocedure recovery following ambulatory surgery places more responsibility on the patient and family. Families require education to support the management of the patient at discharge. Patient and family education begins early with the preanesthesia screening and continues through discharge and into the postoperative follow-up.

PREPARATION FOR RESPONDING TO COMPLICATIONS

Recovery room staff are frequently relied upon to provide an immediate extension of the anesthesia provider role and must be skilled in airway management, cardiovascular manipulation, and drug delivery.[12] For example, perianesthesia nurses acquire skills for determining the need for oral or nasopharyngeal airways and demonstrate competencies when placing an airway. Steps are always taken to prevent complications from happening, but they still occur. The preparation for managing a crisis includes, but is not limited to, the provision of adequate supplies and equipment, as well as proper staff training.

Supplies and Equipment

In the ambulatory setting, supplies and equipment are required for the support of emergency situations. When the pediatric patient is served in the outpatient setting, appropriate age-adjusted equipment must be available. Emergency equipment must include oxygen delivery devices and bag-valve masks, as well as ventilators for full respiratory support. Quick access to crash carts and emergency medications specific for the patient population served, whether adult or pediatric, is crucial. ASPAN's recommended equipment for the day-of-surgery preparation area in phase I, and phase II can be found in Boxes 8.1, 8.2, and 8.3. A fully stocked malignant hyperthermia (MH) emergency cart or a drug box for MH treatment must be available if any of the drugs that might trigger the disorder are used in the ambulatory setting. Every bedside

---

BOX 8.1 Equipment for Day of Surgery/Procedure Preparation Area

1. Each patient bedside will have the following:
   a. Means to deliver oxygen
   b. Means to provide constant and intermittent suction
   c. Means to monitor blood pressure
   d. Capacity to ensure patient privacy
2. The following equipment should be available, as needed:
   a. Task-based lighting
   b. Surgical preparation supplies (e.g., skin wipes, clippers)
   c. Capnography
   d. Emergency airway equipment
   e. Venous thromboembolism prophylaxis equipment
   f. Access to safe patient handling and moving equipment
3. The following equipment should be present in the day of surgery/ procedure preparation area:
   a. Vital sign monitors
   b. Blood glucose monitor
   c. Height and weight scales
   d. Supplemental oxygen
   e. Cardiac monitor
   f. Pulse oximeter
   g. Thermometry
   h. Bag-valve masks (size-appropriate)
   i. Suction
   j. Warming measures or devices
   k. Automated medication cabinet or dispensing device (e.g., Pyxis, Omnicell)
4. A method of calling for assistance in emergency situations shall be provided
5. An emergency cart for adults and pediatrics will be always readily available
6. A defibrillator with adult and pediatric pads/paddles and cardiac pacing capability must be readily available
7. Medications that should be available as needed include, but are not limited to, the following:
   a. Antibiotics
   b. Antiemetics
   c. Analgesics
   d. Anxiolytic agents
   e. Alkalizing agents
   f. Reversal agents
   g. Steroids
   h. Intralipids (fat emulsions)
   i. Glucose and insulin
   j. Antihistamines
8. Vascular access supplies and infusion pumps
   a. Should include adult and pediatric volumetric fluid administration devices, intravascular catheters in adult and pediatric sizes, and devices for intraosseous fluid administration, when appropriate, for the population served
9. Recommended stock supplies should include:
   a. Facial tissues
   b. Gloves
   c. Bedpans and urinals
   d. Syringes, needles, and protective needle devices
   e. Emesis containers
   f. Patient linens
   g. Alcohol wipes
   h. Skin antiseptics
   i. Tongue blades
   j. Denture cups and eyeglass protection and contact lens cases
   k. Personal protective equipment (standard precautions)
   l. A variety of single-use tapes
   m. Dressings
   n. Unit and device cleaning supplies
10. A means to safely transport patients to the operating room or procedure unit
    a. Portable oxygen, suction, cardiac monitoring equipment, and pulse oximetry will be available for those patients requiring such equipment during transport
11. Access to latex-free supplies and equipment
12. Means to store patient personal belongings per facility policy

Day-of-surgery area equipment. Adapted from American Society of PeriAnesthesia Nurses. 2023–2024. *Perianesthesia Nursing Standards, Practice Recommendations and Interpretive Statements.* ASPAN; 2022.

BOX 8.2 Equipment for Phase I Care

The following list of equipment for Phase I Care includes, but is not limited to:

1. Each patient bedside will be equipped with the following:
   a. Various types and sizes of artificial airways
   b. Various means of oxygen delivery
   c. Pulse oximetry
   d. Cardiac monitor
   e. Means to monitor blood pressure
   f. Constant and intermittent suction
   g. Adjustable lighting
   h. Capacity to ensure patient privacy
2. Equipment will be available, as needed, to assess:
   a. Hemodynamic cardiovascular status
   b. Point-of-care bedside testing (blood glucose, laboratory draws)
   c. Arterial blood gases
   d. End-tidal CO_2 (e.g., capnography)
   e. Presence of residual neuromuscular blockade (e.g., peripheral nerve stimulators)
   f. Pulses (e.g., bedside portable ultrasound, Doppler ultrasound)
   g. Urine volume (e.g., bladder scanner)
   h. Age/cognitive-appropriate pain assessment tools
3. A means to monitor patient temperature will be available
   a. A method to warm the hypothermic patient will be available
4. Access to safe patient handling and moving equipment
5. Supplies as recommended by the Malignant Hyperthermia Association of the United States will be available (https://www.mhaus.org/ or 1-800-MHHYPER)
6. Ventilatory support equipment to include, but not be limited to:
   a. At least one ventilator will be always readily accessible. A significant number of ventilators will be available to care for any postanesthesia patient who requires one
   b. Bag-valve masks of appropriate sizes for patient population must be always easily accessible
   c. Noninvasive positive pressure devices
7. A method exists to call for assistance in emergency situations
8. An adult and pediatric emergency cart with:
   a. Supplies necessary for access and hemodynamic monitoring per facility policy
   b. Intubation equipment
   c. IV pole
   d. Emergency medications and equipment
9. A defibrillator with adult and pediatric pads/paddles and cardiac pacing capability must be readily available

10. Recommended stock medications should include, but are not limited to, the following:
    a. Antibiotics
    b. Medications for control of blood pressure and heart rate
    c. Medication to treat respiratory insufficiency
    d. Antiemetics
    e. Reversal agents
    f. Analgesics: opioid and nonopioid
    g. Neuromuscular blocking agents
    h. Steroids
    i. Anxiolytic agents
    j. Intralipids (fat emulsions)
    k. Glucose and insulin
    l. Antihistamines
11. Vascular access supplies/infusion pumps
12. Patient protective devices available to use per hospital policy
13. Stock supplies should include:
    a. Dressings
    b. Facial tissues
    c. Gloves
    d. Bedpans and urinals
    e. Syringes, needles, and protective needle devices
    f. Emesis containers
    g. Patient linens
    h. Alcohol swabs
    i. Skin antiseptics
    j. Ice bags/cooling devices
    k. Tongue blades
    l. Irrigation trays
    m. Urinary catheterization supplies
    n. Personal protective equipment
    o. A variety of single-use tapes
    p. Nasogastric tube supplies
    q. Access to oral hydration supplies, as needed
    r. Unit and device cleaning supplies
14. Access to latex-free supplies and equipment
15. Means to secure patient personal belongings
16. A means to safely transport patients from Phase I Care
    a. Portable oxygen, suction, cardiac monitoring equipment, pulse oximetry, and capnography will be available, as indicated, for those patients requiring such equipment during transport
    b. Access to safe patient handling equipment
17. Automated medication dispensing system unit (e.g., Pyxis, Omnicell)

Equipment for Phase I Care. Adapted from American Society of PeriAnesthesia Nurses. *2023–2024 Perianesthesia Nursing Standards, Practice Recommendations and Interpretive Statements.* ASPAN, 2022.

---

design includes basic equipment such as an oxygen source, pulse oximetry, and cardiac monitoring. Bedside suction must be set up and ready to go at every patient care bay as part of the basic preparation.

Ambulatory sites have various levels of laboratory testing capability. The policies and emergency plan should direct employees regarding testing procedures within the facility. Arrangements should be made in advance for transporting specimens to a laboratory if transfer becomes necessary. Ambulatory settings have contingency plans for unanticipated transfers to a higher level of care. Transfer protocols should include the necessary steps and information on the logistics of patient transfers. Some facilities have prearranged contracts with transport services, while others use the 911 system. Plans should include having the appropriate equipment and staff available for unplanned transfers.

Staff Training

Complications occur on a wide continuum, from the most subtle events to a complete crisis. Early recognition and treatment of small changes in a patient's condition can stop or minimize the degree of complications as they occur. Regular training and drills for emergency situations encourage quality and safety. Maintaining current training requirements such as basic life support (BLS), advanced cardiac life support (ACLS), pediatric advanced cardiac life support (PALS), pediatric emergency assessment, recognition and stabilization (PEARS), or

---

BOX 8.3 Equipment for Phase II Care

The following list of equipment for Phase II Care includes, but is not limited to:

1. The unit will be equipped with the following:
   a. Oxygen delivery system
   b. Access to constant and intermittent suction
   c. Blood pressure monitoring devices
   d. Thermometry
   e. Adjustable lighting
   f. Capacity to ensure patient privacy
2. A cardiac monitor and pulse oximeter will be readily available
3. Bag-valve masks of the appropriate size must be easily accessible at all times
4. Equipment will be available to assess blood glucose
5. Supplies as recommended by the Malignant Hyperthermia Association of the United States will be available (https://www. mhaus.org/ or 1-800-MHHYPER)
6. A method exists to call for assistance in emergency situations
7. An emergency cart will be available at all times
8. A defibrillator with adult and pediatric pads/paddles and cardiac pacing must be readily available for the population served
9. Stock medications include, but are not limited to, the following:
   a. Antibiotics
   b. Antiemetics
   c. Reversal agents
   d. Analgesics: opioids and nonopioids
10. Vascular access supplies/infusion pumps
11. Stock supplies should include:
    a. Dressings
    b. Facial tissues
    c. Gloves
    d. Bedpans and urinals
    e. Syringes, needles, and protective needle devices
    f. Emesis containers
    g. Patient linens
    h. Alcohol wipes
    i. Skin antiseptics
    j. Ice bags and cooling devices
    k. Tongue blades
    l. Urinary catheterization supplies
    m. Personal protective equipment
    n. Access to latex-free supplies and equipment
    o. A variety of single-use tapes
    p. Unit and device cleaning supplies
12. A means to safely transport patients (See Practice Recommendation: Safe Transfer of Care Handoff and Transportation)
    a. Wheelchairs, etc.
    b. Portable oxygen, suction, cardiac monitoring equipment, pulse oximetry, and capnography will be available for those patients requiring such equipment during transport
13. Access to warming measures and devices (See Practice Recommendation: Promotion of Normothermia in the Adult Patient)
14. A means to assess urine volume (e.g., bladder scanner) Automated medication cabinet and dispensing device (e.g., Pyxis, Omnicell)

Equipment for Phase I Care. Adapted from American Society of PeriAnesthesia Nurses. *2023-2024 Perianesthesia Nursing Standards, Practice Recommendations and Interpretive Statements*. ASPAN; 2022.

---

other certifications as required by the facility ensure higher clinical skills for emergency responses. Concurrent practice drills and skills demonstrations help to ensure that crisis situations are handled efficiently. Simulation offers the ability to practice in a realistic environment, and if it includes all disciplines and team members, it provides a pathway between formal education and professional practice that is especially effective for rare but potentially fatal situations, such as MH. A crisis plan should identify the duties and individual roles that should be assigned according to previous training and skills. Training also helps to develop the teamwork, confidence, and role delineation needed during a crisis situation.

Communication failure is one of the contributing factors for complications. Clear, appropriate communication is important for maintaining patient safety. Established tools for handover communications can improve the efficiency of care. The situation, background, assessment, and recommendations (SBAR) report is one proven example. SBAR helps to communicate standardized information that makes reports concise, objective, and relevant (Box 8.4). During the handover process, the receiving person needs to have a chance to ask questions.

In a crisis, it may be difficult to recall the exact steps that need to be performed. Basic emergency first steps, such as starting BLS with good airway management, seem inevitable, but having access to appropriate resources can make a critical situation more manageable. Crisis checklists (also termed cognitive aids or emergency manuals) have been developed to manage relatively rare crisis situations that may occur during any surgical or interventional procedure.[13] These quick reference guides can ensure that best practices are followed and no critical steps are missed, so they should be immediately available and can be

---

BOX 8.4 SBAR

Situation: This includes patient identification data, code status, vital signs, and the chief complaint or the nurse's concern(s).
Background: Data in this section include the patient's mental status, skin condition, and respiratory status.
Assessment: In this section, the clinician defines what she believes to be the problem.
Recommendation: This includes provider orders and recommended actions.

Source: Adapted from Good VS. The critical care environment. In: Good VS, Kirkwood PL, eds. *Advanced Critical Care Nursing*. 2nd ed. Elsevier; 2018; p. 5.

---

lifesaving in a crisis. A safety checklist is shown in Figure 8.3. The perianesthesia nurse must be constantly vigilant about the patient's status and able to identify potential complications and treat any untoward reactions before they escalate.

Evidence-Based Practice: Emergency planning
There are several important steps that staff in the Ambulatory Surgery Center (ASC) can employ to be better prepared for emergency situations. When developing an emergency operation plan (EOP), the team should huddle to identify all potential emergency situations. This may include situations within the facility, related to patient care, or events that may occur within the community but may impact the ASC (e.g., floods, hurricanes). The plan

8 Hemorrhage

Acute massive bleeding

START

1. **Call for help and a code cart**
   - Ask: *"Who will be the crisis manager?"*

2. **Open IV fluids** and **assess for adequate IV access**

3. **Turn FiO$_2$ to 100%** and **turn down volatile anesthetics**

4. **Call blood bank**
   - Activate massive transfusion protocol
   - Assign 1 person as primary contact for blood bank
   - Order blood products (in addition to PRBCs)
     - 1 FFP : 1 PRBC
     - If indicated, 6 units of platelets

5. **Request rapid infuser** (or pressure bags)

6. **Discuss management plan** between surgical, anesthesiology, and nursing teams

7. **Call for surgery consultation**

8. **Keep patient warm**

9. **Send labs**
   CBC, PT/PTT/INR, fibrinogen, lactate, arterial blood gas, potassium, and ionized calcium

10. **Consider ...**
    - Electrolyte disturbances (hypocalcemia and hyperkalemia)
    - Uncrossmatched type O-neg blood if crossmatched blood not availbale
    - Damage control surgery (pack, close, resuscitate)
    - Special patient populations (see considerations below)

DRUG DOSES and treatments

HYPOCALCEMIA treatment

Give calcium to replace deficit (calcium chloride or calcium gluconate)

HYPERKALEMIA treatment

1. Calcium gluconate - or - Calcium chloride	• 30 mg/kg IV • 10 mg/kg IV
2. Insulin	• 10 units regular IV with 1–2 amps D50W as needed
3. Sodium bicarbonate if pH < 7.2	• 1–2 mEq/kg slow IV push

SPECIAL PATIENT POPULATIONS

OBSTETRIC:	TRAUMA:	NON-SURGICAL UNCONTROLLED BLEEDING despite massive transfusion of PRBC, FFP, platelets and cryo:
• Empirical administration of 1 pool of cryoprecipitate (10 cryo units)	Give either...	
• Check fibrinogen (goal is 200 mg/dL)	• Antifibrinolytic tranexamic acid: 1000 mg IV over 10 minutes followed by 1000 mg over the next 8 hours	• Consider giving Recombinant Factor VIIa: 40 mcg/kg IV
< 100 mg/dL — Order 2 more pools of cryoprecipitate	– or –	– Surgical bleeding must first be controlled
100 – 200 mg/dL — Order 1 more pool of cryoprecipitate	• Aminocaproic acid: 4–5 g in 250 mL NS/RL IV over first hour followed by a continuing infusion of 1 g in 50 mL NS/RL IV per hour over 8 hours	– **use with CAUTION** in patients at risk for thrombosis – **DO NOT use** when PH is < 7.2

All resonable precautions have been taken to verify the information contained in this publication. The responsibility for the interpretation and use of the materials lies with the reader. Revised April 2017 (042417.1)

Fig. 8.3 Example of a safety checklist. Source: Chen Y-YK, Arriaga AF. Checklists for safer perioperative care. In: Peden CJ, Fleisher LA, Englesbe M, eds. *Perioperative Quality Improvement.* Elsevier; 2023; Figure 34.2.

should also include an inventory of supplies and a plan for access to materials that may be required (e.g., staffing resources, medications, medical records). Another key component to the EOP is the description of a communication process to define what is shared by whom it is shared via which method. Developing a plan for onboarding, training, and educating staff on the steps to managing emergency situations is also crucial for management of unplanned situations. Lastly, should an adverse event occur, the team should be provided an opportunity to debrief and develop an action plan for improving future responses.

Source: Drummond S, O'Rourke M. Emergency preparedness in ambulatory surgery centers and office-based anesthesia practices. In: Rajan N, ed. *Manual of Practice Management for Ambulatory Surgery Centers.* Springer, 2020;283-293. https://doi.org/10.1007/978-3-030-19171-9_19

POSTOPERATIVE COMPLICATIONS
Postoperative Respiratory Complications

Respiratory events are some of the most common complications. The loss of an airway is one of the scariest of these events. A nurse's assessment of the event and skills in airway management prevent the progression of respiratory issues. Respiratory issues in the PACU occur for a wide variety of reasons. Respiratory incidents account for a significant proportion of adverse events in the recovery area.[3] When a patient arrives in the PACU, the initial airway assessment includes basic airway patency and ventilatory effort, respiratory rate, peripheral oxygen saturation (SpO$_2$), and end-tidal CO$_2$ (ETCO$_2$) when indicated.

The initial assessment is followed by continuous monitoring of the respiratory rate and SpO$_2$ and frequent reassessment of the airway patency. The neuromuscular function, mental status, cardiovascular function, and temperature of the patient and the presence of pain or nausea and vomiting can adversely impact oxygenation and ventilation. These parameters are also assessed initially and periodically. Residual neuromuscular blockade after surgery continues to be a major factor for postoperative pulmonary complications.[14] Hypoventilation is also commonly related to the effects of residual inhalation agents. Perianesthesia nursing staff need to be trained in the implementation of various airway adjuncts and to quickly identify complications such as incomplete neuromuscular blockade reversal, laryngospasm, and stridor.[3]

Airway Obstruction

The most common airway complication seen in the PACU is airway obstruction. Risk factors for airway obstruction come from three main issues: poor muscle tone, anatomic problems, and swelling. Tongue obstruction is one of the most common causes of airway obstruction in the PACU. Poor oropharyngeal muscle tone causes the tongue to fall back and occlude the pharynx. Neuromuscular blockers are implicated the most for poor muscle tone, but any medication causing sedation can have muscle relaxant effects[3] (Figure 8.4). The anatomy of the upper airway puts some patients at a higher risk, including patients with short, very muscular necks and obese patients. Obese patients are at an increased risk because of the additional soft tissue at the back of the tongue. There is an increased risk for patients with a large tongue (e.g., infants,

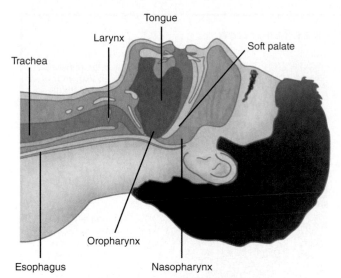

Fig. 8.4 Tongue obstruction. Source: Malamed SF. Unconsciousness: General considerations. In: Malamed SF, ed. *Medical Emergencies in the Dental Office*. 8th ed. Elsevier; 2023; Figure 5.1.

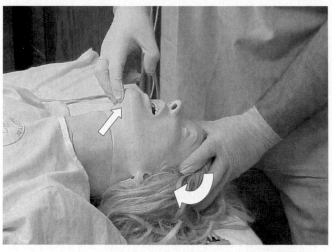

Fig. 8.5 Head tilt and chin lift. Source: O'Brien D. Postanesthesia care complications. In: Odom-Forren J, ed. *Drain's Perianesthesia Nursing: A Critical Care Approach*. 7th ed. Elsevier; 2018; Figure 29.3.

children with Down syndrome). Foreign body obstructions can include teeth, a tonsil sponge, or nasal packing. Secretions, including mucous plugs, blood, and vomit, can also occlude the airway. Improperly placed airways and kinked endotracheal tubes can actually cause an occlusion of the pharynx. Swelling from edema or a hematoma can also be the cause of upper airway obstruction.

Symptoms may present on a continuum and are based on the severity of the obstruction. Patients with obstruction can show signs of snoring, somnolence, dyspnea, activation of accessory muscles, nasal flaring, labored respiration, air hunger, hypoxemia, apprehension, restlessness, or stupor. The heart rate and blood pressure fluctuate, and this can lead to cardiac dysrhythmias due to a lack of oxygen. The airway is a key focus in the immediate phase of recovery, and multiple preventative steps are in place to prevent airway obstruction. Proper management in the operating room, including anesthesia management, ongoing assessments, decreased use of opioids, and proper positioning of the patient, will decrease the risk of airway obstruction. A snoring patient is not someone to ignore. The cause of the obstruction must be immediately addressed. Opening the airway is the simplest way to relieve a basic airway obstruction. A head tilt and chin lift or a jaw thrust is the easiest method of BLS used to open the airway (Figure 8.5)

Placing the patient in a left lateral position helps to maintain the airway. For the obtunded patient, simple airway devices such as nasopharyngeal airways or an oral pharyngeal airway can provide airway support. A small percentage might require tracheal reintubation. If the lingering effects of anesthetic agents are suspected, reversal agents might be appropriate. If the paralytic medication outlasts the reversal medications, the administration of an additional dose of a reversal medication, such as neostigmine and glycopyrrolate or sugammadex, might be required. Excessive sedation related to opioid use can be reversed with naloxone administration, and excessive benzodiazepines can be reversed by flumazenil. Vomit, blood, or mucus can be the causative factor in an obstructed airway. Suctioning and clearing the airway is a priority in those cases. To help reduce swelling and irritability, a nebulizer treatment with racemic epinephrine and lidocaine might be used. A protective airway might need to be placed if swelling or hematoma is preventing oxygen flow (Figure 8.6).

Laryngospasm

While laryngospasm is a very rare complication, it is a true emergency. Spasm of the laryngeal muscle results in a reflex closure of the glottis (vocal cords) and loss of air flow to the lungs. It can present as partial or complete closure of the airway. Laryngospasm can be caused by airway irritations or secretions on the vocal cords during emergence or extubation. Secretions include blood, vomit, or mucus. Other airway irritants that can cause laryngospasm include smoking, chronic obstructive pulmonary disease (COPD), asthma, coughing, and/or an upper respiratory infection. Airway trauma occurring during the placement or removal of an endotracheal tube or laryngeal mask airway (LMA) increases the risk. Even a painful stimulus in a lightly anesthetized patient can trigger a laryngospasm event.

Prevention revolves around avoiding airway irritation. Maintaining hemostasis during surgery, providing oropharynx suctioning before extubation, and minimizing stimulation during extubation are proactive methods of reducing irritation. Providers may administer steroids and/or lidocaine as a preventative measure in high-risk cases. With a partial-closure obstruction, the patient exhibits inspiratory stridor, heard as high-pitched crowing or wheezing sounds, decreased chest compliance, decreased ventilation, and anxiety or panic. Paradoxic chest and/or abdominal movement, along with the absence of breath sounds, indicates a complete laryngospasm event, and the patient is not making any audible sound. In a laryngospasm event, the patient is usually awake and in acute distress.

Treatment for a partial obstruction begins with basic airway management, such as applying a chin lift or jaw thrust, if necessary, maintaining a calm supportive environment, elevating the head of the bed, providing humidified oxygen, and performing suctioning to remove secretions if appropriate. Racemic epinephrine inhalations might be used to help reduce the swelling. Aerosolized lidocaine can be used to reduce irritability, and decadron to reduce inflammation. In complete laryngospasm, the patient has total loss of the airway, and quick actions are required to reverse the situation. Most laryngospasms break with continuous positive pressure ventilation. Grab a bag-valve mask device and provide oxygen at 100% and attempt to break the spasm. If that is unsuccessful, a dose of succinylcholine or another muscle relaxant might be used to break the spasm. Once the spasm breaks, continue to ventilate

Oropharyngeal Airway Insertion

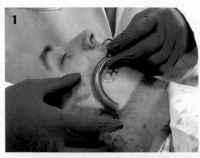
For oropharyngeal airway insertion, first measure. An airway of correct size will extend from the corner of the mouth to the earlobe or the angle of the mandible.

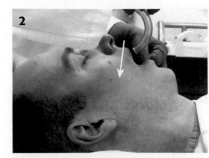
Open the patient's mouth with your thumb and index finger, then insert the airway in an inverted position along the patient's hard palate.

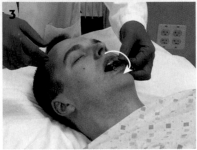
When the airway is well into the mouth, rotate it 180°, with the distal end of the airway lying in the hypopharynx. It may help to pull the jaw forward during passage.

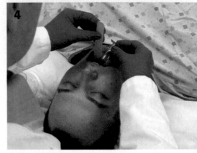
Alternatively, open the mouth widely and use a tongue blade to displace the tongue inferiorly, and advance the airway into the oropharynx. No rotation is required with this method.

NASOPHARYNGEAL AIRWAY INSERTION

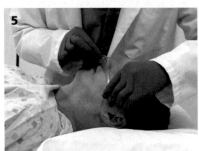
For nasopharyngeal airways, a device of correct size will extend from the tip of the nose to the earlobe.

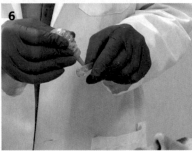
Generously lubricate the airway prior to insertion.

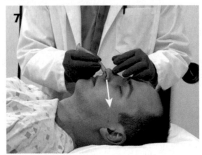
Advance the airway into the nostril and direct it along the floor of the nasal passage in the direction of the occiput. Do *not* advance in a cephalad direction!

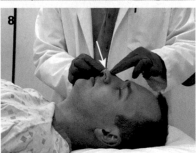
Advance the airway fully until the flared external tip of the device is at the nasal orifice.

Fig. 8.6 Oropharyngeal and nasopharyngeal airway insertion. Source: Driver BE, Reardon RF. Basic airway management and decision making. In: Roberts JR, Custalow CB, Thomsen TW, eds. *Roberts and Hedges' Clinical Procedures in Emergency Medicine and Acute Care*. 7th ed. Elsevier; 2019; Figure 3.5.

the patient until the muscle relaxant wears off and the patient resumes normal respirations. Reintubation might be required to maintain the airway. Corticosteroids and/or lidocaine may be administered to reduce swelling and airway irritation.

Subglottic Edema

Traumatic intubations, an incorrect tube size, movement or coughing while the tube is still present, long procedures, and head and neck surgeries increase the risk of subglottic edema. Symptoms include strider, crowing respirations, and rocking chest movements. Treatment should include humidified oxygen and nebulized mist treatment with racemic epinephrine. Further treatment may include inhalation of a helium–oxygen mixture, administration of dexamethasone, and efforts to calm the patient, including analgesics and having a family member present.[15] Extended or overnight observation might be required for an ambulatory surgical patient depending on the severity of the edema, treatment required, and physiologic response.

Bronchospasm

A bronchospasm is a narrowing or constriction of the bronchial smooth muscle resulting in the closure of small pulmonary airways. An allergic response, asthma, COPD, a history of smoking, aspiration, pulmonary edema, intubation, and endotracheal tube suctioning can trigger a bronchospasm. Signs and symptoms include expiratory wheezing often with shallow respirations, decreased oxygen saturation, cough, dyspnea, tachypnea, and intercostal retractions. Immediate intervention is necessary and may involve increasing the oxygen delivery, considering air humidification, and removing the irritant source. Therapy to resolve the spasm includes using the patient's personal inhaler or administering inhaled aerosol or bronchodilators with albuterol. To relax the airway in a severe response, muscle relaxants, lidocaine, epinephrine, and hydrocortisone may be ordered. With a foreign body aspiration, appropriate methods for removal are implemented as needed.

Aspiration

Prevention measures are key to keeping the incidence of aspiration low, but with a sedated or anesthetized patient there is still a slight risk for occurrence. Aspiration ensues when gastric contents, blood, or foreign bodies (e.g., loose teeth) are inhaled into the lungs. Risk factors are associated with anesthetic techniques, surgical procedures, and patients considered to have a full stomach (e.g., pregnant or obese patients). If an LMA is used, there is an augmented risk of gastric aspiration and airway effects in patients with an increased residual gastric volume, acidic gastric contents, hiatal hernia, or gastroparesis; patients who are unable to protect the airway; patients who have experienced trauma; and patients who have had upper abdominal surgery.

Efforts to minimize the risk include ensuring nothing by mouth (NPO) status for the recommended duration, giving medications to help empty the stomach or decrease the acidity, and placing the sedated or obtunded patient in a side-lying position to protect the airway. Patients present with coughing, wheezing, hypoxia, hypercarbia, and tachypnea. The concurrent cardiac response may include heart rate changes, dysrhythmias, and hypotension. Bronchospasm, hypoxemia, and atelectasis are potential consequences of pulmonary aspiration. A top priority for treatment includes correcting hypoxemia, establishing airway patency, providing for hemostasis, achieving hemodynamic stability, and considering a steroid and antibiotics. Preventative measures help to keep the overall risk low.

Hypoxemia

Hypoxemia occurs when oxygen desaturation is present and the partial pressure of oxygen (PaO_2) is decreasing to less than 60 mm Hg. Risk factors include an inadequate oxygen concentration, hypoventilation, residual effects of the anesthetic agents administered, shivering due to drugs or temperature changes, low hemoglobin levels, surgical procedures that limit ventilation, intrapulmonary shunting, or a ventilation/perfusion mismatch. Sign and symptoms include an oxyhemoglobin saturation of 90% associated with a PaO_2 of less than 60 mm Hg. Patients can present with agitation or somnolence, hypotension or hypertension, bradycardia or tachycardia, and/or premature ventricular contractions.

Lack of treatment can result in cardiac arrest. With the use of standardized pulse oximetry, the incidence of decreasing oxygen saturation is quickly recognized and treated by the nurse. Basic treatment starts with stimulating the patient and increasing the oxygen supply to meet the demand. Then the focus turns to the causative factor. Control shivering and warm the patient if required. If the cause is related to the residual effects of the anesthesia, the patient might require a reversal agent for the paralytic, opioids, or benzodiazepines. Pulmonary issues need to be assessed and treated appropriately.

Hypoventilation

When a patient is hypoventilating and oxygen demands are not being met, the decreased alveolar ventilation results in an increased partial pressure of carbon dioxide ($PaCO_2$). A loss of the central respiratory drive due to anesthetic agents can precipitate respiratory depression. Shivering or inadequate ventilation settings can result in hypoventilation. Patients can become extremely somnolent, with decreased respirations and hypoxemia. The heart rate and blood pressure can be variable. Arterial blood gases show a $PaCO_2$ above 45 mm Hg, and capnography demonstrates an increased expiration of CO_2. After stimulating and ventilating the patient, treatment revolves around correcting the cause and symptoms. The reversal of anesthetic drugs (e.g., opioids, benzodiazepines, neuromuscular blockers), control of shivering, and having optimal ventilator settings are examples of corrective actions.

Pulmonary Embolism

Injury to vessel walls, which occurs with surgery, increases the risk of blood clot formation. A clot becomes a pulmonary embolism when it breaks off and travels to the lung and obstructs the pulmonary vascular bed. The causative agents for pulmonary embolism can be blood clots or a tissue fragment because of venous stasis, hypercoagulability states, and abnormal blood vessel walls that add to clot formation. Obesity, congestive heart failure, immobility, malignancy, and pelvic or long bone fractures or surgery are also risks associated with pulmonary embolism formation. Patients can present with a wide range of symptoms, including no symptoms, and proceed to shock or sudden death. The most common presenting symptom is dyspnea followed by chest pain (classically pleuritic but often dull) and cough. However, many patients, including those with large pulmonary embolisms, have mild or nonspecific symptoms or are asymptomatic.[16] The onset is frequently acute, and in addition to dyspnea, chest or pleuritic pain, and anxiety, can include calf or thigh pain and/or swelling, tachycardia, tachypnea, coughing, wheezing, agitation, restlessness, hypoxia, hemoptysis, hypotension, and dysrhythmias. In acute cases, the cascade of symptoms can progress to congestive heart failure and shock. The majority of patients with pulmonary embolism are hemodynamically stable on presentation.[16] Treatment includes correcting hypoxemia, achieving hemodynamic stability, administering anticoagulation therapy, supporting early mobilization, and applying devices such as sequential or intermittent pneumatic compressions or graduated pressure stockings. Initial testing can include a complete blood count and serum chemistries, arterial blood gases, brain natriuretic peptide, troponin, D-dimer, electrocardiography, and chest radiography. Depending on the severity of the clinical presentation and subsequent care and testing needed, the ambulatory patient is likely to require transfer to a higher level of care.

Pneumothorax

Pneumothorax occurs when air enters the pleural space. With air in the pleural space, negative pressure of the pleural space can destroy tissue and can cause the lung to collapse. In the ambulatory setting, this may be seen more with certain regional blocks, including interscalene, brachial plexus, or intercostal blocks. Other causes include a ruptured pleural bleb, positive pressure ventilation, or surgical procedures invading the pleura. A tension pneumothorax, noted when the intrapleural pressure increases and the lung deflates, causing the heart and great vessels to shift toward the intact lung, is a medical emergency and needs to be treated urgently. Signs and symptoms of pneumothorax include chest pain, dyspnea, diminished breath sounds on the affected side, a tracheal shift, and hyperresonance on the affected side.

Treatment focuses on ensuring oxygenation, elevating the head of the bed, and reinflation of the lung with a chest tube if necessary. The patient's respiratory status and oxygen saturation are monitored, and supplemental oxygen is provided as needed. At this stage, the patient requires both pain control and emotional support. The size of the pneumothorax, the cause of the pneumothorax, and presenting patient symptoms guide treatment. Typically, when the chest x-ray shows a deflation of less than 20%, observation is usually the treatment. When x-rays reveal a deflation of greater than 20% or if the patient is symptomatic even with a deflation of less than 20%, then a chest tube or reinflation might be indicated (Table 8.2).

Pulmonary Edema of a Cardiogenic or Noncardiogenic Nature

There are multiple causes for pulmonary edema. Fluid accumulates in the alveoli owing to increased hydrostatic pressure, decreased interstitial pressure, or increased capillary permeability. Cardiovascular factors that put a patient at risk for pulmonary edema include fluid overload, left ventricular failure, mitral valve dysfunction, or ischemic heart disease. Patients present with tachycardia, dyspnea, tachypnea, confusion, wheezing with rales or rhonchi, and decreased chest wall compliance. Pulmonary infiltrates are observed on chest x-rays. Identification of the cause guides treatment. Oxygenation, diuretics, and fluid restrictions are the priority. Afterload reduction might be considered. Morphine can be useful for relaxing the patient, as well as the pulmonary vascular bed. Reintubation and mechanical ventilation with positive end-expiratory pressure (PEEP) might be required to maintain adequate oxygenation.

TABLE 8.2 Pneumothorax

Spontaneous
Primary
Secondary
COPD
Bullous disease
Cystic fibrosis
Pneumocystis-related
Congenital cysts
Idiopathic pulmonary fibrosis
Pulmonary embolism
Catamenial (menstrual cycle–related)
Neonatal
Traumatic
Penetrating
Blunt
Iatrogenic
Mechanical ventilation
Needle puncture (thoracentesis, fine-needle aspiration of lung nodule, central line insertion)
Postsurgical

Source: Adapted from Wald O, Izhar U, Sugarbaker DJ. In: Townsend CM, Beauchamp RD, Evers BM, Mattox KL, eds. *Lung, Chest Wall, Pleura and Mediastinum.* Elsevier; 2022; Box 58.5.

Negative-pressure pulmonary edema (NPPE), also called noncardiogenic pulmonary edema (NCPE) or postobstructive pulmonary edema, can occur with an upper airway obstruction, a bolus of naloxone, a laryngospasm following extubation, or incomplete reversal of a neuromuscular blocking agent. NPPE usually occurs more often in young healthy patients and is the result of a strong patient's increased inspiratory force when breathing against a closed glottis or laryngospasm.[3] The increase in negative pressure within the chest cavity causes a sharp increase in hydrostatic pressure, which pulls water into the lungs. Pink frothy sputum is a classic sign of NPPE. Other signs and symptoms are restlessness, wheezing, and severe respiratory distress. Treatment of NPPE focuses on ventilatory support with administration of supplemental oxygen, application of a nonrebreather, or use of continuous positive airway pressure (CPAP). If the patient is still unable to be oxygenated, then reintubation with mechanical ventilation including PEEP may be necessary. As appropriate, diuretics and morphine might be administered. A chest x-ray showing signs of pulmonary edema often has a fluffy infiltrate appearance.[3] The patient might require a transfer to an acute care hospital and observation in the intensive care unit. Patients with NPPE typically recover rapidly after the intense initial phase and leave the critical care unit within 24 to 36 hours and fully recover.[15]

Postoperative Cardiovascular Complications

The second major body system significantly affected by anesthesia and surgery is the cardiovascular system. Cardiac events that progress to myocardial ischemia and infarct are the most common perioperative complications leading to an increased length of stay and cost of care.[17] According to Smith et al., acute cardiovascular issues in the ambulatory surgery setting account for 2.9% of adverse events.[1] This risk is more aligned with patients who have a preexisting cardiac disorder. Cardiac emergencies can be fatal; therefore, vigilant monitoring, recognition, and early intervention are important proactive measures.

Hypotension

Hypotension is defined as a blood pressure of less than 20% to 30% of baseline.[15] Hypovolemia is a chief cause of hypotension in the PACU. Fluid limitations or losses from the surgical process such as prolonged preoperative fasting requirements, surgical preps (e.g., bowel), insensible fluid loses during surgery, and blood loss all cause hypovolemia and, potentially, hypotension. Hypotension caused by acute hemorrhage is rare but can occur quickly; it is one of the most serious volume deficits to treat. Excess fluid losses associated with increased urine output can create a negative fluid balance resulting in hypotension. Hypotension can also be caused by myocardial dysfunction from either a primary or secondary cause, a loss of systemic vascular resistance, and cardiac dysrhythmias. Vasodilation from anesthetics or due to a generalized inflammatory response can contribute to hypotension. Shock of a septic, cardiogenic, or neurogenic nature produces hypotension.

Signs and symptoms are based on the severity of hypotension. With mild hypotension, the patient might complain of not feeling well or of feeling light-headed, especially when the head of a stretcher is being elevated or the patient is being helped to sit up. Lowering the head of the stretcher and, if necessary, elevating the patient's legs provides a quick venous return. In a shock situation, symptoms can progress quickly. Disorientation or loss of consciousness, pallor, cool clammy skin, nausea, chest pain, oliguria to anuria, and lactic acidosis can all occur with severe hypotension. Hypotension treatment is based on the cause. If volume loss is the causative factor of mild hypotension, then providing adequate fluid replacement might be all that is necessary for treatment. Fluid challenges with crystalloids and/or albumin, as well as neosynephrine boluses or drips, might be used to modulate the blood pressure. Severe volume loss might require hemostasis and blood replacement. In severe shock cases, the patient needs to be stabilized and transferred to a higher level of care.

Hypertension

A patient may arrive from the operating room in a hypertensive crisis, or the event can occur while the patient is recovering in the PACU. Hypertension is defined as a persistent elevation of systolic blood pressure greater than 140 mm Hg, a diastolic blood pressure greater than 90 mm Hg, or [a condition] requiring an antihypertensive treatment."[15] Patients with a history of hypertension can have exacerbations while in the PACU; they account for the majority of patients experiencing elevated pressures in the PACU.[6] According to Tarrac's report, the hypertension usually occurred within 30 minutes after arrival in the PACU.[6] The elevation is usually benign and short lived; however, it can precipitate myocardial ischemia in the patient with coronary artery disease as a result of stimulation of the sympathetic nervous system.[15] Symptoms are dependent on the degree of hypertension, and often patients are asymptomatic. When addressing hypertension, it is important to focus on identifying and alleviating the cause and not the symptoms. For example, ensure readings are accurate and the correct cuff size is being used. Analgesics, sedatives, bladder decompression, oxygenation, and antihypertensive medications might be indicated. Pharmacologic medications to treat hypertension have varying sites and onsets of action (Table 8.3). Factors leading to postoperative hypertension are listed in Box 8.5.

Cardiac Dysrhythmias

Organizational policies and procedures should direct the treatment of patients who need emergency care. Cardiac dysrhythmias often occur because of anesthetic effects and require minimal

---

BOX 8.5 Factors Leading to Postoperative Hypertension

Preoperative hypertension
Arterial hypoxemia
Hypervolemia
Emergence excitement
Shivering
Drug rebound
Increased intracranial pressure
Increased sympathetic nervous system activity
    Hypercapnia
    Pain
    Agitation
    Bowel distention
Urinary retention

Source: Berg SM, Braehler MR. The postanesthesia care unit. In: Gropper MA, ed. *Miller's Anesthesia*. 9th ed. Elsevier; 2020; Box 80.6.

---

treatment, but a patient can easily have a severe dysrhythmia requiring emergency treatment. Guidelines for BLS, ACLS, and PALS can be followed for the emergency management of lethal dysrhythmias.

Sinus Bradycardia

Sinus bradycardia is common in the PACU, but it is usually benign and resolves without treatment. Young, healthy, athletic patients and sleepy or understimulated patients may present with bradycardia resulting from beta blockers or as a response to anesthetic medications. If the patient develops unstable bradycardia demonstrated by signs such as severe hypotension, acutely altered mental status, signs of shock, ischemic chest discomfort, and acute heart failure, then appropriate treatment is required. Atropine 1 mg by intravenous (IV) push might be used to increase sinus firing and atrioventricular

---

TABLE 8.3 Drugs Used for Treatment of Hypertensive Crisis

Drug	Route	Initial Dose	Onset of Action (minutes)	Duration of Action	Comment
Diazoxide	IV	3–5 mg/kg slow bolus	3–5	5–12 hours	
Sodium nitroprusside	IV	0.25–0.5 µg/kg/min	1–2	Less than 5 minutes	Titrate dose for desired effect
Nitroglycerin	IV	0.25–3 µg/kg/min	2–5	Less than 5 minutes	
Phentolamine	IV	5–15 mg bolus; 200–400 mg/L infusion	Immediate	Less than 15 minutes	Titrate dose for desired effect
Hydralazine	IV	5–10 mg	15–20	4–6 hours	Given slowly when IV
	IM	10–40 mg	30		
Trimethaphan camsylate	IV	10–20 µg/kg/min	1	2–4 minutes	
Propranolol	IV	0.1–0.5 mg slowly, up to 2 mg	10	4–6 hours	May repeat dose
Esmolol	IV	50–300 µg/kg/min	5	20 minutes	Avoid concentration of more than 10 mg/mL
Labetolol	IV	0.25 mg/kg	10	4–6 hours	Give slowly
Nifedipine	Slow IV	10 mg	3	7 hours	Slow infusion while nitroglycerin is prepared
	IV	10 mg (slow)	5–10		
Verapamil	IV	2.5–5 mg	2–5	4–6 hours	

Source: Cosco-Holt L, Burkard JF. The cardiovascular system. In: Odom-Forren J, ed. *Drain's Perianesthesia Nursing: A Critical Care Approach*. 7th ed. Elsevier; 2018; Table 11.5.

conduction for severe sinus bradycardia. The American Heart Association warns that atropine in doses less than 0.5 mg given intravenously may further slow the heart rate.[18] An IV infusion of dopamine 5 to 20 ug/kg/min or epinephrine 2 to 10 µg/min can be used as an alternative to transcutaneous pacing for persistent sinus bradycardia.[18] In the presence of acute coronary ischemia or myocardial infarction, use atropine cautiously, because an atropine-mediated increase in heart rate may worsen ischemia or increase the infarct size.[18] If the sinus bradycardia progresses to a heart block (e.g., Mobitz type II second-degree or third-degree heart block), follow ACLS protocols. Newly identified or chronic cardiac disease might require cardiac consultation.

Sinus Tachycardia and Supraventricular Tachycardia

Self-limiting supraventricular tachycardias (SVTs), with a heart rate of 100 to 140 bpm, are a frequent compensatory response seen in the PACU. At this time, the SVT can be seen as part of the surgical stress response, pain, anxiety, bladder distention, hypovolemic states, anemia, or fever, or as a reflex response to medications such as muscle relaxant reversals or vasoactive drugs. Treatment focuses on the cause. Control anxiety, pain, and fever and provide adequate fluid replacement if needed. Bladder scanning for urinary retention and straight catheterization can be done if required. If the heart rate increases to over 150 bpm and the patient is showing signs of distress such as hypotension, acutely altered mental status, shock, ischemic chest discomfort, or acute heart failure, then emergency treatment is needed. The therapy for narrow QRS tachycardia with a regular rhythm is vagal maneuvers, and expert consultation is considered. If the SVT does not respond to vagal maneuvers, give adenosine 6 mg rapidly by IV push followed by a rapid saline flush. If the SVT does not convert within 1–2 minutes, give a second 12-mg dose of adenosine followed again by a rapid saline flush.[18]

Atrial Fibrillation

In atrial fibrillation, the atria "quiver" chaotically and the ventricles beat irregularly. Chronic atrial fibrillation can be seen in the history of some senior patients, but new-onset atrial fibrillation is a concern in the PACU. Atrial fibrillation poses the risk for atrial thrombi or emboli and subsequent strokes. In the PACU, atrial fibrillation can occur as a result of fluid overload in a cardiac-sensitive patient or could represent a perianesthesia cardiac issue. A rapid uncontrolled ventricular response can lead to physical decompensation and needs to be controlled quickly. If significant signs or symptoms are observed, immediate cardioversion is indicated.

Premature Ventricular Contractions

Premature ventricular contractions (PVCs) are usually benign but can be a reflex response to hypokalemia, acidosis, or hypercarbia. A quick laboratory test can rule out these causes. Hypoxia in a sedated and groggy patient might precipitate PVCs. Stimulation or a stir-up routine and/or oxygen quickly corrects the low oxygen status. PVCs in the presence of severe bradycardia are a compensatory mechanism. Treating the bradycardia should correct the PVCs. Cardiac ischemia can present as PVCs, and if this is a possibility, it should be ruled out. Obtain a 12-lead ECG, check laboratory results, and consult an anesthesiologist and cardiologist if necessary.

Chest Pain or Myocardial Infarction

A patient's subjective complaint of chest discomfort or pain needs to be addressed immediately. The rule of caution always assumes the problem is a cardiac one until proven otherwise. Surgery and anesthesia can compromise the delicate hemostasis between the myocardial oxygen supply and demand in the patient with preexisting cardiac disease. Myocardial infarction (MI) is the most common cardiovascular complication leading to postoperative death.[3] Chest pain can be caused by multiple factors. Patients with a preexisting cardiac disease, debilitation, obesity, or diabetes are at increased risk for chest pain or an MI postoperatively. Hypotension, hypoxemia, anemia, and hypovolemia are factors that compromise the oxygen supply to the heart. Pain, anxiety, fever, and shivering from hypothermia increase the myocardial oxygen demand. Evaluation of the pain is critical to the diagnosis. Assess the pain for characteristics such as inclusion of the jaw, chest, left arm, or back; radiation of the pain to another area such as the neck; or pain that feels like indigestion. In addition to chest pain, patients may present with diaphoresis, nausea, tachypnea, tachycardia, cardiac arrhythmias, or blood pressure fluctuations. Ruling out cardiac issues such as MI or ischemia is at the top of the list. Gas pains sometimes are described as chest pains by patients and can be a result of laparoscopic or colon procedures. Other differential causes to investigate include pneumothorax, pulmonary embolism, reflux esophagitis, peptic ulcer, pancreatitis, or myalgia from depolarizing muscle relaxants. Provide hemodynamic support for the blood pressure and dysrhythmias, provide adequate oxygen and hydration, obtain a 12-lead ECG, institute laboratory testing for cardiac enzymes and serial troponins, and consider morphine for pain and an antianginal (nitroglycerin) and other treatments as appropriate. Potential ischemia patients need to be transferred to an acute care facility for further workup and advanced cardiac care. Rule out pulmonary causes or other reasons for chest pain. Dyspnea, shortness of breath with extensive rales, or diffuse wheezing may indicate pulmonary edema. A pneumothorax after a regional block (e.g., a block done in the upper chest area) or from a procedure that introduced surgical instruments into the intrapleural space can cause the loss of intrapleural negative pressure, and this sometimes presents as chest pain. A chest x-ray can help to rule out a pneumothorax. Other actions might include repositioning the patient for comfort, checking vascular integrity, or providing antacids for noncardiac pain (Table 8.4).

TABLE 8.4 Criteria for Diagnosis of Perioperative Myocardial Infarction

The diagnosis of perioperative MI requires any of the following criteria.

Criterion 1: A typical rise in the troponin level or a typical fall in an elevated troponin level detected at its peak after surgery in a patient without a documented alternative explanation for an elevated troponin level (e.g., pulmonary embolism).

- This criterion requires that one of the following criteria be met:
  - Ischemic signs or symptoms (e.g., chest, arm, or jaw discomfort; shortness of breath; pulmonary edema)
  - Development of pathologic Q waves on an ECG
  - Changes on an ECG indicative of ischemia
  - Coronary artery intervention
  - New or presumed new cardiac wall motion abnormality on echocardiography or new or presumed new fixed defect on radionuclide imaging

Criterion 2: Pathologic findings of acute or healing MI

Criterion 3: Development of new pathologic Q waves on an ECG if troponin levels were not obtained or were obtained at times that could have missed the clinical event

Source: Adapted from Redelmeier DA. Postoperative care and complications. In: Goldman L, Schafer AI, eds. *Goldman-Cecil Medicine.* 26th ed. Elsevier; 2020; Table 405.1.

Postoperative Complications Involving Bleeding

Bleeding occurs with a loss of vascular integrity that results in the loss of intravascular volume. Visible signs of bloody drainage, saturated dressings, or oozing suture lines are obvious signs of bleeding. Not all postoperative bleeding is apparent. Often a nurse sees symptoms pointing to covert bleeding, such as bruising or abnormal skin discoloration, tight casts or dressings, swelling or unanticipated firmness without obvious signs of bruising or bleeding, high levels of uncontrolled pain, or hypotension with compensatory tachycardia. A patient's subjective complaint of drainage in the back of the throat or excessive swallowing after ear, nose, or throat procedures could indicate bleeding. Postprocedural heavy vaginal flow or extreme hematuria also indicates bleeding.

Laparoscopic procedures have the risk for occult bleeding. A laceration or inadvertent burning of abdominal vessels or organs during laparoscopic surgery poses the potential for retroperitoneal bleeding. Intra-abdominal bleeding might not be associated with obvious signs until there is significant blood loss. Prevention of bleeding is achieved by having good surgical hemostasis. Acute bleeds can lead to rapid volume loss and, if untreated, cardiac arrest. Reassure the patient and initiate measures to reduce or stop any additional blood loss. Apply manual pressure or elevate the extremity if possible. Notify the anesthesiologist and surgeon, as treatment revolves around controlling the bleeding and achieving vascular integrity along with volume replacement as appropriate. Increase the intravenous rate to prepare for blood loss replacement with colloids or blood products as appropriate.

Postoperative Complications Related to Anesthesia

Postoperative Nausea and Vomiting

Postoperative nausea and vomiting (PONV) is one of the most common postoperative complaints encountered by patients following anesthesia and surgical procedures. Nausea is a patient's subjective experience of unpleasant flushing or pallor, swallowing, tachycardia, and an urge to vomit. Vomiting is an objective experience, which includes the contraction of abdominal muscles, descent of the diaphragm, opening of the gastric cardia, and expulsion of stomach contents through the mouth. In high-risk patients, the incidence of PONV can be 70% to 80% and the incidence of postdischarge nausea and vomiting (PDNV) is 35% to 50%.[3,19,20] Maras and Bulut conducted a descriptive study that found that 30.6% of patients had PONV and 26.3% had PDNV.[21] Among patients with postdischarge nausea, 26.1% experienced mild nausea, 44.6% moderate nausea, 20.7% significant nausea, and 8.7% severe nausea.[21] PONV is the most commonly reported patient fear before elective surgery, and it is rated by patients as being more debilitating than postoperative pain or the surgery itself. PONV continues to be a serious postoperative complication. It can increase rates of morbidity and mortality and cause electrolyte imbalances or aspiration. Increased costs along with delays in discharges are noted when the patient is converted to a 23-hour admission or has a wound injury or dehiscence. PONV is one of the strongest predictors of a prolonged postoperative stay and unanticipated admissions.

The emetic reflex is triggered in the medullary vomiting center and later in the reticular formation in the brain stem. The emetic centers are stimulated by visceral afferent neurons, vagal afferents, vestibular afferents, visual and cortical inputs, and direct inputs from the chemoreceptor trigger zone (CTZ). The CTZ is located in the medulla and has four major receptors: dopaminergic, histaminic, muscarinic (cholinergic), and serotonergic. Triggering any of these receptors causes nausea and vomiting.

The following risk factors for PONV have been determined by the strongest evidence: female gender, history of PONV, history of motion sickness, nonsmoker, postoperative use or administration of opioids, use of volatile anesthetics, and use of nitrous oxide. Women are two to four times more at risk for PONV, with increases seen during the menstrual cycle and in early pregnancy. Any patient with a history of gastrointestinal irritability, PONV, or motion sickness also has a higher risk of PONV. With a history of motion sickness or other issues indicating a sensitive vestibular system a patient is up to three times more likely to get PONV. Anesthetic agents, including inhalation agents and opioids, are associated with increasing PONV. A patient's preoperative anxiety, if it increases the levels of circulating catecholamine, can increase the risk of PONV. The gastric volume can also play a role in the development of PONV. Gastroparesis or delayed gastric emptying can be seen with diabetic neuropathy, chronic cholecystitis, small bowel obstruction, pregnancy, gastroesophageal reflux disorders, and a full stomach. Swallowing air during mask ventilation or the drainage of fluids, blood, mucus, or gas into the stomach also increase the gastric volume. Obese patients are at a higher risk as some anesthetics are deposited into adipose compartments and cause fat-soluble drugs to metabolize slowly and have delayed elimination. The site of surgery or the type of procedure can also increase the PONV risk. Laparoscopy (related to carbon dioxide irritation), strabismus repair, and intra-abdominal, gastrointestinal, and gynecologic surgeries are some that have been implicated. The duration of surgery could also play a role in PONV development. In the PACU period, pain relief is important. PONV could also be the result of hypotension, seen with hypoglycemia from fasting; sometimes starts with movement; or is due to the premature intake of fluids or food on a sensitive stomach (Figure 8.7).

To reduce the incidence of PONV and PDNV, patients are assessed preoperatively to identify their level of risk. Studies have shown that using a simplified risk factor identification tool provides better discrimination and calibration for the prediction of PONV. The Society of Ambulatory Anesthesia (SAMBA) Consensus Guidelines for the management of PONV state that all patients should be assessed for risk factors, including sex, smoking status, history of PONV and/or motion sickness, and postoperative opioid requirements[22] (Box 8.6). The guidelines identify three evidence-based risk scores useful for the prediction of PONV, PDNV, and postoperative vomiting (POV) in children[22] (Box 8.7). The higher the risk score for each of these assessment tools, the greater the cumulative risk for PONV, PDNV, or POV in children. Figure 8.8 shows the evidence-based algorithm for the treatment of PONV in children and adults.

Prophylactic recommendations include anesthesia-related, pharmacologic, therapeutic, and complementary interventions. Changing anesthesia techniques could include avoiding potent inhalation agents, administering more total intravenous anesthesia or regional anesthesia, using nonsteroidal anti-inflammatory drugs for pain control, using propofol, providing adequate hydration, and, if necessary, emptying the stomach of air, fluid, or blood while the patient is still asleep. Pharmacologic prophylactic interventions are based on the potential trigging mechanism for the patient; high-risk patients could receive a cocktail of different antiemetics to prevent PONV. Antiemetics are listed in Table 8.5, p. 60. If a patient has a low risk of PONV (e.g., 10% to 20%), the patient does not require prophylactic treatment. A patient with a moderate risk of 40% requires one intervention; a patient with a severe risk of 60% requires two interventions;

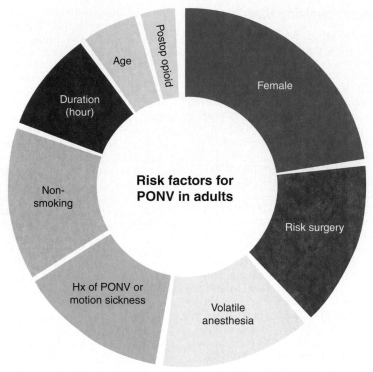

Fig. 8.7 Risk factors for PONV. Figure reused with permission from the American Society for Enhanced Recovery.

BOX 8.6 Adult Risk Factor Scores for PONV

Risk Factor*	Points
Female gender	1
Nonsmoker	1
History of PONV	1
Postoperative opioids	1
Sum	0–4

*Basic PONV risk if no risk factors are present is 10%. Risk increases to 20%, 40%, and 80% for each additional risk factor.
Source: Hooper VD. SAMBA Consensus guidelines for the management of postoperative nausea and vomiting: An executive summary for perianesthesia nurses. *J Perianesth Nurs.* 2015;30(5):377–382. Table 2. https://doi.org/10.1016/j.jopan.2015.08.009

BOX 8.7 Risk Factor Scores for POV in Children

Risk Factors	Points
Surgery > 30 minutes	1
Age > 3 years	1
Strabismus surgery	1
History of POV or PONV in relatives	1
Sum	0–4

Basic POV risk if no risk factors are present is 10%. Risk remains at 10% for one risk factor and increases to 30%, 50%, and 70% for each additional risk factor.
Source: Hooper VD. SAMBA Consensus guidelines for the management of postoperative nausea and vomiting: An executive summary for perianesthesia nurses. *J Perianesth Nurs.* 2015;30(5):377–382. Table 4. https://doi.org/10.1016/j.jopan.2015.08.009

---

and a patient with a very severe risk of 80% requires three interventions.[22]

In the PACU, supplemental oxygen helps if the patient is hypoxemic. Hypotension can contribute to PONV. When the patient is hypotensive, a small dose of ephedrine, 5–10 mg by IV push, can quickly raise the blood pressure. Fluid volume replacement is also helpful. Safety includes positioning the patient to ensure protection of the airway. If the patient is unconscious or there is a possibility of a compromised airway or loss of protective reflexes, position the head down and the body in the left lateral position during active retching and vomiting to facilitate drainage of contents from the oral cavity, decreasing the possibility of aspiration. Left lateral positioning further decreases the possibility, as it protects the vulnerable right main stem bronchus. Elevate the head of the bed 30–45 degrees for patients with abdominal distention or a history of esophageal reflux. Remove or minimize any noxious stimulus if still present. Assess the airway and breathing, auscultate breath sounds, and encourage deep breathing. Monitor for aspiration with vomiting. If adventitious sounds are audible and there is a decrease in oxygen saturation, aspiration should be suspected. The benefit of deep breathing is three-fold. Stirring up the patient facilitates the elimination of inhaled anesthetic agents, minimizes nausea and vomiting, and is a method of distraction. If necessary, perform oral/tracheal suctioning to remove vomitus and clear the airway. Provide comfort and support, apply a cool washcloth, and minimize movement. Provide wound support during episodes of retching or vomiting if applicable. Report excessive or prolonged nausea and vomiting so other causes and treatment options can be investigated.

Complimentary therapies include acupressure, aroma therapy, music therapy, and other distraction techniques. They have had some success in the PACU but require some planning with patients. Control pain but avoid the use of opioids. Slowly advance oral fluids for high-risk patients, beginning with ice chips and sips of water. Remember that the premature intake of oral fluids is an influencing factor for nausea and vomiting.

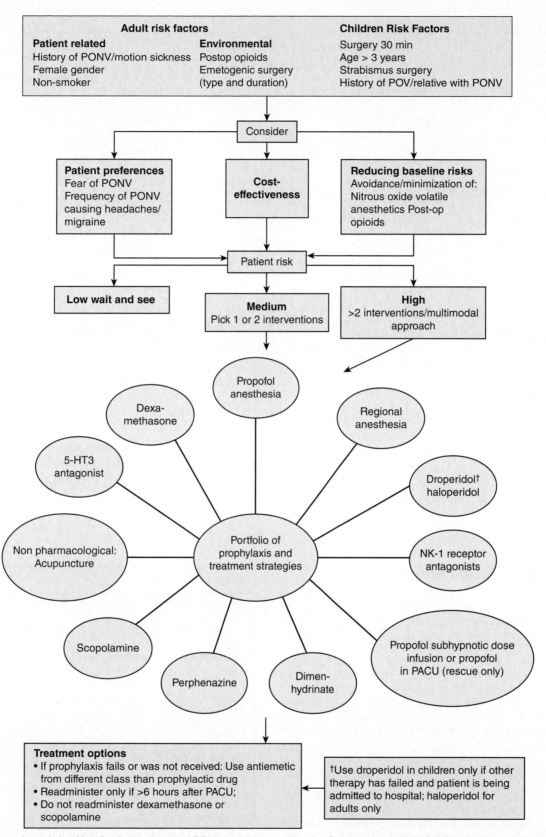

Fig. 8.8 Evidence-based algorithm for the treatment of PONV in children and adults. Source: Hooper VD. SAMBA Consensus Guidelines for the management of postoperative nausea and vomiting: An executive summary for perianesthesia nurses. *J Perianesth Nurs.* 2015;30(5): 377–382, Figure 1.

TABLE 8.5 Drugs for Postoperative and Postdischarge Nausea and Vomiting

Drug	Usual Adult Dose	Comment
5-HT₃ ANTAGONISTS		
Ondansetron	Adult 4–8 mg IV Child 50–100 µg/kg (max 4 mg)	Effective for prevention of both nausea and vomiting; more effective for PONV than PDNV Administer at the end of the procedure
Granisetron	Adult 1 mg IV Child 40 µg/kg up to 0.6 mg	Administer at the end of the procedure
Palonosetron	0.075 mg IV	Long duration may make it effective for PDNV
DOPAMINE ANTAGONISTS		
Droperidol	0.625–1.25 mg IV	Black box warning
Haloperidol	1–2 mg IV	Sedation, extrapyramidal and QT prolongation may occur
Metoclopramide	10–20 mg IV	Contraindicated in patients with gastric obstruction due to prokinetic effects
Prochlorperazine	10 mg IV	Sedation prominent
ANTIHISTAMINES		
Hydroxazine	12.5–25 mg IV	Sedation prominent
Promethazine	12.5–25 mg IV	Sedation prominent
Diphenhydramine	25 mg IV or IM	Sedation prominent
GLUCOCORTICOID		
Dexamethasone	Adult 4–8 mg IV Child 150 µg/kg up to 8 mg	May produce hyperglycemia postoperatively in diabetics
ANTICHOLINERGIC		
Scopolamine transdermal	2.5 cm² patch contains 1.5 mg scopolamine	Long duration may make it effective for PDNV
NEUROKININ 1 ANTAGONIST		
Aprepitant	40 mg PO	Long duration may make it effective for PDNV
Rolapitant	90 mg PO	Approved for chemotherapy-induced nausea and vomiting; should not be taken more than once every 2 weeks

Source: Nagelhout JJ. Additional drugs of interest. In: Naglehout JJ, Elisha S, eds. *Nurse Anesthesia.* 6th ed. Elsevier; 2018; Table 14.7.

Postdischarge Nausea and Vomiting

Nausea and vomiting can continue or occur after discharge. Prior to discharge, patients need to be assessed for their risk and need for prophylaxis for PDNV. If the patient is at risk, consider prophylaxis prior to discharge. If the patient has been treated for PONV, consider a different medication. A scopolamine patch can provide some extended relief, and it may be left on for 24 hours. A P6 acupoint stimulation system can be purchased over the counter and is another option for high-risk patients. Provide patient education, including how to manage PDNV. Rescue treatment may include ondansetron dissolving tablets, promethazine suppositories or tablets, or a scopolamine patch.

Anaphylactic Reactions

Anaphylaxis is a severe, potentially life-threatening allergic reaction. While an anaphylactic reaction is rare, no one can predict if a patient is going to have a severe antigen–antibody reaction from a medication. Box 8.8 shows the differential diagnoses. Anaphylaxis usually occurs within minutes of exposure to an allergen. Triggers such as antibiotics, opioids, latex, neuromuscular blockers, and anesthetic agents have been implicated in perioperative anaphylaxis. The incidence of anaphylaxis during general anesthesia is 1:10,000 to 1:20,000.[23] An anaphylactic reaction triggers the inflammatory process and the initiation of

BOX 8.8 Differential Diagnosis for Perioperative Anaphylaxis

Hypotension and tachycardia
  Anesthesia induction
  Perioperative antihypertensive or tricyclic antidepressant use
  Sepsis
  Hemorrhage or volume depletion
  Myocardial ischemia
  Arrythmia
  Pulmonary embolism
  Systemic mastocytosis
Bronchospasm
  Asthma
  Recent viral infection
  Obesity
  Mucous plugging
  Aspiration
  Difficult intubation
Urticaria and angioedema
  ACE inhibitor use
  C1 esterase inhibitor deficiency
Cold-induced urticaria

Source: Adapted from: Pitlick MM, Volcheck GW. Perioperative anaphylaxis. *Immunol Allery Clin N Am.* 2022;42(1):145–159. Box 1. https://doi.org/10.1016/j.iac.2021.09.002

the complement and arachidonic cascade. Activation of the mast cells and basophils usually occurs in response to immunoglobulin E but can be caused by other immunologic mechanisms or by a direct activation reaction. Mast cells release histamine and vasoactive mediators, causing massive vasodilation and increased capillary permeability.

Signs and symptoms include skin reactions such as urticarial hives, itching, and flushed or pale skin. Swelling and constriction of the airways with angioedema, laryngeal edema, and bronchoconstriction cause wheezing and shortness of breath. Patients can faint or report dizziness, along with hypotension, tachycardia, and dysrhythmias. Gastrointestinal effects could include nausea, vomiting, or diarrhea. The symptoms increase with repeated exposures and are dependent on the severity of the response. If one is unable to stabilize the patient, a total cardiac collapse can occur.

Immediate actions are required once a patient shows signs of an allergic or anaphylactic reaction. The perianesthesia nurse should stop any IV infusions to remove any potential causative agents. A fresh infusion setup of crystalloids (e.g., normal saline) is needed for fluid boluses. The airway and oxygenation must be monitored in the presence of airway edema. Increase the oxygen delivery to 100% and monitor the patient for potential intubation. The patient requires the administration of epinephrine to restore the vascular tone, increase the arterial blood pressure, and provide bronchodilation. Begin with a dose of 0.1 mg/kg for a pediatric patient or 0.2–0.5 mg for an adult patient 1:1000 (1 mg/ml) intramuscularly or 0.05–0.1 mg IV (adult) and titrate to effect per physician orders.[15] If the patient is wheezing, aminophylline or inhaled beta-adrenergic agents (e.g., albuterol) might be administered to relax and open airway passages in the lungs and cause bronchodilation, making it easier to breathe. To combat the effects of histamine, an antihistamine (e.g., diphenhydramine) might be administered. Glucocorticoids could be provided to decrease the inflammatory response. Gastric acid blockers might be given for stomach protection. These patients require emotional care and support. If the patient is not intubated, continue to monitor the oxygenation and ventilation and keep the patient informed as to what is going on. Patients are scared and apprehensive during anaphylactic reactions. Patients who experience perioperative anaphylaxis should be referred to an allergy specialist.

Delayed Awakening or Failure to Awaken

Delayed awakening or failure to awaken is a frightening but fortunately rare condition seen when there is slow or no responsiveness or a failure to return to the neurologic baseline level after the administration of an anesthetic. There are multiple causes for delayed awakening, and making a differential diagnosis is necessary. It is important to know the patient's baseline neurologic status, medical history, and laboratory results. The nurse can help to rule out causes so treatment focuses on the cause. Three quick actions can rule out some concerns. First, check blood glucose levels for hyperglycemia or hypoglycemia and administer insulin or glucose as necessary. Second, since hypothermia delays the metabolism of drugs, monitor the temperature and gradually rewarm the patient if required. Third, provide adequate ventilation and oxygenation to prevent hypercarbia and hypoxia, which can extend sedation. Otherwise, consider prolonged drug effects from neuromuscular blocking agents, opioids, or benzodiazepines. Review the anesthesia record to see which medications were administered. The patient could have an inadequate reversal of a nondepolarizing neuromuscular blocking agent or a pseudocholinesterase deficiency (discussed below). If the paralytic medication outlasts the reversal medications, then the administration of an additional dose

of a reversal medication such as neostigmine with glycopyrrolate or sugammadex might be required. Constricted pupils suggest that an opioid effect is still occurring, and excess sedation could be caused by opioids or benzodiazepines. Naloxone might be needed to reverse the opioids, and flumazenil could be used to reverse the benzodiazepines. Other risk factors include electrolyte imbalance, adrenal excess, neurologic injury such as stroke, seizures, or an intracerebral hemorrhage, myocardial infarction, organ failure, or hypothyroidism. Assess the situation, rule out potential causes, and intervene as appropriate. Continue to provide the patient emotional support and oxygenation and ventilation as needed until recovery occurs.

Pseudocholinesterase Deficiency

Pseudocholinesterase deficiency is a relatively rare condition affecting 1 in 3200 to 5000 patients worldwide.[24] A physiologic deficiency of the enzyme that metabolizes succinylcholine (and in some cases mivacurium) results in a prolonged muscle relaxation response. Normally, the estimated elimination half-life of succinylcholine is 2–4 minutes. There are numerous factors that are known to reduce the functioning levels of pseudocholinesterase. The condition can be acquired related to a disease state such as cirrhosis, hepatitis, cancer, uremia, hypothyroidism, malnutrition, chronic anemia, skin disease, collagen disease, infection, burns, and tetanus.[25] Pregnancy also lowers the enzyme level, and infants under 6 months have a deficiency of pseudocholinesterase. This condition requires confirmation by laboratory testing, which is unreasonable for ASC patients given the limited rates of the event. Preanesthesia assessments include questions related to previous anesthetic experiences to determine if there is a history of the problem. Patients are asked if they or anyone in their family ever had a reaction to anesthesia where they had a delayed awakening. Recovery from succinylcholine should be seen within 10–15 minutes after administration. When this quick recovery is not readily apparent, consider a pseudocholinesterase deficiency. The only course of treatment once the problem is recognized is symptom support until the agent naturally degrades itself. Individuals can remain paralyzed for as long as 8 hours.[25] During this time, the patient has to remain on the ventilator to maintain respirations, have effective gas exchange, and have adequate airway clearance until muscle strength returns. Return of adequate muscle strength can be monitored by a peripheral nerve stimulator.

Recovery takes time, so one aspect of making the patient comfortable is sedation with midazolam or a propofol drip. Provide comfort and emotional support for the patient as needed. While the patient is paralyzed, the patient will be able to hear and feel. During this time, some providers order anxiolytics and pain medications to help mediate the awareness patients experience. Signs such as tachycardia, hypertension, dilated pupils, and/or cool, pale skin may be indications that the patient is experiencing pain. The nurse should continue the appropriate pain management plan. Care of the patient also includes keeping the skin integrity intact, so the patient needs to be turned and repositioned at least every 2 hours. After the crisis, the patient needs to be educated about pseudocholinesterase deficiency. The patient should be tested for it. Because this is an inherited disorder, relatives should also be encouraged to be tested. Depending on the ambulatory setting, these patients might be transferred to an acute care hospital for recovery.

Emergence Delirium

Emergence delirium, also referred to as emergence excitement or emergence agitation, is a transient state of disassociation

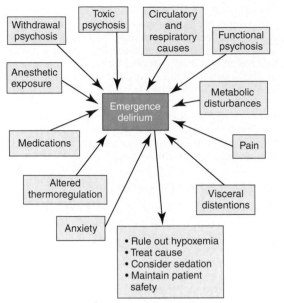

Fig. 8.9 Emergence delirium in the postanesthesia care unit: contributing factors and treatment. Source: Modified from Odom-Forren J, Brady JM. Postanesthesia recovery. In: Naglehout JJ, Elisha S, eds. *Nurse Anesthesia*. 6th ed. Elsevier; 2018; Figure 55.2.

marked by extreme confusion, combativeness, and disorientation while a patient is emerging from anesthesia.[3,26] Causes of emergence delirium include residual preoperative medications, pain, bladder distention, a feeling of suffocation, hypoxia, and preoperative fears.[26] While it is most commonly observed in children (< 30% of cases), nearly 5% of adults are estimated to experience emergence delirium.[3] In a prospective study published in 2006, adult risk factors included preoperative medicating with benzodiazepines, breast or abdominal surgery, and longer procedures under anesthesia.[27] Additionally, inhalational anesthetics and an underlying temperament may contribute to the incidence.[3] Efforts to prevent the occurrence of emergence delirium are aimed at identifying patients at risk and mitigating the experience by addressing and reducing preoperative anxiety, offering proactive pain management, and maintaining minimal stress in the environment (Figure 8.9).

While treating the patient with emergence delirium, safety is the first concern. Generally, the delirium is temporary and gradually resolves over 30–60 minutes. The irrational, agitated, thrashing patient is usually extremely strong when delirious. Several staff members are needed to protect the patient, keep the patient on the stretcher, and avoid patient or staff injury. Use a soft calm voice to reorient the patient and provide a

quiet environment. Loud commands and forceful movements tend to increase the agitation. Persistent delirium may require sedation or anxiolytics to control the symptoms. Physostigmine to reverse central anticholinergic medications may be indicated for protracted delirium. Continue to ensure adequate oxygenation and manage pain until the patient recovers.

Local Anesthetic Systemic Toxicity

Local anesthetic system toxicity (LAST) is a rare but potentially lethal adverse consequence of regional anesthesia. The development of LAST is a result of the accidental injection or absorption of local anesthetics systemically into the vascular system. LAST has an incidence of 1 in 1000 peripheral nerve blocks.[28,29] Wolfe and Spillars reported studies finding 0.3 to 1.8 LAST events per 1000 peripheral nerve blocks.[30] The fullblown LAST cascade can result in a mortality rate of nearly 10% if proper early intervention is not given.[30] Safe administration of local anesthetics includes judicious needle placement with ultrasound guidance, fractionated dosing with frequent aspiration, and observing dose limits. Table 8.6 shows the maximum appropriate dosages.

Organ systems that are primarily disrupted by toxic doses of local anesthetics include the central nervous system (CNS) and cardiovascular system. The degree of LAST is influenced by the site of injection, local anesthetic drug characteristics, and total dosage involved. Overall, the timing of a LAST presentation is highly variable and should be suspected whenever physiologic changes occur after, or simultaneously with, the administration of a local anesthetic.[30] The early and mild CNS effects can include the report of a metallic taste, circumoral numbness, diplopia, and tinnitus. As the level of anesthetic toxicity spreads, increasing CNS excitation occurs, causing progressive light-headedness, agitation, confusion, muscle twitching, and seizures. As the cascade progresses, CNS depression manifests as extreme drowsiness, obtundation, coma, or apnea. Cardiovascular signs may include hypertension initially and then tachycardia and ventricular arrhythmias (e.g., ventricular tachycardia, torsades de pointes, or ventricular fibrillation). Later cardiovascular progression leads to hypotension, bradycardia, and then asystole with respiratory arrest.

LAST should be ruled out in patients who present with altered mental status, neurologic symptoms, or cardiovascular instability after regional anesthesia. When LAST occurs, provide adequate oxygenation and ventilation, hydration, intralipid therapy, and targeted treatment of symptoms (e.g., seizures, hypotension, apnea, cardiac arrest) (Figure 8.10). Early airway management and the prevention of hypoxemia and acidosis have been found to halt the progression of LAST to seizures and cardiovascular compromise.[28] Seizures can be quickly controlled by benzodiazepines or propofol. In a situation requiring ACLS, epinephrine may enhance dysrhythmias

TABLE 8.6 Maximum Dosages and Durations of Various Local Anesthetics

Agent	Onset	Maximum Dosage (mg/kg)		Duration (minutes)	
		Without Epinephrine	**With Epinephrine**	**Without Epinephrine**	**With Epinephrine**
Bupivacaine	Slow	8	10	240	480
Lidocaine	Rapid	4.5	7	120	240
Mepivacaine	Rapid	5	7	180	360
Prilocaine	Medium	5	7.5	90	360
Procaine	Slow	8	10	45	90
Tetracaine	Slow	1.5	2.5	180	60

Source: Wadlund DL. Local anesthetic systemic toxicity. *AORN J*. 2017;106(5):367-377. Table 2. https://doi.org/10.1016/j.aorn.2017.08.015

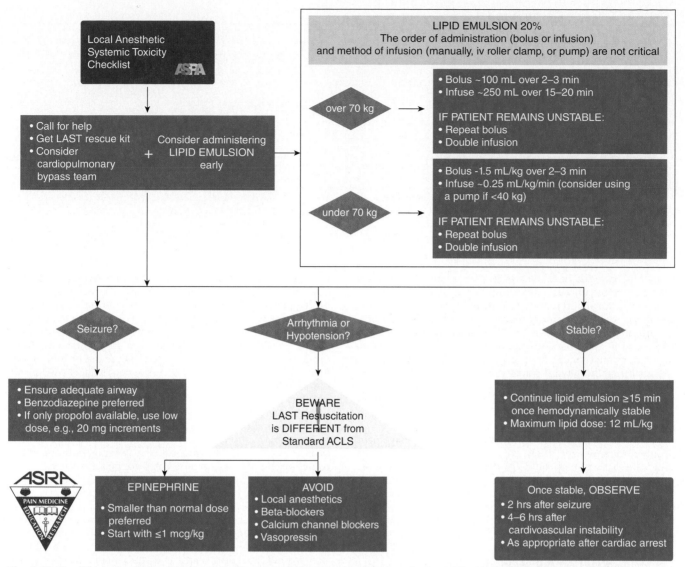

Fig. 8.10 Checklist for treatment of local anesthetic system toxicity. Source: American Society of Regional Anesthesia and Pain Medicine. Checklist for Treatment of Local Anesthetic System Toxicity. 2020. https://www.asra.com/news-publications/asra-updates/blog-landing/guidelines/2020/11/01/checklist-for-treatment-of-local-anesthetic-systemic-toxicity

induced by local anesthetics. Treatment to stop the effects of LAST include the administration of a lipid emulsion (20%) bolus and infusion. Lipid infusion provides a "lipid sink" or pool of lipids that bind with the fat-loving local anesthetic, pulling it out of tissues, and halting and reversing the severe symptoms and consequences of LAST.[28] The dosage for the intralipid bolus is 1.5 mL/kg followed by an infusion of 0.25 mL/kg/min, continued for at least 10 minutes after circulatory stability is attained. If circulatory stability is not attained, consider a second bolus and an increase in the infusion to 0.5 mL/kg/min.[30,31] Ferry and Cook found that education and information about LAST were not readily available for nurses, patients, and families in a local hospital.[32] Increasing knowledge about the treatment of LAST is needed, and training, drills, and competencies in the care of the patient given local anesthetics should be a standard requirement in the ambulatory surgical setting.

Complications of Neuraxial Anesthesia

In addition to LAST, there can be additional risks associated with neuraxial anesthesia and particular anesthetics. Spinal and epidural blocks may be administered in the outpatient setting to provide anesthetic-quality paresthesia (Table 8.7). Common neuraxial complications include transient hypotension, nausea and vomiting, urinary retention, hypothermia, and postdural puncture headaches. More serious complications include LAST, spinal or epidural hematomas, and high spinal blocks.

Spinal hematomas are an extremely rare complication of neuraxial anesthesia. Patients with coagulopathy issues are at the highest risk. The most common presenting symptoms for a neurologically significant hematoma include a progressive motor block, sensory block, or bowel and bladder dysfunction. Back pain is a less common presenting complaint. Hematomas pose a medical emergency and require surgical evacuation within 6–8 hours to prevent permanent neurologic damage.[33] Patients being treated in an ambulatory setting need to be transferred to a medical center for a possible decompressive laminectomy .

During administration of an epidural block, if the needle punctures the dural canal there is the potential for cerebrospinal fluid (CSF) to appear when doing the needle aspiration. If medications for the epidural are injected into the spinal space, the result is a high spinal block. The best treatment is prevention

TABLE 8.7 Differences Between Spinal and Epidural Anesthesia

Characteristic	Spinal Anesthesia	Epidural Anesthesia
Site or mechanism of action	Nerve roots blocked as they pass through the cerebrospinal fluid	Nerve roots blocked outside the cerebrospinal fluid
Site of administration	Lower lumbar area below the termination of spinal cord	Lumbar or thoracic area
Dosage of local anesthetic	Small	Large
Instrument for administration	Needle	Catheter
Ability to repeat dose	No	Yes
Onset	Rapid, intense blockade; may lead to hypotension	Gradual; may have less intense blockade; decrease in blood pressure is more gradual

Source: Nagelhout JJ. Regional anesthesia. In: Odom-Forren J, ed. *Drain's Perianesthesia Nursing: A Critical Care Approach*. 7th ed. Elsevier; 2018; Table 25.1.

by making sure the needle placement for an epidural is in the right area before injection. Injecting a test dose minimizes accidental intravascular injections and spinal injections. Total spinal anesthesia, or a high sensory block, results when the anesthetic spreads up the spinal canal toward the head and causes excessive sensory and motor anesthesia. If a local anesthetic spreads higher than the thoracic spine level (T1), there is a potential for depression of the cervical spinal cord and brain stem. The patient becomes confused, agitated, hypotensive, and nauseated and complains of difficulty breathing. This may progress to upper extremity weakness, pupillary dilation, and cardiopulmonary collapse.[33]

Treatment is aggressive and includes airway management, positive pressure ventilation, volume infusion, and vasopressors. The patient may suffer cardiac arrest and require advanced life support measures. If the patient requires ventilator support until the medication wears off, ensure that the patient is provided emotional support and sedation. Early recognition is critical to the management of total spinal anesthesia and the prevention of permanent injury.

Postoperative Complications Involving Thermoregulation

Unplanned Hypothermia

Maintaining normothermia has been recognized as an important process during surgical procedures to support optimal patient outcomes. The ASPAN practice experts who publish the ASPAN Standards recommend a series of assessments and interventions designed to obtain or maintain continuous normothermia (e.g., a temperature of 96.8 to 100.4°F, or 36 to 38°C) throughout the preoperative, intraoperative, phase I (PACU), and phase II (ambulatory or same-day care unit) periods of care.[34] The clinical sign of hypothermia is a core body temperature of less than 36°C (96.8° F). Li et al. conducted a retrospective study of 2223 patients admitted to the PACU to determine the risk factors for hypothermia. The incidence of hypothermia was found to be 6.01%.[35] The results also suggested that older patients, patients with higher ASA scores, surgical procedures of a longer duration, and the presence of preoperative hypothermia were some of the key risk factors that could trigger hypothermia in the PACU.[35] Unplanned postanesthesia hypothermia is associated with complications such as coagulopathies, increased wound infections, prolonged postanesthetic recovery, and postoperative thermal discomfort.[36] Patients with hypothermia may be shivering and have piloerection and/or cold extremities. Shivering during the

PACU period results in increased myocardial oxygen consumption and patient discomfort. The body's normal mechanism for temperature regulation is altered by anesthetic agents used during surgery. Heat loss during surgery can come from radiation, convection, conduction, or evaporation. Radiative heat loss, in which heat is transferred from the patient's body to other surfaces in the operating room, is the main cause of patient heat loss. Convection occurs when heat is lost to air movement dependent on thermal gradients. Conduction is heat lost from direct contact between objects (e.g., cold sheets, instruments, monitors, IV fluids). Evaporation of bodily fluids during respiration or from skin-prepping solutions also adds to heat loss. Evaporation from open wounds or surgical incisions is another way in which the body temperature may become lowered during surgery. Hypothermia can be seen with anesthetic techniques that cause vasodilation, such as spinal anesthesia during which heat is lost from peripheral vessels, or general anesthesia, during which the use of muscle relaxants and opioids causes vasodilation. General anesthesia can also alter the thermoregulation center at the hypothalamus.

The potential consequences of hypothermia can be shivering, wound infection, cardiac disturbances, delayed emergence from anesthesia, and coagulopathy. The shivering is a normal autonomic response that has the goal of generating heat. However, shivering can increase oxygen requirements and consumption by 400% to 500%. Small doses of meperidine hydrochloride (e.g., 12.5 to 25 mg IV) can effectively suppress shivering. Interventions aimed at decreasing cutaneous heat loss include keeping the patient's skin covered as much as possible and using blanket layering and active surface rewarming. Active rewarming includes using warm airflow devices. Passive rewarming is done with warm cotton blankets, thermal drapes, fluid warmers, and the use of heated, humidified oxygen delivery. During rewarming, monitor the temperature every 30 minutes until normothermia is achieved.

Malignant Hyperthermia

While a malignant hyperthermia (MH) crisis is very rare, it can very quickly turn deadly and is a true anesthetic emergency. MH is more likely to occur in the operating room, and the perianesthesia nurse therefore supports the management of the patient. However, MH may also have a delayed onset, presenting within the first hour and possibly up to 12 hours postoperatively.[37] According to the Malignant Hyperthermia Association of the United States (MHAUS), the exact incidence of MH is unknown.[38] Epidemiologic studies reveal that MH complicates 1 in about 100,000 surgeries in adults and 1 in about 30,000 surgical procedures in children.[38] MH is a hypermetabolic syndrome triggered in genetically susceptible individuals when certain potent volatile inhalation anesthetics or succinylcholine is administered. These agents interfere with the ability of the sarcoplasmic reticulum to control the intracellular movement of calcium. The excessive release of calcium creates a high intracellular level of calcium, and this leads to continuous contractures of the skeletal muscles. This hyperactivity of the skeletal muscles leads to increased oxygen consumption, increased heat production, and increased use of adenosine triphosphate (ATP). Increased use of ATP causes the release of carbon dioxide and lactic acid, which creates an acidotic state. ATP use also causes heat release leading to a rise in body temperature. These actions cause a subsequent interruption of the cell membrane integrity, which allows potassium, magnesium, phosphate, cellular enzymes, and myoglobin to leak into the extracellular fluid.[37-39] Triggering drugs include the depolarizing neuromuscular relaxant succinylcholine and volatile inhalation agents, including desflurane, sevoflurane, isoflurane, enflurane, and halothane. Nitrous oxide is the only safe inhalation agent for an MH-susceptible patient.

The goal with MH is prevention. The pre-assessment history is an important tool for identifying susceptible patients. Personal or family histories of any anesthetic-related complications or deaths, muscle disorders, or episodes of fever or dark-colored urine after a previous surgery are hallmark warning signs. Identification of MH-susceptible patients allows providers to avoid triggering agents to prevent the crisis from developing. These patients can safely have anesthesia using any number of "safe" anesthetic agents and techniques.

Initial signs are increased levels of end-tidal carbon dioxide (EtCO$_2$), masseter spasm or rigidity, and sympathetic hyperactivity presenting as sudden unexplained tachycardia, tachypnea, and profound muscle rigidity. Hypoxemia, respiratory acidosis, metabolic acidosis, cyanosis, tachypnea, and hemodynamic instability quickly follow. Hyperthermia is actually a later sign. MH can cause increases in levels of potassium, magnesium, and phosphate; myoglobinuria; arrhythmias; cardiac instability; left ventricular failure; coagulopathy; and cardiac arrest. Not all cases of MH are fulminant ($\sim$10% reach this level); rather, there is a spectrum or continuum of severities, ranging from an insidious onset with mild complications to an explosive metabolic response with pronounced rigidity, temperature increase, arrhythmias, and, eventually, death.[37-39] Get help! MH requires immediate treatment. Multiple tasks have to be done at the same time, and extra people are needed. The first priority is to discontinue the triggering agents if they have not already been stopped, hyperventilate the patient with 100% oxygen, get additional IV access, and administer massive doses of the muscle relaxant dantrolene sodium, which counteracts the high levels of intracellular calcium.

Treatment for MH also involves focusing on treating the effects of muscle damage. Severe metabolic acidosis is managed by administering sodium bicarbonate (1–2 mEq/kg) for acidosis, utilizing frequent measurements of arterial blood gasses and bicarbonate levels for replacement. Generous fluid resuscitation is provided to sustain the fluid balance and urine output and to flush the kidneys to remove myoglobins and prevent renal failure. Maintain a urine output of at least 2 mL/kg/hour by using IV fluids, mannitol, or furosemide. The shifts in electrolytes need to be monitored and treated. Increasing potassium levels might have to be treated with insulin and glucose to lower them. Calcium chloride might be used to treat cardiac dysrhythmias.

Patient cooling measures must be introduced. Use ice or disposable cold packs placed on the body surface, especially the neck, axilla, and groin areas, and use cooling blankets and chilled IV solutions to initiate immediate patient cooling. Begin invasive cooling measures as needed. A nasogastric tube, rectal tube, and urinary catheters can be placed for lavaging irrigating cooling solutions into the stomach, rectum, and bladder. The patient's condition will continue to change and require diligent monitoring of the hemodynamic status, urine output, and temperature, and laboratory studies need to be continued. Watch for signs of the crisis breaking, a decreased heart rate, a decreased temperature, decreasing EtCO$_2$ levels, and a correction of acidosis. The sequelae to MH crisis can be CNS damage, permanent renal failure, left-sided heart failure, pulmonary edema, disseminated intravascular coagulation, hemorrhage, and cerebral edema, and the MH crisis may recur. Patients in an ambulatory surgical setting require transfer to a tertiary care center as soon as possible. Because MH is exceedingly uncommon, it is important for anesthesia providers and perioperative clinicians to stay abreast of the signs, symptoms, and treatment of MH. Successful management of an MH crisis hinges on advanced preparation for an unexpected MH incident (Figure 8.11).[37] Outpatient preparation is comparable to inpatient preparation except that fewer resources such as medications, personnel, and laboratory testing capabilities may be available. The patient and family members need to be referred to the Malignant Hyperthermia Association of the United States (MHAUS) to register and learn more about MH. The physician or nurse should speak with the family members and give them information concerning MH, such as how to contact MHAUS and where to find website information. The MH Hotline is available 24/7 in the event of an MH crisis: 1-800-644-9737.[38]

Miscellaneous Postoperative Complications

Corneal Abrasion

Corneal abrasion is the most common cause of eye pain with or without visual disturbance in the postoperative period. Its incidence is estimated to range from 0.17% to as high as 44%.[3] Most corneal abrasions acquired intraoperatively are due to lagophthalmos (the inability to close the eyelids properly) and changes in tear production induced by general anesthesia. Other causes include direct trauma from a face mask or dangling badge or chemical injury related to surgical prep solutions. Inadequate taping, sealing, and lubricating of the eyes during general anesthesia and head and neck procedures and lateral or prone positioning in the operating room also increase the risk for corneal abrasions. A natural reflex for some patients is to rub the eyes when emerging from anesthesia, which further increases the risk of corneal abrasions. Another risk factor is the location of pulse oximeter probes on the fingers. Bed linens and IV tubing and other lines, along with nasal cannulas and face mask edges, have been associated with corneal abrasions in the PACU.

Patients with a corneal abrasion present with blurred vision, light sensitivity, tearing, pain, and redness. They complain of the sensation of a foreign body in the affected eye. The anesthesiologist assesses the eye and orders an antibiotic eye ointment for treatment. Do not use topical local anesthesia in the eye or give the patient an eyepatch. Patients should be instructed to use the antibiotic ointment three times per day in the affected eye, applying it in the area between the eye and lower lid. The healing process should take 24–48 hours. During this time, patients should be instructed not to rub the eye, as this delays the healing process. If patients have persistent symptoms beyond 48 hours, they should be advised to contact their ophthalmologist.

Postoperative Vision Loss

Postoperative vision loss (POVL) is a rare condition with several contributing factors. It tends to occur most commonly with spinal fusions and cardiac surgeries.[3] Positioning and

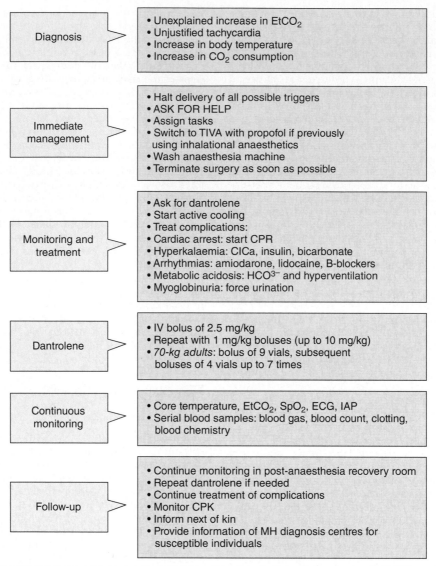

Fig. 8.11 Example of MH crisis management protocol. From Kollman-Camaiora A, Alsina E, Dominguez A, Del Blanco B, Yepes MJ, Guerrero JL, Garcia A: Clinical protocol for the management of malignant hyperthermia. *Rev Esp Anestesiol Reanim.* 2017;64(1):32–40, Figure 2. © 2016 Copyright Elsevier BV. All rights reserved.

hemodynamic functioning can impair the blood flow to the optic nerve, resulting in ischemic optic neuropathy. This neuropathy is the most common cause of permanent POVL and accounts for 89% of cases of POVL following prone spine surgeries.[3] Risk factors for ischemic optic neuropathy include male gender, obesity, prone positioning on a Wilson frame, long surgical procedures and episodes of anesthesia (< 6.5 hours), high intraprocedural blood losses (< 45% of the estimated blood volume), and inadequate colloid fluid administration.[3] Once POVL is suspected, immediate ophthalmologic consultation should be sought.

Other Miscellaneous Postoperative Complications

Maintaining an airway during anesthesia has its own risk of postanesthesia complications. Dental damage can present as a chipped or lost tooth or oral soft tissue trauma, and hoarseness/pharyngitis can be due to intubation or the placement of airway adjuncts. Electrical or chemical burns can be caused by cautery instruments, lasers, or malfunctioning equipment. There are numerous other minor complications that can be

seen in the PACU. Some complications are related to the surgical process, surgical procedure, anesthesia technique, or medications administered.

CHAPTER HIGHLIGHTS

- Appropriate patient selection is a key component of a safe ambulatory surgery experience.
- Staff, patient, and family education allows for realistic expectations, optimal preoperative preparation, and ready mitigation of postoperative complications.

CASE STUDY

Mrs. Paul is a 60-year-old female having a rotator cuff repair. She is allergic to Codeine, Vicodin, and Darvocet all of which cause her to experience depression. She has no latex allergy upon assessment. She has no significant health history. She lives with her husband and has children nearby who can help after her procedure. She is a good candidate for ambulatory surgery. Mrs. Paul arrives for surgery and is taken into the preoperative unit. Her vital signs are blood pressure 149/87 mm Hg, heart rate 71 bpm, respiratory rate 18 breaths per minute, oxygen saturation 99%, and temperature 97°F. An 18-gauge IV catheter is started for an infusion of lactated Ringer solution and kept open. She drank a glass of water earlier in the morning but has now been NPO for over 3 hours. The anesthesia plan includes an interscalene brachial plexus block. Mrs. Paul is anxious, so a low dosage of midazolam is given and cefazolin is ordered as a preoperative antibiotic. The anesthesia team performs the interscalene brachial plexus block in the preoperative area. The patient is monitored during and after the procedure. The patient is resting comfortably with her daughter at the bedside. Soon, however, the daughter says her mom seems to be having trouble breathing. You arrive to find the patient becoming dyspneic with marked sinus bradycardia.

What is going on with the patient? What are your first actions going to be?

The nurse asks for help and grabs the bag-valve mask to provide positive pressure ventilation with 100% oxygen. The crash cart, along with the defibrillator and pacemaker, are brought to the bedside. A 1-mg dose of atropine is given by IV push to treat the bradycardia and the hypotension. The patient is intubated, and the heart rate and blood pressure are stabilized.

What just happened?

A quick review of potential complications from interscalene brachial plexus blocks helped with the differential diagnosis. Potential difficulties included a vertebral artery injection. If this had occurred, signs of CNS toxicity from the local anesthetic would be observed, along with paralysis of the recurrent laryngeal nerve, unilateral Horner syndrome, pneumothorax, cervical epidural or spinal anesthesia (if a local anesthetic was injected into a dural cuff), and paralysis of the phrenic nerve. The respiratory arrest was due to the phrenic nerve being blocked. Mrs. Paul was put on a ventilator and moved to the PACU for closer monitoring. Mrs. Paul and her family were updated throughout the process on how she was doing. Mrs. Paul received some sedation for comfort. She was monitored until the anesthetic wore off and was discharged home later that day.

REFERENCES

1. Smith I, Skues MA, Philip BK. Ambulatory (Outpatient) anesthesia. In: Gropper MA, ed. *Miller's Anesthesia*. 9th ed. Elsevier; 2020:2251-2283.
2. Brull R, Macfarlane AJR, Chan VWS. Spinal, epidural, and caudal anesthesia. In: Gropper MA, ed. *Miller's Anesthesia*. 9th ed. Elsevier; 2020:1413-1449.
3. Berg SM, Braehler MR. The postanesthesia care unit. In: Gropper MA, ed. *Miller's Anesthesia*. 9th ed. Elsevier; 2020:2586-2613.
4. Hines RB, Barash PG, Watrous G, O'Connor T. Complications occurring in the postanesthesia care unit: a survey. *Anesth Analg.* 1992;74(4):503-509. Available at: https://doi.org/10.1213/00000539-199204000-00006.
5. Kluger MT, Bullock MFM. Recovery room incidents: a review of 419 reports from the Anaesthetic Incident Monitoring Study (AIMS). *Anaesthesia.* 2002;57(11):1060-1066. Available at: https://doi.org/10.1046/j.1365-2044.2002.02865.x.
6. Tarrac SE. A description of intraoperative and postanesthesia complication rates. *J Perianesth Nurs.* 2006;21(2):88-96. Available at: https://doi.org/10.1016/j.jopan.2006.01.006.
7. Hadler RA, Neuman MD, Fleisher LA. Risk of anesthesia. In: Gropper MA, ed. *Miller's Anesthesia*. 9th ed. Elsevier; 2020.
8. Portuondo JI, Shah SR, Singh H, Massarweh NN. Failure to rescue as a surgical quality indicator: current concepts and future directions for improving surgical outcomes. *Anesthesiology.* 2019;131(2):426-437. Available at: https://doi.org/10.1097/aln.0000000000002602.
9. Cain CL, Riess ML, Gettrust L, Novalija J. Malignant hyperthermia crisis: optimizing patient outcomes through simulation and interdisciplinary collaboration. *AORN J.* 2014;99(2):301-311. Available at: https://doi.org/10.1016/j.aorn.2013.06.012.
10. Mathis MR, Naughton NN, Shanks AM, et al. Patient selection for day case-eligible surgery: identifying those at high risk for major complications. *Anesthesiology.* 2013;119(6):1310-1321. Available at: https://doi.org/10.1097/aln.0000000000000005.
11. Foley CK. American Society of Anesthesiologists Physical Status Classification as a reliable predictor of postoperative medical complications and mortality following ambulatory surgery: an analysis of 2,089,830 ACS-NSQIP outpatient cases. *BMC Surg.* 2021;21(1):253. Available at: https://doi.org/10.1186/s12893-021-01256-6.
12. American Society of PeriAnesthesia Nurses. *A Competency-Based Orientation Program for the Registered Nurse in the Perianesthesia Setting.* ASPAN; 2019.
13. Chen Y-YK, Arriaga AF. Checklists for safer perioperative care. In: Peden CJ, Fleisher LA, Englesbe M, eds. *Perioperative Quality Improvement.* Elsevier; 2023:204-210.
14. Redelmeier DA. Postoperative care and complications. In: Goldman L, Schafer AI, eds. *Goldman-Cecil Medicine.* 26th ed. Elsevier; 2020:2586-2591.
15. O'Brien D. Postanesthesia care complications. In: Odom-Forren J, eds. *Drain's Perianesthesia Nursing: A Critical Care Approach.* 7th ed. Elsevier; 2018.
16. Clark LH, Gehrig PA, Valea FA. Perioperative management of complications: fever, respiratory, cardiovascular, thromboembolic, urinary tract, gastrointestinal, wound, and operative site complications; neurologic injury; psychological sequelae. In: Gershenson DM, Lentz GM, Valea FA, Lobo RA, eds. *Comprehensive Gynecology.* 8th ed. Elsevier; 2022.
17. Yepuri N, Pruekprasert N, Cooney RN. Surgical complications. In: Townsend CM, Beauchamp RD, Evers BM, Mattox KL, eds. *Sabiston Textbook of Surgery.* 21st ed. Elsevier; 2022.
18. American Heart Association. *ACLS Advanced Cardiovascular Life Support Providers Manual.* American Heart Association; 2020.
19. Finch CP, Parkosweich JA, Perrone D, Weidman KH, Furino L. Incidence, timing, and factors associated with postoperative nausea and vomiting in the ambulatory surgery setting. *J PeriAnesth Nurs.* 2019;34(6):1146-1155. Available at: https://doi.org/10.1016/j.jopan.2019.04.009.
20. Hooper VD. SAMBA Consensus guidelines for the management of postoperative nausea and vomiting: an executive summary for perianesthesia nurses. *J Perianesth Nurs.* 2015;30(5):377-382. Available at: https://doi.org/10.1016/j.jopan.2015.08.009.
21. Maras GB, Bulut H. Prevalence of nausea-vomiting and coping strategies in patients undergoing outpatient surgery. *J Perianesth Nurs.* 2021;36(5):487-491. Available at: https://doi.org/10.1016/j.jopan.2020.10.004.
22. Gan TJ, Belani KG, Bergese S, et al. Fourth consensus guidelines for the management of postoperative nausea and vomiting. *Anesth Analg.* 2020;131(2):411-448. Available at: https://doi.org/10.1213/ANE.0000000000004833.
23. Pitlick MM, Volcheck GW. Perioperative anaphylaxis. *Immunol Allery Clin N Am.* 2022;42(1):145-159. Available at: https://doi.org/10.1016/j.iac.2021.09.002.
24. Drain CB. Neuromuscular blocking agents. In: Odom-Forren J, ed. *Drain's Perianesthesia Nursing: A Critical Care Approach.* 7th ed. Elsevier; 2018.
25. Wijeysundera DN, Finlayson E. Preoperative evaluation. In: Gropper MA, ed. *Miller's Anesthesia.* 9th ed. Elsevier; 2020.
26. Schick L. Perianesthesia Complications. In: Schick L, Windle PE, eds. *PeriAnesthesia Nursing Core Curriculum: Preprocedure, Phase I and Phase II PACU Nursing.* 4th ed. Elsevier; 2021.
27. Lepouse C, Lautner CA, Liu L, Gomis P, Leon A. Emergence delirium in adults in the post-anaesthesia care unit. *Br J Anaesth.* 2006;96(6):747-753. Available at: https://doi.org/10.1093/bja/ael094.
28. Noble KA. Local anesthesia toxicity and lipid rescue. *J Perianesth Nurs.* 2015;30(4):321-335. Available at: https://doi.org/10.1016/j.jopan.2014.03.010.
29. Wadlund DL. Local anesthetic systemic toxicity. *AORN J.* 2017;106(5):367-377. Available at: https://doi.org/10.1016/j.aorn.2017.08.015.

30. Wolfe RC, Spillars A. Local anesthetic systemic toxicity: reviewing updates from the American Society of Regional Anesthesia and Pain Medicine Practice Advisory. *J Perianesth Nurs*. 2018;33(6):1000-1005. Available at: https://doi.org/10.1016/j.jopan.2018.09.005.

31. Collins S, Neubrander J, Vorst Z, Sheffield B. Lipid emulsion in treatment of local anesthetic toxicity. *J Perianesth Nurs*. 2015;30(4):308-320. Available at: https://doi.org/10.1016/j.jopan.2014.03.011.

32. Ferry SL, Cook KR. Local anesthetic systemic toxicity (LAST): increasing awareness. *J Perianesth Nurs*. 2020;35(4):365-367. Available at: https://doi.org/10.1016/j.jopan.2020.02.013.

33. West C. Anesthesia agents & adjuncts. C. Regional anesthesia. In: ASPAN. *A Competency-Based Orientation Program for the Registered Nurse in the Perianesthesia Setting*. ASPAN; 2019.

34. American Society of PeriAnesthesia Nurses. *2023-2024 Perianesthesia Nursing Standards, Practice Recommendations and Interpretive Statements*. ASPAN; 2022.

35. Li C, Zhao B, Li L, Na G, Lin C. Analysis of the risk factors for the onset of postoperative hypothermia in the postanesthesia care unit. *J Perianesth Nurs*. 2021;36(3):238-241. Available at: https://doi.org/10.1016/j.jopan.2020.09.003.

36. Wagner D, Hooper V, Bankieris K, Johnson A. The relationship of postoperative delirium and unplanned perioperative hypothermia in surgical patients. *J Perianesth Nurs*. 2021;36(1):41-46. Available at: https://doi.org/10.1016/j.jopan.2020.06.015.

37. Mullins MF. Malignant hyperthermia: a review. *J Perianesth Nurs*. 2018;33(5):582-589. Available at: https://doi.org/10.1016/j.jopan.2017.04.008.

38. Malignant Hyperthermia Association of United States. *Frequently Asked Questions*. MHAUS; 2023. Available at: https://www.mhaus.org/faqs/.

39. Elsevier. *Clinical Overview. Malignant Hyperthermia*. Elsevier; 2022. Available at: https://www.clinicalkey.com/#!/content/clinical_overview/67-s2.0-031f7e44-bc4d-42a6-8a64-95c2222e17df?scrollTo=%2367-s2.0-031f7e44-bc4d-42a6-8a64-95c2222e17df-f9a9b7cf-d6e2-46e6-8654-653c663dccb9-annotated.

9 General Anesthesia

Denise Faraone Diaz, MSN, BA, RN, CPAN, CAPA

LEARNING OBJECTIVES

A review of the content of this chapter will help the reader to:

1. Apply perianesthesia nursing principles to the care of patients receiving general anesthesia.
2. Demonstrate knowledge of select competencies to safely care for patients receiving general anesthesia.
3. Differentiate among different types of general anesthesia.
4. Recognize potential complications of general anesthesia.

GENERAL ANESTHESIA OVERVIEW

Patients receiving general anesthesia are completely unconsciousness and do not feel pain during surgical procedures. In this state, the patient has lost all protective reflexes and is unable to maintain a patent airway. The perianesthesia registered nurse should be aware of the types and classifications of drugs used to induce and maintain general anesthesia, as well as any potential complications of these drugs. A focused nursing assessment of the patient recovering from general anesthesia can prevent complications and emergencies and promote patient safety in the perianesthesia setting.

Introduction to General Anesthesia

Anesthesia is a temporary state of induced loss of sensation or awareness that can include analgesia, paralysis, amnesia, or loss of consciousness. General anesthesia is a drug-induced loss of consciousness characterized by partial or complete loss of protective reflexes. Patients under general anesthesia are unable to breathe independently and require ventilatory support, and they are unable to be aroused or respond to even painful stimuli.[1] The patient's physical status and type of surgery often determine the need for general anesthesia. The American Society of Anesthesiologists (ASA) Physical Status Classification System is one of several tools available for determining a patient's risk related to the administration of anesthesia.

ASA Physical Status Classification System

The ASA Physical Status Classification System (Figure 9.1) was developed by the American Society of Anesthesiologists (ASA) over 60 years ago. The system is used to assess a patient's preanesthesia co-morbidities. While the classification system alone does not predict perioperative risks, it can be used in conjunction with other indicators, such as the type of surgery and the patient's frailty, to predict risks associated with surgery and anesthesia.

The anesthesia provider assigns an ASA score, also called a physical status (PS) score, based on multiple factors after evaluating the patient on the day of surgery. The ASA PS classification is as follows:

- ASA I denotes a normal healthy patient.
- ASA II denotes a patient with mild systemic disease, such as well-controlled diabetes mellitus or hypertension.

ASA physical status classification scoring system	
ASA physical status 1	A normal healthy patient
ASA physical status 2	A patient with mild systemic disease
ASA physical status 3	A patient with severe systemic disease
ASA physical status 4	A patient with severe systemic disease that is a constant threat to life
ASA physical status 5	A moribund patient who is not expected to survive without the operation
ASA physical status 6	A declared brain-dead patient whose organs are being removed for donor purposes

Fig. 9.1 ASA Physical Status Classification. Brenner P, Kautz DD. Postoperative care of patients undergoing same-day laparoscopic cholecystectomy. *AORN J.* 2015;102(1):15–32.

- ASA III denotes a patient with severe systemic disease, such as poorly controlled diabetes mellitus or hypertension, or a history of myocardial infarction or chronic obstructive pulmonary disease.
- ASA IV denotes a patient with severe systemic disease that is a constant threat to life, such as one with end-stage renal disease not currently undergoing scheduled dialysis.
- ASA V denotes a moribund patient who is not expected to survive without surgical intervention with a condition such as a ruptured abdominal or thoracic aneurysm, an intracranial bleed, or massive trauma.
- ASA VI denotes a patient declared brain-dead who is undergoing surgery to remove organs for donor purposes.

The addition of an "E" to any ASA PS score indicates an emergency surgery.[2]

Stages of Anesthesia

General anesthesia occurs along a continuum that starts with diminished consciousness and pain perception and ends with muscle relaxation and cessation of spontaneous respirations. There are four stages of general anesthesia (Figure 9.2).[3]

Stage I is known as the *stage of anesthesia*. It begins with the initiation of general anesthesia and ends with the loss of consciousness. This stage is the lightest level of anesthesia. During this stage, patients can breathe spontaneously and open their eyes on command, maintain protective reflexes, and respond to stimuli.

Stage II is known as the *stage of delirium*. It begins with the loss of consciousness and ends with the onset of a regular pattern of breathing and loss of the eyelid reflex. In this stage of excitement, untoward responses such as vomiting, laryngospasm, and cardiac arrest can occur.

Stage III is the *stage of surgical anesthesia*. It lasts from the onset of a regular pattern of breathing to the cessation of spontaneous respiration. At this stage, patients do not respond to surgical incision. Stage III is further divided into four planes:

1. The patient enters Plane 1 when respirations become regular. The vomiting reflex gradually diminishes during this plane. Swallowing, retching, and vomiting reflexes disappear in that order during induction and reappear in the same order as the patient emerges from anesthesia.
2. Plane 2 begins when the eyeballs stop moving and become concentrically fixed and ends with the beginning of decreased intercostal muscle activity. During this plane, the threat of laryngospasm disappears.
3. The patient enters Plane 3 when intercostal muscle paralysis occurs, and respirations are solely produced by the diaphragm.
4. Plane 4 lasts from the time of intercostal muscle paralysis to the absence of spontaneous respiration.

Stage IV is the *stage of overdose*. This stage is characterized by medullary depression and circulatory system failure.

INDUCTION AGENTS

Intravenous (IV) agents are commonly used for both the induction and maintenance of general anesthesia. Induction of general anesthesia occurs more quickly and smoothly with the use of IV agents as opposed to inhalation agents.[1] Although IV agents are commonly used to induce general anesthesia in adults, inhalation agents are the preferred method of induction for pediatric patients.

There are several categories of IV induction agents that include sedative and hypnotic agents (including barbiturates and nonbarbiturates), dissociative agents, alpha$_2$ antagonists, and benzodiazepines. The anesthesia provider may choose one or any number of these agents to induce general anesthesia.

	Respiration		Ocular movements	Pupils no pre-med	Eye reflexes	Pharynx larynx reflexes	Lacrimation	Muscle tone	Resp. response incision
	Intercostal	Diaphragm							
Stage I			Voluntary control				Normal	Normal	
Stage II					Lid tone	Swallow / Retch		Tense struggle	
Stage III Plane 1						Vomit			
Plane 2					Corneal	Glottis			
Plane 3					Pupillary light reflex				
Plane 4						Carinal			
Stage IV									

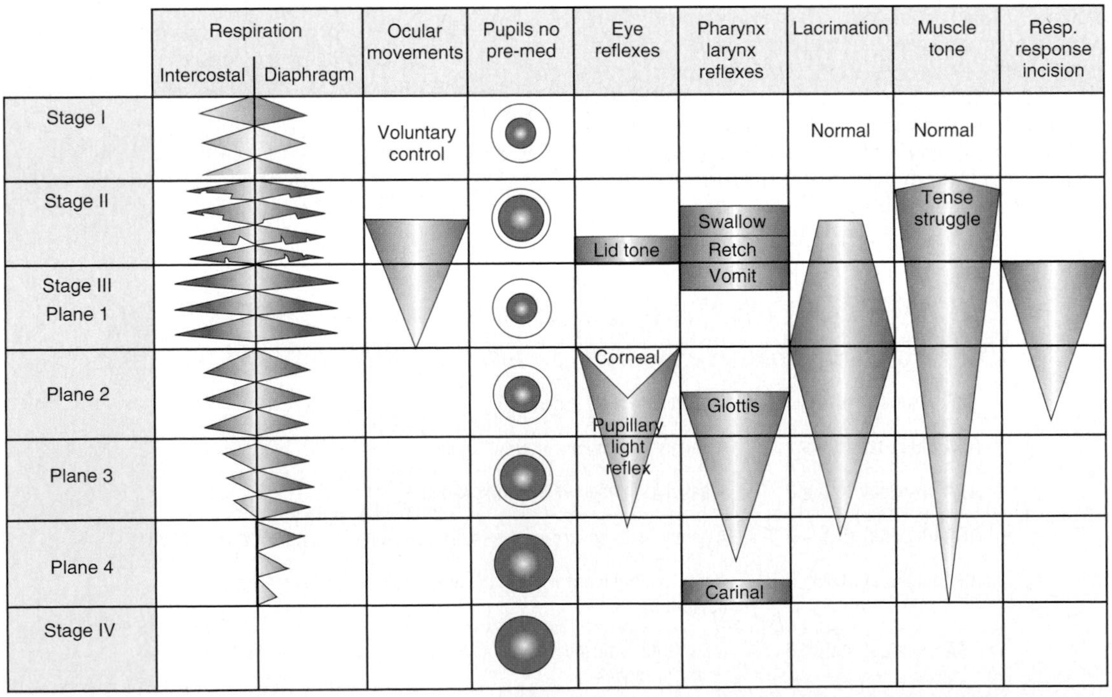

Fig. 9.2 Four stages of general anesthesia. Modified from Odom-Forren J. *Drain's Perianesthesia Nursing: A Critical Care Approach*. 7th ed. Elsevier; 2018; Figure 20.1. Adapted from Gillespie NA: Signs of anesthesia, *Anesth Analg*. 1943;22:275. https://www.clinicalkey.com/nursing/#!/content/book/3-s2.0-B9780323399845000205?scrollTo=%23f0010

Sedative and Hypnotic Agents

Sedative and hypnotic agents are commonly used to induce general anesthesia and can be further categorized as barbiturates and nonbarbiturates. Barbiturate agents, such as thiopental and methohexital, work by decreasing neuronal excitability in the brain. These agents can decrease intracranial pressure because they reduce the cerebral blood flow, and they have little to no analgesic or muscle relaxant effects. Their rapid onset and quick recovery time make them an ideal choice for IV induction, but side effects can include hypotension, respiratory depression, laryngospasm or bronchospasm, and bradycardia.

The nonbarbiturate sedative and hypnotic agents most commonly used to induce general anesthesia include etomidate and propofol.[1] For patients with a history of cardiovascular disease, etomidate is preferred because it is less likely than propofol to cause hypotension. Etomidate carries minimal negative ionotropic effects but can cause nausea and vomiting in some patients. Propofol, a milky-white emulsion, is contraindicated in patients with egg or soy allergies. If administered too quickly, propofol can cause hypotension, and it carries a very high incidence of pain at the injection site. While propofol is less likely than etomidate to cause nausea and vomiting, it does not have any analgesic qualities.

Propofol is an excellent choice for procedures requiring a short period of sedation, such as cardioversion. While it is commonly used for induction, it can be used continuously during surgery and in the postanesthesia care unit (PACU) as an IV infusion with the level of sedation titrated to give the desired effect. When the infusion is discontinued, the patient can be extubated in a short period of time. Long-term use of propofol infusion can result in increased triglyceride levels and can be associated with pancreatitis. Use of propofol infusion in children is not recommended in the PACU due to the possibility of emergence delirium.[1]

Dissociative Agent

The drug ketamine is known as a dissociative agent because it is known to cause vivid hallucinations both during and after surgery. It is an IV induction agent related to phencyclidine (PCP) and lysergic acid diethylamide (LSD). Ketamine has excellent analgesic properties and can be used to manage postoperative pain, particularly in patients with a history of chronic pain. It does not produce respiratory depression, but increased salivary gland secretion is commonly seen.[1,4]

As patients emerge from ketamine, they may experience a phase of vivid dreaming that may include hallucinations, confusion, and irrational behavior, though pediatric patients seem to be less prone to these side effects. Reducing auditory, tactile, and visual stimulation upon the patient's arrival to the PACU may help reduce symptoms. The anesthesia provider may administer the alpha$_2$ agonist dexmedetomidine to reduce these untoward side effects. Because of the increased salivation that typically occurs following administration of ketamine, the PACU nurse should assess for mechanical airway obstruction and respiratory insufficiency.[4]

Alpha$_2$ Agonists

The prototypical alpha$_2$ agonist is clonidine, a drug useful in preventing and treating chronic pain as well as emergence delirium in children. Side effects of clonidine include dry mouth, sedation, bradycardia, and contact dermatitis.[1]

Dexmedetomidine is a newer alpha$_2$ agonist that, like clonidine, provides sedation and analgesia without causing respiratory depression. Because the drug is highly selective for alpha receptors, it can reduce the need for inhalation agents and opioids during induction. While it can be useful to treat delirium associated with ketamine, dexmedetomidine can cause perioperative hypothermia.[4] Continuous IV infusion can cause bradycardia and hypotension; therefore, an infusion should not last longer than 24 hours.[1,4]

Benzodiazepines

When used as induction agents, benzodiazepines produce an excellent hypnotic effect, retrograde amnesia, anxiolysis, and skeletal muscle relaxation. They work by depressing the limbic system without causing cortical depression. The IV benzodiazepines most commonly used for anesthesia induction are midazolam, diazepam, and lorazepam.

Midazolam has become popular as a premedication and as an intraoperative adjunct for inhalation anesthesia. It has excellent hypnotic and muscle-relaxant abilities and is an effective anticonvulsant. Diazepam is useful for allaying apprehension and, like midazolam, also has anticonvulsant properties. Lorazepam is long-acting but has a slow onset and is sometimes used to treat agitation in critically ill patients. The effects of benzodiazepines can be reversed with flumazenil, a benzodiazepine antagonist. The usual reversal dose of flumazenil is 0.4 mg administered slowly in 0.1 mg increments intravenously to avoid the consequences of waking abruptly. Following administration of flumazenil, patients should be monitored for resedation in the PACU.[1]

INHALATION AGENTS

Inhalation agents are used to produce unconsciousness and amnesia. In adult patients, inhalation agents are mainly used for the maintenance of general anesthesia, but these drugs are commonly used for induction in children.

Inhalation agents are typically administered through an anesthesia machine that is essentially a breathing circuit that delivers the agent and oxygen to the patient (Figure 9.3). Inhalation agents are characterized as gaseous or volatile: gaseous agents are in the gaseous state at room temperature, whereas volatile agents are in the liquid state at room temperature.[3]

Gaseous Agent

Nitrous oxide (N_2O) is the only inorganic gas used as an anesthetic agent. It can be odorless or sweet-smelling and can be used in conjunction with a volatile inhalation agent. Nitrous oxide has very good analgesic effects but is associated with a high incidence of postoperative nausea and vomiting (PONV).[1]

Although the N_2O molecule contains oxygen, that oxygen is unavailable for respiration, so oxygen must be administered concurrently. When the delivery of N_2O is stopped, the full amount of the gas can diffuse back into the alveoli, putting the patient at risk of diffusion hypoxia. Therefore, patients must be monitored closely for signs of hypoxia or anoxia upon arrival in the PACU.[3]

Volatile Agents

The most commonly used modern inhalation anesthetic agents include sevoflurane, isoflurane, and desflurane. Sevoflurane is a rapid-acting agent that is not irritating to the respiratory tract. Patients typically emerge quickly from this agent, and therefore there is a need for analgesia in the immediate postoperative period. Because it is sweet-smelling and nonirritating, sevoflurane is the drug of choice for inhalation induction in children. While it is a respiratory depressant, it is not likely to induce arrhythmias, has little effect on the heart rate, and does not depress kidney or liver function.[3]

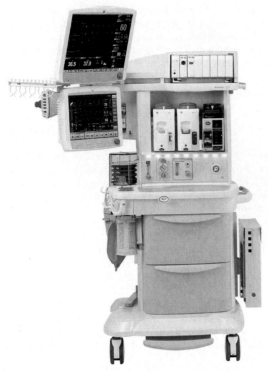

Fig. 9.3 Anesthesia machine. Odom-Forren J. *Drain's Perianesthesia Nursing: A Critical Care Approach.* 7th ed. Elsevier; 2018; Figure 20.2. https://www.clinicalkey.com/nursing/#!/content/book/3-s2.0-B97803 23399845000205?scrollTo=%23f0010)

Neither isoflurane nor desflurane are suitable for mask induction because both have a strong, pungent odor and can cause breath-holding, coughing, and laryngospasm. These agents are used for maintenance anesthesia following induction.[1]

ANESTHESIA ADJUNCTS
Opioids

When used as an IV adjunct to general anesthesia, opioid medications enhance the effectiveness of inhalation agents and manage intraoperative and postoperative pain. Opioids are drugs that contain opium or a derivative of opium, along with synthetic or semisynthetic drugs that have opium-like properties.[5] They can be natural, semisynthetic, or synthetic. Natural opiates are alkaloids, nitrogen-containing base chemical compounds that occur in plants. Semisynthetic opioids are created in laboratories from natural opiates, and fully synthetic opioids are completely manmade. Box 9.1 lists common natural, semisynthetic, and synthetic opioids.[5]

The effects of opioids can last well into the postoperative period, thereby putting the patient at risk of opioid overdose. Potential signs and symptoms of opioid overdose include pinpoint pupils, respiratory depression, hypotension, airway obstruction, and seizures. The opioid antagonist naloxone is used to treat opioid overdose and should be administered slowly to prevent acute pain, hypertension, pulmonary edema, and arrhythmias. A typical naloxone dose of 0.2–0.4 mg reverses the respiratory depression, as well as the analgesic effects, associated with opioid overdose.[1]

Anticholinergics

Anticholinergic agents block acetylcholine and inhibit parasympathetic nerve impulses that control involuntary muscle

BOX 9.1 Natural, Semisynthetic, and Synthetic Opioids

Natural	Morphine
	Codeine
Semisynthetic	Hydromorphone
	Hydrocodone
	Oxycodone
Synthetic	Fentanyl
	Meperidine
	Methadone
	Tramadol

Source: Drain CB. Opioid intravenous anesthetics. In Odom-Forren J: *Drain's PeriAnesthesia Nursing: A Critical Care Approach.* 7th ed. Elsevier; 2018.

movements in the gastrointestinal tract, lungs, and urinary tract. When acetylcholine signals are blocked during surgery, involuntary movements, digestive processes, and mucus production are decreased. Patients who received an anticholinergic agent may experience urinary retention and dry mouth.

Anticholinergic agents used during surgery include atropine, scopolamine, and glycopyrrolate. Atropine counteracts bradycardia and arrythmias while inhibiting the production of respiratory and salivary secretions. It can cause postoperative dysphonia (difficulty speaking). Scopolamine, which can be administered subcutaneously, intramuscularly, or intravenously, is also available as a transdermal patch applied prior to surgery to prevent postoperative nausea and vomiting. The drug inhibits secretions but is less effective at preventing bradycardia and more likely to cause postoperative delirium than atropine. When removing the scopolamine patch, patients must be instructed to avoid touching their eyes after touching the drug as this can cause pupillary dilation. Glycopyrrolate is longer acting than atropine and more effective at reducing salivary and gastric acid secretions.[1]

COMPLICATIONS OF GENERAL ANESTHESIA

A number of complications and emergencies can occur as the patient emerges from general anesthesia. More detailed descriptions of the potential complications can be found in Chapter 8. The most common types of general anesthesia complications seen in the immediate postoperative period include respiratory, cardiovascular, and neurologic complications, as well as postoperative nausea and vomiting (PONV).[6,7]

Respiratory Complications

All general anesthetics and opioid drugs have respiratory depressant effects. Acute postoperative pain can impair the ability to breathe deeply, putting the patient at further risk of respiratory compromise. Respiratory complications following general surgery include airway obstruction, laryngeal edema, laryngospasm, bronchospasm, noncardiogenic pulmonary edema, aspiration, hypoxemia, and hypoventilation.[6,7] Table 9.1 lists the causes, signs and symptoms, and nursing interventions for each of these complications.[6]

Cardiovascular Complications

The anesthetic effects of general anesthesia can alter the cardiac output, leading to cardiovascular complications such as dysrhythmias, postoperative hypertension, and postoperative hypotension.

TABLE 9.1 Respiratory Complications Following General Anesthesia

Complication	Cause	Patient Presentation	Nursing Interventions
Airway obstruction	Relaxed nasal or oropharyngeal muscles, rigid neck muscles, upper respiratory tract secretions, soft tissue obstruction such as the tongue	Stridor, nostril flaring, snoring, tachycardia, decreased breath sounds, intercostal retractions	Airway repositioning, insertion of nasopharyngeal or oropharyngeal airway NOTE: Do not use oropharyngeal airway in a conscious patient as this may cause gagging, vomiting, and laryngospasm
Laryngeal edema	Swelling of laryngeal tissue, allergic reaction	Stridor, hoarseness, intercostal retractions, croup-like cough	Airway repositioning, humidified oxygen, nebulized racemic epinephrine; administer epinephrine, bronchodilators, and antihistamines if result of allergic reaction
Laryngospasm	Reflex contractions of pharyngeal muscles which cause vocal cord spasm: airway emergency	Dyspnea, hypoxia, hypoventilation, absence of breath sounds, hypercarbia, high-pitched "crowing" sound	Positive-pressure mask ventilation with 100% oxygen; patient may require succinylcholine to relax the vocal cords to allow for ventilation
Bronchospasm	Increase in smooth muscle tone in lower airways causing constriction and airway obstruction, inflammation, asthma	Wheezing, shallow respirations, use of accessory muscles, hypertension, tachycardia	Inhaled bronchodilators
Noncardiogenic pulmonary edema	Upper airway obstruction (usually laryngospasm) that causes fluid in interstitial spaces of alveoli; can occur following naloxone administration	Tachypnea, dyspnea, crackles on auscultation	Supplemental oxygen, CPAP or mechanical ventilation with PEEP, pulmonary toileting, administration of morphine and corticosteroids
Aspiration	Passage of regurgitated stomach contents or foreign materials into trachea	Tachypnea, dyspnea, decreased oxygen saturation levels, wheezing, chest pain, tachycardia	Supplemental oxygen, CPAP
Hypoxemia	Respiratory depressant effects of anesthetic agents; more common following abdominal surgery	Decreased oxygen saturation levels	Supplemental oxygen, promotion of deep breathing, use of incentive spirometry
Hypoventilation	Central respiratory depression from anesthetic agents, incomplete neuromuscular blockade reversal	Hypertension, tachycardia, hypoxemia	Supplemental oxygen, repositioning

Source: Gelinas C. Pain and pain management. In Urden JD, Stacy KM, Lough ME: *Critical Care Nursing: Diagnosis and Management*. 9th ed. Elsevier; 2022.

Because general anesthesia lowers the dysrhythmia threshold of the myocardium, patients can experience sinus tachycardia, sinus bradycardia, premature ventricular contractions, supraventricular tachydysrhythmias, and ventricular tachycardia. The American Society of PeriAnesthesia Nurses (ASPAN) recommends that perianesthesia nurses be able to interpret cardiac rhythms.[8] Always refer to advanced cardiac life support (ACLS) guidelines for appropriate dysrhythmia interventions.

Postoperative hypertension is a common occurrence in the postoperative period and is usually related to fluid overload, preexisting hypertension, or heightened activity of the sympathetic nervous system. The stress of surgery, postoperative pain, anxiety or restlessness during emergence, bladder or bowel distention, or hypothermia can increase the sympathetic tone and result in hypertension. Hypoxia or hypercarbia can stimulate the autonomic nervous system, and these factors can occur alone or in combination. Perianesthesia nurses should work to identify and treat the cause of postoperative hypertension.[6,7]

The most common cause of postoperative hypotension is intravascular volume depletion resulting from inadequate replacement of blood loss, insensible loss, third-space fluid loss, and urinary output. More serious causes of postoperative hypotension include reduced preload caused by pulmonary embolism, reduced afterload caused by sepsis or hyperthermia, or reduced myocardial contractility caused by myocardial ischemia and dysrhythmias. Prolonged hypotension can lead to serious ischemic organ damage, so prompt treatment is essential. Patients may require increased IV fluids or vasopressors to maintain perfusion.[6,7]

Neurologic Complications

Most patients exhibit some level of arousal within 15 minutes after anesthesia is complete, but alterations in emergence can manifest as delayed emergence or emergence delirium.

Delayed emergence is defined as a failure to regain consciousness within 20 to 30 minutes after anesthesia is complete. Causes include prolonged action of anesthetic agents, metabolic alterations, or neurologic injury. In most cases, prolonged sedation is the result of residual general anesthetic and can be exacerbated by administration of opioids or benzodiazepines. Hypothermia, advanced age, hepatic dysfunction, and renal disease can also cause delayed emergence. In diabetic patients, fasting or excessive insulin can lead to unconsciousness.

The successful management of delayed emergence depends on careful consideration of the differential diagnosis. Patients may require interventions such as supplemental oxygenation with adequate gas exchange, implementation of warming measures to increase body temperature, assessment of serum electrolyte and blood glucose levels with appropriate replacements and interventions, or administration of reversal agents such as naloxone or flumazenil. Neurologic injury is typically a diagnosis of exclusion, but if all other causes of emergence delirium have been ruled out, the patient may require a neurologic consultation.[6,7]

Emergence delirium occurs when patients emerge from general anesthesia in a state of excitement and display restlessness, disorientation, crying, moaning, or irrational talking. In this extreme form of excitement, the patient may scream, shout, and thrash about wildly. This condition is seen most frequently after tonsillectomy, thyroid surgery, circumcision, hysterectomy, and perineal and abdominal wall procedures.

Causes of emergence delirium include hypoxia, hypercarbia, hyponatremia, pain, urinary bladder and gastric distention, and reaction to anticholinergics or ketamine. Patients who were anxious or fearful prior to surgery are more likely to experience emergence delirium. Young patients and patients undergoing emergency surgery have an increased incidence of postoperative excitation, as do patients with a history of alcoholism, insomnia, depression, or debility.

Management of emergence delirium includes determining a cause, initiating the specific therapy, and protecting patients from injuring themselves. Hypoxia must be first ruled out as the underlying cause. Prevent postoperative anxiety by providing patient support and reassurance prior to surgery. Patients in pain who do not experience relief with opioids may benefit from a short-acting benzodiazepine. A restless patient requires constant, careful observation, and gentle physical restraint may be required to prevent injury.[6,7]

Postoperative Nausea and Vomiting

Postoperative nausea and vomiting (PONV) is a significant cause of postoperative morbidity and patient discomfort and the leading cause of unexpected hospitalization after surgery. Risk factors most strongly associated with PONV include nonsmoker, female sex, history of PONV or motion sickness, postoperative use of opioids, and use of volatile inhalation agents or nitrous oxide during surgery.[6,7]

In the PACU, nausea typically precedes vomiting and is frequently accompanied by excessive salivation, tachypnea, dilated pupils, pallor, sweating, and tachypnea. If retching occurs, the patient may become bradycardic. The perianesthesia nurse should remain with the patient to prevent aspiration should the patient begin vomiting without notice. Encourage patients to remain calm and breathe deeply. Pharmacologic intervention may be required. Box 9.2 lists drugs commonly used to treat PONV.[7]

Evidence-Based Practice: Postoperative shivering

Shivering following anesthesia is among the top five postoperative clinical conditions which also includes postoperative nausea and vomiting, hypoxia, hypothermia, and cardiovascular instability. The incidence of postoperative shivering after general anesthesia is estimated to occur in nearly 66% of cases, despite not always being associated with hypothermia. Patients at risk for postoperative shivering are generally younger, having endoprosthetic surgery, or developed core hypothermia while in the operating room. Shivering not only leads to increase oxygen demands but can lead to hypertension and adversely impact patient satisfaction. Treatment for postoperative shivering includes the application of passive or active warming devices and in some cases, the administration of pharmacologic agents which commonly have demonstrated effective reduction in shivering. These agents include opioids, ondansetron, clonidine, ketamine, and dexmedetomidine. Meperidine 12.5 to 25 mg intravenously is most commonly administered to the adult patient.

Source: Berg SM, Braehler MR. The postanesthesia care unit. In: Gropper MA, ed. *Miller's Anesthesia.* 9th ed. Elsevier, 2020: 2586-2613.

OVERVIEW OF MUSCLE RELAXANTS

Muscle relaxants, also called neuromuscular blocking agents, are used during general anesthesia to block nerve impulses to the muscles and relax the body during surgery. These agents have been in use in clinical anesthesia since the early 1940s and are commonly used to enhance patient care in the PACU, critical care units, and emergency departments. Muscle relaxants are used to facilitation endotracheal intubation, to treat laryngospasm, to paralyze respiratory muscles to prepare for mechanical ventilation, to relax extraocular muscles for ophthalmic surgery, and to support muscle relaxation during surgical procedures.[9]

Physiology of Muscle Relaxants

There are both electric and biochemical factors that affect the activation of skeletal muscle. Conduction occurs when an impulse passes along an axon to a muscle fiber, and transmission occurs when a neurotransmitter substance passes across the neuromuscular junction. The biochemical neurotransmitter involved in the initiation of muscle contraction is acetylcholine.[9] Neuromuscular blocking agents work by blocking the action of acetylcholine in postsynaptic receptor sites in neuromuscular junctions, causing muscle paralysis.[10] Figure 9.4

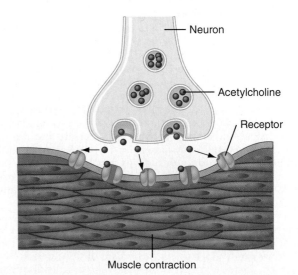

Fig. 9.4 Muscle contraction. Siedlecki SL. Pain and sedation. In: Good VS, Kirkwood PL: *Advanced Critical Care Nursing.* 2nd ed. Elsevier; 2018; p. 773.

BOX 9.2 Pharmacologic Interventions for PONV

Haloperidol	Dolasetron
Prochlorperazine	Granisetron
Promethazine	Palonosetron
Diphenhydramine	Scopolamine
Metoclopramide	Dexamethasone
Ondansetron	Apretitant

Source: O'Brien D. Postanesthesia care complications. In Odom-Forren J: *Drain's PeriAnesthesia Nursing: A Critical Care Approach.* 7th ed. Elsevier; 2018.

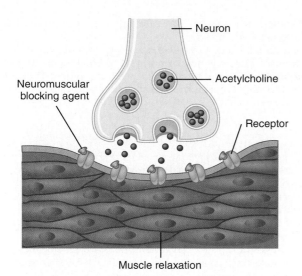

Fig. 9.5 Muscle relaxation. Siedlecki SL. Pain and sedation. In: Good VS, Kirkwood PL: *Advanced Critical Care Nursing.* 2nd ed. Elsevier; 2018; p. 773.

depicts normal muscle contraction, while Figure 9.5 shows how muscle relaxants block the action of acetylcholine.

Neuromuscular blockades are classified as depolarizing or nondepolarizing. Depolarizing muscle relaxants act as acetylcholine receptor agonists that bind to acetylcholine receptors and generate an action potential. Because they are not metabolized by acetylcholinesterase, the binding of this drug to the receptor is prolonged, resulting in an extended depolarization. Nondepolarizing muscle relaxants act as competitive antagonists that bind to receptors and prevent acetylcholine from binding. Their effects can be overcome with reversal agents.[11]

Patients can still feel pain even after a full neuromuscular block is achieved, so general anesthetics and analgesics are given to prevent anesthesia awareness.

Depolarizing Agent

Succinylcholine chloride is the only depolarizing muscle relaxant. The drug is given in bolus form only and is used for rapid-sequence intubation. Succinylcholine should be used with extreme caution as it can cause a rapid elevation in serum potassium levels, increasing the risk of hyperkalemia and cardiac arrest.[10]

Because succinylcholine is a depolarizing agent, anticholinesterase agents are not used to reverse the effects of the drug; doing so would likely increase the degree of neuromuscular blockade. Overdose of succinylcholine chloride is treated by discontinuing the drug and providing airway maintenance and respiratory support until the effects of the drug have worn off.[10] Succinylcholine is a triggering agent for malignant hyperthermia, a rare but potentially life-threatening genetic disorder characterized by sustained muscle contractions.

Nondepolarizing Agents

Nondepolarizing neuromuscular blocking agents can be long-, intermediate-, or short-acting agents.[9,10] The long-acting agent pancuronium bromide has a 1- to 2-hour duration of action and can be used for continuous infusion. It should not be used in patients who cannot tolerate an increased heart rate.[10] Vecuronium bromide, atracurium, and cisatracurium are intermediate-acting agents that peak in 25–35 minutes.[10] Rocuronium is a short-acting agent with a rapid onset and short duration, and these features are not altered in obese patients. Because rocuronium has such rapid effects and a short duration of action, spontaneous recovery from neuromuscular blockade is possible.[9]

Nondepolarizing muscle relaxants are reversed by anticholinesterase drugs that increase the amount of acetylcholine available at the receptor sites, resulting in the return of normal skeletal muscle function. Increased levels of acetylcholine at receptor sites in the heart, lungs, eyes, and gastrointestinal tract can cause bradycardia, bronchospasm, miosis, and increased peristalsis and secretion. Anticholinergic agents such as atropine or glycopyrrolate are often given along with the reversal agent to prevent or minimize these effects.[11]

In 2015, the Food and Drug Administration approved sugammadex for the reversal of neuromuscular blockade. Sugammadex does not have an effect on acetylcholinesterases, so it is not necessary to administer anticholinergic drugs along with this reversal agent. Sugammadex, however, may bind to progesterone; therefore, patients taking contraceptives should be advised to use an additional nonhormonal contraceptive method for 7 days following surgery.[12] Table 9.2 summarizes the characteristics of reversal agents and anticholinergic agents.

Complications of Muscle Relaxants

Patients may experience a prolonged response to neuromuscular blockade due to an overdose; the use of antibiotics; or the presence of temperature changes, an acid–base imbalance, carcinoma, myasthenia gravis, or liver disease.[9] Complications of muscle relaxants include residual paralysis and bradycardia. Residual paralysis, also called compromised ventilation, partial reversal, or reduced train-of-four, occurs when the patient re-experiences the pharmacologic actions of a nondepolarizing

TABLE 9.2 Commonly Used Anticholinesterase, Anticholinergic, and Select Relaxant Binding Agents

Agent	Dosage Range	Onset (minutes)	Duration	Comments
Neostigmine	25–75 µg/kg	5–15	45–90 minutes	Most commonly used reversal agent; may increase incidence of postoperative nausea and vomiting
Edrophonium	500–1000 µg/kg	5–10	30–60 minutes	Not recommended for deep block; rapid onset, short duration
Atropine	15 µg/kg	1–2	1–2 hours	Should be combined with edrophonium because of more rapid onset
Glycopyrrolate	10–20 µg/kg	2	2–4 hours	Less initial tachycardia than atropine; no central nervous system effects; most frequently used
Sugammadex	2–16 mg/kg	1–2	2–16 hours	Selective relaxant binding agent; up to 16 mg/kg has been safely used

Source: Nagelhout J. Neuromuscular blocking agents, reversal agents, and their monitoring. In: Nagelhout JJ, Elisha S: *Nurse Anesthesia.* 6th ed. Elsevier; 2018.

skeletal muscle relaxant administered during surgery. Even with sufficient reversal, residual paralysis can occur for up to 8 hours; it is partly caused by the fading effect of neostigmine. Patients with residual paralysis exhibit a reduction in the ability to sustain a head lift for 5 seconds, phonate or ventilate adequately, or maintain their own airway. Avoid the use of opioids in these patients, as these agents enhance a residual neuromuscular block. The treatment for this complication is neostigmine.[9]

Bradycardia following neuromuscular blockade can occur when the patient has received an atropine–neostigmine combination, as neostigmine has a longer duration than atropine. When other causes of bradycardia, such as pain, hypoventilation, and a full bladder, have been ruled out, the treatment for this complication is glycopyrrolate.[9]

Plasma Cholinesterase Deficiency

Plasma cholinesterase deficiency is a rare disorder that renders patients unable to metabolize succinylcholine, resulting in prolonged skeletal muscle paralysis. The typical response to succinylcholine is skeletal muscle paralysis that lasts 5–10 minutes. Patients with abnormal or deficient plasma cholinesterase may remain apneic and paralyzed for longer than 2 hours.[7] Plasma cholinesterase deficiency can be genetic or acquired. Box 9.3 lists the causes of plasma cholinesterase deficiency.[7]

Because succinylcholine is not reversible, the care for plasma cholinesterase deficiency is supportive, with mechanical ventilation until the patient regains spontaneous respiratory effort. Patients should be counseled to carry identification that indicates they have plasma cholinesterase deficiency and to alert blood relatives that they may also have this genetic variant.[7]

CHAPTER HIGHLIGHTS

- General anesthesia is a state in which patients have lost all protective reflexes and are unable to independently maintain a patent airway.
- There are four stages of general anesthesia; they begin with diminished consciousness and pain perception and end with muscle relaxation and cessation of spontaneous respirations.
- Intravenous induction agents are commonly used for both the induction and maintenance of general anesthesia. There are several categories of IV induction agents.
- Inhalation agents are used to produce unconsciousness and amnesia. These drugs are used for induction in children, but in adults, they are mainly used for the maintenance of anesthesia following induction.
- The primary complications associated with general anesthesia affect the respiratory, cardiovascular, and neurologic systems.

BOX 9.3 Causes of Plasma Cholinesterase Deficiency

Liver disease
Malignancy
Pregnancy
Collagen vascular disease
Malnutrition
Hypothyroidism
Chronic infections, such as tuberculosis

Extensive burn injuries
Organophosphate pesticide poisoning
Uremia
Plasmapheresis

Source: O'Brien D. Postanesthesia care complications. In Odom-Forren J: *Drain's PeriAnesthesia Nursing: A Critical Care Approach.* 7th ed. Elsevier; 2018.

Postoperative nausea and vomiting is another complication of general anesthesia.
- Muscle relaxants, also called neuromuscular blocking agents, are used during general anesthesia to block nerve impulses to the muscles and relax the body during surgery. They work by blocking the action of acetylcholine and causing muscle paralysis.

CASE STUDY

Ciara is a 42-year-old female patient presenting for outpatient surgery for laparoscopic repair of a right inguinal hernia. Her past medical history is significant for allergy-induced asthma, which is being well-controlled with antihistamines, as well as type 2 diabetes mellitus, which is being controlled with diet and exercise. She is allergic to latex, eggs, and cat dander. Her body mass index is 36, categorizing her as obese. She does not smoke or consume alcohol. According to her preoperative anesthesia assessment, Ciara's physical status is ASA II. The plan today is for Ciara to receive general anesthesia with IV opioid pain control in the immediate postoperative period. When she has met the discharge criteria, she will be discharged home with a prescription for an opioid.

Based on her gender and smoking status, which postoperative complication is Ciara at risk of developing? What strategies can be used to prevent this complication? What drugs can be administered to treat this complication in the immediate postoperative period?

Based on her medical history, what respiratory complications is Ciara most at risk of developing? What are the nursing interventions for these complications?

REFERENCES

1. Brown C. Anesthesia, moderate sedation/analgesia. In: Schick L, Windle PE, eds. *PeriAnesthesia Nursing Core Curriculum: Preprocedure, Phase I and Phase II PACU Nursing.* 4th ed. Elsevier; 2021.
2. American Society of Anesthesiologists. *ASA Physical Status Classification System.* 2020. Available at: https https://www.asahq.org/standards-and-guidelines/asa-physical-status-classification-system. Accessed July 3, 2021.
3. Drain CB. Inhalation anesthesia. In: Odom-Forren J, ed. *Drain's PeriAnesthesia Nursing: A Critical Care Approach.* 7th ed. Elsevier; 2018:260-271.
4. Drain CB. Nonopioid intravenous anesthetics. In: Odom-Forren J, ed. *Drain's PeriAnesthesia Nursing: A Critical Care Approach.* 7th ed. Elsevier; 2018:272-283.
5. Drain CB. Opioid intravenous anesthetics. In: Odom-Forren J, ed. *Drain's PeriAnesthesia Nursing: A Critical Care Approach.* 7th ed. Elsevier; 2018:284-296.
6. Gelinas C. Pain and pain management. In: Urden JD, Stacy KM, Lough ME, eds. *Critical Care Nursing: Diagnosis and Management.* 9th ed. Elsevier; 2022;116-139.
7. O'Brien D. Postanesthesia care complications. In: Odom-Forren J, ed. *Drain's PeriAnesthesia Nursing: A Critical Care Approach.* 7th ed. Elsevier; 2018:398-416.
8. American Society of PeriAnesthesia Nurses. *2021-2022 Perianesthesia Nursing Standards, Practice Recommendations and Interpretive Statements.* ASPAN; 2021.
9. Drain C. Neuromuscular blocking agents. In: Odom-Forren J, ed. *Drain's PeriAnesthesia Nursing: A Critical Care Approach.* 7th ed. Elsevier; 2018:297-315.
10. Siedlecki S. Pain and sedation. In: Good VS, Kirkwood PL, eds. *Advanced Critical Care Nursing.* 2nd ed. Elsevier; 2018:746-778.
11. Nagelhout JJ. Neuromuscular blocking agents, reversal agents, and their monitoring. In: Nagelhout JJ, Elisha S, eds. *Nurse Anesthesia.* 6th ed. Elsevier; 2018:140-164.
12. Golembiewski J. Sugammadex. *J Perianesth Nurs.* 2016;31(4):354-357. Available at: https://doi.org/10.1016/j.jopan.2016.05.004.

10 Local and Regional Anesthesia

Denise Faraone Diaz, MSN, BA, RN, CPAN, CAPA

LEARNING OBJECTIVES

A review of the content of this chapter will help the reader to:

1. Apply perianesthesia nursing principles to the care of patients receiving regional or local anesthesia.
2. Demonstrate knowledge of select competencies to safely care for patients receiving regional or local anesthesia.
3. Differentiate among different types of regional and local anesthesia.
4. Recognize potential complications of regional and local anesthesia.

REGIONAL ANESTHESIA OVERVIEW

When compared with general anesthesia, regional anesthesia carries many benefits, including fewer drugs required to induce and maintain anesthesia, a reduced need for an artificial airway device, and overall decreased rates of morbidity and mortality. Regional anesthesia reduces the risk of systemic complications such as respiratory depression, pneumonia, deep vein thrombosis, pulmonary embolism, myocardial infarction, and renal failure. This technique has been shown to preserve immune function and decrease the risk of infection and may positively affect cognitive function and the return of gastrointestinal function.[1] Regional anesthesia includes neuraxial anesthesia, as well as peripheral nerve blocks and local anesthesia.

INTRODUCTION TO NEURAXIAL ANESTHESIA

Neuraxial anesthesia is a type of regional anesthesia in which an anesthetic agent is injected into the area around the nerve roots as they exit the spine or into the cerebrospinal fluid around the spinal cord. Central neuraxial anesthesia includes spinal and epidural blocks. The injections are often preceded by the administration of a local anesthetic or procedural sedation.

Neuraxial Anesthesia: Spinal Anesthesia

Spinal anesthesia is classified as regional anesthesia because it can anesthetize a selected region of the body from pain. As a type of neuraxial anesthesia, it is also called a subarachnoid or intrathecal block. Sensory and motor blockades are achieved when an anesthetic agent is injected into the intrathecal or subarachnoid space and the agent mixes with the cerebrospinal fluid directly at the nerve roots.[1,2] Spinal anesthesia is a single injection into the subarachnoid or intrathecal space. It is limited to the lower lumbar region and is typically used for lower extremity, abdominal, and perineal surgeries.[1]

The vertebral column is composed of 33 vertebrae: 7 cervical vertebrae that support the head and neck; 12 thoracic vertebrae that support the chest muscles; 5 lumbar vertebrae that support the lower back muscles; 5 sacral vertebrae that are fused into one to support the weight of the upper body; and 4 coccygeal vertebrae that are fused into one to support the pelvic muscles.[3] Figure 10.1 depicts the segments of the spinal cord.

The spinal cord lies within the same three membranes that line the cranium, collectively called the meninges. The meninges are supportive tissues that provide a protective covering for the cord and nerve roots. Within the spinal canal, the three membranes are called the dura mater, arachnoid mater, and pia mater. The outermost layer, the dura mater, is a thick, tough membrane that provides most of the protection for the central cord structures. The nerve roots are covered with the dura mater while inside the spinal canal. The arachnoid mater is a thin, spiderweb-like covering that forms the middle layer. Beneath the arachnoid mater is the subarachnoid space, which is filled with cerebrospinal fluid. Along with this fluid, the arachnoid mater protects the spinal cord from shock injuries. Together, the fluid and arachnoid mater are the medium for the interaction with local anesthetics and opioids that occurs during the administration of regional anesthesia. The innermost layer, the pia mater, is thin and is in direct contact with the outer surface of the spinal cord.[4] Figure 10.2 illustrates the linings of the spinal cord.

The spinal cord is a tubular bundle of nerves about 18 inches (20.3 cm) long. In most adults, it extends from the section of the brainstem known as the medulla oblongata to the lower lumbar region of the spine. It ends at the conus medullaris, the terminal end of the spinal cord, in the lumbar, or L1–L2, region. Below L1, the nerve fibers extend out to resemble a horse's tail in a section known as the cauda equina. There are 31 spinal nerves branching off the spinal cord that contain sensory and motor fibers. The sensory fibers enter and exit through the dorsal root, while the motor fibers enter and exit through anterior roots. To avoid spinal cord trauma associated with spinal anesthesia, the provider typically places spinal blocks below L1–L2 to block one section of the nerve roots.[3,4]

Dermatomes are carefully mapped pathways for the sensory portion of spinal nerves.[5] They correspond to bands circling the body containing sensory nerves able to transmit pain, temperature, and touch to the spinal cord. These bands are 1–2 inches wide and arise posteriorly from the spinal column and radiate away laterally, anteriorly, or caudally, like zebra stripes. They are typically numbered according to their point of origin.[3] Figure 10.3 illustrates the distribution of dermatomes on the front and back of the body. Dermatome levels, also called spinal levels, are used to determine the progression of an anesthetic nerve block and identify landmarks helpful for assessing a patient's level of numbness or loss of function. Box 10.1 identifies common landmarks used during dermatome assessment.[3]

After a local anesthetic agent is injected, the nerves become blocked in a certain pattern based on their sensitivity to the agent. Motor nerve fibers are more difficult to anesthetize than

SPINAL CORD SEGMENTS

The spinal cord contains 31 pairs of spinal nerves (part of the peripheral nervous system), which innervate segments of the body, from the back of the head to the feet. It is divided into 8 cervical, 12 thoracic, 5 lumbar, 5 sacral segments, and 1 coccygeal segment.

C1
C2
C3
C4
C5
C6
C7
C8
Cervical

T1
T2
T3
T4
T5
T6
T7
T8
T9
T10
T11
T12
Thoracic

L1
L2
L3
L4
L5
Lumbar

S1
S2
S3
S4
S5
Sacral

Coccygeal

Fig. 10.1 Segments of the spinal cord. (From Windle PE. Neurological. In: Schick L, Windle PE. *PeriAnesthesia Nursing Core Curriculum* E-book; and Figure 20.17 in: Luckmann J: *Saunders Manual of Nursing Care*, Saunders; 1997.)

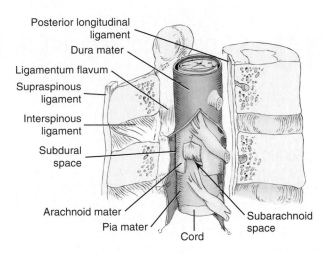

Fig. 10.2 Spinal cord linings. (From Pellegrini JE. Regional anesthesia. Figure 49.5 in: Nagelhout JJ, Elisha S. *Nurse Anesthesia*. 6th ed. Saunders; 2017.)

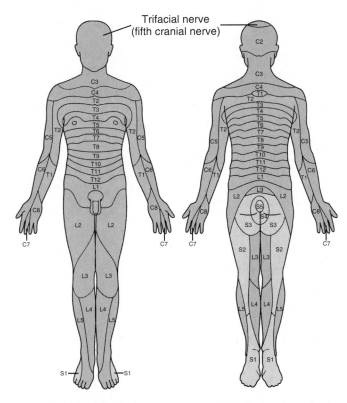

Fig. 10.3 Dermatome levels. (From Pellegrini JE. Regional anesthesia. Figure 49.6 in: Nagelhout JJ, Elisha S. *Nurse Anesthesia*. 6th ed. Saunders; 2017.)

BOX 10.1 Landmarks to Determine Dermatome Level

Neck, C3	Groin, L1
Clavicles, C5	Knees, L4
Nipples, T4	Dorsum of the feet, L5
Xiphoid, T6–7	Lateral ankles, S1
Umbilicus, T10	

Windle, PE. Neurological. Chapter 20 in: Schick L, Windle PE: *PeriAnesthesia Nursing Core Curriculum: Preprocedure, Phase I and Phase II PACU Nursing.* 4th ed. Elsevier; 2021.

sensory nerves, and sensory nerves are more difficult to anesthetize than sympathetic nerves. Nerve fibers are classified by different criteria, such as myelination (thickness of covering), function (sensory or motor), diameter, and conduction velocity. These classifications determine the sequence of blockade. When the anesthetic agent is administered, the blockade occurs in the following sequence: autonomic, sensory, motor. When the anesthetic resolves, function typically returns in the reverse order: motor, sensory, autonomic.[1]

Local anesthetics used for spinal anesthesia can be divided into two groups: amides and esters. Table 10.1 identifies common drugs classified as amides or esters and compares the two groups of local anesthetics.[2] Several factors affect the spread of a local anesthetic in the subarachnoid space, including the dosage, baricity (weight of the drugs), and patient characteristics such as height, weight, and positioning. Baricity refers to the proportional density of the solution to the density of the cerebrospinal fluid. Box 10.2 compares the density of solutions to the density of the cerebrospinal fluid.[6]

Spinal anesthesia may be used alone or in combination with other techniques, such as epidural, general, or intravenous (IV) anesthesia. Such multimodal combinations minimize the side effects of any single technique while maximizing the benefits of blended techniques.[1]

Evidence-Based Practice: Contraindications

There are several contraindications to the administration of a spinal or regional anesthetic. These include a diagnosis of sepsis, bacteremia, observed infection or disrupted skin integrity at the site of the injection, evidence of hypovolemia, known coagulopathies, current anticoagulation therapy use, increased intracranial pressure, and patient refusal.

Source: Hernandez A, Sherwood ER. Anesthesiology principles, pain management, and conscious sedation. In: Townsend CM, Beauchamp RD, Evers BM, Mattox KL, eds. *Sabiston: Textbook of Surgery: The Biological Basis of Modern Surgical Practice.* 21st ed. Elsevier, 2022:315-348.

Neuraxial Anesthesia: Epidural Anesthesia

Epidural anesthesia may not be the first choice for anesthesia in an outpatient setting. Factors that may influence the

TABLE 10.1 Comparison of Amide and Ester Local Anesthetics

	Amides	Esters
Drugs	Bupivacaine Levobupivacaine Lidocaine Mepivacaine Prilocaine Ropivacaine	Benzocaine Chloroprocaine Cocaine Procaine Tetracaine
Metabolism	Metabolized in the liver	Broken down by pseudocholinesterase
Duration	Longer acting because they must be transported to the liver for metabolism	Shorter acting because they are metabolized by hydrolysis and not in the liver
Considerations	Less likely to cause allergic reactions because allergies to amides are rare	More likely to cause allergic reactions because their metabolism releases an antigen that can trigger allergic reactions

Odom-Forren J. *Drain's PeriAnesthesia Nursing: A Critical Care Approach.* 7th ed. Table 24. Elsevier; 2018.

BOX 10.2 Baricity of Local Anesthetic Solutions

Hypobaric solutions	Weigh less than cerebrospinal fluid and tend to rise higher than the injection site (add sterile water)
Hyperbaric solutions	Weigh more than cerebrospinal fluid and sink down from the injection site (add dextrose)
Isobaric solutions	Same density as cerebrospinal fluid and stay at the injection site

The New York School of Regional Anesthesia (NYOSARA). Spinal anesthesia. https://www.nysora.com/techniques/neuraxial-and-perineuraxial-techniques/spinal-anesthesia/

---

decision not to use this approach include the length of time required for the placement and subsequent effect of the epidural and the potential for a prolonged recovery and an adverse impact on the discharge time, as well as the need to void prior to discharge due to the risk for bladder dysfunction. Epidural anesthesia, on the other hand, may be a preferred choice for certain patients and may prevent any sudden hemodynamic shifts observed with spinal anesthesia.

Epidural anesthesia, like spinal anesthesia, is a type of central neuraxial block. Both block the spinal nerve roots, although each type has a different site of administration and mechanism of action. A spinal anesthetic blocks the spinal nerve roots as they pass through the cerebrospinal fluid, resulting in a blockade of sensory, motor, and autonomic impulse transmissions, whereas an epidural anesthetic blocks the spinal nerves outside of the subarachnoid space. Whereas spinal anesthesia is accomplished by the administration of a small dose of local anesthetic into the subarachnoid space, epidural anesthesia requires a larger dose of local anesthetic to allow for diffusion through anatomic barriers, such as the dura mater and less vascularized tissues adjacent to the injection site. With an epidural, the local anesthesia spreads horizontally and vertically within the epidural space.[1]

Spinal anesthesia is a single injection through a needle, however epidural anesthesia is usually administered through a catheter placed through a needle, although single-shot epidurals are possible. The catheter–needle technique allows for repeated dosing and may be used for postoperative analgesia. Unlike spinal anesthesia that is limited to placement in the lower lumbar region below the termination of the spinal cord, epidural catheter placement can occur in the lumbar or thoracic region (see Figure 10.4). Spinal anesthesia is rapidly achieved and produces an intense sensory and motor block, while the onset of epidural anesthesia is gradual and its blockade is less profound.[1] Table 10.2 highlights the differences between spinal and epidural anesthesia.[1]

Neuraxial Anesthesia: Caudal Anesthesia

Caudal anesthesia is commonly used as a regional block in pediatric anesthesia. It can be used for any procedure involving innervation from the sacral, lumbar, or lower-thoracic dermatomes. Caudal anesthesia can be used in conjunction with general anesthesia or solely for postoperative pain management. In the neonate, it is most often placed after induction of general anesthesia prior to the beginning of the surgical procedure.[7] Figure 10.5 demonstrates the placement of a caudal block in a pediatric patient.

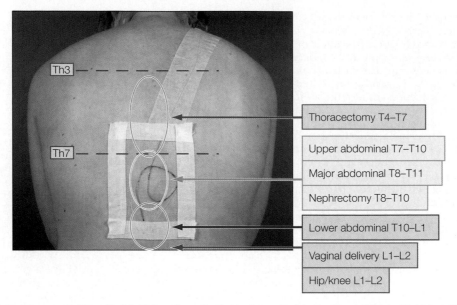

Fig. 10.4 Epidural catheter placement. (From Breivik H. Local anesthetic blocks and epidurals. Figure 37.1 in: McMahon SB, Koltzenburg M. *Wall & Melzack's Textbook of Pain.* 6th ed. Saunders; 2013. Adapted from Breivik H, Shipley M (eds). Plate I in: *Pain Best Practice and Research Compendium.* Elsevier; 2007.)

TABLE 10.2 Differences Between Spinal and Epidural Anesthesia

	Spinal	**Epidural**
Site or mechanism of action	Nerve roots blocked as they pass through the CSF	Nerve roots blocked outside the cerebrospinal fluid
Site of administration	Lower lumbar area below the termination of spinal cord	Lumbar or thoracic area
Dose of local anesthetic	Small	Large
Instrument for administration	Needle	Catheter
Ability to repeat dose	No	Yes
Onset	Rapid, intense blockade; may lead to hypotension	Gradual; may have less intense blockade; decrease in blood pressure is more gradual

Odom-Forren J. *Drain's PeriAnesthesia Nursing: A Critical Care Approach.* 7th ed. Table 25.1. Elsevier; 2018.

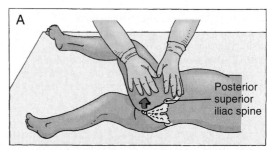

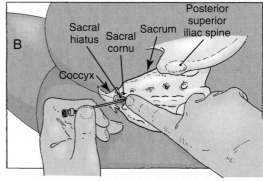

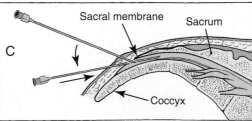

Fig. 10.5 Placement of a caudal block in a pediatric patient. (From Elisha S, Terry KL. Regional anesthesia. Modified from Figure 52.8 in: Nagelhout JJ, Elisha S. *Nurse Anesthesia.* 6th ed. Elsevier; 2018.)

COMPLICATIONS OF NEURAXIAL ANESTHESIA
Postdural Puncture Headache

Postdural puncture headache (PDPH) is a potential complication of spinal anesthesia. A PDPH occurs when the spinal needle inadvertently punctures the dura mater, resulting in a leak of cerebrospinal fluid. This leak decreases the overall volume of cerebrospinal fluid available in the subarachnoid space. Without hydraulic support, the medulla and brainstem drop into the foramen magnum, and this stretches the meninges and pulls on the tentorium. The "pulling" causes a characteristic headache that is exacerbated by movement or the placement of the patient in the upright position.[1,4]

Several factors are known to increase the incidence of PDPH, including the size of the spinal needle, female gender, age less than 40, and history of prior PDPH. These headaches usually occur within several hours to the first or second postoperative day and are typically described as a mild to incapacitating bilateral frontal headache that radiates from behind the eyes and across the head toward the occiput and often into the neck and shoulders. Accompanying symptoms may include nausea, vomiting, loss of appetite, blurred vision, photophobia, loss of hearing acuity, tinnitus, vertigo, and depression. The headache is relieved when the patient is lying down.[1,4]

PDPHs are self-limiting and often resolve in less than 10 days, but prompt treatment can prevent immobility, depression, and patient dissatisfaction. Conservative management includes a horizontal position, adequate hydration, oral analgesics, and caffeine therapy. The definitive treatment for PDPH is an epidural blood patch, which seals the dura mater and increases the cerebrospinal fluid pressure. An epidural blood patch is performed in a manner similar to that of placing an epidural catheter. Between 12 to 15 mL of blood is withdrawn from the patient's vein and slowly injected through the epidural needle into the epidural space. The patient should remain supine for 30 minutes to 1 hour following the procedure, though headache relief is often instantaneous. A repeat blood patch may be attempted in 24 hours.[1,4] Figure 10.5 illustrates how venous blood is injected into the epidural space.

Postoperative Nausea and Vomiting

Although regional anesthesia is associated with a lower incidence of postoperative nausea and vomiting (PONV) than general anesthesia, PONV following spinal anesthesia can occur. Nausea immediately after spinal anesthesia administration is considered a sign of significant hypotension and an ascending block level. PONV is typically treated with fluid administration and vasopressors. Hypotension that precipitates PONV can be avoided prior to initiation of spinal anesthesia with adequate hydration, supplemental oxygen, and premedication with antiemetic drugs.[1,4]

Urinary Retention

Postoperative urinary retention (POUR) is common after spinal anesthesia. The reported incidence of POUR is between 5% and 70%. Spinal or epidural anesthetics block sympathetic fibers and increase the tone of the internal urethral sphincter. Patients suspected of being at risk of POUR (e.g., having a known history of POUR, older adults, surgery involving the pelvis or rectum) should be assessed via portable bladder ultrasound. Catheterization is recommended when the bladder volume exceeds 600 mL to prevent the negative sequelae of prolonged bladder overdistention. Overdistended bladders and urinary retention requiring subsequent catheterization can lead to complications such as urinary tract infections and urethral strictures. Patients deemed at low risk for POUR, with a bladder volume of less than 600 mL, may be sent home with instructions to return if they cannot void.[1,4]

Neurologic Complications

While some patients express a fear of paraplegia resulting from neuraxial anesthesia, the incidence of persistent motor paralysis is exceedingly rare, occurring in less than 1 per 10,000 cases. Permanent neurologic deficits following spinal anesthesia can result from direct needle or catheter nerve injury, drug-related neurotoxicity, anterior spinal artery syndrome, undiagnosed neurologic disease, intraneural or intramedullary injections, the presence of blood in the cerebral spinal fluid (CSF), patient positioning, hematomas, and abscesses. The risk of these complications is reduced using good clinical practice and appropriate anesthetic techniques. Thorough postoperative assessments focusing on early detection, diagnosis, and treatment are essential considering that the reversibility of neurologic complications is often time dependent.[1,4]

Cardiac Arrest

Cardiac arrest associated with neuraxial anesthesia is often sudden and can result in severe neurologic injury and death.

This undesired complication occurs in young, previously healthy patients at an estimated rate of 7 in 10,000 for spinal anesthesia and 1 in 10,000 for epidural anesthesia.[4]

The cause of cardiac arrest during spinal or epidural anesthesia is related to severe bradycardia caused by the reduction of preload resulting from sympathetic blockade. Other factors that increase the risk of developing cardiac arrest include changes in patient positioning and hypovolemia. Efforts to prevent this complication include prophylactic preloading with IV fluids and patient positioning to encourage venous return. Vasopressors may be required to maintain adequate preload. Bradycardia during spinal anesthesia is managed with atropine, ephedrine, or epinephrine.[4]

High Spinal Block

High spinal block occurs when there is an excessive spread of local anesthetic from spinal or epidural anesthesia, resulting in upper extremity sensory and motor changes, nausea and vomiting, loss of consciousness, anxiety, hypotension, bradycardia or asystole, respiratory distress, or apnea. Treatment is dependent on the extent of spread, and the airway, breathing, and circulation are primary considerations. Supplemental oxygen, assistance with a bag-mask-valve device, or intubation may be required. The patient may be aware of the surrounding environment, and verbal reassurance is important to reduce anxiety. Hypotension due to high spinal block is treated with a fluid bolus and vasopressors, and the patient should be repositioned to promote venous return if this is not contraindicated by the surgical procedure. Bradycardia is treated with ephedrine or atropine. In this situation the use of phenylephrine and norepinephrine is avoided, as these drugs can cause reflex bradycardia. Asystole is treated with established advanced cardiovascular life support (ACLS) protocols. High spinal blocks are generally self-limiting and resolve as the concentration of local anesthetic declines.[1]

Cauda Equina Syndrome

Spinal anesthesia is one cause of cauda equina syndrome, a condition that affects the collection of nerves at the end of the spinal cord (cauda equina). The syndrome occurs when there is dysfunction of multiple lumbar and sacral nerve roots of the cauda equina and results in a range of symptoms based on the degree of compression and affected nerve roots.[8] Figure 10.6 lists symptoms of cauda equina syndrome.

When caused by spinal anesthesia, cauda equina syndrome is associated with lidocaine and continuous spinal microcatheters.[1] The treatment of choice is emergency surgery to free up the compressed nerve roots. Without prompt treatment within 48 hours, prospects of recovery are poor. Some patients may experience improvement when treatment is pursued beyond the recommended 48-hour time frame.[1,8]

Spinal or Epidural Hematoma

A spinal subdural or epidural hematoma is an accumulation of blood in the subdural or epidural space that can mechanically compress the spinal cord. It is a rare but devastating complication of neuraxial anesthesia that is more likely to occur in patients with altered homeostasis. Symptoms include low back pain, motor changes, and bowel or bladder dysfunction. Prevention of a poor prognosis requires emergent treatment. Treatment involves emergent decompression and surgery, which should not be delayed beyond eight hours. Patients who take anticoagulation medications should avoid neuraxial anesthesia to prevent this complication.[1] Figure 10.7 shows a spinal hematoma (indicated by arrow) seen on magnetic resonance imaging.

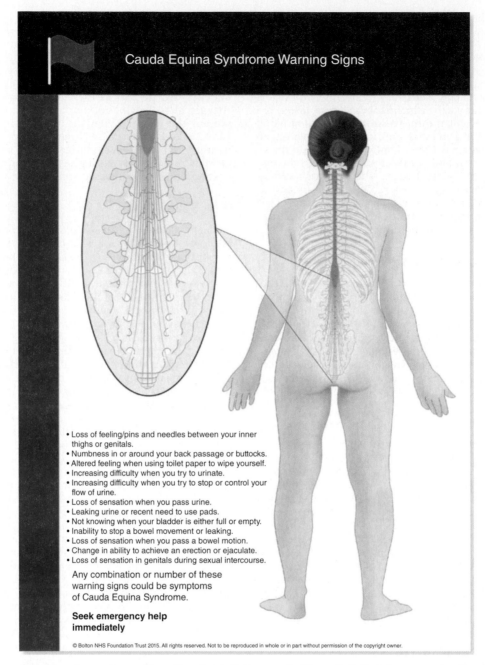

Fig. 10.6 Symptoms of cauda equina syndrome. (From Greenhalgh S, Finucane L, Mercer C, Selfe J. Assessment and management of cauda equina syndrome. *Musculoskel Sci Pract.* 2018;37:69–74. Figure 1. https://www.clinicalkey.com/#!/content/journal/1-s2.0-S246878121830211 X?scrollTo=%231-s2.0-S246878121830211X-gr2.)

INTRODUCTION TO PERIPHERAL NERVE BLOCKS

Peripheral nerve blocks may be used alone or can be combined with general or neuraxial anesthesia and can also be used to manage postoperative pain. There are several advantages to peripheral nerve blocks, including good pain control, decreased nausea and vomiting, a reduction in complications associated with general anesthesia, and a possible reduction in time from the initiation of the procedure to discharge for outpatient procedures. Contraindications to peripheral nerve blocks include patient refusal, a documented allergy to local anesthetics, coagulopathy, and infection at the site of injection.[1] Peripheral nerve blocks can be provided through a single injection or a continuous infusion. Most patients receive procedural sedation before block placement. Table 10.3 lists some types of peripheral nerve blocks and their indications.

Peripheral Nerve Blocks: Ultrasound-Guided Regional Anesthesia

In the United States, the use of ultrasound-guided regional anesthesia is considered the gold standard for the placement of peripheral nerve blocks. This technique allows for accurate needle positioning and monitoring of the distribution of the local anesthetic in real time. Ultrasound imaging can also

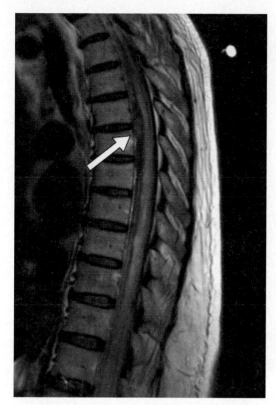

Fig. 10.7 Spinal hematoma on MRI. (From Cooley-Rieders K, Paredes K. Rare pathology leading to diagnostic challenge: A subarachnoid spinal hematoma after catheter cryoablation for atrial fibrillation. *J Cardiol Cases.* 2020;22(1):36–39. Figure 3.)

support the reduction of paresthesia and vascular punctures.[9] Box 10.3 lists the advantages of and Box 10.4 some of the most commonly used terms in ultrasound-guided regional anesthesia.[1,9] Figure 10.8 demonstrates the use of ultrasound-guided regional anesthesia to place a rectus sheath block.

Peripheral Nerve Blocks: Intravenous Regional Anesthesia

Intravenous regional anesthesia is commonly referred to as a Bier block. This type of block is a technically simple, safe, and rapid means of producing surgical anesthesia of the extremity. While the block is best suited for soft-tissue surgical procedures of the hand or wrist lasting one hour or less, it has also been used for lower extremity surgical procedures of the foot and ankle. A tourniquet is inflated to initiate and maintain the block. The tourniquet strategy limits the duration of anesthesia to approximately one hour. Use of a dual-tourniquet

---

BOX 10.3 Advantages of Ultrasound-Guided Regional Anesthesia

Direct visualization of the nerves and adjacent anatomic structures
Observing the local anesthetic spread in real time
Detecting variations in anatomy
Faster onset
Lower incidence of supplemental anesthesia or conversion to general anesthesia
Improvement in block quality
Use of lower, more precise doses of local anesthetics
Possible increase in safety
Less painful administration compared with nerve stimulator techniques
Improved patient satisfaction

Thompson JL. Regional anesthesia: Upper and lower extremity blocks. Chapter 50 in: Nagelhout JJ, Elisha S: *Nurse Anesthesia.* 6th ed. Elsevier; 2018.

BOX 10.4 Terms Associated with the Use of Ultrasound-Guided Regional Anesthesia

Anechoic: Tissue with no reflective index appears gray (fluid-filled structures are anechoic).
Curved Array Probe: Ultrasound waves are transmitted in a fanlike fashion.
Echo: The reflection of acoustic impedance is collected by the probe from the tissue.
Hyperechoic: Tissue with a high reflective index appears brightly (bones and tendons).
Hypoechoic: Tissue with a low reflective index appears dark.
In Axis: Ultrasound beam is oriented to view the nerve in its entirety.
In Plane: Ultrasound beam is oriented to view the needle in its entirety.
Linear Array Probe: Ultrasound waves are transmitted in a straight, frontal direction.
Out of Axis or Off Axis: Ultrasound beam is oriented to view the nerve as a cross section.
Out of Plane or Off Plane: Ultrasound beam is oriented to view the needle as a cross section.

Nagelhout JJ. Regional anesthesia. Chapter 25 in: Odom-Forren J: *Drain's PeriAnesthesia Nursing: A Critical Care Approach.* 7th ed. Elsevier; 2018.

TABLE 10.3 Peripheral Nerve Blocks and Their Indications

Interscalene	Analgesia to the shoulder and upper arm
Supraclavicular	Analgesia to the entire upper extremity distal to the shoulder
Infraclavicular	Analgesia to the elbow and below
Axillary	Analgesia distal to the elbow
Selective blocks at the elbow and wrist	Analgesia to various areas of the wrist and hand
Intercostal	Analgesia to the chest and upper abdominal wall
Transversus abdominis plane	Analgesia to the anterior abdominal wall
Psoas compartment	Anesthesia or analgesia to the entire hip, thigh, and medial aspect of the lower leg
Femoral	Analgesia to the anterior thigh and knee, medial aspect of the lower leg
Fascia iliaca	Analgesia to the hip, femoral shaft, and knee
Sciatic	Analgesia below the knee, sparing the area of the medial side of the lower leg (saphenous distribution)
Popliteal	Analgesia for surgery below the knee, sparing the area of the medial side of the lower leg
Ankle	Anesthesia or analgesia to the foot and distal ankle

Elisha S, Nagelhout J, Plaus K. *Nurse Anesthesia.* 6th ed. Table 50.1. Elsevier; 2018.

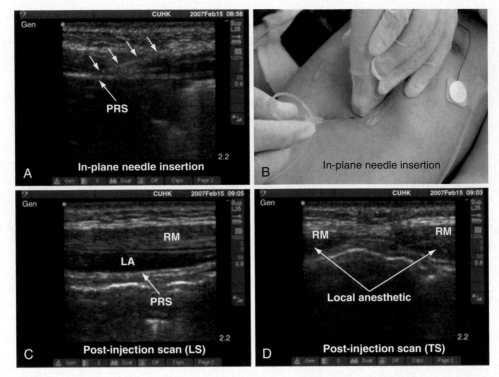

Fig. 10.8 Ultrasound-guided regional anesthesia to place a rectus sheath block. The in-plane needle insertion technique. LA, local anesthetic; LS, longitudinal sonogram; PRS, posterior rectus sheath; RM, rectus muscle; TS, transverse sonogram. (From Karmakar MK, Kwok WH: Ultrasound-guided regional anesthesia. Figure 43.33 in: Cote CJ, Lerman J, Anderson BJ (eds.). *A Practice of Anesthesia for Infants and Children*. 6th ed. Elsevier; 2019.)

system and preoperative and/or intraoperative administration of small doses of opioids may extend this time limit to the maximum tourniquet time of two hours. The greatest risk associated with the Bier block is related to the possibility of an improperly fitted or inflated tourniquet, or tourniquet failure. This could result in a rapid transfer of a large volume of local anesthetic from the extremity to the central circulation, so it is important to have emergency equipment, medications, and monitors immediately available when this block is administered. Because of the rapid onset of the block and the limited duration, it is almost always performed in the operating area, where the emergency items needed are readily available.[9] Figure 10.9 demonstrates the technique of IV regional anesthesia.

COMPLICATIONS OF PERIPHERAL NERVE BLOCKS

General complications associated with regional anesthesia include local anesthetic systemic toxicity (LAST), direct nerve injuries, vascular injury or hematoma, and infection. Box 10.5 lists unexpected outcomes of peripheral nerve blocks.[10]

Local Anesthetic Systemic Toxicity

Local anesthetic systemic toxicity (LAST) is a rare but serious complication that can occur during peripheral nerve block placement when the local anesthetic is inadvertently injected into the vasculature. It can also result from continuous infusion and accumulation of drug metabolites and is more likely to occur with nerve blocks requiring large volumes of injections, such as epidural, axillary, and interscalene blocks. It is estimated that LAST occurs between seven and 20 times in 10,000 peripheral nerve blocks and approximately 4 in 10,000 epidurals. LAST typically occurs within 30 to 50 seconds of injection of a local anesthetic but can occur within hours to days of the initiation of a continuous infusion.[2,11]

The classic typical clinical presentation of LAST occurs when local anesthetics cross the blood–brain barrier and produce signs of central nervous system excitation, such as agitation, tinnitus, circumoral numbness, blurred vision, and a metallic taste in the mouth. These signs can progress to seizures, unconsciousness, coma, and apnea. Cardiovascular toxicity related to LAST can be fatal; it results from the increased plasma concentration of local anesthetics, which blocks sodium channels to the heart. Table 10.4 identifies the cardiac symptoms associated with LAST.[2,11]

Early recognition and treatment are essential to improve patient outcomes and minimize the adverse effects of LAST. Because the pharmacologic treatment of LAST differs from that for other cardiac arrest scenarios, the American Society of Regional Anesthesia and Pain Medicine (ASRA) has developed a checklist to guide practitioners in treating this potentially deadly complication (Figure 10.10).[12]

LAST is an emergency. After calling for help, initial interventions begin, including airway management and ventilation, seizure suppression with benzodiazepines, management of hypotension and bradycardia, and cardiopulmonary resuscitation if the patient becomes unresponsive and pulseless. Follow the American Heart Association's basic and advanced cardiac life support protocols, but avoid the use of vasopressin, calcium channel blockers, beta-blockers, and local anesthetics such as lidocaine. Amiodarone is the preferred treatment for ventricular arrhythmias related to LAST.[2,11,12]

Intravenous Regional Anesthesia

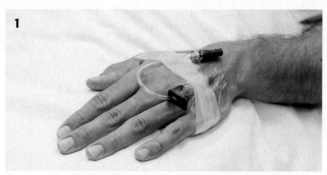

Place an IV catheter or butterfly needle as close to the pathologic site as possible. The site should be at least 10 cm distal to the tourniquet. A dorsal hand vein is ideal.

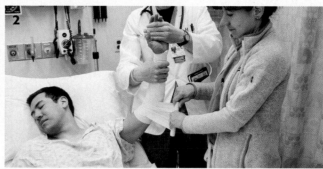

Exsanguinate the extremity by elevating and wrapping it in a distal-to-proximal fashion. Here, an Esmarch bandage is being used.

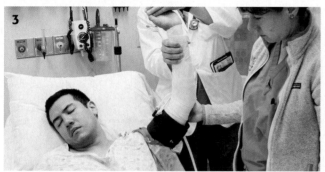

Apply the tourniquet to the patient's arm.

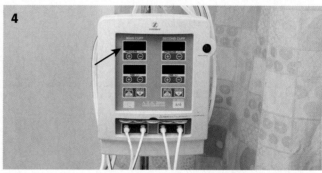

Inflate the tourniquet to 250 mm Hg or 100 mm Hg above systolic pressure. In the leg, inflate the cuff to 300 mm Hg or twice the systolic pressure measured in the arm.

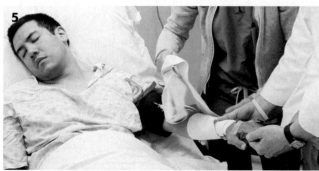

Place the patient's arm by his side and remove the Esmarch bandage. The tourniquet remains inflated.

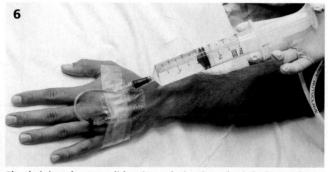

Slowly inject the 0.5% lidocaine solution into the infusion catheter at the calculated dose. See text for details and dosing information.

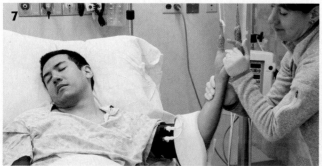

Remove the infusing needle/catheter, and tightly tape the puncture site to prevent extravasation of the anesthetic agent. Perform the procedure, including postreduction films and casting.

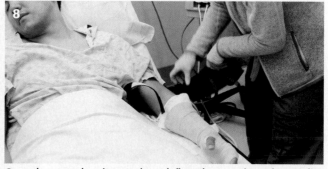

Once the procedure is complete, deflate the tourniquet in a cycling fashion (deflate for 5 seconds, reinflate for 1 to 2 minutes) 2 or 3 times. Then remove the tourniquet.

Fig. 10.9 Intravenous regional anesthesia. (From Roberts JR. Intravenous regional anesthesia. Figure 32.3 in: *Roberts and Hedges' Clinical Procedures in Emergency Medicine and Acute Care.* Elsevier; 2018.)

BOX 10.5 Unexpected Outcomes of Peripheral Nerve Blocks

Inability to insert the catheter
Untimely or erroneous medication administration
Suboptimal analgesia
Adverse medication reactions not recognized
Altered skin integrity from decreased sensory and motor loss
Accidental dislodgement of the catheter delivery system
Leakage from the catheter insertion site
Cracked filter on the delivery system
Inadvertent injection into a blood vessel
Nerve or vessel trauma
Hemorrhage or hematoma
Respiratory distress related to phrenic nerve paralysis, pneumothorax, or medication effect
Local infection at the peripheral nerve block catheter insertion site
Sepsis
Anaphylaxis
Permanent neurologic injuries and damage from insertion
Local anesthetic systemic toxicity

Williams, K. Peripheral nerve blocks: Assisting with insertion and pain management. In: Wiegand DL, ed. *AACN Procedure Manual for High Acuity, Progressive, and Critical Care.* 7th ed. Elsevier; 2017.

TABLE 10.4 Cardiac Complications Associated with Local Anesthetic Systemic Toxicity

Early Changes	Late Changes	Fatal Effects
Early changes include prolonged PR intervals and QRS complexes and signs of cardiac excitement, including: • Hypertension • Tachycardia • Ventricular arrhythmias	Early cardiovascular changes quickly progress to severe cardiac depression, including: • Bradycardia • Hypotension • Decreased cardiac output • Asystole • Cardiac collapse	Patients may experience fatal effects sooner if they have received a cardiac inhibitory drug, such as: • Beta-blockers • Calcium channel blockers • Digitalis

Nagelhout JJ. Local anesthetics. In: Odom-Forren J: *Drain's PeriAnesthesia Nursing: A Critical Care Approach.* 7th ed. Elsevier; 2018.

The current recommended therapy for treating LAST is lipid emulsion therapy, also known as lipid rescue or lipid resuscitation. Because local anesthetics are lipophilic, they bind with lipids and in this way are removed from the tissues, reversing the toxicity. Although propofol is a lipid-based medication, it is not a substitute for 20% lipid emulsion.

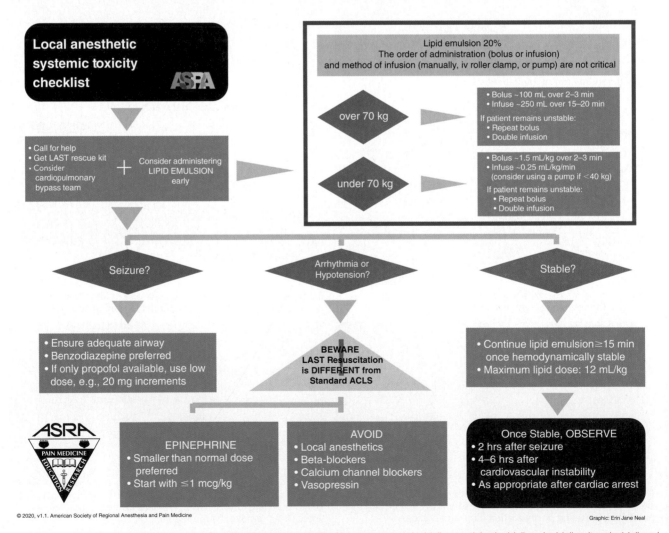

Local anesthetic systemic toxicity checklist ASRA

• Call for help
• Get LAST rescue kit
• Consider cardiopulmonary bypass team

+ Consider administering LIPID EMULSION early

Lipid emulsion 20%
The order of administration (bolus or infusion) and method of infusion (manually, iv roller clamp, or pump) are not critical

over 70 kg
• Bolus ~100 mL over 2–3 min
• Infuse ~250 mL over 15–20 min
If patient remains unstable:
• Repeat bolus
• Double infusion

under 70 kg
• Bolus ~1.5 mL/kg over 2–3 min
• Infuse ~0.25 mL/kg/min (consider using a pump if <40 kg)
If patient remains unstable:
• Repeat bolus
• Double infusion

Seizure?
• Ensure adequate airway
• Benzodiazepine preferred
• If only propofol available, use low dose, e.g., 20 mg increments

Arrhythmia or Hypotension?
BEWARE
LAST Resuscitation is DIFFERENT from Standard ACLS

Stable?
• Continue lipid emulsion ≥15 min once hemodynamically stable
• Maximum lipid dose: 12 mL/kg

EPINEPHRINE
• Smaller than normal dose preferred
• Start with ≤1 mcg/kg

AVOID
• Local anesthetics
• Beta-blockers
• Calcium channel blockers
• Vasopressin

Once Stable, OBSERVE
• 2 hrs after seizure
• 4–6 hrs after cardiovascular instability
• As appropriate after cardiac arrest

ASRA PAIN MEDICINE EDUCATION RESEARCH

© 2020, v1.1. American Society of Regional Anesthesia and Pain Medicine

Graphic: Erin Jane Neal

Fig. 10.10 Local anesthetic systemic toxicity checklist. (Available at: https://www.asra.com/guidelines-articles/guidelines/guideline-item/guidelines/2020/11/01/checklist-for-treatment-of-local-anesthetic-systemic-toxicity.)

BOX 10.6 ASRA Guidelines for Lipid Emulsion Therapy to Treat LAST

For patients over 70 kg: Bolus 100 mL over 2–3 minutes; then infuse 250 mL over 15–20 minutes; may repeat bolus and double infusion if patient remains unstable

For patients under 70 kg: Bolus 1.5 mL/kg over 2–3 minutes; then infuse 0.25 mL/kg/min; may repeat bolus and double infusion if patient remains unstable

American Society of Regional Anesthesia and Pain Medicine. Checklist for treatment of local anesthetic systemic toxicity. https://www.asra.com/guidelines-articles/guidelines/guideline-item/guidelines/2020/11/01/checklist-for-treatment-of-local-anesthetic-systemic-toxicity.

Patients who do not respond to lipid therapy require cardiopulmonary bypass.[2] Box 10.6 lists ASRA's guidelines for lipid emulsion therapy.[12]

INTRODUCTION TO LOCAL INFILTRATION

For immediate short-term pain relief, local anesthesia is administered as a single injection into a surgical wound before suturing or stapling. For long-term pain relief, local anesthesia is administered continuously through an indwelling catheter placed at the end of surgery. Wound catheters are commonly inserted in subcutaneous, fascial, intra-articular, pleural, and periosteal areas.[2,11]

Lidocaine is preferred for local anesthesia because it is more potent, less irritating, and longer lasting than other local anesthetic agents. Epinephrine can be added to lidocaine to prolong the duration of local anesthesia, provide hemostasis, slow anesthetic absorption, and increase the level of anesthetic blockade.[2,11,13] Table 10.5 lists anesthetic agents commonly used for local infiltration. Sustained-release and tumescent anesthesia are forms of local infiltration.

Local Infiltration: Sustained-Release Local Anesthesia

The local anesthetic bupivacaine is available in a sustained-release formula that does not require an indwelling catheter for administration. Liposomal bupivacaine injectable suspension is encapsulated in foam and administered as a single dose into the surgical site. Administration requires slow injection with frequent aspiration to minimize inadvertent vascular injection. This anesthetic choice begins to work slowly, impacting pain, temperature sensation, touch, proprioception, and finally muscle tone. The slow release of analgesia into the tissues provides extended pain relief for up to 72 hours.[11]

TABLE 10.5 Uses and Dosages, Onset and Duration, and Other Features of Local Anesthetics

Esters	Uses and Dosages	Onset and Duration	General Comments
Procaine (Novacain)	*Topical:* 10% to 20% *Infiltration:* 0.25% to 0.5% *Nerve block:* 1% to 2% *Maximum dose:* 5–6 mg/kg plain (400 mg); 8.5 mg/kg with epinephrine (600 mg)	*Onset:* Slow for infiltration and nerve block; fast for spinal block *Duration:* 30 min plain; 60 min with epinephrine Introduced in 1905	• Introduced in 1905 • Limitations include short duration, low potency, and poor stability • Undergoes rapid hydrolysis to PABA; less than 50% excreted unchanged in the urine • Not commonly used for surgical anesthesia in the operating room
Chloroprocaine (Nesacaine)	*Infiltration:* 1% *Nerve block:* 1% to 2% *Epidural block:* 2% to 3% *Maximum dose:* 11 mg/kg plain (800 mg); 15 mg/kg with epinephrine (1000 mg)	*Onset:* Fast (6–12 min) *Duration:* 30 min plain; 60 min with epinephrine	• Not topically active • Short-duration ester manufactured in preservative-free and preservative-containing solution (sodium bisulfate and methylparaben) • Not administered for spinals due to the risk of neurotoxicity • Preservative-free solutions should be used for epidurals • Twelve-fold more potent than procaine • One of the safest local anesthetics in terms of systemic toxicity • Hydrolyzed to inactive metabolites and excreted in the urine
Cocaine	*Topical:* 4% to 20% *Maximum dose:* 3 mg/kg	*Onset:* Fast *Duration:* 10–55 min	• Moderate-duration ester • Vasoconstrictor and used topically only • Inhibits reuptake of norepinephrine and dopamine; may cause constriction of coronary arteries • Limitations include toxicity, sympathetic stimulation, and abuse potential • Partially metabolized in the liver and by ester hydrolysis
Tetracaine (Pontocaine)	*Topical:* 0.5% to 1% *Infiltration:* 0.1% to 0.25% *Maximum dose:* 1.5 mg/kg plain (100 mg); 2.5 mg/kg with epinephrine (200 mg)	*Onset:* Slow *Duration:* (Topical) 55 min; (Spinal) 1–1.5 hours plain; (Spinal) 2–3 hours with epinephrine	• Potent, long-acting ester developed in 1930 • May be used topically • Most commonly used for spinal anesthesia • Cerebrospinal fluid does not contain pseudocholinesterase enzymes and must be absorbed systemically to be metabolized • Metabolized slower than other esters

Continued

TABLE 10.5 Uses and Dosages, Onset and Duration, and Other Features of Local Anesthetics—cont'd

Esters	Uses and Dosages	Onset and Duration	General Comments
AMIDES			
Lidocaine (Xylocaine)	*Topical:* 2% to 4% *Nerve block:* 1% to 2% *Epidural:* 1% to 2% *IRVA:* 0.5% *Maximum dose:* 4.5 mg/kg plain (300 mg) for other blocks; 7 mg/kg with epinephrine (500 mg); (Topical) 3 mg/kg (less due to rapid absorption); (IRVA) 250 mg	*Onset:* Fast; (Topical) 2–4 min *Duration:* 1–2 hours plain; 2–6 hours with epinephrine for nerve block and infiltration; 1–1.5 hours for spinal or epidural anesthesia	• Moderate-duration amide introduced in 1948 • One of the most common and versatile local anesthetics in current use; rapid onset, intense analgesia, good penetration, and stable • Not commonly used for spinal anesthesia due to risk of transient neurologic symptoms • Metabolized by oxidative dealkylation in the liver; liver disease may reduce elimination and place the patient at risk for toxicity
Mepivacaine (Carbocaine)	*Infiltration:* 0.5% to 1% *Nerve block:* 1% to 2% *Maximum dose:* 4.5 mg/kg plain (300 mg); 7 mg/kg with epinephrine (500 mg)	*Onset:* Fast *Duration:* 45–90 min plain; 2–6 hours with epinephrine	• Moderate-duration amide introduced in 1957 • Similar to lidocaine except slightly longer duration, less toxicity, and less localized vasodilation
Ropivacaine (Naropin)	*Epidural:* 0.1% to 0.2% (analgesia); higher concentrations for anesthesia *Nerve block:* 0.5% to 1% *Maximum dose:* 200 mg	*Onset:* Fast *Duration:* 2–6 hours	• Rapid-onset, long-duration amide local anesthetic that has many advantages over bupivacaine; introduced in 1996 • A single enantiomer with a lower risk of toxicity than bupivacaine, which makes it a primary choice for peripheral nerve blocks and epidurals • Less motor blockade at lower doses than bupivacaine, making it an ideal agent for epidural analgesia • Clearance is higher and elimination half-life is shorter than for bupivacaine • Metabolized by cytochrome P-450 system in the liver; less than 1% is excreted unchanged • Unique in its ability to cause localized vasoconstriction, which eliminates the need to add epinephrine
Bupivacaine (Sensorcaine; Marcaine)	*Infiltration:* 0.1% to 0.25% *Nerve block:* 0.25% to 0.5% *Spinal:* 0.5% to 0.75% *Epidural:* 0.125% for analgesia; higher concentrations for anesthesia *Maximum dose:* 2.5 mg/kg plain (175 mg); 3 mg/kg with epinephrine (225 mg)	*Onset:* Slow *Duration:* 2–4 hours plain; 3–7 hours with epinephrine	• Potent, long-duration local anesthetic introduced in 1973; widely used but limited by reports of cardiotoxicity • Produces profound sensory analgesia with minimal motor blockade at low doses • Development of less toxic, potent long-acting amides has reduced its use for peripheral nerve blocks and epidurals • Commonly used for spinal anesthesia • Primarily metabolized in the liver
Levobupivacaine (Chirocaine)	Concentrations used are similar to bupivacaine *Maximum dose:* 2.5 mg/kg plain; 3.2 mg/kg with epinephrine (150 mg)	*Onset:* Slow *Duration:* 4–11 hours	• Long-duration S-enantiomer of bupivacaine; because it is a pure isomer, it exhibits less toxicity than bupivacaine • Exhibits many of the same characteristics of bupivacaine in terms of potency, onset, and duration

Nagelhout JJ. Local anesthetics. In: Odom-Forren J, ed. *Drain's Perianesthesia Nursing: A Critical Care Approach.* 7th ed. Table 24.3. Elsevier; 2018.

Local Infiltration: Tumescent Local Anesthesia

Tumescent local anesthesia is used to provide analgesia for liposuction procedures. It combines lidocaine, sodium bicarbonate, and epinephrine diluted in normal saline solution. The term *tumescent* refers to the physical appearance of tissues after the instillation of large volumes of this anesthetic agent.[8] This approach can be used with opioids if liposuction is performed on a large area.[11]

COMPLICATIONS OF LOCAL INFILTRATION

Although there are few complications associated with local infiltration, an allergic reaction can occur, particularly in response to lidocaine.[13] Increased risk of chondrotoxicity can occur when bupivacaine is used in a catheter placed directly in a joint. Local infiltration poses no risk of LAST.[11]

Complications of indwelling catheter use, which can prevent the patient from receiving an adequate dose of analgesia, include catheter blockage, breakage, or migration away from the intended area. Site infection is a rare but potential complication.[11] Lidocaine with epinephrine should only be used in vascular areas and never in areas supplied by end arteries, including the nose, ears, digits, and penis.[1] Local and regional anesthetic techniques carry many benefits for patients undergoing outpatient ambulatory surgery and can reduce complications and contribute to quicker recovery times.

CHAPTER HIGHLIGHTS

- Regional anesthesia can decrease the risk and incidence of complications related to general anesthesia.
- Neuraxial anesthesia involves injecting an anesthetic agent into the area around the nerve roots as they exit the spine or into the cerebrospinal fluid directly around the spinal cord.
- Spinal anesthesia is a single injection into the subarachnoid space that results in sensory and motor blockade. It is limited to the lower lumbar region.
- Epidural anesthesia blocks spinal nerves outside of the subarachnoid space and is administered through a catheter placed through a needle that allows for repeated dosing or postoperative pain management. Epidural placement can occur in the lumbar or thoracic region.
- Caudal anesthesia is the most commonly used regional block in pediatric anesthesia.
- Peripheral nerve blocks can be used alone or in combination with general or neuraxial anesthesia.
- Local anesthetic systemic toxicity (LAST) is a rare but life-threatening complication of epidural anesthesia and peripheral nerve blocks. Emulsion therapy is the treatment for LAST.
- Local infiltration is a technique that is useful for both short- and long-term pain relief following surgery.

CASE STUDY

Manuelo is a 72-year-old male presenting for outpatient surgery for hemorrhoidectomy. His past medical history is significant for hypertension; chronic obstructive pulmonary disease, for which he uses oxygen at night; and severe postoperative nausea and vomiting following prior abdominal surgery for a small bowel obstruction. He took his betablocker this morning as per his preoperative instructions, and his baseline blood pressure upon arrival was 104/52 mm Hg. He has no known drug allergies. His body mass index is 27. He does not smoke and consumes approximately two alcoholic drinks per week. The plan today is for Manuelo to receive spinal anesthesia with IV opioid pain control in the immediate postoperative period. When he has met all discharge criteria, he will be discharged home with a prescription for an opioid.

Based on his past medical history, why did the anesthesia provider choose to administer spinal anesthesia? What immediate assessments should you perform upon Manuelo's arrival to the PACU? Based on your knowledge of spinal anesthesia, what are your concerns regarding his hemodynamic status? What strategies can be employed to prevent hemodynamic complications related to spinal anesthesia in this patient?

REFERENCES

1. Nagelhout JJ. Regional anesthesia. In: Odom-Forren J, ed. *Drain's PeriAnesthesia Nursing: A Critical Care Approach*. 7th ed. Elsevier; 2018:329-346.
2. Nagelhout JJ. Local anesthetics. In: Odom-Forren J, ed. *Drain's PeriAnesthesia Nursing: A Critical Care Approach*. 7th ed. Elsevier; 2018:316-328.
3. Windle PE. Neurological. In: Schick L, Windle PE, eds. *PeriAnesthesia Nursing Core Curriculum: Preprocedure, Phase I and Phase II PACU Nursing*. 4th ed. Elsevier; 2021:446-498.
4. Pellegrini JE. Regional anesthesia: spinal and epidural anesthesia. In: Nagelhout JJ, Elisha S, eds. *Nurse Anesthesia*. 6th ed. Elsevier; 2018:1015-1041.
5. Mondor EE. Trauma. In: Urden JD, Stacy KM, Lough ME, eds. *Critical Care Nursing: Diagnosis and Management*. 9th ed. Elsevier; 2022;791-830.
6. The New York School of Regional Anesthesia (NYOSARA). *Spinal Anesthesia*. Available at: https://www.nysora.com/techniques/neuraxial-and-perineuraxial-techniques/spinal-anesthesia/. Accessed July 10, 2021.
7. Elisha S, Terry KL. Neonatal anesthesia. In: Nagelhout JJ, Elisha S, eds. *Nurse Anesthesia*. 6th ed. Elsevier; 2018:1092-1116.
8. American Association of Neurological Surgeons. *Cauda Equina Syndrome*. Available at: https://www.aans.org/en/Patients/Neurosurgical-Conditions-and-Treatments/Cauda-Equina-Syndrome. Accessed July 10, 2021.
9. Thompson JL. Regional anesthesia: upper and lower extremity blocks. In: Nagelhout JJ, Elisha S, eds. *Nurse Anesthesia*. 6th ed. Elsevier; 2018:1042-1063.
10. Williams K. Peripheral nerve blocks: assisting with insertion and pain management. In: Wiegand DL, ed. *AACN Procedure Manual for High Acuity, Progressive, and Critical Care*. 7th ed. Elsevier; 2017:948-957.
11. Nagelhout JJ. Local anesthetics. In: Nagelhout JJ, Elisha S, eds. *Nurse Anesthesia*. 6th ed. Elsevier; 2018:110-127.
12. American Society of Regional Anesthesia and Pain Medicine. *Checklist for Treatment of Local Anesthetic Systemic Toxicity*. Available at: https://www.asra.com/guidelines-articles/guidelines/guideline-item/guidelines/2020/11/01/checklist-for-treatment-of-local-anesthetic-systemic-toxicity. Accessed July 11, 2021.
13. Denke NJ. Wound Management. In: Sweet V, ed. *Sheehy's Emergency Nursing: Principles and Practice*. 7th ed. Elsevier; 2020:93-111.

11 Procedural Sedation

Sylvia J. Baker, MSN, RN, CPAN (retired), FASPAN

LEARNING OBJECTIVES

A review of the content of this chapter will help the reader to:

1. Define procedural sedation.
2. Describe responsibilities of the perianesthesia registered nurse during procedural sedation.
3. List the common medications used during procedural sedation.
4. Identify assessment considerations for the patient receiving procedural sedation.
5. State the monitoring requirements for the patient receiving procedural sedation.

OVERVIEW

As the types of procedures being performed in the ambulatory setting increases, it is becoming more important than ever for perianesthesia nurses to know how to monitor patients following these procedures so that they can be returned to a timely functional preprocedural status. Procedural sedation is one of the methods on the continuum of sedation, which ranges from general to deep to moderate to minimal levels, and it is a cost-effective way of providing safe and comfortable care for patients. The perianesthesia nurse who participates in any phase of caring for patients receiving procedural sedation must be knowledgeable about the nursing roles and responsibilities to be learned for delivering care to that group of patients.

Definition of Procedural Sedation

Procedural sedation, formerly known as conscious sedation and at times referred to as moderate sedation, is a drug-induced depression of consciousness in which patients respond purposefully to verbal commands either given alone or accompanied by light tactile stimulation. The patient can maintain a patent airway and adequate spontaneous ventilations. During procedural sedation, cardiovascular function is usually maintained.[1]

> "Procedural sedation is provided by non-anesthesia providers for the purpose of reducing anxiety and pain during noninvasive and minimally invasive procedures while also assuring patient safety. Sedation can describe several drug-induced states during a continuum. Because sedation is a continuum, it is not always possible to predict how an individual patient may respond. Hence, practitioners should be able to rescue a patient who enters a deeper than intended level of sedation. The level of sedation is independent of the route of medication administration."[2]

Four levels of sedation are described in Table 11.1. It is vital to note that by definition, procedural sedation requires that the patient be maintained in the phase of moderate sedation as much as possible. Since sedation occurs on a continuum, however, the possibility exists that the patient may progress to a deeper, unintended level of sedation. For this reason, it is *imperative* that one nurse be solely responsible for monitoring the patient throughout the procedure.

Procedural sedation can be a very efficient means of providing care to patients while they are undergoing any number of procedures in the ambulatory and outpatient settings. Examples of ambulatory procedures include endoscopic procedures, biopsies (e.g., breast or skin), cardiac catheterization procedures, and some pain clinic procedures, to name a few.

Selecting Patients for Procedural Sedation

Not all patients are appropriate for procedural or moderate sedation, just as not all procedures can be successful when this form of sedation is used. Many invasive procedures require deeper sedation in order for the appropriate relaxation of the patient to be achieved, such as some biopsies or laparoscopic procedures. Patient selection for procedural sedation should be criteria driven. It is the responsibility of the physician to assess the patient to determine whether procedural sedation is appropriate. Patients who may not meet the criteria for procedural sedation include individuals who are unable to cooperate and follow the commands of the monitoring nurse and/or provider. A patient with an American Society of Anesthesiologists (ASA) physical status classification as medically unstable (e.g., ASA score of III to VI) is not suitable for procedural sedation, and an anesthesia care provider needs to be consulted in these types of situations (Box 11.1).

ROLES AND RESPONSIBILITIES OF PERIANESTHESIA NURSES IN PROCEDURAL SEDATION

Prior to any procedure, obtaining informed consent is the responsibility of the care provider. One aspect of informed consent is to let the patient ask questions about the procedure and have them answered. A focused history and physical examination need to be documented in the medical record. The record should be updated for any changes on the day of the procedure. At a minimum, the provider's presedation assessment should include an airway assessment, a history of previous adverse sedation or anesthetic events, a medical history that includes difficulties with the airway, and a determination of the patient's ASA physical status classification. The sedation plan that was discussed with the patient or guardian should also be reviewed.

During the pre-procedure period, the perianesthesia nurse must identify the patient using two patient identifiers, as described by The Joint Commission. Appropriate patient identification is one measure to aid in ensuring patient safety. A baseline set of vital signs, confirmation that the patient has had nothing by mouth (NPO) as requested, and the patient's medical history must be reviewed and documented. The preprocedure nurse also needs to establish venous access.

TABLE 11.1 Levels of Sedation

Level	Description	Airway Function	Ventilatory/Cardiovascular Functions	Responsiveness
Level 1	Minimal sedation (anxiolysis)	Airway reflexes are not impaired	Ventilatory and cardiovascular functions are unaffected	Responds normally to verbal commands. Cognitive function and physical coordination may be impaired
Level 2	Moderate sedation (conscious sedation)	No interventions are required to maintain the patient's airway	Spontaneous ventilation is adequate. Cardiovascular function is usually maintained	Induced depression of consciousness during which patients respond appropriately to verbal commands either alone or accompanied by light tactile stimulation
Level 3	Deep sedation/analgesia	May require assistance to maintain a patent airway	Ability to independently maintain ventilatory function may be impaired and spontaneous ventilation may be inadequate. Cardiovascular function is usually maintained	Induced depression of consciousness during which patients cannot be easily aroused but respond purposefully following repeated or painful simulation
Level 4	General anesthesia	Often require assistance in maintaining a patent airway	Ability to independently maintain ventilatory function is often impaired. Positive-pressure ventilation may be required because of depressed spontaneous ventilations or drug-induced depression of neuromuscular function. Cardiovascular function may be impaired	Induced loss of consciousness during which patients are not arousable, even by painful stimulation

American Society of Anesthesiologists. *Continuum of Depth of Sedation: Definition of General Anesthesia and Levels of Sedation.* 2019. https://www.asahq.org/standards-and-guidelines/continuum-of-depth-of-sedation-definition-of-general-anesthesia-and-levels-of-sedationanalgesia

---

BOX 11.1 ASA Physical Status Classification System

ASA PS Classification	Definition	Examples, Including but Not Limited to:
ASA I	A normal healthy person	Healthy, nonsmoking, no or minimal alcohol use
ASA II	A patient with mild systemic disease	Mild diseases only without substantive functional limitations. Examples include (but are not limited to) current smoker, social alcohol drinker, pregnancy, obesity (30 < BMI < 40), well-controlled DM/HTN, mild lung disease
ASA III	A patient with severe systemic disease	Substantive functional limitations; one or more moderate to severe diseases. Examples include (but are not limited to) poorly controlled DM or HTN, COPD, morbid obesity (BMI ≥ 40), active hepatitis, alcohol dependence or abuse, implanted pacemaker, moderate reduction of ejection fraction, ESRD undergoing regularly scheduled dialysis, premature infant PCA < 60 weeks, history (> 3 months) of MI, CVA, TIA, or CAD/stents
ASA IV	A patient with severe systemic disease that is a constant threat to life	Examples include (but are not limited to) recent (< 3 months) MI, CVA, TIA, or CAD/stents, ongoing cardiac ischemia or severe valve dysfunction, severe reduction of ejection fraction, sepsis, DIC, ARD, or ESRD not undergoing regularly scheduled dialysis
ASA V	A moribund patient who is not expected to survive without the operation	Examples include (but are not limited to) ruptured abdominal/thoracic aneurysm, massive trauma, intracranial bleed with mass effect, ischemic bowel in the face of significant cardiac pathology or multiple organ/system dysfunction
ASA VI	A declared brain-dead patient whose organs are being removed for donor purposes	

The addition of "E" denotes emergency surgery: An emergency is defined as existing when a delay in treatment of the patient would lead to a significant increase in the threat to life or body part.

ARD, acute respiratory distress; *BMI*, body mass index; *CAD*, coronary artery disease; *COPD*, chronic obstructive pulmonary disease; *CVA*, cerebrovascular accident; *DIC*, disseminated intravascular coagulation; *DM*, diabetes mellitus; *ESRD*, end-stage renal disease; *HTN*, hypertension; *MI*, myocardial infarction; *PCA*, postconceptional age; *TIA*, transient ischemic attack

Marley RA, Sheets SA. Preoperative evaluation and preparation of the patient. Table 20.18 in: Nagelhout JJ, Elisha S. *Nurse Anesthesia.* 6th ed. Elsevier; 2018.

Complying with the universal protocol is also an important part of the preprocedure process, including the marking of the surgical site as appropriate. Nursing staff need to ensure that the patient has a responsible individual available to escort the patient home and provide care after the procedure. The ASA promotes a "Statement on Nonoperating Room Anesthetizing Locations."[4] This statement addresses anesthesia care involving anesthesia personnel for procedures intended to be performed in locations outside an operating room. The topics addressed in this statement are having the necessary space and lighting available; having the needed supplies, general equipment, and emergency equipment at hand; and having "adequate staff trained to support the anesthesiologist."[2]

Staff should ensure that emergency equipment is readily available and functioning properly. The list of equipment includes, but is not limited to, a setup for oxygen and suctioning, cardiac monitor, blood pressure monitor, pulse oximeter, capnograph, bag-valve mask for respiratory resuscitation, code cart, and reversal medications (e.g., naloxone and flumazenil). A privileged and credentialed provider and perianesthesia nursing staff who have demonstrated competence in procedural sedation must be present during the procedure and take part in universal protocol procedures (e.g., time out). The provider should also re-evaluate the patient immediately prior to initiating the procedure.

During the procedure, one registered nurse is solely responsible for caring for and monitoring the patient; this includes unrestricted, immediate visual and physical access to the patient. Immediately preceding the procedure, the patient should be assessed for the level of consciousness, ventilatory status, oxygenation status, heart rate and rhythm, blood pressure, and respiratory rate. These measurements need to be documented at the onset of the procedure and every five minutes during the procedure. The monitoring nurse must be proficient at recognizing and reporting any changes in the electrocardiogram (ECG) and unplanned level of consciousness.

Sedation occurs due to a dose-related continuum, is variable, and depends on each patient's response to the various drugs administered. The provider must be physically present during the administration of sedation. The ASA recommends that an individual be present in the procedure room who has the knowledge and skills to recognize and treat airway complications. This includes the recommendation that at least one individual present throughout the procedure has successfully completed training in advanced cardiac life support.

The ASA, in a 2018 recommendation, stated that direct observation of the patient is required throughout the entire procedure.[3] The patient's sedation level is monitored by assessing the clinical signs and patient's responsiveness to verbal commands and/or tactile stimulation. The use of an objective scale (e.g., ASA Continuum of Sedation Scale, Ramsay Sedation Scale, Modified Ramsay Sedation Scale), as outlined by the individual organization's policies, adds clarity to the patient's condition during the procedure. The frequency with which vital signs are taken and sedation is scored is dependent upon organizational policy (e.g., typically every five minutes depending on the patient's response).

To promote patient safety, all syringes need to be labeled for content and dosage or concentration.

Lines of communication should be open and respectful. The nursing staff should immediately alert the provider if the patient's oxygen levels decrease or carbon dioxide levels increase. If a patient is unresponsive or does not demonstrate adequate spontaneous respirations, the practitioner must be immediately notified and urgent interventions initiated.

Following the procedure, the patient is monitored every 15 minutes, or per facility guidelines, until objective discharge criteria are met. These criteria may be defined as having vital signs within 20% of baseline, a patent airway and intact protective reflexes, a baseline level of orientation, an ability to answer simple questions, and acceptable pain levels. All criteria should be assessed and documented. Discharge criteria may also be influenced by individual organizations and must be developed in conjunction with statutory, regulatory, and professional organizational standards.[1] Age variations may be noted when considering the length of time for observation, especially in the pediatric population; infants born preterm (< 36 weeks' gestation) may need to be monitored for respiratory depression for an additional 12 hours following a procedure. If reversal medications were administered during the procedure, the patient should be monitored for an additional two hours to monitor the potential for re-sedation and respiratory depression.

ASSESSMENT OF PATIENTS FOR PROCEDURAL SEDATION

Patients who are diagnosed with or are at risk for obstructive sleep apnea (OSA) should have specific assessments completed prior to sedation. Because sedative medications cause relaxation of the head and neck musculature, as well as a decreased level of consciousness, patients should be assessed using a standardized tool such as the commonly used STOP-BANG tool. Table 11.2 lists the available screening tools for OSA.

STOP-BANG is an acronym for eight criteria that help practitioners assess a patient's risk for OSA: **s**noring (louder than talking), being **t**ired (or fatigued during the daytime), **o**bserved (has anyone observed apnea during sleep?), blood **p**ressure (having been treated for hypertension), **B**MI calculator (> 35 kg/m²), **a**ge (> 50 years old), **n**eck circumference (> 17 inches or 40 cm), and **g**ender (male). Each of the criteria is given one point for an affirmative response.[5] A score of zero to 2 indicates that the patient has a low risk for OSA; 3–4 an intermediate risk for OSA; and 5–8 a high risk for OSA. The risk is also high if a patient answers "yes" to two or more of the four STOP questions *and* is a male, or has a body mass index (BMI) of greater than 35 kg/m², or has a neck circumference of 17 inches (43 cm) and is male or of 16 inches (41 cm) and is female. Higher scores indicate an increased risk for airway obstruction with sedation. An anesthesiology consult should be considered for patients with a score over five. (Figure 11.1).

A vital aspect of the assessment prior to procedural sedation is the airway. Knowing the airway anatomy augments the care provided to the patient. Whenever a patient has an abnormal airway, the provider should recognize the potential for the patient to be at an increased risk for obstruction and desaturation during sedation. Patients who present with a considerable history of stridor, significant snoring, sleep apnea, advanced rheumatoid arthritis, dysmorphic facial features, Down syndrome, and/or upper respiratory tract infections are at increased risk for airway obstruction during sedation. The provider must be prepared should mask ventilation or intubation become necessary.

An airway examination also includes an assessment of the patient's mouth opening, typically using the Mallampati classification. The Mallampati score is determined by the ability to visualize the soft palate, uvula, and faucial pillars when the patient opens the mouth and protrudes the tongue as far as possible.[6] There are four classifications. Grade 1, or Mallampati 1, indicates that the faucial pillars, uvula, and soft and hard palates are readily visible when the airway is open.

TABLE 11.2 Common Screening Tools for Obstructive Sleep Apnea

Tool	Domains	Indications
Lausanne NoSAS	Neck circumference Body mass index Sex Age Snoring	Score ≥ 8 indicates high risk of OSA
No-Apnea	Neck circumference Age	Score ≥ 3 indicates high risk of OSA
Epworth Sleepiness Scale (ESS)	Is there dozing or sleeping when: Sitting and reading Watching TV Sitting inactive in a public place, such as a meeting or theatre Riding as a passenger in a car for an hour without a break Lying down to rest in the afternoon when circumstances permit Sitting and talking to someone Sitting quietly after a lunch without alcohol Sitting in a car, stopped for a few minutes in traffic	Score ≥ 9 indicates daytime sleepiness
STOP	Snoring Tiredness (fatigue) Observed apnea High blood pressure	Score ≥ 2 indicates high risk for OSA
STOP-BANG	Snoring Tiredness Observed apnea Pressure (hypertension) BMI (>35 kg m^{-2}) Age (> 50) Neck (circumference > 40 cm) Gender (male)	Score ≥ 3 indicates high risk for OSA
Berlin	Eleven problems in three groups Severity of snoring Daytime sleepiness High blood pressure or obesity	Two or more of the three groups scoring positive indicates high risk for OSA

Zheng Z, Sun X, Chen R, et al. Comparison of six assessment tools to screen for obstructive sleep apnea in patients with hypertension. *Clin Cardiol.* 2021;44(11):1526–1534. https://doi.org/10.1002%2Fclc.23714

Stop		
1. Snoring—Do you *snore* loudly (louder than talking or loud enough to be heard through closed door)?	Yes	No
2. Tired—Do you often feel *tired*, fatigued, or sleepy during the daytime?	Yes	No
3. Observed—Has anyone *observed* you stop breathing while you sleep?	Yes	No
4. Blood pressure—Are you now being or have you been treated for high *blood pressure*?	Yes	No
Bang		
BMI → 35 kg/m²?	Yes	No
Age → 50 years?	Yes	No
Neck circumference (measured around the Adams apple) Male—shirt collar ≥17 inches (43 cm)? Female—shirt collar ≥16 inches (41 cm)?	Yes	No
Gender—male	Yes	No
A high risk of *obstructive* sleep apnea is defined as a score of 3 or more; low risk of obstructive sleep apnea, a score of <3.		

Fig. 11.1 STOP-BANG sleep apnea questionnaire. (Marley RA. Respiratory. Table 18.2 in: Schick L, Windle PE: *PeriAnesthesia Nursing Core Curriculum* E-book. From Chung F, Yegneswaran B, Liao P, et al. STOP questionnaire: A tool to screen patients for obstructive sleep apnea. *Anesthesiology* 2008;108:812–821.)

Grade 2 indicates that the uvula is partially covered while the soft and hard palates remain visible. Grade 3 suggests that the uvula is nearly completely covered, which indicates a narrowing of the airway. Finally, Mallampati 4 scores indicate that only the hard palate is visible, and the airway is covered by the back of the tongue. Grades 1 and 2 are considered adequate exposure and grades 3 and 4 inadequate exposure. Grades 3 and 4 may indicate that an anesthesia care consult is needed (Figure 11.2 and Box 11.2).

COMMON MEDICATIONS USED TO PRODUCE PROCEDURAL SEDATION

Medications used to produce sedation are ordered by the provider, whether that person be an anesthesia provider or a duly credentialed practitioner who is performing the procedure. The major classifications of medications utilized during moderate sedation are benzodiazepines and opioids.

Benzodiazepines include midazolam (Versed) and diazepam (Valium). These drugs aid in promoting anxiolysis and sedation. Benzodiazepine dosing guidelines are individualized and titrated to effect. When titrating benzodiazepines to effect, the administrator needs to monitor the patient until somnolence, nystagmus, and/or slurred speech are observed in the patient. Benzodiazepines should not be administered via rapid injection.

When caring for the healthy patient, small increments of midazolam (0.5 mg) are administered over 2 minutes. Patients may respond to as little as 0.25–0.5 mg, and this suggests that dosing is very individualized (e.g., the same dose that obliterates one patient's respiratory drive may have no effect on another). The initial intravenous (IV) dose should not exceed 2.5 mg. Patients who are elderly, debilitated, or chronically ill or have a reduced pulmonary reserve require smaller incremental doses of midazolam (0.25–0.5 mg) administered over 2 minutes. If additional dosing is required, it is imperative to wait 2–3 minutes to appropriately evaluate the patient response to dosing. For this group of patients, it is wise to follow the adage "start low and go slow."

Diazepam's recommended dosage prior to a planned procedure is 1–2 mg IV, titrated over 1 minute. Additional 1-mg increments may be given over several minutes during the procedure. Caution must be exercised when administering diazepam concurrently with opioids.

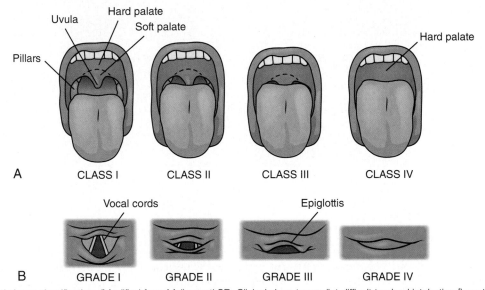

Fig. 11.2 Mallampati airway classification. (Modified from Mallampati SR: Clinical signs to predict difficult tracheal intubation [hypothesis]. *Can Anaesth Soc J* 30:316, 1983. Found in: Brown C. Anesthesia, moderate sedation/analgesia. Figure 14.1 in: Schick L, Windle PE, eds. *Perianesthesia Nursing Core Curriculum: Preprocedure, Phase I and Phase II PACU Nursing.* 4th ed. Elsevier; 2021.)

BOX 11.2 Airway Assessment Parameters: Normal and Abnormal Examinations

Assessment	Normal Examination	Abnormal Examination
Mouth opening	Opens mouth normally (adults: greater than two finger widths or 3 cm)	Inability to open mouth normally
Hyomental distance	Normal chin length (adults: length of chin is greater than two finger widths or 3 cm)	Small or recessed chin
Neck mobility	Normal neck flexion and extension without pain/paresthesia	Neck has limited range of motion Significant obesity of the face/neck
Mallampati classification	Able to visualize at least part of the uvula and tonsillar pillars with mouth wide open and tongue out (patient sitting)	Inability to visualize at least part of the uvula or tonsils with mouth open and tongue out (patient sitting) High-arched palate Tonsillar hypertrophy

Should patients require reversal of the sedative effect of benzodiazepines, flumazenil (Romazicon) can be used as it is a benzodiazepine antagonist. Flumazenil specifically reverses the central nervous system effects of benzodiazepines. The duration and degree of flumazenil's reversal action is dependent upon the amount of benzodiazepine administered and plasma diazepine concentration. The initial dose of flumazenil is 0.2 mg administered over 15 seconds. If the desired level of consciousness is not achieved within 45 seconds, a second dose of 0.2 mg may be administered. Flumazenil may be repeated at 60-second intervals to a maximum of four additional doses (or 1 mg). Flumazenil's onset of action is 1–2 minutes, and an 80% response is achieved within 3 minutes of administration. The patient must be monitored for the potential of re-sedation. The terminal half-life of flumazenil is 40–80 minutes; therefore it is imperative to monitor patients for prolonged sedation or re-sedation[7] (Table 11.3).

Common opioids used during procedures requiring sedation include fentanyl and morphine. Opioids provide analgesia and sedation by altering the perception and response to pain when they become bound to specific receptor sites located within the central nervous system. The practitioner will notice that the patient has become myopic and bradycardic and is experiencing some degree of hypotension. Respiratory depression is the most common side effect of opioid administration, and when opioids are administered in conjunction with benzodiazepines, the respiratory system,

TABLE 11.3 Comparison of Common Medications Utilized During Procedural Sedation

Medication	Dosage	Onset	Duration	Notes
Midazolam (Versed)	Child 6 mo to 5 yr IV 0.05–0.1 mg/kg (total dose of 0.6 mg/kg may be necessary) Child 6–12 yr IV 0.025–0.05 mg/kg (total dose of 0.4 mg/kg may be necessary) Adult < 55 yr 200–350 μg/kg over 20-30 seconds Adult > 55 yr IV (ASA I/II) IV 150–300 μg/kg over 20–30 seconds	PO: 10–30 minutes IM: 15 minutes, peak 30 minutes to 1 hour, duration 2–3 hours IV: 1.5–5 minutes, duration 2 hours	1–5 hours half-life	Metabolized in liver; excreted by kidneys Half-life may be extended in obese patients Respiratory depression/apnea may be increased in geriatric patients Amnesia occurs teach patient and family that patient may not recall events
Diazepam (Valium)	Child > 6 mo: IM/IV 0.04–0.3 mg/kg Adult: IM/IV 2-5 mg	PO: 30 minutes, peak 2 hours, duration up to 24 hours IM: 15–30 minutes, duration 1–1.5 hours IV: Immediate, duration 15–60 minutes	1–12 days half-life	Metabolized by liver; excreted by kidneys Do not dilute or mix with other products
Fentanyl	Anesthesia: Child > 12 yr/Adult: 1–2 μg/kg IV slow push (over 2 minutes) titrated in 25-μg increments Analgesia: Child >12 yr/Adult: 50-100 μg every 60-120 minutes	IM: 7–15 minutes, peak 30 minutes, duration 1–2 hours IV: 1 minute, peak 3–5 minutes, duration 0.5–1 hour	2–4 hours half-life	Metabolized by liver; excreted by kidneys May cause chest wall rigidity, especially if administered too quickly Dilute with 5 mL or more sterile water or 0.9% NaCl through Y-tube or 3-way stopcock at 0.1 mg or less/1–2 minutes
Morphine	0.05–0.2 mg/kg titrated in 1 to 2-mg increments	IM: 30 minutes, peak 30–60 minutes IV: rapid onset, peak 20 minutes	4–5 hours	Metabolized by liver; excreted by kidneys
Meperidine (Demerol)	0.5–1 mg/kg titrated in 25-mg increments	PO: 15 minutes, peak 1.5 hours IM: 10 minutes, peak 30–60 minutes IV: immediate onset, peak 5–7 minutes	3–4 hours half-life	Metabolized by liver; excreted by kidneys
Propofol (Diprivan)	Child 2 mo to 16 years (maintenance: IV 125–300 μg/kg/min) Child > 3 yr or ASA I or II IV inductions: 2.5–3.5 μg/kg over 20–30 seconds when not premedicated or lightly premedicated Adult < 55 and ASA I/II IV: 40 mg q10 sec until induction onset, maintenance 100–200 μg/kg/min	IV: 15–30 seconds	Half-life: 1–8 minutes; terminal half-life 3–12 hours	Nurse administration varies from state-to-state nurse practice act Metabolized by liver; excreted by kidneys Pain at administration site Package insert states this should be used only by individuals trained in anesthesia Watch for ECG changes Results in lower incidence of post procedure nausea and vomiting Allows for quicker patient discharge MUST monitor and support airway No known reversal agent

Compiled from Skidmore-Roth L. *Mosby's 2023 Nursing Drug Reference*. 36th ed. Elsevier; 2023.

11

which demonstrates subtle yet important signals regarding the level of sedation, should be closely observed.

Fentanyl (Sublimaze) is a synthetic narcotic analgesic 100 times more potent than morphine. A usual dose of fentanyl is 1–3 µg/kg, which has a duration of 30–60 minutes. Fentanyl should not be administered too quickly as it may cause chest wall rigidity, which may prohibit ventilatory assistance. Morphine is a prototype of other opioids with a rapid onset and a 4-hour duration. Many patients exhibit histamine release upon administration, as may be observed by an inflammatory response along the injected vein.

The opioid antagonist naloxone (Narcan) should be readily available during (and after) procedural sedation. Naloxone is a nonselective competitive antagonist at all opioid receptor sites. Naloxone has a short duration of action of approximately 30–45 minutes. Administration of naloxone should be slow to avoid the side effects of pulmonary edema, hypertension, arrhythmias, pain, projectile vomiting, and convulsions. Titration of naloxone can be accomplished by diluting the vial of 0.4 mg in 9 mL of 0.9% NaCl (making a total dose of 10 mL). Administer 2.5 mL (0.1 mg) over 15–30 seconds; wait 45 seconds to assess for the patient's response; and then repeat to a total dose of 0.4 mg, should that be necessary. Because the half-life of naloxone is 45 minutes, the potential for re-sedation exists; therefore, the patient needs to be observed and monitored for two additional hours following reversal to ensure adequate respiratory and ventilatory functions.

EMERGENCY INTERVENTIONS FOR PROCEDURAL SEDATION

Personnel involved with procedural sedation should demonstrate airway management knowledge, competencies, and skills. These criteria should be assessed and validated during orientation to the department, as well as regularly per institutional policy (e.g., annually), to help maintain airway management skills. Methods for airway stabilization include verbal and physical stimulation, repositioning of the airway using jaw support or jaw thrust, and bag-valve-mask assistance. Any time that a maneuver is required to correct hypoventilation for the patient, notification of the patient condition needs to be given to the provider. In many organizations, the use of end-tidal carbon dioxide (EtCO$_2$) monitoring is standard during procedural sedation. According to the ASA's practice guidelines for moderate and procedural sedation, a review of the findings of randomized control studies suggests that routine use of EtCO$_2$ monitoring is an adjunct tool to help observe the depth, frequency, and effectiveness of respirations.[8] Using capnography as an assessment tool during procedural sedation is associated with fewer hypoxic events and the sufficient maintenance of oxygen saturation[8] (Figure 11.3).

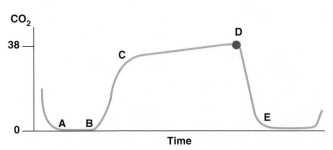

Fig. 11.3 Essentials of the normal capnographic waveform. (Modified from and reprinted by permission of Nellcor Puritan Bennett LLC, Boulder, CO, part of Covidien. *Continuous End-Tidal Carbon Dioxide Monitoring: ClinicalKey for Nursing.*)

Evidence-Based Practice: Capnography and Sedation
In the 2018 version of the Practice Guidelines for Moderate Procedural Sedation and Analgesia, the task force convened to develop the guidelines also established clinical criteria upon which the guidelines are based. Following the conduct of a meta-analysis of randomized clinical trials, the task force identified a notable reduction in hypoxemic events observed when using end-tidal carbon dioxide monitoring compared to sedation monitoring without the use of capnography. As a result of the meta-analysis, the task force strongly recommended the use of capnography in the setting of procedural sedation unless hindered by the nature of the patient, the type of procedure, or the availability of equipment.

Source: American Society of Anesthesiologists Committee on Standards and Practice Parameters. Practice Guidelines for Moderate Procedural Sedation and Analgesia 2018: A Report by the American Society of Anesthesiologists Task Force on Moderate Procedural Sedation and Analgesia, the American Association of Oral and Maxillofacial Surgeons, American College of Radiology, American Dental Association, American Society of Dentist Anesthesiologists, and Society of Interventional Radiology. *Anesthesiology.* 2018;128(3):437-479. https://doi.org/10.1097/ALN.0000000000002043

The availability of reversal medications is crucial for averting and mitigating any respiratory issues that may arise due to sedation medications. The availability of flumazenil to reverse the effect of any benzodiazepines and of naloxone for narcotics is necessary. The knowledge of the pharmacologic implications of agents used for sedation, as well as of agents used for reversals, should be incorporated into competencies for any staff member administering medications during a procedure. The potential for a patient to achieve an unintended level of sedation is often cited as the reason that a member of the procedural sedation team should have advanced cardiac life support knowledge while providing care to the patient. The ASA also recommends that an individual with advanced life support skills be readily available.[8]

PRIORITIES FOR AMBULATORY NURSES CARING FOR PROCEDURAL SEDATION PATIENTS

Since many ambulatory procedures occur in an environment that is providing rapid and episodic care, the perianesthesia nurse working in the ambulatory setting must establish a prompt and meaningful relationship with the patient. Establishing a rapport with the patient helps in establishing trust between patient and provider and provides support that can reduce anxiety. Preprocedure education includes reinforcement of NPO requirements and a discussion of the need for a responsible individual to provide transportation home.

ASPAN standards recommend that patients meet discharge criteria prior to discharge.[9] Discharge criteria need to be established in concert with the protocol for anesthesia and the efforts of providers and supported by the facility. When considering discharge criteria, not only should the type of sedation and analgesia be considered, but also the complexity of the patient's status, the procedure, and any procedure-specific criteria. Prior to discharge, patients should be able to return to their preprocedure level of mobility. Pain control and education regarding adjuvant pain control methods should be made available. Methods of discarding unused medications properly need to be included in teaching about discharge. Utilization of the teach-back method has been proven to be an excellent way for the nurse to determine if the patient and family have the information needed for a safe and optimal recovery. Patients also need to know to whom and to what facility they should report if they have any untoward effects or outcomes from their procedure or sedation.

One of the steps in preprocedure assessment is determining what mode of transportation the patient has available for going home. This information needs to be verified following the procedure. If the patient's transportation plans fail, alternate plans should be considered. In some situations, the patient may need to be admitted for an extended stay. This decision must be made collaboratively and include the provider or perhaps a care manager who can facilitate finding community support for transportation and post procedure support. All patients need to be given information on following up after their procedures. This allows them to ask any questions about clarification of their care and to assess for any signs of potential complications. The follow-up may be in the form of a phone call, a questionnaire, or an office appointment. The timing of this follow-up is determined by facility policies and procedures. When a perianesthesia nurse understands the sedation continuum, the procedures for airway maintenance, and the interactions that can occur among medications and is fully able to vigilantly monitor the patient, the nurse can provide safe patient care before, during, and after procedural sedation.

CHAPTER HIGHLIGHTS

- Procedural sedation is a drug-induced depression of consciousness allowing patients to respond purposefully to verbal commands either given alone or accompanied by light tactile stimulation.
- The perianesthesia nurse caring for the patient having procedural sedation must be trained to be prepared to respond to potential emergencies.
- Both benzodiazepines and opioids are commonly used to produce sedation.
- Airway management resulting from over-sedation is a priority for the perianesthesia nurse responsible for monitoring the patient.

CASE STUDY

Peter P. Eder is scheduled for a procedure requiring moderate sedation at your facility. As you admit Mr. Eder, you review his pre-procedure history and ask about his airway. Peter reports that his wife has told him for years that he snores loudly virtually every night, but he has never undergone a sleep study. Peter's neck circumference is 17.5 inches. You notice that he has some limitation when asked to extend his neck, and you are not able to visualize his posterior oropharynx. What will be your first action once you have this information?

During the procedure, Peter experiences a level of airway obstruction that requires you, as the monitoring nurse, to reposition his airway, increase his oxygen delivery rate to 6 L per minute, and vigorously stimulate him. Even with these maneuvers, he continues to be extremely somnolent, and you provide jaw support. The administration of flumazenil is ordered by the provider. Your nursing colleague provides flumazenil 0.2 mg as a rapid bolus. How do you anticipate Mr. Eder will respond to this treatment?

Because you administered flumazenil during Mr. Eder's procedure, you monitor his vital signs and level of arousability (including level of consciousness) for 2 hours. Why is this considered best practice?

Mr. Eder has demonstrated that he will not suffer any issues of re-sedation, and he is now ready for discharge. What are the important topics to cover with Mr. Eder? What is one way of ensuring that he fully understands your instructions?

REFERENCES

1. Brown C. Anesthesia, moderate sedation/analgesia. In: Schick L, Windle PE, eds. *Perianesthesia Nursing Core Curriculum: Preprocedure, Phase I and Phase II PACU Nursing.* 4th ed. Elsevier; 2021: 238-248.
2. American Society of PeriAnesthesia Nurses. Practice Recommendation 7: the role of the registered nurse in the management of patients undergoing procedural sedation. In: *2021-2022 Perianesthesia Nursing Standards, Practice Recommendations and Interpretive Statements.* ASPAN; 2020:73-77.
3. American Society of Anesthesiologists. *Continuum of Depth of Sedation: Definition of General Anesthesia and Levels of Sedation.* 2019. Available at: https://www.asahq.org/standards-and-practice-parameters/statement-on-continuum-of-depth-of-sedation-definition-of-general-anesthesia-and-levels-of-sedation-analgesia.
4. American Society of Anesthesiologists. *Statement on Nonoperating Room Anesthetizing Locations.* 2018. Available at: https://www.asahq.org/standards-and-practice-parameters/statement-on-nonoperating-room-anesthetizing-locations. Accessed September 16, 2022.
5. Lakdawala L. Creating a safer perioperative environment with an obstructive sleep apnea screening tool. *J Perianesth Nurs.* 2011;26(1): 15-24. Available at: https://doi.org/10.1016/j.jopan.2010.10.004.
6. Brown C. Chapter 14: Anesthesia, moderate sedation/analgesia. In: Schick L, Windle PE, eds. *Perianesthesia Nursing Core Curriculum: Preprocedure, Phase I and Phase II PACU Nursing.* 4th ed. Elsevier; 2021:241.
7. Romazicon. Roche Laboratory. NDA 20-073/S-016. 2007. Available at: https://www.accessdata.fda.gov/drugsatfda_docs/label/2007/020073s016lbl.pdf.
8. Anesthesiology. *Practice Guidelines for Moderate Procedural Sedation and Analgesia 2018.* March 2018. Available at: https://pubs.asahq.org/anesthesiology/article/128/3/437/18818/Practice-Guidelines-for-Moderate-Procedural.
9. American Society of PeriAnesthesia Nurses. *2021-2022 Perianesthesia Nursing Standards, Practice Recommendations and Interpretive Statements.* ASPAN; 2020.

12   Principles of Pain Assessment and Multimodal Analgesia

Antoinette A. Zito, MSN, CPAN, FASPAN

LEARNING OBJECTIVES

A review of the content of this chapter will help the reader to:

1. Define the different types of pain encountered postoperatively.
2. List comprehensive tools utilized to conduct a pain assessment.
3. Define multimodal analgesia.
4. Identify risks associated with opioid use in pain management.
5. Describe the importance of patient education in a successful pain management plan.

OVERVIEW

The majority of surgeries in the United States occur in an outpatient or same-day setting. Along with minor procedures once done in the hospital setting, surgeries once defined as major routinely occur in outpatient settings. For example, a healthy patient presenting for a total knee replacement historically would have had surgery in a hospital setting with an anticipated stay of several days. Today, it is common to have a joint replacement in an ambulatory center with discharge to home on the same day. The increased complexity of outpatient procedures performed brings a renewed focus on postoperative pain management. Conventional pain management strategies used in an inpatient setting may not be practical in an ambulatory setting. Ambulatory surgical patients require effective analgesia to facilitate same-day discharge and ensure a safe transition home.

Pain is an anticipated aspect of the postoperative experience and is a normal response to surgery. Because pain is one of the criteria used to assess the feasibility of performing surgery on an outpatient basis, it is important to assess the role that pain and pain management plays in an individual's overall recovery period. Pain levels vary widely amongst patients, and preexisting physical and psychological conditions can influence an individual's pain experience.

After surgery, the goals of pain management include relief from suffering, prevention of complications, and optimization of functional outcomes. Effective pain management plays a critical role in the success of ambulatory surgery, yet it remains one of the most challenging areas for the perioperative team. Inadequate postoperative pain control is associated with limited physical mobility, delayed ambulation, delayed recovery, increased length of stays, decreased patient satisfaction, and the development of persistent postoperative pain, or chronic pain.[1-5] Postoperative pain is one of the most frequent reasons for unplanned admissions after surgery.[3,4]

DEFINITION AND CLASSIFICATION OF PAIN

It is important to understand the concept of pain to plan interventions and improve pain management strategies. Pain is a complex phenomenon that has physiologic, psychological, and social components. It is a multifactorial experience that varies from patient to patient. There have been many attempts to define and describe pain throughout the years. As more information and evidence are discovered, new knowledge brings a deeper understanding of the complexity of pain. A widely used definition was created in 2020 by the International Association for the Study of Pain (IASP). The attempt at and subsequent creation of the definition was a result of the collaboration of a multinational, multidisciplinary task force. The definition of pain from the IASP is, "Pain is an unpleasant sensory and emotional experience associated with, or resembling that associated with, actual or potential tissue damage."[6] The definition also includes six key summaries that were added to further encompass essential concepts that define pain. (Box 12.1). It is difficult to appreciate the complexity of the definition, and further classification is often sought.

Pain can be broadly categorized based on many factors. These may include the cause or origin of the pain, the type of pain, and the occurrence or duration of pain. There is no universal system for pain classification as it is often difficult to define and categorize. Exploring and understanding the source, type, and duration of pain can assist with planning and targeting pain management interventions. It is important to acknowledge the individual response to pain and that types of pain can and do overlap and occur concurrently. The following are traditionally used categorizations of pain.

Acute Pain

Acute pain is commonly associated with tissue damage, inflammation, or a disease process. It is time limited and has a recent onset and a short duration. In general, acute pain typically lasts less than three months and is directly associated with a specific tissue insult (e.g., surgery) or injury. The pain is occurring in response to an underlying cause. Acute pain is considered to be the body's protective response to a known stressor. While there is no consensus on the exact time limit of acute pain, it has a relatively short duration and gradually resolves during the healing process.[7]

Chronic Pain

In contrast to acute pain, chronic pain is of a longer duration than the typical three months; in some cases it may last a lifetime, and it can have multifactorial contributors.[7] It is often difficult to determine the onset. The pain can be associated with underlying co-morbidities and other factors that contribute to pain. Chronic pain can be defined as a syndrome, or a condition characterized by a group of symptoms. The pain can be continuous or intermittent and can be a result of a past injury or surgery, an underlying pathophysiologic condition, or an unknown cause. Chronic pain can be a result of unresolved acute pain. Patients can experience both chronic and acute pain concurrently.[7]

Nociceptive Pain

Nociceptive pain is the most common type of pain and one that is considered "normal" as it follows the pathway of pain conduction. It is a protective mechanism and the body's response to harmful stimuli. Nociception includes the processes of transduction, transmission, perception, and modulation, and these phases highlight the normal pain processing pathway (Figure 12.1).[7] Nociceptive pain can be further divided into somatic pain, which originates in the periphery and superficial areas, and visceral pain, which originates in internal

organs. Nociceptive pain can be localized or radiating and is often described as sharp, dull, aching, or throbbing. The source of pain is identifiable and usually a result of trauma, a known or unknown injury, or an inflammatory response. Examples of nociceptive pain include pain from burns, contusions, lacerations, or an underlying disease process (e.g., appendicitis, surgical procedures).[7]

Neuropathic Pain

Neuropathic pain is defined as pain resulting from damage to or the abnormal functioning of the neurologic processing system. Because it results from nerve damage or dysfunction and does not follow the common nerve pathways, the source of pain can be difficult to determine. There are peripheral and central mechanisms identified in the pathophysiology of neuropathic pain.[7] It is often described as burning, electric shock–like, shooting, numbness, or tingling. Some simply describe it as nerve pain. Attempting to categorize this type of pain can be limiting as it is processed and perceived differently from patient to patient. Nevertheless, common conditions associated with neuropathic pain include diabetic neuropathy, neuralgias, phantom limb pain, and postherpetic neuralgia.[4]

Persistent Postoperative Pain

The development of chronic pain is a major complication following surgery. Persistent postoperative pain (PPP), also known as chronic postoperative pain (CPOP), is an unanticipated surgical outcome and can significantly affect the quality of life of the patient. Although there is no consensus on one definition of PPP or CPOP, most definitions include the following factors: the presence of pain that develops after surgery or increases in its intensity, pain lasts at least two to three months, pain that was not present before surgery, and pain for which other causes and problems have been excluded.[5,8,9] Although the exact mechanism for developing PPP is not clearly understood, there are risk factors associated with its development, including certain types of surgical procedures, genetic factors, and uncontrolled postoperative pain (Figure 12.2).[9,10]

PAIN ASSESSMENT

Pain is an individualized and multidimensional experience; therefore, a personalized, comprehensive pain management

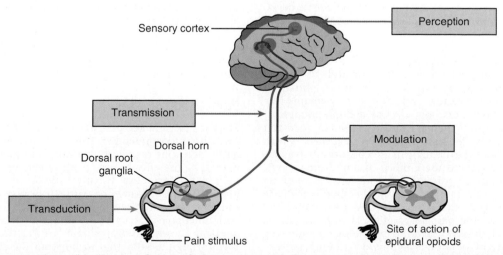

Fig. 12.1 Pain sensory pathway. (Modified from Colwell AQ. Pain management. Figure 31.1 in: Odom-Forren J. *Drain's Perianesthesia Nursing: A Critical Care Approach*. 7th ed. Elsevier; 2018.)

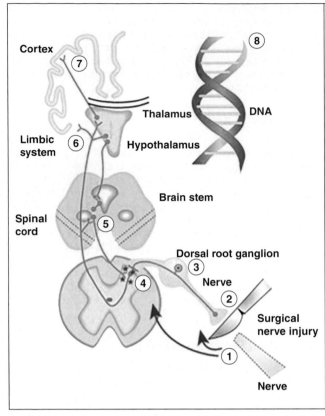

How Surgery (Wound) Can Lead to Chronic Pain

1. Denervated schwann cells and infiltrating macrophages distal to nerve injury produce local and systemic chemicals that drive pain signaling.

2. Neuroma at site of injury is source of ectopic spontaneous excitability in sensory fibers.

3. Changes in gene expression in dorsal root ganglion after excitability, responsiveness, transmission, and survival of sensory neurons.

4. Dorsal horn is site of altered activity and gene expression, producing central sensitization, loss of inhibitory interneurons, and microglial activation, which together amplify sensory flow.

5. Brainstem descending controls modulate transmission in spinal cord.

6. Limbic system and hypothalamus contribute to altered mood, behavior, and autonomic reflexes.

7. Sensation of pain generated in cortex (past experiences, cultural inputs, and expectations converge to determine what patient feels).

8. Genomic DNA predispose (or not) patient to chronic pain and affect their reaction to treatment.

Fig. 12.2 Persistent postsurgical pain. (Kehlet H, Jensen TS, Woolf CJ. Persistent postsurgical pain: Risk factors and prevention. *Lancet.* 2006;367(9522):1618–1625. https://doi.org/10.1016/S0140-6736(06)68700-X.)

plan is crucial and contributes to the success of ambulatory surgery. Ideally, this plan begins during preoperative preparation at the time the decision for surgery is made, whether only hours or months prior to the surgery. Patients who receive preoperative pain education are more likely to feel prepared to manage their pain postoperatively.[11] During this time, expectations about pain and plans for the management of pain are discussed with the patient, family, surgeon, and anesthesiologist. Multimodal pain management planning is an important component of the patient experience that should not be minimized.

A comprehensive pain assessment is essential for the development of an effective individualized pain management plan. The processing of pain has both a physiologic and psychological component; therefore, acquiring a comprehensive medical history and physical assessment that addresses the whole person is integral to creating the plan and establishing the patient's recovery goals prior to surgery. It is important to review the patient's objective and subjective symptoms, the presence of underlying diseases, the use and effectiveness of medications and complementary therapies used for pain and other conditions, and the patient's previous experiences with pain. Attitudes about the use of opioids, a history of substance misuse, and beliefs about the efficacy of nonpharmacologic interventions are also important to explore. Assessment of the presence of pain preoperatively is essential as there is evidence that this may be a predictor of postoperative pain levels.[12]

Intraoperatively, the pain assessment is ongoing and is based on clinical observations and physiologic monitoring according to the type of anesthesia provided. Postoperatively, the ongoing pain assessment requires a practical approach. Assessments, interventions, and evaluations take place frequently, often every few minutes, depending on the intervention.[7] These frequent assessments support the evaluation of the effect of pain treatment, including the patient's comfort level, physiologic response, and hemodynamic stability.[7]

Pharmacologic and nonpharmacologic methods are utilized to target the source of pain and offer comfort measures. The patient's self-report remains the gold standard for pain assessments.[6,13] Due to the sedative qualities of anesthetic and analgesic agents used by an anesthesia provider for the perianesthesia patient, self-reporting may not always be possible. Nonverbal indicators of pain also serve as reliable assessments of the presence of pain in those circumstances where patients are unable to communicate. Pain assessment tools vary within different facilities, and the perianesthesia nurses should be trained to utilize the tools supported by facility policy. It is imperative to select and use the correct assessment tool for the clinical situation encountered.

Pain Assessment Tools

The use of a validated pain assessment tool to establish baseline data is recommended. This baseline assessment helps to guide decisions regarding treatment for pain, as well as to determine the effectiveness of the treatment intervention.[14] Pain scales vary but usually consist of both subjective and objective measures of pain. Common components of the tools measure the presence, intensity, location, quality, and functional impact (e.g., ability to move self in bed, ability to breathe deeply) of pain.[14-16] Practice experts recommend using the same tool throughout the course of patient care for the purpose of continuity and the ability to monitor reporting trends.[14] Figure 12.3 shows examples of pain

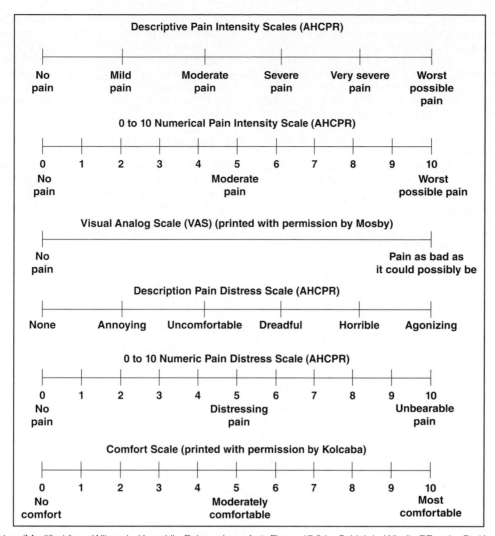

Fig. 12.3 Pain scales. (Modified from Wilson L, Kane HL. Pain and comfort. Figure 17.2 in: Schick L, Windle PE, eds. *PeriAnesthesia Nursing Core Curriculum: Preprocedure, Phase I and Phase II PACU Nursing.* 4th ed. Elsevier; 2021.)

scales. The appropriate tool should be selected based on the individual patient characteristics, including developmental stage and language and cognitive status.

Surgical pain is not the only source of postoperative pain. Limiting the pain assessment to simply a numerical score can lead the nurse to overlook alternative contributing factors. A holistic approach to postoperative patient assessment may reveal other sources of discomfort and appropriate treatment interventions. For example, some patients may experience pain related to intraoperative positioning. In some situations, simply moving or repositioning the patient provides ample relief of stated discomforts. Previously existing conditions such as back pain may be aggravated. Perhaps the patient only needs to void. Patients with anxiety and fear may find comfort and reassurance from the knowledge that the nurse is at the bedside.[1]

An acceptable level of pain for the individual patient is established as part of the baseline data. Pain management is a right of every surgical patient. An often-understated factor is the importance of the practitioner's attitudes and beliefs about pain. Personal biases can interfere with effective pain assessment and management.[15] Even the best tools cannot compensate for the undertreatment of pain due to provider behaviors. Nurses at the bedside who coordinate and implement the treatment of pain and evaluate pain have an inherent responsibility to examine their beliefs so they can best advocate for the patient and ensure that pain management needs are met for all surgical patients.

PREEMPTIVE, PREVENTIVE, AND MULTIMODAL ANALGESIA

As the science of pain management has evolved, several concepts have been instituted into practice. Because they have the same goals of using conventional pain management strategies, providing relief of pain, and promoting comfort, these approaches have had an increased focus on the prevention of adverse effects associated with traditional monotherapy pain management. The combination of preemptive, preventive, and multimodal analgesia is especially effective in the ambulatory surgery setting.

Preemptive Analgesia

Preventing pain before it begins is the underlying theory of preemptive analgesia. The word *preempt* means to forestall or prevent something from happening. The first studies supporting the theory of preemptive analgesia were published in

1986.[17,18] Preemptive analgesia is treatment that begins before surgery and prevents the establishment of central sensitization caused by both the incisional injury and the accompanying inflammatory response during the initial postoperative period.[17] Preemptive analgesia is practiced in many settings, although there is no consensus regarding the timing of the intervention or which is the most appropriate intervention for a particular procedure. Importantly, although preemptive analgesia is initiated prior to surgery, supplemental forms analgesia can also be provided throughout the perioperative period. Preemptive analgesia can take the form of preoperatively consumed oral medications, local or topical anesthetics, or preoperative peripheral nerve blocks, to name a few.

Preventive Analgesia

If the goal of preemptive analgesia is to prevent pain, the use of preventive analgesia involves a wider approach.[18] Preventive analgesia focuses on the prevention of pain and does not reflect the timing of the interventions (e.g., in preemptive analgesia, the timing is before an incision is made). Preventive analgesia can reduce postoperative pain, just as preemptive analgesia can, but preventive analgesia can be given at any time in the perioperative period. The two terms are often confused, but each type of analgesia has a specific purpose and is often incorporated into a broader pain management plan. For example, preemptive analgesia is administered just prior to a surgical event to minimize the pain response, whereas preventive analgesia can be administered beginning the day before surgery, during surgery, and following surgery to help attenuate postoperative pain.

Multimodal Analgesia

Multimodal analgesia (MMA) has become the cornerstone of pain management in the perianesthesia setting. MMA involves the use of a variety of anesthetic techniques and medications targeting different mechanisms of action and different areas of the nervous system.[13] Because pain is complex and the causes are multifactorial, this approach combines multiple interventions to target and treat pain (Figure 12.4). Multimodal interventions include both pharmacologic and nonpharmacologic methods.

The evidence in support of the goals of MMA continues to grow and includes the desire to provide adequate analgesia while reducing the side effects associated with monotherapy

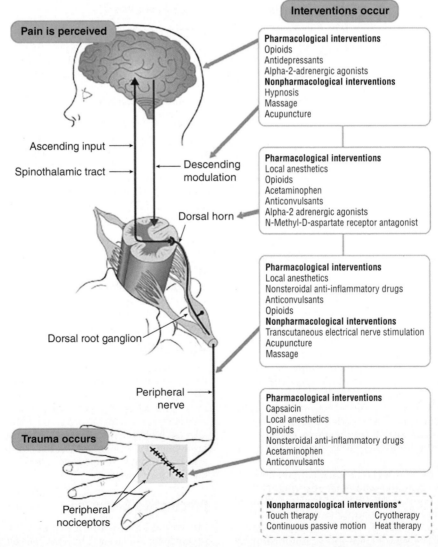

Fig. 12.4 Multimodal analgesia. (Manworren RCB. Multimodal pain management and the future of a personalized medicine approach to pain. *J AORN*. 2015;101(3):307–318. Figure 1.)

approaches. Components of MMA include local and/or regional anesthetic techniques, pharmacologic agents that become activated at various pain receptor sites (e.g., based on their mechanisms and durations of action), and the reduction or the elimination of opioids. Anesthesia plans can also incorporate nonpharmacologic interventions when appropriate, such as cold or heat therapy or elevation and positioning of the patient.

Multimodal analgesia is an essential component of enhanced recovery and aligns with the American Society of Perianesthesia Nurses (ASPAN) standards and guidelines.[19] MMA is individualized to the patient and to the procedure. Many of the MMA techniques can be broadly applied to all perioperative patients unless contraindicated.[20]

Evidence-Based Practice: Multimodal Analgesia

For more than two decades now the practice of multimodal analgesia has emerged as the standard of care for management of surgical pain. Multimodal analgesia is defined as the combination of two or more analgesic techniques or agents to block the pain impulses along particular targets of the nociceptive pathways. The combinations may include typical nonopioid analgesics such as acetaminophen and nonsteroidal anti-inflammatory drugs, adjuvant analgesics such as glucocorticoids and gabapentinoids, and local anesthetics by local infiltration or peripheral blocks. The use of multimodal analgesia as a methodology to manage pain concurrently supports the reduction of opioid-based treatment of pain.

Source: O'Neill A, Lirk P. Multimodal Analgesia. *Anesthesiol Clin.* 2022; 40(3): 455-468. https://doi.org/10.1016/j.anclin.2022.04.002

OPIOID THERAPY FOR PAIN MANAGEMENT AND THE OPIOID EPIDEMIC

The heightened regulatory focus on treating pain more aggressively led to an increase in the amounts of opioids prescribed for both acute and chronic pain. In the last 2 decades, however, overdoses and unintentional deaths in the United States due to opioids have continued to rise.[21] From 1999 to 2019, close to a half million people died from an overdose involving opioids, obtained either legally through a prescription or illegally from unregulated sources.[21] In the United States, this increase in deaths due to opioid overdose and opioid use disorder (OUD) coincided with increases in the prescribing of opioid medications for pain management.[22] Opioid misuse and OUD have led to a serious threat to public health known as the opioid epidemic.[23] Better pain management, that is, management that is not based on opioid monotherapy, is one initiative of the federal plan to combat the opioid epidemic.[23]

Pain is an expected outcome of surgery, and prior to MMA, opioids were predominantly used to manage surgical pain. Although opioids are an acceptable intervention for pain management following surgery, they are not without risks. As new information came to the forefront about opioids and their role in the epidemic, a closer look at opioid use for postoperative pain management was warranted. Historically, prior to MMA, surgeons prescribed opioids (often in excess amounts), which contributed to addiction, diversion, and misuse.[24]

Many patients receive their first dose of opioids following a surgical procedure. As a result, there has been an increased focus on this patient population.[25] The Centers for Disease Control and Prevention (CDC) has provided treatment recommendations for postsurgical pain.[26] Specifically, if a patient requires opioids, the CDC suggests prescribing only a three-day prescription of shorter-acting opioids combined with nonopioid analgesics to facilitate weaning of the opioids.[26] Although the problem of opioid misuse and abuse is multifactorial, working together to reduce the incidence of unintentional deaths from opioids is the responsibility of all healthcare providers. Areas of opportunity include the modification of prescribing practices, patient and prescriber education, proper disposal of unused medications, and alternatives to the use of opioids. Research supports assessing and identifying patient characteristics that pose risk factors for OUD and limiting the length of time a patient remains on opioids postoperatively.

Provider-targeted strategies can further support limiting the amount of opioids prescribed. Clinical guidelines and care pathways for pain management are available for providers that use specific evidencebased pain management recommendations for the type of surgery done. PROcedure-SPECific Pain ManagemenT (PROSPECT), led by a group of anesthesiologists and surgeons who wished to provide perioperative care guidance for specific operative procedures, is one example of an evidence-based strategy.[27]

All states have prescription monitoring programs enabling prescribers to view individual patient prescription histories.[28] There are legal limitations that vary by state as to the quantity of opioids dispensed and the number of refills that are allowed without additional authorization. These strategies focus on decreasing the amount of opioids available for use and misuse.[29] According to the National Safety Council, 33% of prescription opioid users do not know that they are taking opioids.[28] Patients require information about the medications they are prescribed and the risks of using them, including dependence and addiction, side effects, and associated adverse effects. Education about the use of opioids for postoperative pain and an awareness of the risks involved may lead to shared decision making and patient autonomy.

Lastly, providing information regarding the safe storage and disposal of unused medications is essential for patient and community safety. Over 50% of people who have misused prescription opioids reported that they got them from friends or relatives.[30] Safe storage, including locking up and/or disposing of unused medications, is an important step for reducing opioid availability.[31] Today, healthcare institutions have begun to provide information regarding safe use of these medications and how they can be disposed of properly at the time they are prescribed or dispensed. Research has shown that increasing the perianesthesia nurse's consistency in providing patient and family education regarding safe opioid storage and disposal practices after ambulatory surgery discharge is warranted.[31] Decreasing the number of available unused opioids can lower the incidence of medication diversion, misuse, and abuse.

The majority of patients for whom opioids are prescribed do not misuse them.[22] Most patients who receive opioids do not suffer adverse or long-term effects. Opioids are still an effective part of an MMA treatment plan for relief of severe postoperative pain and have a principal role in pain management.[26] The risks associated with the use of opioids should be communicated, and patients should be involved in the decision whether or not to assume that risk. There is a growing body of knowledge about the characteristics that place some patients at a higher risk for persistent opioid use, which can lead to OUD.[29] Identifying high-risk individuals preoperatively and individually tailoring a plan to reduce or eliminate opioids for them is an important step. Creation of an individualized perioperative pain management plan can mitigate the opioid risk while providing alternatives for effective pain control in the postoperative patient.

BOX 12.2 Best Practice Recommendation

Practice experts from the American Pain Society, the American Society of Regional Anesthesia and Pain Medicine, and the American Society of Anesthesiologists' Committee on Regional Anesthesia published the clinical practice guideline on the management of postoperative pain. The panel recommended that clinicians provide patient- and family-centered education to the patient related to treatment options for the management of postoperative pain. In addition, the panel strongly recommended documentation of both the plan for postoperative pain management and the goals. Evidence indicates that patients receiving individualized education benefit from fewer opioid requirements, reduced preoperative anxiety, fewer requests for sedatives, and a reduced length of stay after surgery.

Educational interventions can range from single episodes of face-to-face instruction or provision of written materials, videos, audiotapes, or Web-based educational information, Additionally, more intensive educational interventions may include monitored exercise and group education classes. Individualized approaches to preoperative education include provision of information that is "age-appropriate, geared to the person's and family's level of comprehension, general health literacy, and cultural and linguistic competency, and supported by timely opportunities to ask questions and receive authoritative and useful answers."

Chou R, Gordon DB, de Leon-Casasola OA, et al. Management of postoperative pain: A clinical practice guideline from the American Pain Society, the American Society of Regional Anesthesia and Pain Medicine, and the American Society of Anesthesiologists' Committee on Regional Anesthesia, executive committee, and administrative council. *J Pain.* 2016;17(2):131–157. https://doi.org/10.1016/j.jpain.2015.12.008

PATIENT EDUCATION ABOUT PAIN CONTROL

Education and the setting of expectations are integral parts of a patient's surgical experience. They are especially important with respect to the management plan for the treatment of postoperative pain. Ideally, patient education begins preoperatively and continues throughout the perioperative process. Patients who have received both preoperative and postoperative education regarding pain expectations and management options use fewer postoperative opioids (Box 12.2).[11,13] The education given should include clear instructions about pain management, such as using the pain assessment tool, identifying and treating sources of discomfort associated with the particular planned surgical event, the reasons for and methods for taking the medication prescribed, the nonpharmacologic therapies that may be used, and when to report pain.[13]

Patients' unrealistic expectations about pain can leave them unprepared to manage postoperative pain. Reviewing and setting realistic expectations, focusing on the functional recovery aspects of the pain management, and setting and reinforcing functional pain goals are fundamental components of perianesthesia patient education. Both verbal and written instructions are included as part of the comprehensive postoperative summary provided for the patient and family prior to discharge.

CHAPTER HIGHLIGHTS

- Effective pain management is essential to the success of ambulatory surgery.
- Pain is a personalized experience that has a physiological, psychological, and behavioral component.
- There are a variety of pain assessment tools in use and should be individualized based on the unique needs of each patient.
- The gold standard for pain assessment is the patient's self-report of pain.
- Multimodal analgesia combines agents and nonpharmacological methods to provide pain control.
- The opioid epidemic is a threat to public health and safety.

CASE STUDY

Randy is a 22-year-old male presenting to the ambulatory surgery center for a right knee arthroscopy. He was involved in a motorcycle crash approximately 4 months ago and has had persistent pain in his right knee. He is otherwise healthy. His medical history is unremarkable. His medications include acetaminophen 500 mg to be taken as needed that he takes occasionally and oxycodone 10 mg taken as needed that was prescribed by his family physician following the crash.

What are significant findings in Randy's health history that may impact his pain management needs?

What might Randy expect as part of his pain management plan?

Randy is given a postoperative prescription for additional oxycodone. What type of education should accompany the medication?

REFERENCES

1. Gan TJ. Poorly controlled postoperative pain: prevalence, consequences, and prevention. *JPain Res.* 2017;10:2287-2298. Available at: https://doi.org/10.2147/JPR.S144066.
2. Institute of Medicine (US) Committee on Advancing Pain Research, Care, and Education. *Relieving Pain in America: A Blueprint for Transforming Prevention, Care, Education, and Research.* Washington (DC): National Academies Press (US); 2011. Available at: https://doi.org/10.17226/13172.
3. Raeder J. Procedure-specific and patient-specific pain management for ambulatory surgery with emphasis on the opioid crisis. *Curr Opin Anaesthesiol.* 2020;33(6):753-759. Available at: https://doi.org/10.1097/aco.0000000000000922.
4. Rana MV, Desai R, Tran L, Davis D. Perioperative pain control in the ambulatory setting. *Curr Pain Headache Rep.* 2016;20(3):18. Available at: https://doi.org/10.1007/s11916-016-0550-3.
5. Richebé P, Capdevila X, Rivat C. Persistent postsurgical pain: pathophysiology and preventative pharmacologic considerations. *Anesthesiology.* 2018;129(3):590-607. Available at: https://doi.org/10.1097/aln.0000000000002238.
6. Raja S, Carr D, Cohen M, et al. The revised International Association for the Study of Pain definition of pain: concepts, challenges, and compromises. *Pain.* 2020;161(9):1976-1982. Available at: https://doi.org/10.1097/j.pain.0000000000001939.
7. Colwell AQ. Pain Management. In: Odom-Forren J, ed. *Drain's Perianesthesia Nursing: A Critical Care Approach.* 7th ed. Elsevier; 2018.
8. Thapa P, Euasobhon P. Chronic postsurgical pain: current evidence for prevention and management. *Korean J Pain.* 2018;31(3):155-173. Available at: https://doi.org/10.3344/kjp.2018.31.3.155.
9. Gulur P, Nelli A. Persistent postoperative pain: mechanisms and modulators. *Curr Opin Anaesthesiol.* 2019;32(5):668-673. Available at: https://doi.org/10.1097/aco.0000000000000770.
10. Kehlet H, Jensen TS, Woolf CJ. Persistent postsurgical pain: risk factors and prevention. *Lancet.* 2006:367(9522):1618-1625. Available at: https://doi.org/10.1016/s0140-6736(06)68700-x.
11. Khorfan R, Shallcross ML, Yu B, et al. Pre-operative patient education and patient preparedness are associated with less postoperative use of opioids. *Surgery.* 2020;167(5):852-858. Available at: https://doi.org/10.1016%2Fj.surg.2020.01.002.

12. Garimella V, Cellini C. Postoperative pain control. *Clin Colon Rectal Surg.* 2013;26(3):191-196. Available at: https://doi.org/10.1055%2Fs-0033-1351138.
13. Chou R, Gordon DB, de Leon-Casasola OA, et al. Management of postoperative pain: a clinical practice guideline from the American Pain Society, the American Society of Regional Anesthesia and Pain Medicine, and the American Society of Anesthesiologists' Committee on Regional Anesthesia, executive committee, and administrative council. *J Pain.* 2016;17(2):131-157. Available at: https://doi.org/10.1016/j.jpain.2015.12.008.
14. Card EB, Wells N, Mesko P, et al. Perianesthesia nurses pain management practices: Findings and recommendations from a national descriptive study of members of the American Society of Perianesthesia Nurses. *J Perianesth Nurs.* 2021;36(2):128-135. Available at: https://doi.org/10.1016/j.jopan.2020.07.007.
15. Wells N, Pasero C, McCaffery M. Improving the quality of care through pain assessment and management. In: Hughes RG, ed. *Patient Safety and Quality: An Evidence-Based Handbook for Nurses.* Agency for Healthcare Research and Quality (US); 2008 [chapter 17]. Available at: www.ncbi.nlm.nih.gov/books/NBK2658/.
16. Wilson L, Kane HL. Pain and comfort. In: Schick L, Windle PE, eds. *PeriAnesthesia Nursing Core Curriculum: Preprocedure, Phase I and Phase II PACU Nursing.* 4th ed. Elsevier: 2021.
17. Kissin I. Preemptive analgesia. *Anesthesiology.* 2000;93(4):1138-1143.
18. Rosero EB, Joshi GP. Preemptive, preventive, multimodal analgesia: what do they really mean? *Plast Reconstr Surg.* 2014;134(4 suppl2):85S-93S. Available at: https://doi.org/10.1097/prs.0000000000000671
19. American Society of Perianesthesia Nurses. *2021-2022 Perianesthesia Nursing Standards, Practice Recommendations and Interpretive Statements.* ASPAN; 2020.
20. Mariano ER, Schatman ME. A commonsense patient-centered approach to multimodal analgesia within surgical enhanced recovery protocols. *J Pain Res.* 2019;12:3461-3466. Available at: https://doi.org/10.2147/jpr.s238772.
21. Centers for Disease Control and Prevention. *Understanding the Opioid Overdose Epidemic.* CDC; 2022. Available at: www.cdc.gov/opioids/basics/epidemic.html#combatting-the-epidemic.
22. National Academies of Sciences, Engineering, and Medicine. *Pain Management and The Opioid Epidemic: Balancing Societal and Individual Benefits and Risks of Prescription Opioid Use.* The National Academies Press; 2017. Available at: https://doi.org/10.17226/24781.
23. U.S. Department of Health & Human Services. *Overdose Prevention Strategy.* DHHS; 2022. Available at: https://www.hhs.gov/overdose-prevention/.
24. Neuman MD, Bateman BT, Wunsch H. Inappropriate opioid prescription after surgery. *Lancet.* 2019;393(10180):1547-1557. Available at: https://doi.org/10.1016/s0140-6736(19)30428-3.
25. Hasak JM, Roth Bettlach CL, Santosa KB, et al. Empowering postsurgical patients to improve opioid disposal: a before and after quality improvement study. *J Am Coll Surg.* 2018;226(3):235-240.e3. Available at: https://doi.org/10.1016/j.jamcollsurg.2017.11.023.
26. Centers for Disease Control and Prevention. *Postsurgical Pain.* CDC; 2022. Available at: https://www.cdc.gov/acute-pain/postsurgical-pain/index.html.
27. Lee B, Schug SA, Joshi GP, Kehlet H. Procedure-Specific Pain Management (PROSPECT) - an update. *Best Pract Res Clin Anaesthesiol.* 2018;32(2):101-111. Available at: https://doi.org/10.1016/j.bpa.2018.06.012.
28. National Safety Council. *Addressing the Opioid Crisis.* NSC; 2021. Available at: https://www.nsc.org/home-safety/safety-topics/opioids.
29. Centers for Disease Control and Prevention. *Prescription Drug Monitoring Programs (PDMPs).* CDC; 2021. Available at: https://www.cdc.gov/drugoverdose/pdmp/index.html.
30. Brummett CM, Waljee JF, Goesling J, et al. New persistent opioid use after minor and major surgical procedures in US adults. *JAMA Surg.* 2017;152(6):e170504. Available at: https://doi.org/10.1001/jamasurg.2017.0504.
31. Odom-Forren J, Brady J, Rayens MK, Sloan P. Perianesthesia nurses' knowledge and promotion of safe use, storage, and disposal of opioids. *J Perianesth Nurs.* 2019;34(6):1156-1168. Available at: https://doi.org/10.1016/j.jopan.2019.04.005.

12

13 Pharmacologic Interventions for Pain Management

Antoinette A Zito, MSN, CPAN, FASPAN

LEARNING OBJECTIVES

A review of the content of this chapter will help the reader to:

1. Identify analgesic strategies to address postoperative pain.
2. List appropriate analgesic techniques utilized in the ambulatory surgery patient.
3. Identify common pharmacologic interventions used for pain management.
4. Identify nursing implications associated with pharmacologic agents.

OVERVIEW

The goal of an effective pain management plan is to reduce and/or control the patient's pain with minimal side effects and maximum physical functioning and to support early mobilization. Whenever possible, a multimodal approach incorporating both pharmacologic and nonpharmacologic methods is used. Pharmacologic agents are the central components for the treatment of postoperative pain. A variety of medications are used to target different levels of the pain neuropathway by way of varied mechanisms of action. Box 13.1 shows a multimodal pain management plan.

The different types of pain are discussed in Chapter 12. Ambulatory surgery requires a focused approach so that patients can be discharged to go home on the day of the procedure. A comprehensive pain assessment and an individualized approach guide the pain management plan. The type of surgical procedure being done, the anticipated severity of pain based on the procedure planned, the expectations for pain management, and the physiologic makeup of the patient are all contributing factors to the overall pain management plan. Patients requiring highly complex surgeries and/or those with extremely multifaceted pain management needs may be excluded from the ambulatory surgery setting.

The following pharmacologic interventions are typically utilized in the ambulatory surgery setting. An increased focus on the best practice for effective acute perioperative pain management has resulted in the development of evidence-based guidelines.[1] This chapter does not provide an exhaustive list of the medications and techniques available, but it discusses here the most common pharmacologic interventions used with ambulatory surgery (Table 13.1).

Anesthetic Techniques and Administration

The type of drug, the site of action targeted, and any adverse effects that may occur require careful consideration for every patient. Many medications act in different areas of the central nervous system, and prescribers therefore use a multimodal approach to avoid opioids as much as possible. In light of the opioid epidemic in the United States, the focus has shifted from the historical reliance on opioid monotherapy as the first line of treatment for postoperative pain to multimodal therapies. The use of a variety of analgesic medications targeting different mechanisms of action along pain pathways is the current best practice. Multimodal therapies may have a synergistic effect resulting in reduced opioid requirements and more effective pain management (Figure 13.1).[1]

The route of medication administration can vary in the perianesthesia setting. Initiating oral agents for pain management postoperatively is often the preferred first route of administration when feasible.[2] This is a common approach when administering preemptive or preventive medications in the preoperative phase of care. During intraoperative and postoperative phases, depending on the immediate postoperative presentation of the patient, the intravenous (IV) route is highly efficient.[2] Clinicians are cautioned to avoid using an intramuscular injection for analgesic administration because the injection can cause pain, the absorption of the medication is unreliable, and this route has not demonstrated an advantage over the others.[3] Local analgesics can also be administered topically and intradermally, although the rate of absorption may be inconsistent and unpredictable.

Local/Regional Anesthesia

Local and regional forms of anesthesia are routinely used in the ambulatory surgery setting and are reviewed in greater detail in Chapter 10. These techniques can be a crucial part of the initial analgesic plan. In some cases, the entire surgical procedure can be performed using only local or regional anesthesia as the primary anesthetic technique.

Local infiltration refers to the administration of a local anesthetic targeting a small area of the body. This infiltration results in numbness or a loss of sensation in the skin, tissue, and local nerves, minimizing or eliminating pain. The local anesthetic agent works by blocking conduction at the nociceptor pain receptors and prevents signals or impulses from reaching the brain. Local infiltration can be accomplished by a single injection or several injections and is most often administered by the surgeon directly at the operative site.

There are two groups of local anesthetics, amides and esters. The clinical differences between the two groups are based on their molecular structures (Table 13.2). Local anesthetics have minimal side effects, and complications are rare unless the agents are inadvertently absorbed intravascularly. A local anesthetic can have an approximate duration of action of 8–12 hours, and because it is a single anesthetic technique, it allows the patient to remain fully awake for the procedure. The absorption of the local anesthetic is dependent on the medication, dose, and location of application; any additives to the medication; and the physiologic features of the patient.[2,4]

Neuraxial and peripheral nerve blocks are also discussed in Chapter 10 and are mentioned here as a common part of a multimodal pain management plan. The local anesthetic agent is injected near a specific nerve or bundle of nerves, resulting in the loss of sensation and, sometimes, movement, so that anesthesia can be obtained in a larger distribution of

BOX 13.1 Example of Multimodal Pain Management (Pharmacologic-Only) Plan

PREOPERATIVE PHASE

Acetaminophen 1000 mg morning of surgery with sips of water
Celecoxib 400 mg po once

INTRAOPERATIVE PHASE

Regional anesthesia per anesthesia provider
Liposomal bupivacaine infiltrated at site by surgeon
Fentanyl 100–200 μg evaluated by effect

POSTOPERATIVE PHASE

Acetaminophen 1000 mg IV every 6 hours
Ketorolac 30 mg IV postoperatively
Oxycodone 5–10 mg po every 6 hours for breakthrough pain
(prescription provided)

Adapted from O'Neill A, Lirk P. Multimodal analgesia. *Anesthesiol Clin*. 2022;40(3):455–468. https://doi.org/10.1016/j.anclin.2022.04.002; and Pitchon DN, Dayan AC, Schwenk ES, Baratta JL, Viscusi ER. Updates on multimodal analgesia for orthopedic surgery. *Anesthesiol Clin*. 2018;36(3):361–373. https://doi.org/10.1016/j.anclin.2018.05.001

Step 3 **Strong opioid**
e.g. morphine, hydromorphone, oxycodone, buprenorphine, fentanyl, methadone

Step 2 **Weak opioid**
e.g. codeine, dihydrocodeine, tramadol

Step 1 **Non-opioid**
e.g. aspirin, ibuprofen, diclofenac, COX-2 inhibitors, paracetamol

- The World Health Organization (WHO) guidelines advocate that when pain occurs, there should be prompt oral administration of drugs, administered in accordance with steps 1–3.
- To maintain freedom from pain, drugs should be taken 'by the clock' every 3–6 hours, rather than 'on demand' and each patient should receive tailored pain management.
- This 3-step approach of administering the right drug in the right dose at the right time is inexpensive and 80–90% effective.

Fig. 13.1 World Health Organization pain ladder. (From Ramaswamy S. Patients in pain. In: Glynn M, Drake WM, eds. *Hutchinson's Clinical Methods*. 25th ed. Elsevier; 2023.)

TABLE 13.1 Common Classes of Pain Medications

Nonopioid Analgesics	Opioid Agents
Acetaminophen	Morphine
NSAIDs	Hydrocodone
Aspirin	Oxycodone
Ibuprofen	Hydromorphone
Naproxen	Oxymorphone
Meloxicam	Fentanyl
Celecoxib	Tramadol
Antidepressants	
Amitriptyline	
Antiepilpetics	
Gabapentin	
Pregabalin	
Ketamine	
Glucocorticoids	
Local Anesthetics	

Adapted from Queremel Milani DA, Davis DD. Pain management medications. [Updated July 4, 2022]. In: StatPearls [Internet]. Treasure Island (FL): StatPearls Publishing; 2022. Available from: https://www.ncbi.nlm.nih.gov/books/NBK560692/

TABLE 13.2 Differences Between Amides and Esters

	Amides	Esters
Metabolism	Liver; can result in high blood levels if rapidly absorbed	Catalyzed by plasma and tissue enzymes through hydrolysis; rapid process
Allergic reactions	Rare	Uncommon but higher allergy potential
Duration	Longer acting; lipophilic and protein bound	Shorter acting

Adapted from Nagelhout JJ. Local anesthetics. Table 24.2 in: Odom-Forren J, ed. *Drain's PeriAnesthesia Nursing: A Critical Care Approach*. 7th ed. Elsevier; 2018.

nerves. This technique can be used as the sole form of anesthesia and is commonly used for procedures on the upper and lower extremities. Current and advancing technology allows for the greater application of nerve block techniques.

Each agent's pharmacokinetic properties provide certain advantages (Table 13.3). The greatest advantage of local anesthesia is pain control without generalized involvement of the central nervous system.[5] This allows for minimal compromise in individuals with co-morbidities who may be unable to tolerate more invasive anesthetic approaches. Local and regional anesthesia can also facilitate improved patient throughput in an ambulatory setting because pain is one of the most common reasons for delayed discharge.[6,7] Local anesthetic systemic toxicity (LAST) resulting from intravascular absorption of the anesthetic can occur with any of the agents given and is a rare but serious complication of local anesthesia[2,4] (see Chapter 10). A local anesthetic is considered a safe alternative to general anesthesia and plays an important role in a multimodal anesthetic plan.

TABLE 13.3 Characteristics of Local Anesthetics

Potency	Drug	Onset	Duration of Action
Low	Procaine (Novocaine)	Slow	60–90 minutes
	Chloroprocaine (Nesacaine)	Fast	30–60 minutes
Intermediate	Mepivacaine (Carbocaine)	Fast	120–140 minutes
	Lidocaine (Xylocaine)	Fast	90–120 minutes
High	Tetracaine (Pontocaine)	Slow	3–10 hours
	Bupivacaine (Marcaine, Sensorcaine)	Slow	3–20 hours
	Ropivacaine (Naropin)	Slow	3–10 hours

Nagelhout JJ. Local anesthetics. Table 10.3 in: Nagelhout JJ, Elisha S, eds. *Nurse Anesthesia*. 6th ed. Elsevier; 2018.

PHARMACOLOGIC CLASSES OF COMMONLY USED DRUGS FOR PAIN MANAGEMENT

Acetaminophen

Acetaminophen, also known as APAP or paracetamol, has both analgesic and antipyretic properties. It is one of the most frequently used and cost-effective analgesics in the United States. Acetaminophen works by targeting nociceptive pain (e.g., the most common type of pain related to inflammation or injury) and inhibiting the generation of the prostaglandins responsible for inflammatory responses. Acetaminophen is available without a prescription in a variety of preparations. It is commonly used to treat mild to moderate pain and to temporarily reduce fever. Acetaminophen is recommended as part of a pain management plan for adults and children when there are no contraindications to its use, such as severe liver disease.[3] Routes of administration include oral, rectal, and intravenous; currently, the evidence for which route is more effective remains inconclusive; however, the most common route is oral. Acetaminophen can be given preoperatively as part of a preemptive pain management plan, intraoperatively, or postoperatively.

Adverse effects of acetaminophen are rare, but because the drug is metabolized in the hepatic system, hepatotoxicity can occur. This is most common with high doses, chronic use, the concurrent use of alcohol, and overdose and in patients with known liver disease. Also, acetaminophen can be found in other medications such as certain cold medications and combination prescription drugs. These combination drugs can cause patients to unknowingly ingest higher doses of acetaminophen than intended. Patients should be cautioned NOT to take the dosage prescribed for their postoperative pain control with any other product containing acetaminophen. The maximum daily adult dose of acetaminophen in all forms is 4000 mg in healthy adults. In 2011, the makers of acetaminophen sold as the Tylenol Extra Strength brand voluntarily lowered the maximum daily dosage on the label from 4000 mg to 3000 mg with messaging suggesting that healthcare professionals use discretion when recommending a maximum of 4000 mg daily.[8]

NonSteroidal Anti-inflammatory Drugs

Surgical procedures result in an inflammatory response and enhance the nociceptive pain response.[2,3,9] Nonsteroidal anti-inflammatory drugs (NSAIDS) are nonopioid analgesics designed to target the inflammatory response by limiting the generation and release of the prostaglandins responsible for inflammation and pain. They also have antipyretic properties.

NSAIDS can be used for the mild or moderate pain associated with surgical inflammation and also play a key role in multimodal pain management plans. They are utilized frequently in ambulatory enhanced recovery after surgery (ERAS) protocols.[10,11] NSAIDS are classified as either nonselective or COX-2–specific medications. They can be administered orally, intravenously, or topically.

Nonselective NSAIDS

Nonselective NSAIDS work by inhibiting the synthesis of both the cyclooxygenase 1 (COX-1) and cyclooxygenase 2 (COX-2) enzymes, which inhibit prostaglandin production.[12] COX-1 is found in nearly all tissues in the body. Its most important functions are protecting the gastric mucosa, controlling renal function, and assisting with platelet aggregation.[5,12] The earliest drug recognized in this class was aspirin. Aspirin is also classified as a salicylate and is an irreversible inhibitor of cyclooxygenase. It has an antiplatelet action that is beneficial to many patients with cardiovascular disease.

Nonselective NSAIDS inhibit both COX-1 and COX-2 synthesis and provide an anti-inflammatory effect. Certain drugs in this class also block the protective properties of cyclooxygenase, and this can increase the risk of adverse effects, such as gastrointestinal discomfort and gastric ulcers, bleeding, impaired renal function, myocardial infarction, and stroke.[12] Drugs in this class include naproxen, meloxicam, ibuprofen, and ketorolac.

Selective COX-2 Inhibitors

COX-2–specific inhibitors, or second-generation anti-inflammatory drugs, were developed specifically to target COX-2 enzymes. This action provides an anti-inflammatory response and reduces adverse gastrointestinal effects.[12] These selective drugs can be administered prior to surgery, as well as postoperatively, and have been shown to be effective in pain control.[10] Benefits include less gastrointestinal ulceration and the reduced inhibition of platelet production. Risks include an increase in cardiovascular events, including myocardial infarction and thromboembolism.[7] Adverse effects of selective NSAIDS must be weighed against the benefits in the individual pain management plan. Recommendations include taking the lowest dose for the shortest period since renal and cardiovascular side effects are uncommon with short-term use.[13,14]

Topical NSAIDS treat localized musculoskeletal pain with minimal systemic absorption. Because such a low percentage of these drugs is absorbed systemically, the risk of adverse effects and drug interactions is decreased. One common agent is diclofenac gel, and others are available in the form of creams, sprays, and solutions. Patients are advised to apply the topical NSAID directly over a painful joint or muscle. They are not used directly over surgical sites.

Ketamine

Ketamine is classified as an *N*-methyl-D-aspartate (NMDA) antagonist. It has been available for decades and was initially used as a sole anesthetic for trauma cases due to its limited cardiovascular depression. Ketamine was also an ideal induction agent for patients with reactive airway disease. Ketamine in nonanesthetic doses has more recently been used for the treatment of acute pain, chronic pain, and depression. As an NMDA antagonist, ketamine is currently gaining favor for postoperative pain management as a single agent and as an adjuvant to opioid analgesics. Ketamine can be administered intravenously, intranasally, subcutaneously, and topically as a spray. Adverse effects include mind-altering properties, including feelings of inebriation, confusion, dissociation, perceptual disturbances, and dizziness.[15] Some side effects are reported to be dose dependent. Lower doses of ketamine that manage pain and have minimal side effects are also associated with a decrease in opioid use.[11,15]

Evidence-Based Practice: Ketamine
Once reserved for anesthesia and induction, ketamine can be used at sub-anesthetic doses to produce analgesia. Either as a constant infusion or intermittent dosing, ketamine can reduce postoperative pain scores and increase the amount of time that a patient may require rescue analgesics. Side effects are minimal and often not associated with lower doses. These include nausea, vomiting, dreaming, hallucinating, and dissociation. Patients with known histories of psychosis and post-traumatic stress disorders, cardiovascular disease, and liver anomalies should not receive this adjunct medication.

Source: Silverstein WK, Juurlink DN, Zipursky JS. Ketamine for the treatment of acute pain. *CMAJ*. 2021;193:E1663. https://doi.org/10.1503/cmaj.210878

Glucocorticoids

Local tissue injury and subsequent inflammation are expected outcomes of surgical procedures. The analgesic effect of glucocorticoids (steroids) is aimed at inhibiting prostaglandins, which are responsible for the body's inflammatory response to the surgical injury of tissues. Studies support that a single dose of dexamethasone either preoperatively or intraoperatively can generate positive effects. These positive responses include reduced postoperative pain, the consumption of lower amounts of opioids, and a decreased postanesthesia length of stay.[16] Although dexamethasone has been associated with mild increases in blood glucose postoperatively, its benefits make it a frequent component of multimodal pain management plans.

Additional Adjuvant Pharmacologic Agents

As the practice of pain management continues to evolve, a variety of pharmacologic agents are being used as adjuvant agents in multimodal pain management plans for ambulatory surgery patients. These include α-2 adrenergic agonists, gabapentinoids (antiepileptics), lidocaine, and antidepressants.

Alpha-2 agonists have an anti-nociceptive effect that results from the stimulation of the α-2 receptors in the spinal cord and supraspinal region.[11,14] Their analgesic properties make them appropriate adjuvant agents for multimodal plans. Clonidine and dexmedetomidine are two α-2 agonists that are used in perioperative pain management. Their use is associated with decreased opioid consumption following surgery, with dexmedetomidine being more effective in this regard.[14] Common side effects include bradycardia, hypotension, dizziness, blurred vision, dry mouth, and sedation.[11,14]

Gabapentinoids block calcium channels and thereby inhibit central sensitization. They have both anticonvulsant and nociceptive blocking characteristics.[5,17] Drugs in this class include gabapentin and pregabalin. The use of gabapentinoids for the treatment of chronic neuropathic pain is well established. Gabapentinoids are used as adjuvants for acute postoperative pain and have demonstrated effectiveness in the prevention of chronic postsurgical pain.[18] Gabapentin is commonly prescribed as an anticonvulsant or an antiepileptic drug. Side effects include sedation. These medications are common components of multimodal pain management plans.

Lidocaine is commonly used for its antiarrhythmic effects. This drug also has anti-hyperanalgesic, anti-inflammatory, and analgesic effects. Lidocaine has again seen limited use in the area of acute pain management. More research is needed to demonstrate its benefit in an ambulatory surgery patient population.

Antidepressant medications are classified based on their chemical structure, and many types have been used successfully for the treatment of chronic pain. These include tricyclic antidepressants and selective serotonin reuptake inhibitors. Although these medications have been thought to be potential additions to the field of acute postsurgical pain management, their safety and efficacy have not been consistently demonstrated in studies focusing on acute pain management.[19,20] Research is ongoing to substantiate the routine use of these medications for acute pain management.

Opioids

The class of opioids is one of the oldest classes of drugs used for the management and treatment of pain. Initially, opioids were used to treat coughs, pain, and a variety of maladies. For many years, opioids were the cornerstone of postoperative pain management. The potency of opioids, both pure and synthetic, is measured against that of the standard drug in this class, morphine. Opioids primarily work by acting at the *mu* and *kappa* opioid receptors in the central and peripheral nervous systems.[5,17]

When the *mu* receptors are activated, the physiologic response includes analgesia, euphoria, respiratory depression, and sedation.[5,17] Unintended respiratory depression and unwanted sedation are most concerning in the postoperative setting. Other adverse effects include constipation, orthostatic hypotension, hyperalgesia, urinary retention, nausea, vomiting, pruritis, and the risk for persistent use and addiction. Long-acting opioids are not recommended for use postoperatively due to the risk of misuse and the prevalence of substance use disorders. When necessary, opioids are incorporated in limited doses in a multimodal pain management regime following ambulatory surgery. Many providers strive for opioid-sparing options.

CHAPTER HIGHLIGHTS

- Considerations for the drug chosen for pain management include mechanism of action, duration of action, and route of administration.
- A multimodal approach to promote pain management is the standard of care in postsurgical pain protocols.
- Combining different agents that act on different receptor sites is the key to a successful pain management plan.
- Consideration is given to the individual needs of the patient, the type of surgery being done, and the postoperative needs of the patient.
- An opioid-only approach is no longer considered the standard of care.

CASE STUDY

Emilia R., age 65, presents to the ambulatory surgery center for elective right total hip arthroplasty. She is extremely healthy. Her only documented diagnosis is osteoarthritis of the right hip. She is planning for a same-day discharge. She has participated in a preoperative prehabilitation consultation to optimize her physical conditioning. A complete physical examination, medical history, and pain assessment have been completed. She has received acetaminophen 1000 mg and celecoxib 400 mg by mouth preoperatively. Upon arrival at the ambulatory surgical center, the anesthesiologist administered an ultrasound-guided fascia iliaca regional block with 0.2% ropivacaine used as a local anesthetic.

Intraoperatively, Emilia received a spinal anesthetic with 1.7 mL of 0.75% bupivacaine. The surgeon injected a local infiltration of 30 mL of 0.5% ropivacaine at the surgical site prior to wound closure. Emilia received midazolam 1 mg in the operating room.

Postoperatively, Emilia was awake and alert with partial resolution of the spinal anesthetic. Ice bags were placed on the operative site. She had an uneventful postoperative course and received no further analgesic medication in the PACU. She was transferred to phase II, where she was able to fully participate in the physical therapy session once the spinal anesthesia had resolved, demonstrating safety with ambulation. She received ketorolac 30 mg intravenously prior to discharge and voided without difficulty. Emilia was safely discharged to go home, where she continued to take acetaminophen 1000 mg every 6 hours. In addition, she had a prescription for oxycodone 5–10 mg every 6 hours as needed for breakthrough pain.

What information does this patient need to have regarding her postoperative pain management plan?

- Should she be told when to take the next dose of acetaminophen and how to proceed with around-the-clock dosing?
- Is she likely to also have a schedule for taking an oral NSAID?
- Should this patient be advised to take opioids preemptively prior to a physical therapy session "in case of pain?"
- Which nonpharmacologic interventions should be recommended for enhancing comfort? Rest? Elevation? Ice?
- What education does Emilia need regarding unused opioids?

REFERENCES

1. Mariano ER, Dickerson DM, Szokol JW, et al. A multisociety organizational consensus process to define guiding principles for acute perioperative pain management. *Reg Anesth Pain Med.* 2021;47(2):118-127. Available at: https://doi.org/10.1136/rapm-2021-103083.
2. Pasero C. Pain management. In Odom-Forren J, ed. *Drain's Peri-Anesthesia Nursing: A Critical Care Approach.* 7th ed. Elsevier; 2018.
3. Chou R, Gordon DB, de Leon-Casasola OA, et al. Management of postoperative pain: a clinical practice guideline from the American Pain Society, the American Society of Regional Anesthesia and Pain Medicine, and the American Society of Anesthesiologists' Committee on Regional Anesthesia, executive committee, and administrative council. *J Pain.* 2016;17(2):131-157. Available at: https://doi.org/10.1016/j.jpain.2015.12.008.
4. Brown C. Anesthesia, moderate sedation/analgesia. In: Schick L, Windle PE, eds. *PeriAnesthesia Nursing Core Curriculum: Preprocedure, Phase I and Phase II PACU Nursing.* 4th ed. Elsevier; 2021:250.
5. Rosenthal LD, Burchum JR, eds. *Lehne's Pharmacotherapeutics for Advanced Practice Nurses and Physician Assistants.* 2nd ed. Elsevier; 2021.
6. Raeder J. Procedure-specific and patient-specific pain management for ambulatory surgery with emphasis on the opioid crisis. *Curr Opin Anaesthesiol.* 2020;33(6):753-759. Available at: https://doi.org/10.1097/aco.0000000000000922.
7. Rana MV, Desai R, Tran L, Davis D. Perioperative pain control in the ambulatory setting. *Curr Pain Headache Rep.* 2016;20(3):18. Available at: https://doi.org/10.1007/s11916-016-0550-3.
8. Johnson & Johnson Consumer, Inc. McNeil Health Care Division. Tylenol for Healthcare Professionals. *Adult Dosing Charts.* Available at: www.tylenolprofessional.com/adult-dosage. Accessed November 6, 2021.
9. Brown EN, Pavone KJ, Naranjo M. Multimodal general anesthesia: theory and practice. *Anesth Analg.* 2018;127(5):1246-1258. Available at: https://doi.org/10.1213/ane.0000000000003668.
10. Charipova K, Gress KL, Urits I, Viswanath O, Kaye AD. Maximization of non-opioid multimodal analgesia in ambulatory surgery centers. *Cureus.* 2020;12(9):e10407. Available at: https://doi.org/10.7759/cureus.10407.
11. Kaye AD, Urman RD, Rappaport Y, et al. Multimodal analgesia as an essential part of enhanced recovery protocols in the ambulatory settings. *J Anaesthesiol Clin Pharmacol.* 2019;35(suppl 1):S40-S45. Available at: https://doi.org/10.4103/joacp.joacp_51_18.
12. Dahlen L, Oakes JM. A review of physiology and pharmacology related to acute perioperative pain management. *AANA J.* 2017; 85(4):300-308.
13. Helander EM, Menard BL, Harmon CM, et al. Multimodal analgesia, current concepts, and acute pain considerations. *Curr Pain Headache Rep.* 2017;21(1):3. Available at: https://doi.org/10.1007/s11916-017-0607-y.
14. Jafra A, Mitra S. Pain relief after ambulatory surgery: progress over the last decade. *Saudi J Anaesth.* 2018;12(4):618-625. Available at: https://doi.org/10.4103/sja.sja_232_18.
15. Radvansky BM, Shah K, Parikh A, Sifonios AN, Le V, Eloy JD. Role of ketamine in acute postoperative pain management: a narrative review. *Biomed Res Int.* 2015;2015:749837. Available at: https://doi.org/10.1155/2015/749837.
16. Waldron NH, Jones CA, Gan TJ, Allen TK, Habib AS. Impact of perioperative dexamethasone on postoperative analgesia and side-effects: systematic review and meta-analysis. *Br J Anaesth.* 2013;110(2): 191-200. Available at: https://doi.org/10.1093/bja/aes431.
17. Burchum JR, Rosenthal RD, eds. *Lehne's Pharmacology for Nursing Care.* 11th ed. Elsevier; 2021.
18. Clarke H, Bonin RP, Orser BA, Englesakis M, Wijeysundera DN, Katz J. The prevention of chronic postsurgical pain using gabapentin and pregabalin: a combined systematic review and meta-analysis. *Anesth Analg.* 2012;115(2):428-442. Available at: https://doi.org/10.1213/ane.0b013e318249d36e.
19. Wong K, Phelan R, Kalso E, et al. Antidepressant drugs for prevention of acute and chronic postsurgical pain: early evidence and recommended future directions. *Anesthesiology.* 2014;121(3):591-608. Available at: https://doi.org/10.1097/aln.0000000000000307.
20. Gilron I. Antidepressant drugs for postsurgical pain: current status and future directions. *Drugs.* 2016;76(2):159-167. Available at: https://doi.org/10.1007/s40265-015-0517-4.

14 Nonpharmacologic Interventions for Pain Management

Helen C. Fong, DNP, RN, CPAN, PHN, FASPAN

LEARNING OBJECTIVES

A review of the content of this chapter will help the reader to:

1. Determine the best available evidence on the effectiveness of nonpharmacologic interventions to reduce pain.
2. Identify terms, definitions, and general information associated with nonpharmacologic therapies.
3. Identify the role of nurses in the preoperative and postoperative phases while using nonpharmacologic interventions.

OVERVIEW

Pain is inevitable after surgery. The International Association for the Study of Pain defines *pain* "as an unpleasant sensory and emotional experience with actual or potential tissue damage."[1] Patients who undergo surgical procedures are generally prescribed postoperative pharmaceutical remedies for pain control. In addition to pharmacologic therapies, many patients accept nonpharmacologic methods for supporting their optimal comfort and relief of operative pain.[2] These methods include physical, biologic, and cognitive therapies. Examples include massage, acupuncture, heat or cold devices, relaxation techniques, meditation, essential oils, and therapeutic touch, to name a few.[2]

The use, abuse, and misuse of opioids that have contributed to the recent opioid crisis serve as an additional impetus for the application of nonpharmacologic therapies in the setting of acute postoperative pain. An estimated 50,000 opioid overdose deaths were reported in 2019,[3] and 10.1 million people reportedly misused opioids.[4] The Centers for Disease Control and Prevention (CDC) analyzed the 2016 National Health Interview Survey data[3] and estimated that 20.4% (~50 million) U.S. adults had chronic pain and about 8% suffered from high-impact chronic pain.[5] About 50% of patients diagnosed with chronic pain attributed the origin to acute care settings, such as surgical facilities.[6] Chronic pain and reliance on pharmaceutical approaches have been factors in the rise in opioid substance use disorder (SUD).[7] As a result of the growing concern about opioid misuse, healthcare providers are directing patients toward nonpharmacologic interventions to help manage pain.[7]

Beginning in January 2018, The Joint Commission (TJC) recommended that all accredited facilities adopt nonpharmacologic therapies for pain management (Box 14.1).[6] The CDC also recommended alternative pain interventions to help mitigate the potential for opioid abuse.[8] The CDC and TJC have provided guidelines for pain management that include nonpharmacologic means to help reduce opioid misuse, abuse, and overdoses[9] (Box 14.2). Nonpharmacologic methods have demonstrated great benefits for postoperative pain

and acute pain not related to surgery.[6] Reports suggested that 49% of patients who were receiving treatment for SUD also used nonpharmacologic strategies to provide pain relief.[10] These findings support the importance of integrating nonpharmacologic pain management interventions in the plan of care.[5]

EFFICACY OF NONPHARMACOLOGIC INTERVENTIONS

Colwell reports that most patients want to be offered alternative methods of self-management pain strategies for their health.[2] The Mayo Clinic joined the Agency for Healthcare Research and Quality to conduct systematic reviews of nonpharmacologic methods for chronic pain management.[7] The systematic reviews identified a variety of professional occupations with access to training in the use of and delivery of nonpharmacologic pain interventions (e.g., athletic trainers, yoga instructors, massage therapists, physical therapists, nurses, chiropractors).[7] The study also showed how education, policies, and practices can either be a barrier to or a facilitator of effective collaborative forms of nonpharmacologic pain management and cited the value of team-based care.[7] For example, Pollack and colleagues suggested that while many professions provide alternative therapies, primary care providers, as well as patients and consumers, may lack knowledge of the services available in the community to support nonopioid and nonpharmacologic treatment of both acute and chronic pain.[7]

Pain is an unpleasant multidimensional experience.[11] As a complex event, pain impacts several factors in a person's life, including physical, psychological, and emotional components. Accordingly, it is important that pain strategies address these components by employing a combination of physical, psychological, and behavioral approaches.[7,11] The effects of nonpharmacologic interventions can be unpredictable but may offer other benefits to patients.[2] Research has shown that complementary therapies enable patients to relax, thus reducing anxiety and stress.[2] Colwell indicated that the integration of nonpharmacologic therapies enhanced coping strategies, which in turn enabled patients to experience greater control and management of acute pain.[2]

Tick, along with other members of the Pain Task Force of the Academic Consortium for Integrative Medicine and Health, reviewed evidence-based nonpharmacologic therapies in the context of comprehensive pain care.[6] These evidence-based strategies are considered both safe and effective with regard to postsurgical pain.[6] Examples include acupuncture, massage, osteopathic and chiropractic manipulation, meditative movements such as tai chi and yoga, mind–body behavioral interventions, dietary components, and a self-care/self-efficacy strategy.[6] Studies have shown that evidence-based nonpharmacologic therapies such as acupuncture, yoga, tai chi, qigong, and the Alexander technique are effective in managing pain.[7,12]

BOX 14.1 The Joint Commission's Requirement and Rationale for the Use of Nonpharmacologic Interventions

Requirement: EP 2: The hospital provides nonpharmacologic pain treatment modalities.

Rationale: While evidence for some nonpharmacologic modalities is mixed and/or limited, these modalities may serve as a complementary approach for pain management and potentially reduce the need for opioid medications in some circumstances. The hospital should promote nonpharmacologic modalities by ensuring that patient preferences are discussed and, at a minimum, providing some nonpharmacologic treatment options relevant to their patient population. When a patient's preference for a safe nonpharmacologic therapy cannot be provided, hospitals should educate the patient on where the treatment may be accessed postdischarge. Nonpharmacologic strategies include, but are not limited to, physical modalities (e.g., acupuncture therapy, chiropractic therapy, osteopathic manipulative treatment, massage therapy, and physical therapy), relaxation therapy, and cognitive-behavioral therapy.

The Joint Commission. R3 Report: Requirement, Rationale, Reference. 2017;11:1–7. Page 2. https:// www.jointcommission.org/-/media/tjc/documents/resources/pain-management/r3_report_issue_11_pain_assessment_2_11_19_rev.pdf?db5web&hash515B5F09539D1CE9DBA629DB9FDAF0756&hash515B5F09539D1CE9DBA629DB9FDAF0756

BOX 14.2 Nonpharmacologic and Nonopioid Solutions for Pain Management

Evidenced-based, nonopioid treatment options to consider for treating pain.

Behavioral/Cognitive Interventions/Psychological

- *Meditation techniques* utilized with mindfulness-based reduction (MBSR) have been shown to be effective for pain reduction and strong continued patient compliance.
- *Progressive muscle relaxation* can assist in regulating neurosystems found in muscle tension and situational stress commonly seen with pain.

Environmental-based Interventions

- *Lighting* alterations can create an environment that supports muscle relaxation.
- *Music therapy* has been associated with a statistically significant reduction in opioid and nonopioid analgesic use.

Physical Interventions

- *Acupuncture* was recommended as a first-line treatment in lower back pain by the American College of Physicians.
- *Massage therapy* has been shown to be effective in adult and pediatric populations with minimal risks of side effects.
- *Spinal manipulation* has shown improvement in pain for patients experiencing chronic lower back pain, shoulder pain, and migraines.

The Joint Commission. Non-pharmacologic and non-opioid solutions for pain management. *Quick Safety*. 2018;44:1–2. https:// www.jointcommission.org/-/media/tjc/newsletters/qs-nonopioid-pain-mgmt-8-15-18-final2.pdf, CDC

Nonpharmacologic therapies can be applied as monotherapy approaches or can be used as complementary therapies in combination with contemporary pain management methods.[6] The benefits of these therapies include, but are not limited to, their ability to reduce pain, anxiety, depression, and nausea and vomiting, promote sleep, improve a patient's sense of well-being, and support a patient's motivation to be involved in the recovery of health.[6]

COMPLEMENTARY ALTERNATIVE MEDICINE AND INTEGRATIVE MEDICINE

Nonpharmacologic interventions are considered components of complementary and alternative medicine (CAM).[13] CAM is a term used to describe therapies that are based on certain beliefs, theories, and practices that are not elements of standard medical care. Many of the traditional CAM practices are considered natural and holistic remedies derived primarily from Eastern medicine and beliefs.[14] Healing systems and beliefs have evolved over time and in various cultures.[15] For example, ayurvedic medicine, which started in India, believes that healing includes the cleansing of the body, mind, and spirit, while traditional Chinese medicine believes that health is a balance of energy known as yin and yang.[14] CAM practices include, but are not limited to, tai chi, yoga, acupuncture, massage, osteopathic manipulation, reiki, and hypnosis.[1,7,12,14] CAM, when combined with standard medical treatment, is referred to as integrative medicine.[6,7,14]

According to the Johns Hopkins pain clinic, an estimated 38% of adults and 12% of children use CAM.[16] Some CAM therapies have undergone thorough evaluations and been found to be safe and effective, such as yoga, acupuncture, and meditation.[12] The ability of nonpharmacologic therapies to produce the desired outcome, which is reduced postoperative pain and discomfort, can be difficult to predict, and for many, further study is required.[2] The National Center for Complementary and Integrative Health funds and conducts a wide range of studies focusing on the utilization and effects of CAM. For more detailed resources, visit https://www.nccih.nih.gov.

FIVE CATEGORIES OF NONPHARMACOLOGIC INTERVENTION

Nonpharmacologic methodologies can be grouped into five basic categories, each of which has its own approach to nonpharmacologic pain management (Table 14.1).[7,14,16] Since pain is multifaceted, it is important to understand which minimally invasive, nonpharmacologic modalities will help reduce the pain while minimizing the intake of oral medications, particularly opioids.[7]

Behavioral Health and Cognitive Modalities

Behavioral health approaches to pain and comfort management address the emotional, behavioral, social, and cognitive factors affecting a patient's response to pain.[7,11] Pain is processed in the brain. The gate control theory of pain, which is based on the transmission of a pain impulse through the dorsal horn of the spinal cord, explains the clinical and scientific rationales for the way that pain is perceived.[14] Psychological factors, including thoughts and emotions, are an integral part of pain processing.[17] This knowledge of the psychology of pain opens new avenues for pain control. The nerve pain gate can be closed by impulses in the brain to prevent the pain signal from reaching the brain and being experienced as pain.[17] These

TABLE 14.1 Basic Categories of Nonpharmacologic Pain Management Interventions

Modality	Examples	Therapeutic Action
Behavioral health (cognitive)	Breathing Distraction Mindfulness Psychotherapy	Supports the engagement of patients to learn healthy responses to pain
Biofield (energy therapies)	Reiki Therapeutic touch	As a popular therapy, the biofield approach uses the manipulation of energy fields to reestablish balance and health
Biologic	Aromatherapy Cannabis Dietary approach Essential oils Herbal supplements Homeopathy	Dietary and herbal approaches aim to balance the nutritional well-being of the body
Body-based (physical)	Cold therapy Exercise and physical therapy Heat therapy Massage Positioning	Body-based therapies support the body's effort to heal by stimulating the natural production of pain-relieving physiologic chemicals
Body–mind	Biofeedback Hypnosis Meditation Prayer Tai chi Yoga	Allows for physical and mental relaxation, which helps lower the pain experience

Adapted from Johns Hopkins Medicine. Types of complementary and alternative medicine. What are different types of CAM? 2022. https://www.hopkinsmedicine.org/health/wellness-and-prevention/types-of-complementary-and-alternative-medicine; Pollack SW, Skillman SM, Frogner BK. *The health workforce delivering evidence-based non-pharmacological pain management.* February 2020. https://depts.washington.edu/fammed/chws/wp-content/uploads/sites/5/2020/02/Non-Pharmacological-Pain-Management-FR-2020.pdf ; and Yazici G, Erdogan Z, Bulut H, et al. The use of complementary and alternative medicines among surgical patients: A survey study. *J PeriAnesth Nurs.* 2018;34(2):322–329. https://doi.org/10.1016/j.jopan.2018.04.007

impulses can be categorized as sensory (physical being and activities), cognitive (thoughts), and emotional (feelings). Poor body mechanics and inactivity keep pain gates open, while increasing activities and relaxation techniques stimulate the inhibition of pain signal transmission, improve circulation, reduce suffering, and enhance sleep quality.[12] Patients who always worry about pain and focus on negative thoughts are best directed to use their imagination, sense of play, and focus on relaxation.[12] Breathing techniques, guided imagery, distraction, mindfulness, stress reduction strategies, and music therapy work well for these patients.[1,7,12] These modalities allow patients to relax and not focus on the pain. Behavioral and cognitive strategies are also effective for patients experiencing depression, anxiety, and stress.[12] Guided imagery allows patients to imagine scenes, pictures, or experiences to help the body heal.[12] A recent meta-analysis revealed a positive correlation between the use of guided imagery preoperatively and the reduction of anxiety and postoperative pain.[18] For guided imagery suggestions, see Box 14.3.

Biofield Modalities

Energy medicine, also known as biofield therapy, embraces the belief that the body has energy fields that can be used for healing

BOX 14.3 Common Interactive Guided Imagery Suggestions and Questions

Allow an image to form.
What do you notice about it?
What are you aware of?
What are you experiencing?
What would you like to notice yourself having?
What would you like to say to it?
What sensations are you aware of?
Let me know when you are ready to move on.

Rossman ML. Guided imagery and interactive guided imagery. Table 94.4 in: Rakel D, Minichiello VJ, eds. *Integrative Medicine.* 5th ed. Elsevier; 2023.

and wellness.[1,2,19] Biofield practitioners believe that human beings are open energy systems and that the flow of energy between people is continuous and natural.[19] Therapists use energy therapy by placing their hands in and through these energy fields to facilitate healing during treatment.[12,19] Examples include therapeutic touch, reiki, and tai chi.[2] Reiki techniques originated 3000 years ago and are believed to balance energy and bring harmony to the body, mind, and soul.[19] Reiki involves the movement of the therapist's hands over energy fields in the body, employing a light touch over clothing. This touch begins with the head and moves down to the body, front and back.[12,19] In certain circumstances, reiki has been shown to reduce stress, minimize anxiety, and promote relaxation.[19]

Biologic Modalities

Vitamins, herbs, and essential oils fall in the category of biologic modalities.[2] Biologic modalities use items found in nature, such as dietary supplements, plants, or parts of plants. Cannabis, herbs, and spices such as turmeric, cinnamon, and ginger are among the many available biologic possibilities.[12] Special foods or particular diets can also help alleviate pain.[12] Homeopathy is based on the belief that very small doses of natural substances will trigger the body to heal itself. Arnica, derived from a medicinal preparation of the arnica plant, is often used postoperatively by patients to treat aches, pains, and bruises.[20] Limited studies indicate that some herbal therapies should be discontinued prior to surgery due to potential complications. Refer to Table 14.2 for a brief summary and see Figure 14.1.

Evidence-Based Practice: Homeopathic Arnica Montana
Homeopathy is a common form of complementary or integrative therapy that uses products produced from plant, mineral, or animal sources. These products, in the form of sugar pellets, ointments, gels, drops, tablets, or creams, are used based on the theory that diseases can be cured by substances that produce similar symptoms in people using the lowest possible dose to create the maximum effect. A meta-analysis published by Gaertner et al., found that the advertised benefits of Arnica montana including the prevention or treatment of pain and excessive bleeding, could be effective. The conclusion of the analysis is that the effects of the homeopathic remedy, Arnica, were comparable to that of anti-inflammatory agents.

Gaertner K, Baumgartner S, Walach S. Is homeopathic Arnica effective for postoperative recovery? A meta-analysis of placebo-controlled and active comparator trials. *Front Surg.* 2021;8:680930. https://doi.org/10.3389/fsurg.2021.680930

TABLE 14.2 Clinically Important Effects, Perioperative Concerns, and Recommendations for Perioperative Discontinuation of 11 Commonly Used Herbal Medicines

Herbs (Common Names)	Pharmacologic Effects	Perioperative Concerns	Discontinue Before Surgery
Echinacea (purple coneflower root)	Activation of cell-mediated immunity	Allergic reactions Decreases effectiveness of immunosuppressants Potential for immunosuppression with long-term use	No data
Ephedra (ma huang)	Increases heart rate and blood pressure through direct and indirect sympathomimetic effects	Risk of myocardial ischemia and stroke from tachycardia and hypertension Ventricular arrhythmias with halothane Long-term use depletes endogenous catecholamines and may cause intraoperative hemodynamic instability Life-threatening interaction with monoamine oxidase inhibitors	24 hours
Garlic (ajo)	Inhibits platelet aggregation (may be irreversible) Increases fibrinolysis Equivocal antihypertensive activity	May increase risk of bleeding, especially when combined with other medications that inhibit platelet aggregation	7 days
Ginger	Antiemetic Antiplatelet aggregation	May increase risk of bleeding	No data
Ginkgo (duck-foot tree, maidenhair tree, silver apricot)	Inhibits platelet-activating factor	May increase risk of bleeding, especially when combined with other medications that inhibit platelet aggregation	36 hours
Ginseng (American ginseng, Asian ginseng, Chinese ginseng, Korean ginseng)	Lowers blood glucose Inhibits platelet aggregation (may be irreversible) Increased prothrombin time/partial thromboplastin time in animals	Hypoglycemia May increase risk of bleeding May decrease anticoagulant effect of warfarin	7 days
Green tea	Inhibits platelet aggregation Inhibits thromboxane A2 formation	May increase risk of bleeding May decrease anticoagulant effect of warfarin	7 days
Kava (awa, intoxicating pepper, kawa)	Sedation Anxiolysis	May increase sedative effect of anesthetics Increase in anesthetic requirements with long-term use unstudied	24 hours
Saw palmetto (dwarf palm, *Sabal*)	Inhibits 5*a*-reductase Inhibits cyclooxygenase	May increase risk of bleeding	No data
St. John's wort (amber, goat weed, hardhay, hypericum, Klamath weed)	Inhibits neurotransmitter reuptake Monoamine oxidase inhibition unlikely	Induction of cytochrome P450 enzymes; affects cyclosporine, warfarin, steroids, and protease inhibitors; may affect benzodiazepines, calcium channel blockers, and many other drugs Decreased serum digoxin levels Delayed emergence	5 days
Valerian (all heal, garden heliotrope, vandal root)	Sedation	May increase sedative effect of anesthetics Benzodiazepine-like acute withdrawal May increase anesthetic requirements with long-term use	No data

Shen S, Chen LL. Anesthetic implications of complementary and alternative therapies. Table 33.1 in: Gropper MA. *Miller's Anesthesia.* 9th ed. Elsevier; 2020.

Body-based (Physical) Modalities

Massage, acupuncture, chiropractic therapy, and application of heat and cold are considered body-based (physical) modalities.[1,2,12] These methods provide comfort and relief by targeting specific parts of the body using the hands, needles, and heat and/or cold products.[2,12] Massage therapy involves manipulation of the soft tissues of the body by kneading, rubbing, tapping, or stroking.[1,12] Chiropractic therapy practitioners address the function of the central nervous system through manual manipulation of the spine, joints, and skeletal system to allow the body better support for healing itself.[1,7,12] A reflexologist applies pressure to specific points on the hands, feet, or ears to keep the body energy balanced and provide relief to other parts of the body.[12] Acupuncture involves stimulating certain energy pathways on the body with a thin needle to promote health, lessen disease symptoms, or eradicate treatment side effects.[12] This acupoint stimulation inhibits the nociception signals and induces analgesic effects by improving the natural flow of energy through the body.[11]

Body–Mind Modalities

Body–mind therapies combine body movements, mental focus, and breathing to help the body and mind to relax.[1,2,12] Examples of these modalities include meditation, biofeedback, hypnosis, yoga, the Alexander technique, and tai chi.[1,2,12] Meditation focuses on intentional breathing and/or

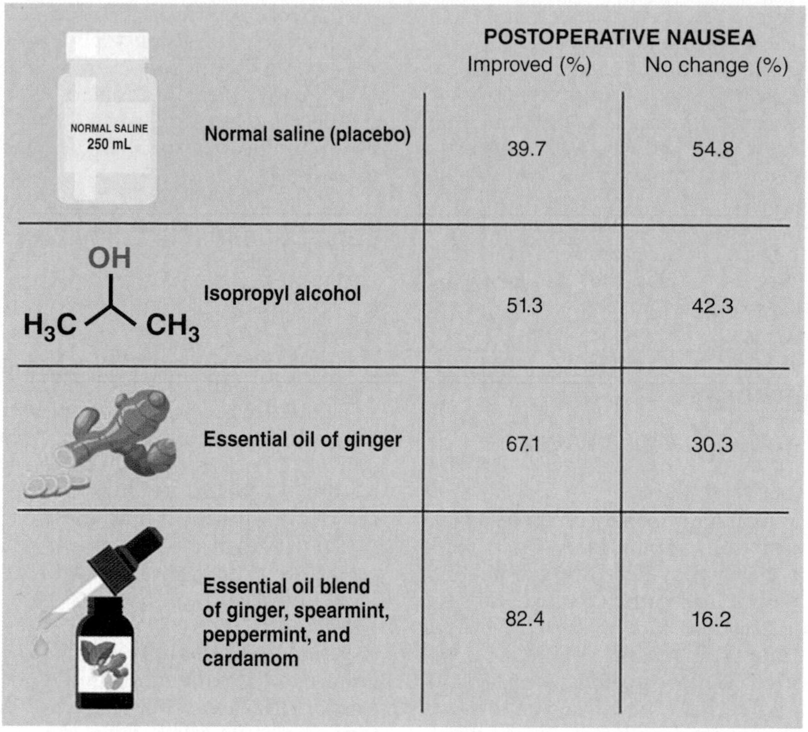

		POSTOPERATIVE NAUSEA	
		Improved (%)	No change (%)
	Normal saline (placebo)	39.7	54.8
	Isopropyl alcohol	51.3	42.3
	Essential oil of ginger	67.1	30.3
	Essential oil blend of ginger, spearmint, peppermint, and cardamom	82.4	16.2

Fig. 14.1 Comparison of the effectiveness of isopropyl alcohol, essential oil of ginger, and essential oil blend aromatherapy for treating postoperative nausea in 301 ambulatory surgery patients. (Alcohol, ginger, and essential oil blend aromatherapy for postoperative nausea. *AORN J.* 2020;111(5):P22.)

the repetition of words or phrases to quiet the mind.[2,12] Biofeedback uses simple electrical sensors attached to various areas of the body. These sensors allow a person to be aware of body functions such as the heart rate, muscle tension, and breathing.[1,12] For example, studies on biofeedback have shown a reduction of recurrent headaches, including the intensity of the headaches, for as long as six months.[1]

Hypnosis is conducted in a controlled environment, usually facilitated by a trained therapist. Using verbal repetition and mental imaging the patient enters a relaxed state and focuses on certain feelings, ideas, or suggestions to aid in healing.[12] Yoga, originally a spiritual practice, is a system of stretches and special poses or body movements that incorporate focused breathing.[12] This mindfulness practice focuses on meditation and stretching, which help decrease stress and pain intensity through the gaining of body awareness.[7] The Alexander technique instructs patients in how to release muscle tension through improved posture and movement.[6,7] Tai chi is a low-impact exercise that uses slow, gentle movements combined with aerobic exercise, meditation, and deep breathing. Performed by a choreographed sequence of movements and positions, tai chi can help improve balance, reduce pain, and improve overall well-being.[7,12]

APPLICATION OF NONPHARMACOLOGIC INTERVENTIONS IN AMBULATORY SURGERY CENTERS

Not all of the nonpharmacologic interventions previously described can be utilized in the ambulatory surgery setting. Some therapies need time and space for implementation, such as biofeedback, yoga, and tai chi, and are not appropriate for implementation in the ambulatory pathway. However, certain techniques, such as meditation, therapeutic touch, and massage, can be implemented in preoperative, as well as postoperative, environments.

PREOPERATIVE STRATEGIES
Preoperative Preparation and Assessment

Preoperative assessments should include a discussion of the patient's knowledge and use of CAM. Documentation of the patient's reliance on nonpharmacologic methods to manage pain can be applied to the pain and comfort management plan. Anxiety and pain, when left unaddressed, impose harmful effects on the body.[2] The negative impact of unrelieved pain affects the extended release of stress hormones such as cortisol, catecholamines, and glucagon.[2] In response, the body also decreases the levels of both insulin and testosterone.[2] Perianesthesia nurses in preoperative units provide education to prepare the patient for techniques to manage both anxiety and postoperative discomfort. For example, teaching the patient about deep breathing as a basic tool to help reduce preoperative anxiety can promote relaxation in the preoperative period, as well as during the postoperative phase.[2,14]

Additional techniques for supporting the anxious patient preoperatively can be implemented by the nurse and patient in the preanesthesia unit. With approval of the anesthesia team, many of the nonpharmacologic methods patients incorporate into their approach to managing discomfort can be implemented at the clinical bedside. Examples include the use of aromatherapy, music, distraction, and focused breathing exercises.

Education on Pain and Pain Management

The preoperative nurse has an important role during patient preparation for surgery. Nurses educate patients about pain and pain expectations before pain is experienced and help patients to establish realistic pain management goals.[2,19] In addition, the perianesthesia nurse prepares the patient by reviewing both the pharmacologic and nonpharmacologic treatment options. In a study published by O'Donnell in 2015, preoperative teaching related to pain, including nonpharmacologic means, was shown to reduce the intensity of postoperative pain, minimize the side effects reported by patients, and increase patient utilization of nonpharmacologic methods of dealing with pain.[21] For an example of a patient education tool, refer to Box 14.4. This tool can easily be modified to focus on the nonpharmacologic therapies a patient may choose.

POSTOPERATIVE STRATEGIES
Practical Strategies for Nonpharmacologic Interventions

Certain nonpharmacologic interventions require time, space, and certified practitioners to be administered. These techniques are generally not routinely provided in an ambulatory setting. Examples include yoga, acupuncture, and tai chi. However, there are certain strategies such as early mobilization (physical therapy) and bedside massage that can be implemented to help the patient achieve an improved level of comfort while in the recovery period. These interventions are very easy to incorporate into the nursing daily practice.[2] Simple nursing interventions, such as ensuring the proper body alignment of the patient through optimal positioning and frequent repositioning, can help prevent or relieve pain.[21,22] Nurses can initiate the use of the pillows to support the extremities or back, raise limbs to reduce swelling, and ultimately provide comfort. In addition, the application of heat or cold gel packs can alleviate pain and provide comfort by decreasing the sensitivity to pain and easing muscle spasms and joint and muscle aches.[2,21,22] Cold therapy relieves pain faster and longer.[1,11,19] Cold therapy applications can decrease bleeding and edema.[19] Heat therapy and/or active warming are responsible for pain relief in more than 40% of patients.[1,11,19]

Caring Communication and Presence

Postoperative nurses also have an important role in providing nonpharmacologic intervention in the ambulatory setting in spite of the short time a patient spends in a postoperative unit.[2] A nurse's caring, nonjudgmental, and reassuring communication, whether verbal or nonverbal, substantially contributes to good pain control.[2] The nurse's unique role in supporting pain management is vital in the delivery of effective and safe care and optimal patient outcomes.[2] Nurses at the bedside use assessment and monitoring skills, as well as the knowledge of drug delivery.[2] The constant presence of perianesthesia nurses as they tailor the application of a pain management intervention to the individual needs of their patients is the hallmark of high-quality pain control.[2]

Sometimes a simple touch provides a therapeutic caring gesture to the patient.[19] Simply touching a patient, no matter how briefly, can convey a sense of caring. This connotation of caring adds a sense of compassion and sincerity to the patient's overall experience. In addition, attention to the environment of care also helps create a calm and relaxed encounter. Even making a simple adjustment to the temperature, light, or noise level of a unit and minimizing interruptions can do wonders for improving comfort and relaxation.[2]

GENERAL CONSIDERATIONS

The perianesthesia registered nurse has the responsibility to assess the needs and preferences of the patient regarding pain management. Nonpharmacologic strategies may be sufficient for mild to moderate pain but should not be a substitute for pharmacologic care when patients are experiencing severe pain.[2,11] During the assessment and reassessment of pain, the perianesthesia registered nurse uses prudent discernment, expresses concern when patients report their pain, and acts appropriately to relieve the pain. A multimodal approach to managing pain incorporates pharmacologic as well as nonpharmacologic interventions to achieve optimal comfort. Table 14.3 offers some nursing care considerations.

CHAPTER HIGHLIGHTS

- Several studies show the effectiveness of nonpharmacologic interventions for supporting a pain management plan.
- The Joint Commission has included nonpharmacologic interventions as part of the therapeutic methods for reducing pain.
- The five categories of nonpharmacologic interventions are behavioral (cognitive), biofield (energy), biologic, body-based (physical), and body–mind.
- Preoperative strategies include a thorough preoperative assessment, education on pain and pain management, and an introduction to nonpharmacologic techniques.
- Postoperative strategies include caring communication and the introduction of practical strategies for implementing nonpharmacologic interventions.

BOX 14.4 Patient Education Information Form

What You Need to Know About Postoperative Pain

Pain control after surgery is very important. When your pain is controlled, you sleep better, eat better, and return to normal activities sooner. You may recover more quickly from your surgery and get back to work sooner. The following information will help you understand how to manage your pain after surgery.

1. Take pain medication as directed. The best time to take medication is when the pain first begins. If pain is worse with activity, such as walking or going to the bathroom, take the medication on a regular schedule.
2. Manage side effects early. Some medications cause constipation or nausea. Take medications with food to avoid nausea and also take a stool softener daily to prevent constipation.
3. Report side effects, such as severe nausea, vomiting, or constipation.
4. Comfort measures, such as heat, ice, massage, relaxation, walking, or listening to music, may help.
5. Communicate with your provider if your pain is not controlled. You may need different medication or a stronger dose to relieve your pain.
6. Be sure to make a postoperative visit and discuss any problems with your pain management.

O'Donnell KF. Preoperative pain management education: A quality improvement project. *J Perianesth Nurs*. 2015;30(3):221–227. Table 1. https://doi.org/10.1016/j.jopan.2015.01.013

TABLE 14.3 Nursing Care Considerations

Types of Physical Interventions	Intervention Examples	Purpose	Care Considerations
Cold Therapy	Use of conventional cold pack, waterproof ice bag, or commercial cold therapy device(s)	Effective for surgical incisions, headache, muscle spasms, low back pain	Avoid tissue damage by providing appropriate protective covering Inspect skin to assess for potential tissue damage
Distraction	Music, deep breathing, digital devices, family visitation	Promotes relaxation, relieves stress, reduces pain	The care environment may not support this technique May not help when pain is too intense
Elevation/Repositioning	Raise the limb on pillows or foam support devices	Reduces swelling and eases pain	Monitor circulation and sensation
Heat Therapy	Use of hot packs layered by towels	Useful in muscle aches, spasms, low back pain	Avoid tissue damage by providing appropriate protective covering Inspect skin for potential skin damage
Vibrations/ Massage	Handheld and stationary vibrators; light massage	Relieves pain by causing numbness, paresthesia Promotes relaxation of muscles, tendons, and joints May change character of sensation from sharp to dull	May aggravate pain if touch is too intense or the patient has a hyper-sensitivity condition such as chronic pain syndrome

Adapted from Tick H, Nielsen A, Pelletier KR, et al. Evidence-based nonpharmacologic strategies for comprehensive pain care: The Consortium Pain Task Force White Paper. *Explore (NY)*. 2018;14(3):177–211. https://doi.org/10.1016/j.explore.2018.02.001; and Yazici G, Erdogan Z, Bulut H, et al. The use of complementary and alternative medicines among surgical patients: A survey study. *J PeriAnesth Nurs*. 2018;34(2):322–329. https://doi.org/10.1016/j.jopan.2018.04.007

CASE STUDY

Hai Lun Chang is a 15-year-old female patient with autism spectrum disorder who was admitted to the ambulatory surgery center (ASC) for a right knee arthroscopy.

Mrs. Chang (Hai Lun's mom) told the preoperative nurse that her daughter has heightened sensitivities to many situations. She especially has a heightened sensitivity to pain. This would be her second surgery, and her mom wanted this experience to be better for her. During her first surgery, Hai Lun had a hard time expressing her discomfort. As a result, her initial recovery experience was extremely difficult. The only thing that helped her calm down was having someone conduct reiki therapy. For this surgery, Mrs. Chang requested that a certified reiki practitioner be brought in to help Hai Lun both preoperatively and postoperatively to help cope with pain. Hai Lun knows the reiki practitioner and is amenable to having the therapy. The session took 20 minutes in the preoperative unit and unfortunately delayed the start of the surgery. Following the procedure, Hai Lun was brought to the recovery room. As soon as she had a stable airway and was awake, the postoperative nurse called Mrs. Chang into the recovery room. The nurse had positioned Hai Lun with pillows under her right knee. An ice pack was also placed on her knee. The postoperative nurse was informed that Hai Lun loved to listen to music. Mrs. Chang gave Hai Lun her iPad and played her favorite music playlist. Again, Mrs. Chang requested that the reiki therapist be summoned to come in and do the reiki therapy. The postoperative nurse allowed the therapist to come in and provided privacy so she could do the reiki therapy.

Here are a few questions to ponder with this scenario: What nonpharmacologic interventions were offered to Hai Lun? Should the preoperative nurse have asked for the credentials of the reiki practitioner before allowing her to do the reiki therapy? What was the nurse's understanding of how reiki works? What were the nonpharmacologic interventions that the postoperative nurse offered in the recovery phase?

REFERENCES

1. Mu PF, Chen YC, Cheng SC. The effectiveness of non-pharmacological pain management in relieving chronic pain for children and adolescents. *JBI Lib Syst Rev*. 2009;7(34):1489-1543. Available at: https://doi.org/10.11124/01938924-200907340-00001.
2. Colwell AQ. Pain Management. In: Odom-Forren J, ed. *Drain's PeriAnesthesia Nursing: A Critical Care Approach*. 7th ed. Elsevier; 2018:431-450.
3. National Institute of Health: National Institute of Drug Abuse. *Overdose Death Rates*. Available at: https://nida.nih.gov/research-topics/trends-statistics/overdose-death-rates.
4. Substance Abuse and Mental Health Services Administration (SAMHSA). *Key Substance Use and Mental Health Indicators in the United States: Results from the 2019 National Survey on Drug Use and Health*. PEP20-07-01-001. 2020. Available at: https://www.samhsa.gov/data/sites/default/files/reports/rpt29393/2019NSDUHFFRPDFWHTML/2019NSDUHFFR1PDFW090120.pdf.
5. Dahlhamer J, Lucas J, Zelaya C, et al. Prevalence of chronic pain and high-impact chronic pain among adults–United States, 2016. *Morb Mortal Wkly Rep*. 2018;67(36):1001-1006. Available at: https://www.cdc.gov/mmwr/volumes/67/wr/mm6736a2.htm.
6. Tick H, Nielsen A, Pelletier KR, et al. Evidence-based nonpharmacologic strategies for comprehensive pain care: The Consortium Pain Task Force White Paper. *Explore (NY)*. 2018;14(3):177-211. Available at: https://doi.org/10.1016/j.explore.2018.02.001.
7. Pollack SW, Skillman SM, Frogner BK. *The Health Workforce Delivering Evidence-Based Non-Pharmacological Pain Management*. Feb 2020. Available at: https://depts.washington.edu/fammed/chws/wp-content/uploads/sites/5/2020/02/Non-Pharmacological-Pain-Management-FR-2020.pdf.
8. Centers for Disease Control and Prevention. *Nonopioid Therapies*. 2022. Available at: https://www.cdc.gov/opioids/patients/options.html.
9. The Joint Commission. Non-pharmacologic and non-opioid solutions for pain management. *Quick Safety*. 2018;44:1-2. Available at: https://www.jointcommission.org/resources/news-and-multimedia/newsletters/newsletters/quick-safety/quick-safety-44-nonpharmacologic-and-nonopioid-solutions-for-pain-management/#.Y4bD6MvMLtw.
10. Lewei AL, Bohnert ASB, Jannausch M, Goesling J, Ilgen MA. Use of non-pharmacological strategies for pain relief in addiction treatment patients with chronic pain. *Am J Addict*. 2017;26: 564-567. Available at: https://doi.org/10.1111/ajad.12600.

11. Mota M, Cunha M, Santos MR, Silva D, Santos E. Non-pharmacological interventions for pain management in adult victims of trauma: a scoping review protocol. *JBI Database System Rev Implement Rep.* 2019;17(12):2483-2490. Available at: https://doi.org/10.11124/jbisrir-2017-004036.

12. National Institutes of Health. *National Center for Complementary and Integrative Health (NCCIH).* 2019. Available at: https://www.nih.gov/about-nih/what-we-do/nih-almanac/national-center-complementary-integrative-health-nccih.

13. Bagheri H, Salmani T, Nourian J, et al. The effects of inhalation aromatherapy using lavender essential oil on postoperative pain of inguinal hernia: a randomized controlled trial. *J PeriAnesth Nurs.* 2020;35(6):642-648. Available at: https://doi.org/10.1016/j.jopan.2020.03.003.

14. Yazici G, Erdogan Z, Bulut H, et al. The use of complementary and alternative medicines among surgical patients: a survey study. *J PeriAnesth Nurs.* 2018;34(2):322-329. Available at: https://doi.org/10.1016/j.jopan.2018.04.007.

15. Tang SK, Tse MMY, Leung SF, Fotis T. The effectiveness, suitability, and sustainability of non-pharmacological methods of managing pain in community-dwelling older adults: a systemic review. *BMC Public Health.* 2019;19(1):1488. Available at: https://doi.org/10.1186/s12889-019-7831-9.

16. Johns Hopkins Medicine. *Types of Complementary and Alternative Medicine. What are different types of CAM?* 2022. Available at: https://www.hopkinsmedicine.org/health/wellness-and-prevention/types-of-complementary-and-alternative-medicine.

17. Freudenrich C. *How Pain Works. Gate Control Theory of Pain.* 2022. Available at: https://science.howstuffworks.com/life/inside-the-mind/human-brain/pain4.htm.

18. Alvarez-Garcia C, Yaban ZS. The effects of preoperative guided imagery interventions on preoperative anxiety and postoperative pain: a meta-analysis. *Complement Ther Clin Pract.* 2020;38:101077. Available at: https://doi.org/10.1016/j.ctcp.2019.101077.

19. Wilson L, Kane HL. Pain and comfort. In: Schick L, Windle PE, eds. *PeriAnesthesia Nursing Core Curriculum: Preprocedure, Phase I and Phase II PACU Nursing.* 4th ed. Elsevier; 2021:312-331.

20. Cummings KC, Keshock M, Ganesh R, et al. Preoperative management of surgical patients using dietary supplements: Society for Perioperative Assessment and Quality Improvement (SPAQI) Consensus Statement. *Mayo Clin Proc.* 2021;96(5):1342-1355. Available at: https://doi.org/10.1016/j.mayocp.2020.08.016.

21. O'Donne\ll KF. Preoperative pain management education: a quality improvement project. *J Perianesth Nurs.* 2015;30(3):221-227. Available at: https://doi.org/10.1016/j.jopan.2015.01.013.

22. Gumus K, Musuroglu S, Ozlu ZK, Tasci O. Determining the use of nonpharmacologic methods by surgical nurses for postoperative pain management and the influencing professional factors: a multicenter study. *J PeriAnesth Nurs.* 2020;35(1):75-79. Available at: https://doi.org/10.1016/j.jopan.2019.04.011.

15 Phases of Care: Preoperative Preparation and Optimization of the Ambulatory Surgery Patient

Ronda E. Dyer, MSN, BSPA, RN, CPAN, CAPA, CNE

LEARNING OBJECTIVES

A review of the content of this chapter will help the reader to:

1. Identify factors that put patients at risk for complications when undergoing anesthesia.
2. Select appropriate screening tools to quantify patient risk factors.
3. Describe appropriate preoperative testing based on specific patient conditions and risk factors.
4. Describe risk factors that may make patients inappropriate for surgery in the ambulatory surgery setting.

OVERVIEW

Patient selection, preparation, and evaluation are crucial in the ambulatory surgery center (ASC). As technologic modes, surgical techniques, and anesthetic approaches evolve, it is possible to perform more procedures on an outpatient basis. Still, some patients are not candidates for successful outpatient procedures due to their baseline status or co-morbidities. Others do not have the support system or caregivers needed to recover at home. The key for the ASC team is to identify potential challenges, determine if risks can be mitigated, optimize the patient status, and educate patients regarding transportation, home assistance, medications, supplies, and equipment. Many ASC programs have established patient selection criteria to ensure that risks are minimized and that the patient requiring anesthesia for surgeries or procedures is provided care in the safest environment possible (Figure 15.1).

The design of preoperative clinics varies across the country and is based on community needs, surgical programming, and clinical resources. Some clinics provide medical co-management of the surgical patient, while others have created entire multidisciplinary teams to help patients become optimized for their surgeries. These services include weight management, smoking cessation, educational sessions (e.g., "joint camp" for arthroplasty candidates), and hospitalist services for medical clearances and referrals.

Forty years ago, a cholecystectomy required a week of hospitalization. Ten years ago, the idea of outpatient total hip or knee replacement was just on the horizon. Today, outpatient thyroidectomies, hysterectomies, and mastectomies are all becoming more commonplace. As these more complex and invasive surgeries are refined with new technologies and techniques, and as anesthetic options expand, surgery centers adopt processes to ensure that patients can experience safe surgical procedures. This includes a team approach to selecting and optimizing the patients beginning in the surgeon's office.

Once the surgeon and patient agree that a surgery is to be scheduled, the planning begins. Patient preferences regarding surgical location or timing are considered. The surgeon must have privileges at the desired facility. If the surgery is expected to be covered by insurance, the process of obtaining required payer authorization begins. The insurer is a driving factor as it is likely to require that the surgery be performed in a contracted facility. Patients who go elsewhere may pay a significant portion out of pocket.

Facility policies and scopes of service define what procedures may or may not be performed and if any patients are unable to be accommodated. Obviously, an orthopedic procedure would not be scheduled at an eye center. However, even sites that can do orthopedic procedures may not have the equipment or supplies to do, for instance, a total knee replacement. Additionally, facilities may have policies regarding age or weight limitations. They may be unable to accommodate young children because pediatric procedures may require specialized staff and equipment, ranging from surgical instruments to supplies such as pediatric airways and splints, that the ASC does not have. Gurneys, surgical tables, and wheelchairs may not be rated for extreme weights, and this can limit the ability to care for obese patients.

PATIENT SELECTION
Chronic Conditions

Many patient factors must also be considered. Not all patients are candidates for outpatient procedures, and some require the precaution of having outpatient procedures performed at a hospital rather than an ASC. This decision may be made by the surgeon or after additional assessment during the preanesthesia evaluation. Patients who have debilitating co-morbidities such as chronic obstructive pulmonary disease (COPD) requiring continuous oxygen, class IV congestive heart failure (CHF), or Class III obesity are easily identified as being at risk for complications when needing larger procedures or those requiring general anesthesia (Tables 15.1, 15.2, and 15.3). However, other risks may be less obvious.

Age and Frailty

Although age over 70 has been shown to be a factor associated with increased hospitalization after ambulatory surgery, it is noted that co-morbidities must also be considered.[1] A 50-year-old patient with multiple chronic conditions may be much more medically at risk than a healthy octogenarian. Much

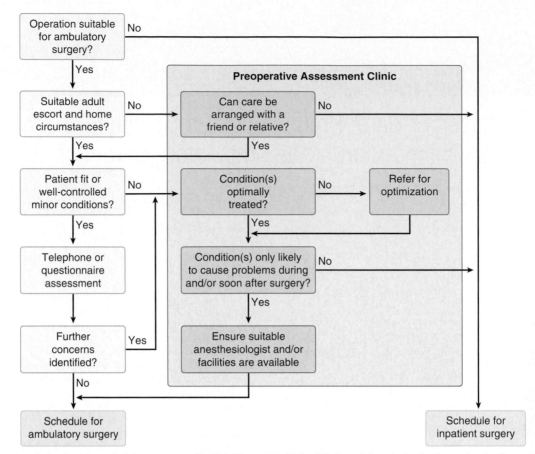

Fig. 15.1 Sample criteria chart for ambulatory surgery. (Smith I, Skues MA, Philip BK. Ambulatory (outpatient) anesthesia. Figure 72.1 in: Gropper MA. *Miller's Anesthesia*. Elsevier; 2020.)

TABLE 15.1 New York Heart Classification of Cardiovascular Disease

Class	Functional Capacity (Limitation of Physical Activity)	Objective Assessment (Evidence of Cardiovascular Disease)
I	None	None
II	Slight	Minimal
III	Marked	Moderately severe
IV	Inability to carry on any activity without symptoms	Severe

Harward MP. General medicine and ambulatory care. Table 2.3 in: Harward MP, ed. *Medical Secrets*. 6th ed. Elsevier; 2019.

research is being conducted to identify simple bedside screening tools that enable surgeons to screen patients for outpatient procedure appropriateness. Current literature focuses on frailty screening tools that identify those patients at higher risk for complications, including an unplanned admission, postoperative infection, or mortality. There are more than a dozen different frailty scales originating with the 70-item Canadian Study of Health and Aging Frailty Index.[2] The 11-point modified Frailty Index (mFI-11) has demonstrated a reliable association with poor surgical outcomes,[3] but more recent research shows the 5-point modified Frailty Index (mFI-5) to be as effective as the mFI-11 (Box 15.1).[2,4]

The mFI-5 evaluates patients for diabetes, hypertension, CHF, COPD, and functional status limiting independence. "The 5 comorbidities comprising the mFI-5 are easily obtained through the patient history, making it a practical clinical tool for identifying high-risk patients, informing preoperative counseling, and improving value-based health care."[4] Individual studies have been done validating its use for many orthopedic and spine surgeries, general breast and urologic surgeries, trauma repair surgeries, and even surgeries for brain tumors. "Frailty index will be a valuable preoperative risk assessment tool for the acute care surgeon."[5]

PREOPERATIVE COORDINATION

The surgeon ensures that the patient has been informed about the surgical plan, risks, and benefits. Education and preparation begin in the office. The patient should be provided a list of any needed equipment or supplies, special dietary requirements or foods, or over-the-counter medications needed for recovery from the procedure. There should also be a discussion about any needed support or assistance, such as the need for transportation when going home from surgery and someone to stay with the patient if sedation or anesthesia is planned. Patients need time to acquire needed supplies and arrange for assistance.

Patients need to be informed about time off work and any expected limitations following surgery. They should be aware of anticipated follow-up visits and ideally have these appointments prescheduled. Information about expected postoperative

TABLE 15.2 ASA Physical Status Classification

ASA Physical Status Classification	Definition	Adult Examples (including but not limited to)	Pediatric Examples (including but not limited to)	Obstetric Examples (including but not limited to)
ASA I	A normal healthy patient	Healthy, nonsmoking, no or minimal alcohol use	Healthy (no acute or chronic disease), normal BMI percentile for age	
ASA II	A patient with mild systemic disease	Mild diseases only without substantive functional limitations. Current smoker, social alcohol drinker, pregnancy, obesity (30 < BMI < 40), well-controlled DM/HTN, mild lung disease	Asymptomatic congenital cardiac disease, well-controlled dysrhythmias, asthma without exacerbation, well-controlled epilepsy, non–insulin-dependent DM, abnormal BMI percentile for age, mild/moderate OSA, oncologic state in remission, autism with mild limitations	Normal pregnancy, well-controlled gestational HTN, controlled pre-eclampsia without severe features, diet-controlled gestational DM
ASA III	A patient with severe systemic disease	Substantive functional limitations; one or more moderate to severe diseases. Poorly controlled DM or HTN, COPD, morbid obesity (BMI ≥ 40), active hepatitis, alcohol dependence or abuse, implanted pacemaker, moderate reduction of ejection fraction, ESRD undergoing regularly scheduled dialysis, history (>3 mo) of MI, CVA, TIA, or CAD/stents	Uncorrected stable congenital cardiac abnormality, asthma with exacerbation, poorly controlled epilepsy, insulin-dependent DM, morbid obesity, malnutrition, severe OSA, oncologic state, renal failure, muscular dystrophy, cystic fibrosis, history of organ transplantation, brain/spinal cord malformation, symptomatic hydrocephalus, premature infant PCA < 60 weeks, autism with severe limitations, metabolic disease, difficult airway, long-term parenteral nutrition, full-term infants < 6 weeks of age	Preeclampsia with severe features, gestational DM with complications or high insulin requirements, a thrombophilic disease requiring anticoagulation
ASA IV	A patient with severe systemic disease that is a constant threat to life	Recent (<3 mo) MI, CVA, TIA, or CAD/stents, ongoing cardiac ischemia or severe valve dysfunction, severe reduction of ejection fraction, shock, sepsis, DIC, ARDS, or ESRD not undergoing regularly scheduled dialysis	Symptomatic congenital cardiac abnormality, congestive heart failure, active sequelae of prematurity, acute hypoxic-ischemic encephalopathy, shock, sepsis, DIC, automatic implantable cardioverter-defibrillator, ventilator dependence, endocrinopathy, severe trauma, severe respiratory distress, advanced oncologic state	Preeclampsia with severe features complicated by HELLP or other adverse event, peripartum cardiomyopathy with ejection fraction < 40, uncorrected/decompensated heart disease, acquired or congenital
ASA V	A moribund patient who is not expected to survive without the operation	Ruptured abdominal/thoracic aneurysm, massive trauma, intracranial bleed with mass effect, ischemic bowel in the face of significant cardiac pathology or multiple organ/system dysfunction	Massive trauma, intracranial hemorrhage with mass effect, patient requiring ECMO, respiratory failure or arrest, malignant hypertension, decompensated congestive heart failure, hepatic encephalopathy, ischemic bowel or multiple organ/system dysfunction	Uterine rupture
ASA VI	A declared brain-dead patient whose organs are being removed for donor purposes			

ARDS, acute respiratory distress syndrome; BMI, body mass index; CAD, coronary artery disease; COPD, chronic obstructive pulmonary disease; CVA, cerebrovascular accident; DIC, disseminated intravascular coagulation; DM, diabetes mellitus; ECMO, extracorporeal membrane oxygenation; ESRD, end-stage renal disease; HTN, hypertension; MI, myocardial infarction; OSA, obstructive sleep apnea; PCA, postconceptional age; TIA, transient ischemic attack.

Source: Pardo MC. Preoperative evaluation. Table 13.16 in: Pardo MC, ed. *Miller's Basics of Anesthesia*. 8th ed. Elsevier; 2023.

TABLE 15.3 Adult Body Mass Index Categories

Body Mass Index	Considered
Below 18.5	Underweight
18.5 to 24.9	Healthy weight
25.0 to 29.9	Overweight
30 or higher	Obesity
40 or higher	Class 3 obesity

Data from: Centers for Disease Control and Prevention (CDC). *Defining Adult Overweight & Obesity.* CDC; 2021. https://www.cdc.gov/obesity/adult/defining.html

---

BOX 15.1 Modified 5-Item Frailty Index

Items
1. Diabetes mellitus: noninsulin, insulin, or oral
2. Congestive heart failure within 30 days before surgery
3. Hypertension requiring medication
4. History of chronic obstructive pulmonary disease or pneumonia
5. Functional health status before surgery; partially dependent or totally dependent

Adapted from: Traven SA, Horn RW, Reeves RA, Walton ZJ, Woolf SK, Slone HS. The 5-factor modified frailty index predicts complications, hospital admission, and mortality following arthroscopic rotator cuff repair. *Arthroscopy.* 2020;36(2):383–388. https://doi.org/10.1016/j.arthro.2019.08.036

---

pain should be provided, along with pain management plans. Some physicians provide prescriptions at the preoperative visit to reduce stress on the day of surgery. However, many are hesitant to provide opioid prescriptions that might be misused or abused before surgery or to prescribe medications ahead of time in case the procedure is cancelled.

A key factor is communication between the surgical center and the partnering surgeons' offices. Patients become frustrated if they receive conflicting information about their procedures. If the office has given a patient a date and time for surgery and they are later changed by the surgery center (or vice versa), this affects the patient's plan for time off work, transportation, and home assistance. Likewise, if information about the length of the procedure, supplies needed, preoperative preparation, diet, or medications vary, patients become very confused and dissatisfied with the process. Continuity and standardization are keys to a seamless process and satisfied patients.

Many surgery centers provide handouts or pamphlets that answer frequent questions and can be given to the patient at the surgeon's office. This can include information about the process, calls, and contacts they will have with surgery center staff, required testing, and basic information about the facility processes and routines. Patients often have caller identification and are hesitant to answer unknown numbers, and they are even more hesitant when an unknown caller begins asking personal questions. Communicating in advance about expected calls from the surgery center scheduling department, patient registration department, preanesthesia testing center, and preoperative staff allows patients to feel more comfortable with the process.

Historically, patients were scheduled for surgery by the surgeon's office, arrived at the surgery center or hospital on the day of surgery, and, upon evaluation by an anesthesia provider, were determined to need an additional workup, which resulted in delays or cancellations. Currently, the trend is to have preadmission evaluations performed by anesthesia providers or nurses under their direction. Preanesthesia evaluation clinics are becoming commonplace and increasingly are conducting services by telephone. In fact, one study showed telemedicine visits to be as effective as other contact methods while resulting in greater patient satisfaction.[6]

Evidence-Based Practice: Prehabilitation
The practice of prehabilitation can include interventions to improve physical conditioning, nutrition, and the psychological status of a patient prior to undergoing surgery. Based on a systematic review of studies aimed at prehabilitation, researchers agree that there is evidence suggesting that preoperative therapies such as exercise and weight management programs can reduce the rates of complications and unplanned admissions. In addition, patients who have undergone prehabilitation methods have lower lengths of stay and improved functional recoveries. Further studies can help delineate the benefits of prehabilitation based on the amount of time spent with preoperative preparation as well as the types of interventions and the surgery types and the specific outcomes.

Source: McIsaac DI, Gill M, Boland L, et al. Prehabilitation in adult patients undergoing surgery: an umbrella review of systematic reviews. *Br J Anaesth.* 2022;128(2):244-257. https://doi.org/10.1016/j.bja.2021.11.014

PREOPERATIVE EVALUATION AND TESTING
History

The preadmission evaluation includes a review of the patient's prior medical, surgical, and anesthetic history, along with the results of preoperative tests and medications, to identify and allow the mitigation of potential risks with the goal of reducing delays and cancellations.[7] Surgery centers can realize additional efficiency through the use of integrated documentation, which avoids the duplication of efforts by the admitting staff on the day of surgery and expedites the day-of-surgery admission process. If a history has been obtained by the preanesthesia testing center, nurses on the day of surgery can inquire about any changes without repeating the comprehensive interview.

A complete history helps to establish the American Society of Anesthesiologists (ASA) physical status classification and evaluate the anesthesia risk (see Table 15.2). History gathering includes a review of prior surgeries, including prior reactions to anesthesia. A patient or family history of malignant hyperthermia (MH) or delayed awakening is vitally important due to the genetic disposition for MH and pseudocholinesterase deficiency. A personal history of postoperative nausea and vomiting (PONV) or postdischarge nausea and vomiting (PDNV) influences the use of prophylactic treatment for prevention, as well as anesthetic and pain management plans.

Any known history of a difficult intubation or respiratory complications needs to be communicated to the anesthesia team. When the evaluation is done in person, the Mallampati airway classification scoring system can be used to assess the risk of a difficult airway (Figure 15.2).

Cardiac Screening

Patients often choose not to mention medical conditions or events that they feel are irrelevant for the planned procedure.

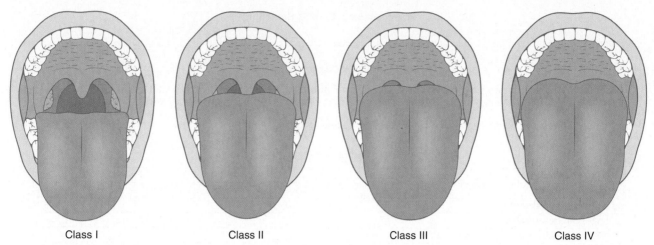

| Class I | Class II | Class III | Class IV |

Fig. 15.2 Mallampati airway classification. Class I: The soft palate, fauces, uvula, and tonsillar pillars are visible. Class II: The soft palate, fauces, and uvula are visible. Class III: The soft palate and base of the uvula are visible. Class IV: The soft palate is not visible. (Liaonitkul M, Infosino A. Airway management. Figure 16.4 in: Pardo MC, ed. *Miller's Basics of Anesthesia*. 8th ed. Elsevier; 2023.)

They may fail to disclose a myocardial infarction or a cerebrovascular accident that completely resolved. Yet, because the anesthetic experience has a significant impact on the cardiovascular system, this is vital information. "Patients who have had a myocardial infarction (MI) within 6 months before surgery have a recurrence rate of 54.5% during or after the surgical procedure."[8] More recent studies indicate that the number has fallen to 26%, with those who have had a more recent MI having a greater risk. Yet, even with improvements in the rate of risks, it has been shown that major cardiac events account for nearly half of perioperative deaths and that the mortality rate is 26% for those having had a perioperative MI.[9] Additionally, the patient who experienced an MI within the prior six months is at increased risk for a perioperative cerebrovascular accident (CVA), which carries an eight-fold increase in mortality.[10]

Cardiac screening may include asking whether the patient sees a cardiologist and investigating why the patient is taking blood thinners or cardiac or antihypertensive medications. Many patients will say they do not have high blood pressure when, in fact, they do but it is controlled by antihypertensive medications. The Revised Cardiac Risk Index (RCRI) is a simple tool originally based on the 2014 American College of Cardiology/American Heart Association guidelines related to the perioperative cardiovascular evaluation and management of patients undergoing noncardiac surgery (Figure 15.3). The RCRI tool assists in the identification of patients who may require further cardiac evaluation prior to undergoing surgical procedures. The tool consists of two sections, one measuring the surgical risk and the second estimating the functional status.

The surgical risk portion includes six items: an elevated risk for surgery, a history of ischemic heart disease, a history of CHF, a history of cerebrovascular disease, preoperative treatment with insulin, and a preoperative serum creatinine level greater than 2 mg/dL/176.8 µmol/L. High-risk surgeries are defined as either emergent, aortic, peripheral vascular, or prolonged procedures. For each identified risk factor, the patient receives one point. Each increase in points is associated with an increased risk of complications. A patient with zero points has a class I risk, one point has a class II risk, two points has a class III risk, and three to six points has a class IV risk.[10]

The second portion of the cardiac risk screening is the functional status assessment. Researchers evaluated certain activities of daily living to determine how they compared with exercise in terms of oxygen consumption. "Functional capacity is expressed in terms of metabolic equivalents (METs)."[10] Activities rated as requiring 4 METs include climbing one flight of stairs, walking briskly on level ground, and performing heavy housework such as mopping or vacuuming. Patients who cannot do these activities without associated symptoms of fatigue, shortness of breath, or angina are at an increased risk of perioperative cardiac events. Patients with a class III or IV surgical risk or a functional status of 4 or fewer METs are reviewed by the anesthesia provider for consideration of additional testing or clearance by a cardiologist.[10]

Additional cardiac concerns to be noted include the presence of CHF, dysrhythmias, atrial fibrillation, heart murmurs, or hypertension and any prior interventions such as cardiac stents, valve replacements, pacemakers, or automatic internal defibrillators (AICDs). The anesthesiologist may request electrocardiograms (ECGs) or cardiac clearance for these patients. Patients taking blood thinners because of atrial fibrillation or the presence of artificial valves need instructions about whether and/or when to stop and restart therapy. Depending on the medication, they may require laboratory work to evaluate the coagulation status. Diuretic therapy may result in electrolyte imbalances requiring laboratory work and/or an intervention such as potassium replacement. CHF patients may require a chest x-ray to assess for pulmonary infiltrates or edema. Bovie electrosurgery or cautery should be avoided if the patient has an AICD. If cautery is required, the AICD can be turned off with an external defibrillator available for emergency intervention.[11] Table 15.4 lists the cardiac risk estimates based on the type of surgery.

Pulmonary Screening

A thorough pulmonary history and assessment are vital to identify any potential risks for the perianesthesia patient. The volatile anesthetic agents rely on the respiratory system for delivery and removal. In addition, sedatives, opioids, and nearly all the anesthetic agents cause respiratory depression. "In fact, 70% to 80% of the morbidity and mortality in the PACU is postulated to be associated with some form of respiratory dysfunction."[8] Therefore, it is important that the pulmonary status of the patient be known and any deficits optimized prior to surgery.

Patients should be asked about any preexisting respiratory conditions, including COPD, asthma, obstructive sleep apnea

Pre-anesthesia Cardiac Screening

Planned procedure: _____   Surgeon: _____

Lee's Revised Cardiac Risk Index

High risk: Major emergency surgery, major vascular surgery, prolonged surgery with large fluid shifts
Moderate risk: Carotid endarterectomy, head and neck surgery, intraperitoneal or intrathoracic surgery, orthopedic surgery, prostate surgery
Low risk: Cataract removal, endoscopy, breast surgery, superficial procedures

Score one point for each applicable area

Clinical variable	Points
High-risk surgery	
Coronary artery disease	
Congestive heart failure	
History of cerebrovascular disease	
Insulin treatment for diabetes mellitus	
Preoperative serum creatinine > 2.0 mg/dL	
Total points:	

Score interpretation (% risk of surgical complications):

0 points = class I (0.4%)   2 points = class III (6.6%)
1 point = class II (0.9%)   3 points = class IV (11.0%)

Functional Status Assessment

Metabolic equivalents	Activity	Surgical risk
</= 4 METs	Patient may be able to perform activities of daily living such as eating, dressing, toileting, walking in the house, light housework. Patient unable to walk > 2 blocks on level ground without stopping due to symptoms such as angina or dyspnea.	Poor
> 4 METs	Patient is able to perform heavy housework (mopping, vacuuming), yard work, walk up hill > 2 blocks, climb 1 flight of stairs, ride a bicycle, or golf without stopping due to symptoms such as angina or dyspnea	Moderate to excellent

For any patient with Lee's cardiac risk indicator of class III or class IV, or any patient with a </= 4 METs on the functional status assessment, contact anesthesia for review and consideration of need for additional testing or cardiac clearance.

Anesthesia recommendations:

❏ Referral for cardiac clearance   ❏ No clearance needed

Comments: _____
_____
_____

Fig. 15.3 Revised Cardiac Risk Index. (Data from: Fleisher LA, Fleischmann KE, Auerbach AD, et al. 2014 ACC/AHA guideline on perioperative cardiovascular evaluation and management of patients undergoing noncardiac surgery: A report of the American College of Cardiology/American Heart Association Task Force on practice guidelines. *J Am Coll Cardiol.* 2014;64(22):e77–137.)

TABLE 15.4 Surgical Cardiac Risk Estimates Based on Type of Surgery

Low Risk: Less than 1%	Intermediate Risk: 1% to 5%	High Risk: Greater than 5%
Superficial surgery	Intraperitoneal: splenectomy, hiatal hernia repair, cholecystectomy	Aortic and major vascular surgery
Breast		Open lower limb revascularization or amputation or thromboembolectomy
Dental	Carotid symptomatic (CEA or CAS)	Duodenopancreatic surgery
Endocrine: thyroid	Peripheral arterial angioplasty	Liver resection, bile duct surgery
Eye	Endovascular aneurysm repair	Esophagectomy
Reconstructive	Head and neck surgery	Repair of perforated bowel
Carotid asymptomatic (CEA or CAS)	Neurologic or orthopedic: major (hip and spine surgery)	Adrenal resection
Gynecologic: minor		Total cystectomy
Orthopedic: minor (meniscectomy)	Urologic or gynecologic: major	Pneumonectomy
Urologic: minor (transurethral resection of the prostate)	Renal transplant	Pulmonary or liver transplant
	Intrathoracic: nonmajor	

Zaydfudim VM, Hu Y, Adams RB. Principles of preoperative and operative surgery. Table 10.2 in: Townsend CM, Beauchamp RD, Evers BM, Mattox KL, eds. *Sabiston Textbook of Surgery.* 21st ed. Elsevier; 2022.

(OSA), recent cough, influenza, coronavirus disease (e.g., CO-VID-19), bronchitis, or pneumonia. A history should be gathered regarding smoking tobacco, vaping, or using marijuana. If the assessment is conducted in person, it should include the observation of breathing patterns and auscultation of breath sounds. If it is done by phone, the nurse may note mid-sentence pauses for breaths, audible wheezing, or frequent coughing, which may indicate respiratory problems. Patients should be queried about inhalers prescribed and the frequency of their use and whether home oxygen, nebulizers, or continuous positive airway pressure (CPAP) or bilevel positive airway pressure (BiPAP) is used.[11]

Patients with preexisting or chronic respiratory conditions are asked about symptoms, severity, exercise tolerance, and triggering factors. The anesthesia provider may request additional testing, such as a chest x-ray or pulmonary function tests, and/or clearance from the patient's pulmonologist. The anesthetic plan may need to be altered to avoid anesthetic gases, and the decision may be made to opt instead for a regional block or total intravenous anesthesia (TIVA) to reduce respiratory complications. Use of steroids within the prior 6 months should be documented. The frequent or recent use of corticosteroids may necessitate the administration of perioperative steroids to compensate for steroid-induced adrenal insufficiency. If the patient is experiencing acute respiratory infection, the surgery will likely be cancelled until the patient has recovered.[11]

Obstructive Sleep Apnea

Obstructive sleep apnea (OSA) can pose significant problems for the perianesthesia patient receiving sedatives, muscle relaxants, and opioids. These individuals frequently experience periods of apnea owing to airway occlusion while sleeping. Added respiratory depression related to medications produces a situation in which patients are less likely to rouse when the obstruction occurs, resulting in the increased potential for hypoxic episodes and even death. It is important for the team to be aware if the patient has a known history of sleep apnea and to have a CPAP or BiPAP available for use. Depending on the facility policy related to fire safety and infection control, patients may be asked to bring their OSA equipment and may be excluded from the outpatient setting if they admit to noncompliance with their OSA treatment plan.

Unfortunately, it is estimated that as many as 80% of OSA patients are undiagnosed.[11] These individuals are at even more risk, as they can experience airway risks without protective equipment. This is especially true once they are discharged home with opioid medications for pain management. A simple screening can identify the OSA risk (Figure 15.4). The STOP-BANG questionnaire asks eight simple questions, with each affirmative answer scoring one point. Points are scored for those who snore loudly; experience daytime fatigue; are observed having apnea episodes; have hypertension, a body mass index (BMI) over 35 kg/m^2, age over 50 years, or a large neck

STOP-Bang
Screening for Sleep Apnea

Have you been diagnosed with sleep apnea by a sleep study?   Yes ☐   No ☐

Have you received treatment for sleep apnea, such as CPAP or Bi-PAP?   Yes ☐   No ☐

Please answer the following four questions with a *yes* or *no* answer:

1) Do you snore loudly (louder than talking or loud enough to be heard through closed doors)?
   Yes ☐   No ☐

2) Do you often feel tired, fatigued, or sleepy during daytime?
   Yes ☐   No ☐

3) Has anyone observed you stop breathing during your sleep?
   Yes ☐   No ☐

4) Do you have or are you being treated for high blood pressure?
   Yes ☐   No ☐

FOR STAFF USE ONLY, DO NOT WRITE BELOW THIS LINE

5) Is the BMI ≥35 kg/m^2?
   Yes ☐   No ☐

6) Is the patient ≥50 years of age?
   Yes ☐   No ☐

7) Is the neck circumference greater than 15.7 inches (40 cm)?
   Yes ☐   No ☐

8) Is the patient male?
   Yes ☐   No ☐

Total number of questions answered YES: _____   Is the patient at high risk for OSA? Yes ☐   No ☐

High risk of OSA: Yes to >3 items

Fig. 15.4 STOP/BANG questionnaire for obstructive sleep apnea. (Wijeysundera DN, Finlayson E. Preoperative evaluation. Figure 31.8 in: Gropper MA, ed. *Miller's Anesthesia*. 9th ed. Elsevier; 2020.)

circumference (> 43 cm for males or > 41 cm for females), and/or are male. Patients who score more than four points are at high risk. and those who score between three and four points are at intermediate risk.[12] The anesthesia team may modify the treatment plan for these patients by avoiding excess sedation and employing regional anesthesia, nerve blocks, and/or multimodal anesthesia with nonopioid therapy for pain.

Postoperative adverse respiratory events (PAREs) are certainly not limited to the adult population. Many children are diagnosed with asthma, which predisposes them to an increased risk of PAREs. Additionally, an alarming and growing number of children are obese, with some data indicating a prevalence as high as 21% in the United States.[13] The presence of obesity in children, much like adults, puts them at risk of OSA, as well as impaired lung function. In fact, in a review, it was found that "significant associations between obesity and overall PAREs were identified in all studies that tested this association."[13] This population was found to have higher rates of asthma and OSA and therefore have a greater risk for bronchospasm and hypoxemia in the postoperative setting.[13] Thus, the anesthesia team must be made aware of the risk factors to allow for additional planning for a safe anesthesia experience.

Patients who smoke are known to have an increased risk of COPD, heart disease, hypertension, peripheral vascular disease, hypoxia, poor tissue healing, wound dehiscence, and a hyperreactive airway.[11] In fact, those who smoke a half-pack a day have a six times greater risk of postoperative pulmonary complications.[8] Elevated levels of carboxyhemoglobin result in decreased oxygenation. Smokers experience a greater risk of bronchospasm and laryngospasm, especially during induction, intubation, and extubation.[11] The damaged mucociliary transport system makes them more prone to bronchitis and pneumonia.

Patients who smoke need to be instructed to stop as soon as possible before surgery. Cessation for 2 weeks allows the mucociliary transport to return to nearly normal functioning.[8] As with other pulmonary co-morbidities, the anesthesia team attempts to avoid intubation and inhalation anesthesia to increase safety. Patients may require optimization with nebulizer treatments on the day of surgery.

Diabetes Mellitus

Patients with diabetes mellitus now comprise nearly 10% of the U.S. population and present special considerations for the perianesthesia setting. This group is often overweight and has the associated obesity risk factors. In addition, they suffer a significantly increased risk of cardiovascular, cerebrovascular, and peripheral vascular disease. They may experience renal insufficiency or failure, which can alter their medication metabolism, and they may have problems related to neuropathies.[11] Because of the multitude of risks and co-morbidities, preoperative testing should include a complete blood count, basic metabolic panel, and ECG.[14] Additionally, "hyperglycemia in the perioperative period is associated with several adverse outcomes, including wound infection, pneumonia, sepsis, and cardiovascular events."[11]

The management of diabetes is constantly evolving, with the development of new therapies and tools for monitoring. Ideally, the diabetic patient is scheduled early to avoid prolonged periods of fasting. The patient should be given clear instructions regarding the management of medications preoperatively. Some may have had a consultation with their endocrinologist for this guidance, but most often, the surgery center policies or anesthesia team provide this direction. Diabetic medications are generally continued the day before surgery, with the exception of metformin if contrast dye is expected to be used. Adjustments are made to the evening dose of long-acting basal insulin, which may be reduced by 50% to 75% to reduce the perioperative risk of hypoglycemia.[15] The day-of-surgery dosage of insulin may be reduced or held depending on anesthesia preference. The blood glucose is monitored throughout the day to allow for the identification and treatment of hypoglycemia or hyperglycemia.[11] "For patients taking insulin or a sufonylurea, it is desirable that the blood glucose level be greater than 100 mg/dL before the start of surgery. If the blood glucose is greater than 180 mg/dL, a supplemental correction dose of rapid-acting insulin is often administered."[15]

Renal Function

Those with renal failure or chronic kidney disease experience fluid and electrolyte imbalances, acid–base balance disruption, dysregulation of blood pressure, and anemia related to the impaired production of erythropoietin. They often have co-morbidities such as diabetes mellitus, hypertension, and cardiovascular disease. They do not normally metabolize many of the anesthetics, often are slow to recover, and are at increased risk of requiring hospital admission following surgery. In addition, they are highly susceptible to postoperative infections. This population is generally not considered appropriate for treatment in outpatient-based ASCs.[11] Any patient identified in the preanesthesia department as having renal disease or showing significant increases in blood urea nitrogen or creatinine levels on laboratory testing should have their case reviewed by the anesthesiologist.

Because of the impact on coagulation, medication metabolism, and nutritional status of liver failure, cirrhosis, acute hepatitis, or advanced liver disease, these diseases generally render a patient inappropriate for outpatient-based ambulatory surgery.[11] Preanesthesia testing should include a complete blood count, complete metabolic panel, and prothrombin time and partial thromboplastin time.[14] Patients with a history of chronic hepatitis or significant alcohol or drug abuse should be evaluated for potential liver damage, which could alter the plan for procedures in the ambulatory surgery setting.

Medication Reconciliation

The history gathering must include medication reconciliation, including all prescription and over-the-counter medications (e.g., herbals, nutritionals, and supplements). Prescription medications are generally taken until the day of surgery except for anticoagulants, which may be stopped by the surgeon or anesthesia provider. Patients should be instructed on which medications to take on the day of the procedure following an organizational protocol. These generally include cardiac medications, beta-blockers, calcium channel blockers, anticonvulsants, chronic pain medications, and medications used to treat Parkinson disease.

Over-the-counter and herbal medications should be stopped 1 to 2 weeks before surgery. Many patients believe herbals, nutritionals, and supplements are all natural and harmless. The actions and interactions of many have not been studied or are not fully understood. Some, such as melatonin, kava kava, valerian, and St. John's wort, are known to have interactions with anesthesia resulting in increased sedation. Others such as feverfew, garlic, ginger, ginko, and vitamin E can cause an increased risk of bleeding.[11]

Diagnostic Testing

Preoperative laboratory and diagnostic testing may be ordered by the surgeon or the anesthesia provider, or both. Routine tests ordered for all patients regardless of age, condition, history, or planned procedure are not appropriate. Studies have demonstrated that as much as 50% of the ordered testing is not necessary and results in 18 billion dollars wasted annually. The American Society of Anesthesiologists (ASA) has created a *Practice Advisory of Preanesthesia Evaluation*, which outlines the appropriate indications for selective testing.[14] Tests should be indicated by information gleaned from the medical record, patient interview, or physical assessment, or based on the type of procedure planned for the purpose of identifying or assessing conditions that may affect the anesthesia plan and assist the provider in forming a safe anesthesia plan.[14] Based upon the ASA recommendations, an algorithm can be created to guide nurses or anesthesia providers who are completing the preanesthesia assessment regarding testing that may be advised (Figure 15.5).

Allergies

Allergies to food and drugs should be assessed, including the type and severity of reaction. Allergies to foods may indicate risks for cross-sensitivities. For instance, egg allergies are often associated with a sensitivity to propofol. "Allergies to banana, kiwi, peaches and water chestnuts may have a link with latex allergies."[11] The increasing prevalence and severity of latex allergies have prompted most institutions to eliminate latex products. The entire surgical team should be made aware

Pre-anesthesia Ancillary Studies

Condition	CBC	PT/PTT/INR	BMP	CMP	EKG	CXR	Other
Age							
Age >40 and smokes or has BMI >36	×		×		×		
Age > or = 60	×		×		×		
Medical conditions							
AIDS	×	×	×		×	×	
Autoimmune diseases	×		×		×		
Blood disorders	×	×					
Diabetes mellitus	×		×		×		
Dyspnea, orthopnea, productive cough	×		×		×	×	
Heart (CHF, MI, CAD, angina, arrhythmia, etc)	×		×		×	×	
HIV	×			×			
Hypercholesterolemia	×		×		×		
Hypertension	×		×		×		
Kidney disease	×	×	×		×		
Liver disease	×	×		×			Add CXR if cirrhosis
Organ transplant	×		×		×		
Pulmonary disease	×		×		×	×	
Seizures	×		×		×		
Thyroid disease				×	×		TSH
Treatments							
Dialysis patient							K⁺/HemoCue DOS
Radiation or chemo in last 3 months	×		×		×		
Substance use							
Smokes						×	
Drug or alcohol abuse	×	×		×	×		
Current medications							
Amniodorone							Thyroid panel
Anticonvulsants (ie: Dilantin, depakote, phenobarbital)							Drug level
Warfarin (coumadin)	×	×					
Digoxin							Dig level
Diuretic			×				
Platelet inhibitors (ie: Plavix, brilinta, or effient)							Platelet function
Other considerations							
Female of childbearing age							Urine HCG DOS
Major procedure	×						T&C

[1]**Major procedures:** Major urologic procedure, major abdominal surgery, major vascular surgery, total joint replacement, hysterectomy

Recommendations are cumulative, based on patient condition. For example, if a patient having a hysterectomy has renal failure, is on dialysis, and smokes, the kidney disease, dialysis, smoker, and major procedure tests would be ordered.

Fig. 15.5 Preanesthesia testing per ASA guidelines. (Data from: Apfelbaum JL, Connis RT, Nickinovich DG, et al. Practice advisory for preanesthesia evaluation: An updated report by the American Society of Anesthesiologists Task Force on Preanesthesia Evaluation. *Anesthesiology*. 2012;116(3): 522–538. https://pubmed.ncbi.nlm.nih.gov/22273990/.)

of any known latex allergy so the safety of all supplies and equipment can be ensured.

PREOPERATIVE INSTRUCTIONS

The final preoperative instructions will include the date, time, and location to which the patient reports on the day of surgery. Remind patients to bring any needed documents, such as identification or insurance cards and advance directives, if they are not on file. Patients should be reminded to provide the name and phone number of the responsible adult who will be driving them home. Specific instructions regarding any premedications should be reviewed, along with dietary and intake restrictions.

NPO Status

The NPO instructions should be given according to facility policy or at a minimum according to ASA standards. These include 2 hours for clear liquids, 4 hours for full liquids, and 6 hours for solid foods (Table 15.5). Patients should be reminded that NPO includes no gum, hard candy, or water. Tobacco users should be instructed to refrain for at least 8 hours if they have not already stopped.[11]

Patients should be encouraged to wear comfortable clothing with specific considerations for the type of procedure. For instance, no pullover tops for head or eye surgery. Loose oversized tops for shoulder surgery and loose-fitting pants for foot or leg surgery to allow room for splints, casts, or bulky dressings. Jewelry should be left at home to avoid burns associated with the use of cautery and to avoid liability related to loss or damage. Makeup should be avoided as it can injure the eyes and interfere with the clinician's assessment of skin color. Specific instructions such as bowel preps should be reviewed, along with reminders about the use of antibacterial soap for the preop shower.[11] Patients should be reminded not to shave the operative areas due to risk of nicks, which can increase the risk of infection. Any required hair removal will be performed by staff using clippers.

Day-of-Surgery Preparation

When patients arrive on the day of surgery, they are often anxious and nervous. The nurse immediately begins putting them at ease with introductions and an overview of the plan for the day. The patient's support person or family member may be allowed in the preoperative area as per facility policy. Patients with special needs and minors will have a parent or guardian present. Patient identification and understanding of the planned procedure are confirmed, and preparation for the procedure begins. Following organizational policy, patients are asked to change into gowns and remove any jewelry. Glasses, dentures, hearing aids, and/or prosthetics may need to be removed as per needs of the type of procedure or anesthesia and facility policy. Cautionary arm bands such as "allergy" or "do not use extremity" are applied.

If the organization does not have a preanesthesia testing center or preoperative clinic, the previously described history review, medication reconciliation, and screening are completed. If this work has already been completed, the admitting nurse reviews the data and adds information such as height and weight, times of the last medication doses, times of the last food or drink, and any new changes since the interview. The responsible adult planning to drive the patient home and provide home care is identified and confirmed.

Venous access is established according to organizational protocols. When selecting the size and site for an intravenous (IV) line, the nurse considers the surgical site, surgical position, complexity of surgery, and patient concerns. A history of mastectomy, significant surgery, fistula or shunt for dialysis, scarring, or trauma all limit the use of an extremity. The anesthesiologist may be consulted if site selection is unclear. For instance, the patient having a right arm surgery who has previously had a left mastectomy with lymph node resection may require that an IV line be placed in the foot or the external jugular vein.

The height, weight, and vital signs are obtained, and any additional testing such as urine pregnancy tests for women of child-bearing age and fingerstick blood glucose tests for diabetic patients are performed. The physical assessment is completed, including auscultation of heart and lung sounds, assessment for edema and peripheral pulses, and assessment of the skin, especially in the surgical area.

Patients should be screened for potential postoperative nausea and vomiting (PONV). Patients who have a history of PONV or motion sickness, females, nonsmokers, and those having abdominal surgery are at increased risk and benefit from premedication by the anesthesia provider. Those with multiple risks may benefit from the additional application of a scopolamine patch. Some facilities may use additional measures such as acupressure or aromatherapy per protocols.[11]

Hair removal, chlorhexidine skin cleansing, and/or betadine nasal swabs for prevention of surgical site infections are performed according to facility protocols. Any ordered preoperative medications such as acetaminophen or nonsteroidal anti-inflammatory agents or scopolamine patches are administered. The timing of prophylactic antibiotics is coordinated with the surgical team to ensure compliance with the former Surgical Care Improvement Project standards of administration within one hour of incision (Box 15.2).[11] If needed, insulin for the correction of hyperglycemia is given and glucose levels are closely monitored.

Patients are instructed on the use of pain scores determined by the facility and any symptoms to report postoperatively. Ideally, postoperative home care instructions are given to the patient and/or care provider prior to sedation. This allows for better understanding and recollection and gives the patient the opportunity to ask questions. The use of anticipated equipment, drains, or catheters can be demonstrated, with the patient having the opportunity to verify understanding using the teach-back approach or return demonstrations. Any written material should be at the 5th-grade reading level to meet health literacy goals.[11]

A current history and physical examination are required and must be updated within 24 hours of the procedure. Consents are obtained according to facility policy and following all state and federal regulations. It is the responsibility of the surgeon and anesthesia provider to ensure that consent has

TABLE 15.5 ASA Preoperative Fasting Guidelines

Ingested Substance	Minimum Fasting Period
Clear liquids	2 hours
Breast milk	4 hours
Infant formula	6 hours
Nonhuman milk	6 hours
Solid food	6 hours

Hernandez A, Sherwood ER. Anesthesiology principles, pain management, and conscious sedation. Table 14.7 in: Townsend CM, Beauchamp RD, Evers BM, Mattox KL, eds. *Sabiston Textbook of Surgery*. 21st ed. Elsevier; 2022.

BOX 15.2 Surgical Care Improvement Project Process Measures for Prevention of Infection

SCIP INF 1: Prophylactic antibiotic received within 1 hour before surgical incision.SCIP INF 2: Prophylactic antibiotic selection for surgical patients.SCIP INF 3: Prophylactic antibiotics discontinued within 24 hours after end time of surgery (48 hours for patients for cardiac surgery).SCIP INF 4: Patients for cardiac surgery with controlled, 6:00 a.m. postoperative serum glucose.SCIP INF 6: Surgery patients with appropriate hair removal.SCIP INF 9: Urinary catheter removed on postoperative day 1 or 2 with day of surgery being day 0.

SCIP INF 10: Surgery patients for whom either active warming was used intraoperatively for the purpose of maintaining normothermia or who had at least one body temperature equal to or greater than 96.8°F (36°C).

Sturm L. Infection prevention and control in the PACU. Box 5.1 in: Odom-Forren J, ed. *Drain's PeriAnesthesia Nursing: A Critical Care Approach.* 7th ed. Elsevier; 2018.

been obtained after risks and benefits have been explained. The nurse may obtain and witness the signature on the consent form only after the function of obtaining provider informed consent is complete. The nurse signature is only validating that the signature of the patient was witnessed. Some facilities require separate anesthesia consents. Some procedures, such as elective sterilization or any experimental procedures, require specific additional consents. The perianesthesia and surgical nurses are responsible for ensuring that patients are not taken to surgery without the required consents. If consents are missing, incomplete, or incorrectly completed, this must be corrected prior to transport to surgery.[11]

In some facilities, anesthesia providers may place peripheral nerve blocks or regional anesthesia in the preoperative setting. This increases efficiency by reducing the time in the operating suite and allows additional time for the block to become effective. If the facility does not have a block team, the perianesthesia nurse may assist with this procedure. As with any procedure, a time-out should be performed and documented ensuring the presence of consent and the correct patient, procedure, and site prior to beginning. The nurse may be asked to assist with positioning and monitoring of the patient.

Before the patient is transferred to surgery, the admitting nurse provides hand-off to the surgical nurse. The facility should have a standardized hand-off tool to ensure consistent communication. Findings of the patient history and assessment; special needs such as sensory deficits, assistive devices, or language barriers; any abnormalities noted; any medications or treatments administered and those ordered; and the presence of required documentation are communicated. The hand-off must allow the opportunity for the receiving nurse to ask questions.[11]

CHAPTER HIGHLIGHTS

- Patient selection, preparation, and evaluation are crucial to the ASC.
- Optimal patient outcomes depend on criteria-driven patient selection tools.
- Patients with preoperative co-morbidities, if optimized (e.g., medically managed), may be considered for the outpatient setting.
- Preoperative laboratory and diagnostic testing should be selective, based on criteria rather than routine.

CASE STUDY

Geneva is a 34-year-old married mother of three young children. Since her last pregnancy and delivery over 8 months ago, she has been experiencing dysfunctional uterine bleeding, and her gynecologist has recommended an endometrial ablation in the outpatient surgery center. Geneva presents to the preoperative clinic for her nursing assessment and education. During the nursing interview, she discloses that she was told by her primary care nurse practitioner that she was "prediabetic," but she did not have the money or time to adhere to home testing. Additionally, she disclosed that her husband had recently lost his job due to alcoholism, he could no longer drive due to a recent arrest, and the family was experiencing food insecurity. At the time of the interview, her BMI was determined to be 43 kg/m². The clinic staff noted that she had difficulty staying focused during the interview, and she admitted she often woke up extremely tired.

- What red flags may influence the decision to keep her surgery in the outpatient setting?
- What preoperative laboratory testing may be indicated?
- Given her disclosure of food insecurity, financial struggles, and lack of support from her spouse, what steps should the preoperative nurse take to provide Geneva support?

REFERENCES

1. De Oliveira Jr GS, Holl JL, Lindquist LA, Hackett NJ, Kim JY, McCarthy RJ. Older adults and unanticipated hospital admission within 30 days of ambulatory surgery: an analysis of 53,667 ambulatory surgical procedures. *J Am Geriatr Soc.* 2015;63(8):1679-1685. Available at: https://doi.org/10.1111/jgs.13537.
2. Subramaniam S, Aalberg JJ, Soriano RP, Divino CM. New 5-factor modified frailty index using American College of Surgeons NSQIP data. *J Am Coll Surg.* 2018;226(2):173-181. Available at: https://doi.org/10.1016/j.jamcollsurg.2017.11.005.
3. Wahl TS, Graham LA, Hawn MT, et al. Association of the modified frailty index with 30-day surgical readmission. *JAMA Surg.* 2017;152(8):749-757. Available at: https://doi.org/10.1001/jamasurg.2017.1025.
4. Traven SA, Horn RW, Reeves RA, Walton ZJ, Woolf SK, Slone HS. The 5-factor modified frailty index predicts complications, hospital admission, and mortality following arthroscopic rotator cuff repair. *Arthroscopy.* 2020;36(2):383-388. Available at: https://doi.org/10.1016/j.arthro.2019.08.036.
5. Farhat JS, Velanovich V, Falvo AJ, et al. Are the frail destined to fail? Frailty index as predictor of surgical morbidity and mortality in the elderly. *J Trauma Acute Care Surg.* 2012;72(6):1526-1530. Available at: https://doi.org/10.1097/ta.0b013e3182542fab.
6. Mullen-Fortino M, Rising KL, Duckworth J, Gwynn V, Sites FD, Hollander JE. Presurgical assessment using telemedicine technology: Impact on efficiency, effectiveness, and patient experience of care. *Telemed J E Health.* 2019;25(2):137-142. Available at: https://doi.org/10.1089/tmj.2017.0133.
7. Lew E, Pavlin DJ, Amundsen L. Outpatient preanaesthesia evaluation clinics. *Singapore Med J.* 2004;45(11):509.
8. Odom-Forren J, ed. *Drain's PeriAnesthesia Nursing: A Critical Care Approach.* 7th ed. Elsevier; 2018.
9. Larsen KD, Rubinfeld IS. Changing risk of perioperative myocardial infarction. *Perm J.* 2012;16(4):4-9. Available at: https://doi.org/10.7812/tpp/12-033.
10. Fleisher LA, Fleischmann KE, Auerbach AD, et al. 2014 ACC/AHA guideline on perioperative cardiovascular evaluation and management of patients undergoing noncardiac surgery: a report of the American College of Cardiology/American Heart Association Task Force on practice guidelines. *J Am Coll Cardiol.* 2014;

64(22):e77-e137. Available at: https://doi.org/10.1016/j.jacc.2014.07.944.

11. Schick L, Windle PE, eds. *PeriAnesthesia Nursing Core Curriculum: Preprocedure, Phase I and Phase II PACU Nursing.* 4th ed. Elsevier; 2021.

12. Carr SN, Reinsvold RM, Heering TE, Muckler VC. Integrating the STOP-Bang questionnaire into the preanesthetic assessment at a military hospital. *J PeriAnesth Nurs.* 2020;35(4):368-373. Available at: https://doi.org/10.1016/j.jopan.2020.01.014.

13. Kiekkas P, Stefanopoulos N, Bakalis N, Kefaliakos A, Konstantinou E. Perioperative adverse respiratory events in overweight/ obese children: systematic review. *J PeriAnesth Nurs.* 2016;31 (1):11-22. Available at: https://doi.org/10.1016/j.jopan.2014.11.018.

14. Apfelbaum JL, Connis RT, Nickinovich DG, et al. Practice advisory for preanesthesia evaluation: an updated report by the American Society of Anesthesiologists Task Force on Preanesthesia Evaluation. *Anesthesiology.* 2012;116(3):522-538. Available at: https://doi.org/10.1097/ALN.0b013e31823c1067.

15. Simha V, Shah P. Perioperative glucose control in patients with diabetes undergoing elective surgery. *JAMA.* 2019;321(4):399-400. Available at: https://doi.org/10.1001/jama.2018.20922.

16 Phases of Care: Phase I: Immediate Postoperative Care

Denise Faraone Diaz, MSN, BA, RN, CPAN, CAPA

LEARNING OBJECTIVES

A review of the content of this chapter will help the reader to:

1. Prioritize elements of the initial postanesthesia assessment.
2. Demonstrate knowledge of interventions to achieve optimal patient outcomes in Phase I postanesthesia care.
3. Recognize signs of adequate oxygenation and ventilation in the postanesthesia patient.
4. Describe criteria for progression to Phase II postanesthesia care.

INTRODUCTION TO PHASES OF CARE

Perianesthesia nursing occurs on a continuum, or through phases of care, as the patient is physically moved from the preanesthesia holding or admitting area to the operating room or procedural room and then to the postanesthesia care unit (PACU). Postanesthesia recovery involves the management of patients who have received anesthesia, analgesia, or sedation regardless of their physical location. The primary purpose of postanesthesia recovery is to critically assess and stabilize these patients while working to prevent and detect complications. Phase I PACU care focuses on providing immediate postanesthesia nursing care and transitioning the patient to the intensive care setting, the inpatient setting, or Phase II outpatient care.[1] The focus of Phase II is to ultimately prepare the patient for discharge to home.[2]

PHASE I POSTANESTHESIA CARE UNIT

The primary purpose of the Phase I postanesthesia care unit (PACU) is to provide the perianesthesia nurse the opportunity for conducting a critical evaluation of and the stabilization of patients after procedures. The emphasis during this phase of care is on the anticipation and prevention of complications of anesthesia or the surgical procedure or intervention. A knowledgeable and skillful perianesthesia registered nurse should fully assess the patient upon admission to and discharge from the PACU, as well as at frequent intervals throughout the postanesthesia period. Assessment is a continuous and complete process incorporating sound, prudent nursing judgment and the use of therapeutic interventions. The Phase I PACU nurse gathers assessment data from the direct observation of the patient, as well as from the physician and other healthcare personnel, the medical record, and the care plan.[3]

TRANSITION FROM THE OPERATING ROOM TO THE POSTANESTHESIA CARE UNIT

Before the patient is transferred from the operating room to the PACU, the PACU nurse should be notified not only to expect the patient but of any special needs or required equipment, such as the patient's isolation status or the need for a ventilator.[1] Advanced preparation allows for safe transition of care. The patient should be assigned based on patient classification and recommended staffing. Table 16.1 identifies the patient classification and staffing guideline recommendations from the American Society of PeriAnesthesia Nurses.[2]

Evidence-Based Practice: Laidlaw Versus Lions Gate Hospital

In 1966, a very unfortunate postanesthesia care event occurred. A 44-year-old woman underwent general anesthesia for the excision of her gallbladder. At the time there were two nurses assigned to the unit. One nurse had gone for a coffee break leaving the second nurse alone. The postoperative gallbladder patient was the fourth patient who arrived in the unit and was soon followed by a fifth patient. While the lone nurse was attempting to address the fifth patient's restlessness, the 44-year-old woman became apneic and hypoxic, a condition leading to permanent brain injury. The judge in this case went on to make the most profound statement concerning the postanesthesia care unit.

"From this point of view, it is my opinion that this is the most important room in a hospital and the one in which the patient requires the greatest attention because it is fraught with the greatest potential dangers to the patient. This known hazard carries with it in my opinion a high degree of duty owed by the hospital to the patient. As the dangers or risks are ever-present, there should be no relaxing of vigilance if one is to comply with the standard of care required in this room."

Source: Laidlaw v. Lions Gate Hospital. (1969). CanLII 704 BC SC. http://canlii.org/en/bc/bcsc/doc/1969/1969canlii704/1969canlii704.pdf

---

The foundation of perianesthesia nursing is to provide safe, high-quality care for the surgical patient. Clear and thorough communication to the PACU nurse is essential. The transfer of patient care from the anesthesiology, surgical, and operating room personnel to the perianesthesia nurse includes a complete, structured verbal report at the time of transfer, with time allowed for the receiving nurse to ask questions.[4] Box 16.1 includes some elements that should be included in handoff reports.[2,4] In order to anticipate possible side effects or untoward complications, the perianesthesia nurse should receive comprehensive communications about all anesthetic techniques and agents used during surgery.[4]

ADMISSION TO THE PHASE I POSTANESTHESIA CARE UNIT

Admitting a patient to the Phase I unit should be a collaborative effort between the anesthesia provider and the PACU nurse. The immediate priority is evaluating and ensuring the adequacy of respiratory and circulatory function. The PACU nurse performs an initial assessment to identify signs and

TABLE 16.1 Recommended Staffing in the Postanesthesia Care Unit Based on Patient Classification

	Recommended Staffing	Patient Classification
Class 1:2	One perianesthesia nurse to two patients	Two conscious patients, stable and free of complications but not yet meeting discharge criteria Two conscious patients, stable and younger than 8 years of age, with family or competent support staff present but not yet meeting discharge criteria One unconscious patient, hemodynamically stable, with a stable airway, and older than 8 years of age; one conscious patient, stable and free of complications
Class 1:1	One nurse to one patient	From the time of PACU admission until all critical elements are met: Initial assessment is complete Patient has a stable and secure airway Patient is hemodynamically stable Patient is free from agitation, restlessness, or combative behaviors The 1:1 ratio should also be maintained when: Active interventions are needed to maintain a patent airway There is evidence of airway obstruction or respiratory distress The patient is unconscious and is 8 years of age or younger When the patient has contact precautions, the nurse must have sufficient time to don and remove personal protective equipment and wash hands between patients
Class 2:1	Two nurses to one patient	One critically ill, unstable patient

McLaughlin MF. Postoperative/postprocedure assessment. Chapter 37 in: Schick L, Windle PE: *PeriAnesthesia Nursing Core Curriculum: Preprocedure, Phase I and Phase II PACU Nursing.* 4th ed. Elsevier; 2021.

BOX 16.1 Elements of Handoff Report to the Perianesthesia Nurse

Patient's name, medical record number, date of birth, age, weight/body mass index
Gender identity, sex at birth, and preferred pronouns as applicable
Pertinent medical history, including allergies, precautions, sensory deficits, and physical limitations
Procedure performed, including name of surgeon, estimated blood loss, surgical site information (drains, catheters, dressings)
Type and tolerance of anesthesia or sedation
Operative complications
Family/significant other name, contact information, or location
Invasive lines, including peripheral intravenous lines, arterial lines, and other invasive monitoring lines
Anticipatory Phase I needs, including radiologic imaging, laboratory work, procedure-specific testing, immediate orders, or frequency of vital signs if different from PACU routine

McLaughlin, MF. Postoperative/postprocedure assessment. Chapter 37 in: Schick L, Windle PE: *PeriAnesthesia Nursing Core Curriculum: Preprocedure, Phase I and Phase II PACU Nursing.* 4th ed. Elsevier; 2021; and Schick L. Assessment and monitoring of the perianesthesia patient. Chapter 26 in: Odom-Forren J: *Drain's PeriAnesthesia Nursing: A Critical Care Approach.* 7th ed. Elsevier; 2018.

BOX 16.2 Signs and Symptoms of Inadequate Oxygenation

Respiratory signs
- Shallow, rapid respirations or normal, infrequent respirations
- Tachypnea
- Dyspnea
- Snoring (obstructive)
- Oxyhemoglobin saturation less than 90%

Neurologic signs
- Anxiety, restlessness, inattentiveness
- Altered mental status, confusion
- Dimmed peripheral vision
- Seizures
- Unresponsiveness

Skin signs
- Diaphoresis
- Cyanosis

Cardiac signs
- Early: tachycardia
- Increased cardiac output
- Increased stroke volume
- Increased blood pressure
- Late: bradycardia, hypotension
- Dysrhythmias

Odom-Forren J, Brady JM. Postanesthesia recovery. Chapter 55 in: Nagelhout JJ, Elisha S: *Nurse Anesthesia.* 6th ed. Elsevier; 2018.

---

causes of inadequate oxygenation or ventilation.[1,2] Box 16.2 identifies signs and symptoms of inadequate oxygenation.[1] Any evidence of respiratory compromise requires immediate intervention.

Electrocardiographic (ECG) monitoring is used in Phase I to determine the cardiac rate and rhythm and any deviation from preoperative or intraoperative findings that should be evaluated. Blood pressure measurements are used to determine the adequacy of organ perfusion. If a patient is decompensating physiologically, any necessary invasive monitoring, such as an arterial line, is initiated.[1] Any evidence of cardiocirculatory compromise requires immediate intervention.

The anesthesia provider should be active during the patient's transfer and stabilization in the PACU and may assist with initiating oxygen therapy, maintaining or verifying airway adequacy, and assessing circulatory status to ensure a smooth transfer of care. After the patient is initially stabilized, the anesthesia provider should provide handoff communication to the PACU nurse.[1,2]

PHASE I PACU ASSESSMENT

Once the PACU nurse has received the handoff from the anesthesia provider, a more thorough physical assessment is performed. Because the patient's condition can quickly change, the PACU nurse should maintain vigilance at the bedside and perform a thorough assessment.[1,2] The goals of the PACU assessment are shown in Box 16.3.[1]

A systematic assessment of the patient's total condition can
be made from head to toe or by a system review, whichever the
individual nurse prefers. These methods are essentially identical, and because each body system has an integral function, all
observations are interrelated. Throughout the patient's stay in
the Phase I PACU, the ongoing assessment and documentation
should include, but not be limited to, the vital signs, pain assessment, intake and output, neurologic assessments, including neurovascular, sensory, and motor assessments, medication management, safety needs, and subsequent interventions.[3]

Phase I PACU Assessment: Assessment of Major Body Systems

The major body systems assessment is a methodical evaluation of the body systems that are most affected by anesthesia
and the surgical procedure. After the patient is admitted to the
PACU, the perianesthesia nurse assesses the cardiorespiratory
stability by evaluating the respiratory rate, depth of ventilation, breath sounds, oxygen saturation level, end-tidal carbon
dioxide (if appropriate), type of oxygen delivery system, and
presence of any artificial airway. The heart is auscultated for
the quality of heart sounds, the presence of any adventitious
sounds, and any irregularities in rate or rhythm. Peripheral
pulses are evaluated for strength and equality, and the body
temperature, skin color, and skin condition are assessed.[1,2]

The neurologic system assessment evaluates the level of
consciousness, orientation, sensory and motor function,
and pupil size, equality, and reactivity. The patient is
assessed for the ability to follow commands and move
extremities purposefully and equally. The renal system assessment focuses on fluid intake and output, including intraoperative fluid totals and inspection of all output devices,
including drains, catheters, and tubes. The perianesthesia
nurse should note and document the amount, color, and
consistency of all drainage. Examination of the surgical site
includes the status of dressings. The patient is also assessed
for pain or discomfort, such as nausea, with appropriate
interventions administered.[1,2]

Phase I PACU Assessment: Ongoing Assessments

An ongoing assessment of the patient receiving Phase I care
identifies the progress in recovery from anesthesia and any
residual effects and allows for periodic reexamination to assess physiologic trends. An ongoing clinical nursing assessment is used to determine the patient's needs, deficits, and
challenges, diagnose actual or potential problems, plan and
implement appropriate interventions, and evaluate patient
outcomes.[2] An ongoing assessment should evaluate the
respiratory and cardiovascular functions, mental status, including any acute changes in neurologic function, and pain.[1]
Table 16.2 lists the patient outcomes for the Phase I PACU.

TABLE 16.2 Postanesthesia Care Unit Phase I Patient Outcomes

Potential and Actual Problems (Nursing Diagnoses)	Outcome Goals (Patient Will Be Able To)	Nursing Interventions	Resources
Alteration in oxygenation/ ventilation Potential for aspiration Ineffective breathing patterns or respiratory depression related to sedation, anesthesia, positioning, and/or pain Increased secretions PONV	Maintain normal respiratory parameters (rate, depth, ease, clarity of breath sounds) Encourage deep breaths/use of incentive spirometer Maintain clear airway Avoid aspiration: head of bed elevated, dysphagia screening prior to oral liquids Maintain adequate oxygenation of tissues Encourage early mobility	Understanding of effects of anesthetics, analgesics, sedatives, and muscle relaxants and associated drug interactions Practice airway maintenance techniques Continuously assess oxygenation and ventilation Administer oxygen per protocol Identify preexisting respiratory disease and individualize care appropriately Request that patient breathe deeply frequently Position patient to provide optimal respiratory function Report abnormal symptoms to anesthesiologist and surgeon	Physiologic monitoring equipment at each bedside, to include continuous pulse oximetry; end-tidal carbon dioxide if available and clinically indicated Adequate staffing patterns to ensure proper nurse-to-patient ratio Immediate access to anesthesia provider Comprehensive anesthesia report before transfer of patient ASPAN Perianesthesia Nursing Standards, Practice Recommendations and Interpretive Statements Facility policies regarding interventions for cardiovascular and respiratory problems Oxygen and suction at each bedside Immediate access to emergency medications and equipment: crash cart, resuscitator bag-valve mask, ventilator, airway maintenance supplies

Continued

TABLE 16.2 Postanesthesia Care Unit Phase I Patient Outcomes—cont'd

Potential and Actual Problems (Nursing Diagnoses)	Outcome Goals (Patient Will Be Able To)	Nursing Interventions	Resources
Cardiovascular instability Potential for altered mental status Potential alterations in tissue perfusion	Maintain normal cardiovascular parameters, avoiding extremes in blood pressure and/or heart rate Return to baseline neurologic function/mental status Demonstrate normal parameters of peripheral circulation	Maintain normal cardiovascular parameters, avoiding extremes in blood pressure and/or heart rate Return to baseline neurologic function/mental status Demonstrate normal parameters of peripheral circulation	Maintain normal cardiovascular parameters, avoiding extremes in blood pressure and/or heart rate Return to baseline neurologic function/mental status Demonstrate normal parameters of peripheral circulation
Altered skin integrity related to surgical wound Potential for infection at surgical site	Experience appropriate and uncomplicated wound healing	Assess surgical site throughout PACU Phase I stay Use aseptic technique when changing bandages Avoid constricting bandages at surgical site	Standard precautions Personal protective equipment and sterile dressing supplies Antibiotics as ordered
Altered skin integrity related to pressure points or positioning	Avoid skin breakdown related to pressure, tape, and constricting bandages	Perform comprehensive skin assessment upon admission to Phase I PACU; document abnormal finding and reassess prior to transfer, more frequently as needed Position patient using appropriate padding to avoid pressure points Assess full body for pressure areas	Nonallergenic tape Padding, pillows, and foam for protection
Anxiety related to unfamiliar surroundings, separation from family/significant other, and potential diagnosis or surgical outcome	Express reduced anxiety Display calm demeanor Verbalize needs related to family Provide emotional support	Minimize sights, sounds, or other areas of PACU Phase I whenever possible Encourage family presence in PACU Phase I as appropriate and per institutional policy Provide emotional support and answers to patient's questions within boundaries of nursing Monitor and oversee patient care while patient is vulnerable to environment	Separate PACU Phase I critical care patients and patients undergoing treatments from preoperative and PACU Phase II patients Policy allowing families and responsible adult caregiver to visit in PACU Phase I
Altered thought process and/or memory loss related to sedation or anesthesia	Display or verbalize appropriate orientation to surroundings and situation Avoid self-injury related to altered thought patterns	Provide frequent affirmation of orientation to time, place, and events Assess patient's orientation	Pharmaceutical literature outlining effects of anesthesia and sedative medications Predetermined PACU Phase I discharge criteria that include assessment of mental status
Alteration in comfort: pain	Express acceptable comfort level	Assess and administer appropriate analgesics; evaluate effectiveness Position patient for comfort Apply nonpharmacologic/complimentary interventions as ordered/appropriate Provide positive reinforcement and encourage philosophy of wellness throughout process Encourage appropriate pace for increased activity	Analgesic medications Positioning and support of body areas Breathing exercises Positive reinforcement of comfort
Alterations in comfort: PONV	Express acceptable comfort level Avoid vomiting and retching	Assess for presence of protective reflexes: cough, gag, and swallow Encourage appropriate pace for oral intake of fluids Administer antiemetics as needed Provide positive reinforcement and encourage philosophy of wellness throughout process Use complementary therapies if acceptable to patient	Antiemetic medications IV fluids Literature related to reducing gastrointestinal symptoms Appropriate food and beverages (avoid acid-producing juices and spicy or difficult-to-digest foods)
Self-care deficit	Display sufficient level of alertness and self-care for discharge to Phase II or to a nursing unit	Provide comprehensive nursing care modified to patient's abilities Assess patient for ability to turn, move, and call for assistance before transfer	Level of consciousness scale PACU Phase I discharge criteria

TABLE 16.2 Postanesthesia Care Unit Phase I Patient Outcomes—cont'd

Potential and Actual Problems (Nursing Diagnoses)	Outcome Goals (Patient Will Be Able To)	Nursing Interventions	Resources
Actual or perceived loss of privacy, confidentiality, or dignity	Express satisfaction with level of privacy and confidentiality provided Maintain dignity and sense of self-esteem	Support patient's right to privacy, confidentiality, and dignity Provide privacy and ensure confidentiality Provide curtains, blankets, and clothing that covers patient Allow patient as much decision-making as is possible in the PACU Phase I setting	Surroundings that are friendly, family focused, private, and apart from the view of other patients and staff
Risk of hemorrhage	Maintain hemodynamic stability Avoid hypertension	Ensure availability of IV solutions Observe surgical site for signs of bleeding and report to physician Administer anxiolytic and/or antihypertensive medications as ordered	Access to blood bank for rapid availability of blood products if needed Antihypertensive agents Anxiolytic medications IV fluids and supplies
Alterations in health that can complicate postanesthesia care	Provide honest preoperative information about any existing medical factors Comply with instructions to optimize medical status before the day of surgery Experience no complications related to prior medical status	Encourage patient to provide complete and accurate information regarding health status and practices before surgery that may be influential in the perianesthesia setting Assess patient's physical status frequently Use active listening and observe for clues to patient's health status Review record and receive comprehensive report from anesthesia provider Individualize patient care related to prior health status	Structured preoperative time frame for physical and historical assessment Books and literature on patient assessment and various medical conditions Primary care physician available to assist in optimizing patient's health status before and after surgery
Risk of injury related to environment, equipment, positioning, medications, and emergence delirium	Remain free from allergic reactions, burns, skin breakdown or pressure points, falls, or nerve or joint injuries Complete PACU Phase I experience without complications or injury	Observe patient at all times Reinforce patient's orientation to time Identify symptoms of emergence delirium and intervene appropriately Position patient according to acceptable standards of care and individual needs using proper body mechanics for staff and patient Ensure that side rails remain in up position Lock bed or stretcher wheels at all times while patient is on bed or stretcher Keep only the current chart (if applicable) at the bedside Check the emergency alarm system and emergency equipment regularly	Patient record ASPAN Perianesthesia Nursing Standards, Practice Recommendations and Interpretive Statements Manufacturer's instructions for proper use of equipment Appropriate positioning supplies: pillows, padding, and foam sheeting Ongoing program of preventive maintenance of equipment Ongoing safety programs for employees Policy on enacting Safe Medical Devices Act Soft restraint policy
Hypothermia Discomfort related to cold	Maintain normal body temperature Avoid shivering Verbalize comfort with temperature	Assess and document patient's temperature on admission and periodically in PACU Phase I Maintain normothermia: keep patient covered as fully as possible, including head and neck areas; apply warm blankets or use forced air warming equipment, especially for patients at high risk for hypothermia (infants and frail elderly)	ASPAN Perianesthesia Nursing Standards, Practice Recommendations and Interpretive Statements Cabinets for warming blankets and solutions Warm forced air and heating blankets Thermometers
Hypothermia Discomfort related to cold	Express comfort	Mouth care Give ice chips or sips of water initially per provider orders/dysphagia screening	Provider orders

McLaughlin MF. Postoperative/postprocedure assessment. Table 37.1 in: Schick L, Windle PE: *PeriAnesthesia Nursing Core Curriculum: Preprocedure, Phase I and Phase II PACU Nursing*. 4th ed. Elsevier; 2021.

Ongoing Assessments: Respiratory

During Phase I PACU care, the perianesthesia nurse should continually assess the patient for common respiratory complications, including upper airway obstruction, laryngospasm, hypoxemia, atelectasis, hypoventilation, bronchospasm, and aspiration. Table 16.3 lists the causes and interventions for these complications.

Ongoing Assessments: Cardiovascular

During Phase I PACU care, the perianesthesia nurse initiates continuous cardiac monitoring and observes for signs of myocardial ischemia, including ECG changes, chest pain, changes in skin color, diaphoresis, and gastrointestinal complaints, such as nausea, pain, or heartburn. Dysrhythmias seen in the PACU are usually transient and rarely require intervention.[1]

Other cardiovascular assessments include the presence of hypotension or hypertension. Hypotension in the PACU is usually caused by hypovolemia secondary to the inadequate replacement of intraoperative fluid and blood loss. Initial treatment includes restoring the circulating volume, but the patient should be assessed for active bleeding from the surgical site. Pain is the leading cause of hypertension and tachycardia in the PACU and should be treated as indicated. Other causes of postoperative hypertension include shivering, agitation, and urinary retention.[1]

Ongoing Assessments: Mental Status

Postoperative mental status changes may be associated with poor anesthetic outcomes. The perianesthesia nurse should perform frequent mental and behavioral status assessments.[1]

Any acute change in mental status should be immediately reported to the anesthesia provider as the patient may need to be evaluated for a stroke or other neurologic injury. Stroke assessment includes observing facial symmetry, evaluating speech, and assessing for pronator drift. Additional assessment findings should include the level of orientation, pupillary response, movement, and muscle strength.[5]

Some patients emerge from anesthesia in a state of excitement, characterized by restlessness, disorientation, crying, moaning, irrational talking, and inappropriate behavior. In the extreme form of excitement known as *emergence delirium*, the patient screams, shouts, and wildly thrashes. Postoperative delirium or emergence excitement is defined as responsive or unresponsive agitation. Figure 16.1 identifies factors that contribute to emergence delirium. The incidence is higher in children, the elderly, and patients with a history of substance use or psychiatric disorders. Patients who are emotional prior to surgery are at increased risk of developing emergence delirium. Treatment is focused on identifying the cause, such as hypoxia or urinary retention, and treating it appropriately. The PACU nurse must always maintain patient safety and should notify the anesthesia provider if the condition persists.[5]

Delayed awakening occurs when patients awaken from anesthesia more slowly than expected. Medication effects are the most common cause of delayed awakening, though metabolic problems such as hypoglycemia, hypocalcemia, hyponatremia, and hypermagnesemia can contribute to the condition. Other factors contributing to delayed awakening include hypovolemia, hypothermia, neurologic injury, hypercarbia, and hypoxemia. Treatment consists of thorough assessments and quick identification of the cause or causes with appropriate interventions. Oxygenation and ventilation, along with adequate cardiac output, must be maintained, and metabolic

TABLE 16.3 Respiratory Complications in Phase I PACU

Complication	Signs and Symptoms	Interventions
Upper airway obstruction	Obstruction occurs when the tongue falls back, occluding the pharynx and blocking the flow of air into and out of the lungs. Signs and symptoms of an upper airway obstruction include snoring, but patients are usually somnolent and may be difficult to arouse.	Stimulate the patient to take deep breaths and reposition the airway. Placement of an oral or a nasal airway may be required. Never insert an oral airway in a conscious patient as this may cause gagging or vomiting.
Laryngospasm	Respiratory emergency caused by a reflex closure of the glottis (intrinsic muscles) or the larynx (extrinsic muscles). Symptoms include agitation, decreased oxygen saturation, absent breath sounds, and acute respiratory distress. Incomplete obstruction may manifest as a crowing sound or stridor.	Immediate treatment includes jaw thrust maneuver and positive pressure ventilation. If ineffective, a subparalytic dose of IV succinylcholine may be given by the anesthesia provider. Reintubation is undesirable and should be used only if severe airway edema is present or if the obstruction persists despite treatment interventions.
Hypoxemia	Low arterial oxygen pressure characterized by low pulse oximetry reading. Patient may exhibit agitation, somnolence, hypertension, hypotension, tachycardia, or bradycardia.	Administer supplemental oxygen as needed and encourage the patient to take deep breaths. May require use of incentive spirometry.
Atelectasis	Usually the result of bronchial obstruction caused by secretions or decreased lung volumes.	Use of humidified oxygen, coughing and deep breathing, postural draining, and increased mobility.
Hypoventilation	Decreased respiratory rate caused by anesthetic agents. More common with upper abdominal surgery.	Administer supplemental oxygen and stimulate patient to take deep breaths as needed.
Bronchospasm	Can result from aspiration, pharyngeal or tracheal suctioning, or allergic response. More common in patients with asthma and chronic obstructive pulmonary disease.	Management includes administration of beta-2 agonists, anticholinergics, and epinephrine. Steroids may be helpful in patients with asthma.
Aspiration	Foreign matter enters the airway, causing cough, obstruction, atelectasis, bronchospasm, and pneumonia. May cause hypertension, tachycardia, and dysrhythmias.	In the absence of complete upper airway obstruction, interventions are supportive and include supplemental oxygen and repositioning for patient comfort.

Odom-Forren J, Brady JM. Postanesthesia recovery. Chapter 55 in: Nagelhout JJ, Elisha S: *Nurse Anesthesia*. 6th ed. Elsevier; 2018.

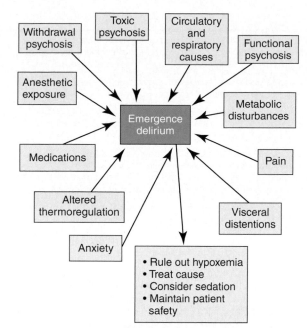

Fig. 16.1 Factors contributing to emergence delirium. Modified from Odom-Forren J. Figure 29.7 in: *Drain's PeriAnesthesia Nursing: A Critical Care Approach.* 7th ed. Elsevier; 2018.

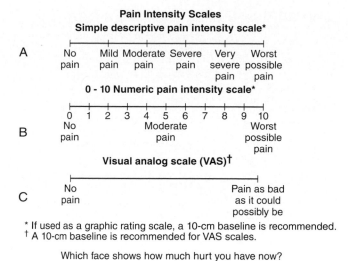

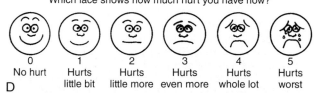

Fig. 16.2 Examples of pain assessment tools. Modified from Nagelhout JJ, Elisha S. Figure 55.3 in: *Nurse Anesthesia.* 6th ed. Elsevier; 2018.

abnormalities should be corrected. If hypothermia is the suggested cause, warming measures are instituted with appropriate temperature monitoring. Neurologic evaluation may be needed if other causes of delayed arousal have been excluded.[5]

Ongoing Assessments: Pain

A primary goal of Phase I PACU care is the relief of surgical pain with minimal side effects. Patients should be assessed on admission to the PACU and then at frequent intervals using a verbal rating scale or visual analog scale for the severity of pain (Figure 16.2). When prioritizing the pain assessment, the patient's self-report is the most important measure of pain, but other pain assessment tools include behavioral signs, such as crying or agitation, and physiologic indicators, such as elevated vital signs. In some cases, a proxy pain rating by someone who knows the patient well may be most helpful in evaluating the patient's postoperative pain. Uncontrolled postoperative pain is a major source of preoperative fear, can impede mobility and recovery, and is a major source of dissatisfaction in surgical patients.[1] The perianesthesia nurse should continually assess the patient's pain, provide appropriate interventions, and reassess the effectiveness of those interventions. The anesthesia provider should be notified if interventions are ineffective.

DISCHARGE FROM PHASE I PACU

A patient can be discharged from the Phase I PACU to an inpatient unit or to the Phase II PACU for continued care. Discharge to Phase II can occur physically by changing the location of the patient or can be simply documented while the patient remains in the same physical location. A patient is ready for discharge from Phase I when the patient has met the preestablished discharge criteria approved by the anesthesia department. Box 16.4 shows the common Phase I PACU discharge criteria.

A patient who has recovered from the effects of anesthesia is ready for transfer to Phase II in the PACU when the vital

---

BOX 16.4 Phase I PACU Discharge Criteria

Regular respiratory pattern
Respiratory rate appropriate for age
Absence of restlessness and confusion
Vital signs within preoperative range
Pulse oximetry level as indicated by unit policy or equal to preoperative level
Ability to maintain patent airway
Surgical stability of operative site or system

Odom-Forren J, Brady JM. Postanesthesia recovery. Chapter 55 in: Nagelhout JJ, Elisha S: *Nurse Anesthesia.* 6th ed. Elsevier; 2018.

---

signs are stable, pain is manageable and tolerable, and no surgical complications have arisen. The patient should be oriented and able to call for assistance if needed, and the surgical site should be dry and intact. The PACU nurse should discharge the patient when the patient meets the medically approved discharge criteria, and the anesthesia provider should see the patient prior to discharge.[1,6]

The PACU nurse should never immediately discharge a patient from Phase I after the patient has received an initial dose of an opioid medication. Patients with a history of obstructive sleep apnea may be especially sensitive to opioids, and for them, discharge to Phase II may be delayed to assess for pain relief and the adverse side effects of opioid drugs. The PACU nurse should document the pain assessment and management for the ongoing evaluation of pain intensity and treatment effectiveness. A proper handoff should be made from the Phase I PACU nurse to the Phase II PACU nurse to ensure a smooth transition in care.[6]

A patient's discharge from the Phase I or Phase II PACU may be delayed for clinical or nonclinical reasons. Nonclinical

TABLE 16.4 Clinical Reasons for Delayed Discharge from PACU

Pain	Patients should be able to express an acceptable comfort level. Perform multimodal nursing interventions, such as administering analgesics as ordered, positioning for comfort, and using nonpharmacologic interventions. Notify the surgical team of worsening pain or pain that is unrelieved by interventions.
Postoperative nausea and vomiting	Patients should be able to express an acceptable comfort level and should be free from vomiting and retching. Intervene by administering antiemetics as ordered and limiting oral intake.
Inadequate oxygenation	Patients should have a patent airway and normal respiratory parameters, be free from hypoxia or dyspnea, and be able to perform effective coughing and deep breathing exercises. Intervene by administering oxygen, as needed; encouraging coughing and deep breathing exercises; and positioning for optimal lung expansion. Notify the anesthesia provider of unresolved abnormal symptoms.
Inability to void	Based on type of surgical procedure and surgeon preference, the patient may be required to void prior to discharge home. Follow your unit's policy for the acceptable amount of urine output as well as indications for bladder scanning and nonpharmacologic interventions to encourage voiding. Notify the surgical team if the patient cannot void.

McLaughlin, MF. Postoperative/postprocedure assessment. Chapter 37 in: Schick L, Windle PE: *PeriAnesthesia Nursing Core Curriculum: Preprocedure, Phase I and Phase II PACU Nursing.* 4th ed. Elsevier; 2021.

reasons include lack of availability of patient transport or reliable transportation home, lack of availability of inpatient beds, and staffing issues. The most common clinical reasons for delayed discharge are summarized in Table 16.4.[2]

The standard of care requires that the Phase I PACU nurse assess and evaluate every perianesthesia patient. Assessment and evaluation continue throughout each phase of recovery to ensure a safe transfer of care and to adequately prepare the patient for discharge from the Phase I PACU.

CHAPTER HIGHLIGHTS

- Perianesthesia nursing occurs along a continuum of levels or phases of care wherever the patient is located physically.
- Phase I care focuses on providing immediate postanesthesia care and transitioning the patient to the next phase of care.
- The primary purpose of Phase I care in the PACU is to stabilize patients after procedures and prevent complications from anesthesia or the surgical intervention.
- A thorough handoff is required at all phases of care to ensure patient safety and a smooth transition along the perianesthesia continuum.
- Phase I PACU nurses perform an initial assessment as well as ongoing assessments to monitor the patient for complications.
- Once all preestablished discharge criteria have been met, the patient may progress from Phase I recovery to the next phase of care.

CASE STUDY

Melody is a 26-year-old female patient presenting for outpatient surgery for the removal of a right breast mass. Her past medical history is significant for substance use disorder. She admits to drinking 12 to 24 ounces of alcohol daily and has most recently used IV drugs 2 days ago. She smokes cigarettes and occasionally vapes. She has no known drug allergies. She does not take any prescribed medications. The plan today is for Melody to receive general anesthesia with local infiltration at the incision site with IV opioid pain control in the immediate postoperative period. When she has met all discharge criteria, she will be discharged to go home with a prescription for an NSAID drug.

Which elements of Melody's past medical history should the anesthesia provider note during the handoff report? Based on this history, what assessments should the Phase I PACU nurse perform immediately upon Melody's arrival at the PACU? What complications is Melody most at risk of developing during Phase I recovery? What strategies can be employed to minimize these complications? What clinical factors could likely contribute to a delayed discharge for Melody?

REFERENCES

1. Odom-Forren J, Brady JM. Postanesthesia recovery. In: Nagelhout JJ, Elisha S, eds. *Nurse Anesthesia.* 6th ed. Elsevier; 2018:1147-1166.
2. McLaughlin MF. Postoperative/postprocedure assessment. In: Schick L, Windle PE, eds. *PeriAnesthesia Nursing Core Curriculum: Preprocedure, Phase I and Phase II PACU Nursing.* 4th ed. Elsevier; 2021:859-895.
3. Schick L. Assessment and monitoring of the perianesthesia patient. In: Odom-Forren J, ed. *Drain's PeriAnesthesia Nursing: A Critical Care Approach.* 7th ed. Elsevier; 2018:357-384.
4. Ball KA. Transition from the operating room to the PACU. In: Odom-Forren J, ed. *Drain's PeriAnesthesia Nursing: A Critical Care Approach.* 7th ed. Elsevier; 2018:347-356.
5. O'Brien D. Postanesthesia care complications. In: Odom-Forren J, ed. *Drain's PeriAnesthesia Nursing: A Critical Care Approach.* 7th ed. Elsevier; 2018:398-416.
6. O'Brien D. Patient education and care of the perianesthesia patient. In: Odom-Forren J, ed. *Drain's PeriAnesthesia Nursing: A Critical Care Approach.* 7th ed. Elsevier; 2018:385-397.

17 Phases of Care: Phase II and Extended Care

Hazel Marie Barmore Wiegert, MAN, BSN, RN, CPAN, CAPA

LEARNING OBJECTIVES

A review of the content of this chapter will help the reader to:

1. Describe the care given in Phase II and extended care.
2. Describe situations that would prevent the patient from being discharged and necessitate extended care and/or patient admission.

OVERVIEW

Postanesthesia care in Phase II and the extended care of patients is discussed in this chapter. Information is presented on the criteria for entering Phase II care, as well as the occasional need for extended care environments. The Phase II unit is typically considered the setting in which an ambulatory surgery patient prepares for discharge to home, although in a hybrid unit, all phases of care from preoperative preparation to immediate postanesthesia Phase I recovery to Phase II predischarge care may occur in the same patient care bay. Extended care, formerly known as Phase III care, is required when the patient needs additional observation or nursing interventions following discharge from Phase I or Phase II. Phases of care are levels of care, not necessarily specific units.[1] This is often true in newly designed ambulatory care centers.

PHASE II POSTANESTHESIA CARE

When patients are close to meeting the discharge criteria for Phase I in the postanesthesia care unit (PACU), they are getting ready to be moved to the next phase of care, known as Phase II. Phase II care is usually provided in a separate area from Phase I care, although many outpatient surgical centers have hybrid units combining phases of care. Patients meeting Phase II criteria are more awake and nearly ready to be discharged from the facility. In addition to patients transferred from Phase I, Phase II may include patients who are fast-tracked from the operating room or are received from areas such as interventional radiologic imaging, endoscopic procedures, cardiovascular laboratory interventions, or electroconvulsive therapy. This area also admits patients from home who will be having special procedures in the operating room or those having other special procedures depending on the facility. The Phase II unit is truly multifunctional.

Perianesthesia nurses need to be able to function well in this environment using their organizational skills and working autonomously. Nurses competently evaluate the physiologic needs, behavioral and cognitive needs, and safety needs of patients. "Phase II nurses must have strong clinical assessment skills and expertise in teaching and can be relied on to heed details that may affect patient recovery at home."[2] Staffing needs can change throughout the day depending on the complexity and acuity of patients, patient census, skill mix of the staff, and nursing competencies.

Phase II Staffing

Staffing recommendations for Phase II and extended care are found in ASPAN's *2023–2024 PeriAnesthesia Nursing Standards, Practice Recommendations and Interpretative Statements* (Box 17.1).[1] Although Phase II is not technically termed a critical care area in the strictest sense, during Phase II patients can be in a delicate physiologic state after anesthesia and invasive procedures. Occasionally, patients can have complications and deteriorate quickly without warning. It is recommended that the Phase II nurse be trained in advanced cardiac life support (ACLS) and pediatric advanced life support (PALS) as appropriate to the population served.

Phase II Equipment

The design of Phase II should include enough space for family-oriented practices. It is important to allow family members to join the patient as soon as possible. This allows for the caregiver to participate in the care of the patient and receive discharge instructions. Equipment and supplies are diverse. ASPAN's *2023–2024 PeriAnesthesia Nursing Standards, Practice Recommendations and Interpretative Statements* offers a list of recommended supplies during Phase II care (Box 17.2).[1] Supplies required for extended care are determined by the facility and are based on the patient population and level of care required by the patient.

Phase II Assessments

The Phase II perianesthesia nurse has significant responsibilities in the care of an ambulatory surgical patient. The nurse must constantly monitor and assess patients who have had a wide variety of procedures and anesthetic approaches. In Phase II, there are two different patient care goals. The first is to provide for any immediate physical needs of the patient. The second is to support and encourage the patient as the patient prepares for self-care upon discharge. The most basic nursing assessments include a review of the patient's physical and mental conditions. Postoperative clinical assessments are often focused and based on the surgical procedure, underlying patient conditions, and the patient's response to any interventions. Simultaneously, the perianesthesia nurse remains prepared for emergencies, provides education and encouragement, promotes a sense of wellness, and includes family members in the plan of action. All these actions are focused on the safe discharge of patients to their home settings.

During Phase II, culturally-sensitive patient care and family-centered care are necessary. If English is not the primary language of the patient and/or caregiver, interpreter services must be available. Knowledge of a patient's and caregivers' cultural beliefs and practices supports best outcomes. These beliefs and practices are typically related to health maintenance, treatment of illnesses, pain issues including responses to patients and treatment of pain, hygiene and modesty norms, and ethical values. Cultural influences of a community determine how a patient and family view the care of the sick and

BOX 17.1 Patient Classification/Staffing Recommendations for Phase II Care

Class 1:3 One Nurse to Three Patients
Examples include, but are not limited to:
   a. Age over 8 years
   b. Eight years and under with family present
Class 1:2 One Nurse to Two Patients
Examples include, but are not limited to:
   a. Eight years of age and under without family or support healthcare team members present
   b. Initial admission to Phase II
Class 1:1 One Nurse to One Patient
Example includes, but is not limited to:
   a. Unstable patient of any age requiring transfer to a higher level of care.

American Society of PeriAnesthesia Nurses. *2023–2024 Perianesthesia Nursing Standards, Practice Recommendations and Interpretive Statements.* ASPAN; 2022. Page 52.

seriously ill and their trust in the modern healthcare system.

In terms of clinical assessments, the stability of vital signs, including cardiovascular and respiratory parameters, need to be determined for discharge readiness. The integrity of the surgical site should also be evaluated frequently for potential bleeding or swelling. Progression of ambulation is encouraged, with particular attention given to the patient who has had regional anesthesia, including a nerve block to the lower extremity or a spinal or epidural block. These patients are particularly susceptible to falls and injuries. Oral intake, particularly of fluids, may be encouraged but is often not necessary.

Pain Issues

Poorly controlled postoperative pain often warrants an extended period of observation and clinical care following outpatient surgery. Analgesics play an important role in providing comfort. The use of other non-narcotic medications and treatments helps to potentiate the ability to decrease pain and promote comfort. Multimodal analgesia incorporating agents such as gabapentin, nonsteroidal anti-inflammatory medications, parenteral acetaminophen, and low-dose ketamine is becoming more common. Other nonpharmacologic alternatives include, but are far from limited to, the application of ice, heat, and/or essential oils. Although stays in extended care are shorter than inpatient stays, patients in extended care often require several additional hours during which they can rest and receive appropriate comfort measures.

Postoperative Nausea and Vomiting

Patients at high risk for postoperative nausea and vomiting (PONV) may also require additional time during which preventative and treatment interventions can be applied. Undertreated PONV causes delays in discharge, increases costs of care, and may contribute to unplanned admissions. NPO times can be shortened depending on the facility policies, adoption of enhanced recovery after surgery (ERAS) principles, and the agreement of the surgical and anesthesia providers. Current guidelines recommend multimodal prophylaxis in patients with known risk factors for PONV.[3] Long NPO times can cause

BOX 17.2 Equipment for Phase II Care

The following list of equipment for Phase II Care includes, but is not limited to:
1. The unit will be equipped with the following:
   a. Oxygen delivery system
   b. Access to constant and intermittent suction
   c. Blood pressure monitoring devices
   d. Thermometry
   e. Adjustable lighting
   f. Capacity to ensure patient privacy
2. A cardiac monitor and pulse oximeter will be readily available
3. Bag-valve masks of the appropriate size must be easily accessible at all times
4. Equipment will be available to assess blood glucose
5. Supplies as recommended by the Malignant Hyperthermia Association of the United States will be available (https://www.mhaus.org/ or 1-800-MHHYPER)
6. A method exists to call for assistance in emergency situations
7. An emergency cart will be available at all times
8. A defibrillator with adult and pediatric pads/paddles and cardiac pacing must be readily available for the population served
9. Stock medications include, but are not limited to, the following:
   a. Antibiotics
   b. Antiemetics
   c. Reversal agents
   d. Analgesics: opioids and nonopioids
10. Vascular access supplies/infusion pumps
11. Stock supplies should include:
   a. Dressings
   b. Facial tissues
   c. Gloves
   d. Bedpans and urinals
   e. Syringes, needles, and protective needle devices
   f. Emesis containers
   g. Patient linens
   h. Alcohol wipes
   i. Skin antiseptics
   j. Ice bags/cooling devices
   k. Tongue blades
   l. Urinary catheterization supplies
   m. Personal protective equipment
   n. Access to latex-free supplies and equipment
   o. A variety of single-use tapes
   p. Unit and device cleaning supplies
12. A means to safely transport patients
   a. Wheelchairs, etc.
   b. Portable oxygen, suction, cardiac monitoring equipment, pulse oximetry, and capnography will be available for those patients requiring such equipment during transport
13. Access to warming measures/devices
14. A means to assess urine volume (e.g., bladder scanner)
15. Automated medication cabinet/dispensing device (e.g., Pyxis, Omnicell)

Adapted from American Society of PeriAnesthesia Nurses. *2023–2024 Perianesthesia Nursing Standards, Practice Recommendations and Interpretive Statements.* ASPAN; 2022. Pages 69–70.

dehydration, thus increasing PONV. The intravascular volume status should be near euvolemia for the best patient outcomes, as both hypovolemia and hypervolemia can be detrimental to the patient.[4]

BYPASSING PHASE I CARE

Bypassing Phase I, or fast-tracking patients from the operating room or a special procedural area directly to Phase II, is dependent on the anesthesia provider and the patient's needs and assessment. Particularly in the ambulatory outpatient setting, anesthesia drugs and techniques are chosen for fast action and resolution.[5] This implies that patients may meet discharge criteria from the Phase I level of care before they actually leave the operating room. The criteria should include, but are not necessarily limited to, the following: the patient is awake or easily arousable and oriented, is hemodynamically stable, is breathing room air and maintaining baseline oxygen saturations, has minimal pain, has minimal nausea, and has no active bleeding at the surgical site, and all signs of neuromuscular blocking agents have resolved.[1,5] Upon arrival at Phase II, the medical report and handover of care is given by the anesthesia provider and circulating nurse to the Phase II nurse. A patient who has met the discharge criteria but is received into the Phase I PACU can potentially create delays in care and discharge when Phase I care is initiated. When the patient in the operating room meets the same discharge criteria used for moving a patient from the Phase I PACU to the Phase II unit, the patient can directly and safely be transferred from the operating room to Phase II care. Depending on the patient assessment and facility policy, the process toward discharge continues.

EXTENDED CARE

Perianesthesia extended care is an extended period of observation following surgery that usually results in discharge less than 23 hours postoperatively from the hospital-based or free-standing ambulatory surgery center (ASC). There are several reasons that some patients need extended care. These may include the need for additional pain management, treatment for PONV, and a failure of the discharge plan (e.g., lack of a designated driver). Some independent patients lack a social support system because they live alone or claim to have no family or friends to help them. In some social situations, it is possible that the spouse or other responsible individual is unwilling or physically unable to support care for the patient. For a list of risk factors and predictors for unanticipated admissions see Box 17.3.

The patient's home may not be conducive for postoperative care. The postoperative needs of the patient may be complicated, such as the need to address specific types of complex wound care strategies or the management of drains or indwelling urinary catheters. The patient may not be emotionally able to leave in a timely manner due to personal coping deficits, such as depression, anxiety, denial of medical problems, orientation, or memory problems. Age should not be a factor for additional assisted care. "The goal of assisted care is to meet the needs of the patient and responsible adult while avoiding an unplanned, unnecessary, and costly inpatient hospital stay whenever possible."[6]

Depending on the facility, patients who need to stay longer than the designated hours of the unit may need to be transferred to an in-house status or temporarily cared for in a designated unit until discharge. In some clinical settings, the Phase II staff stay until the last patient is discharged. In some metropolitan areas, patients may be discharged to a hotel that is usually close to the surgical or procedural center. Some

practices employ a nurse to check on these patients and provide limited care. These patients do need to have a responsible individual with them at the hotel.

DISCHARGE CRITERIA FOR PHASE II CARE AND EXTENDED CARE

Planning for an appropriate discharge begins when the patient consents to a surgical procedure and continues throughout the procedural encounter. This planning includes a safe arrangement for transport home, confirmation of a responsible individual to assist with home care, attainment of necessary supplies or equipment, and home preparation with attention to potential postoperative limitations in mobility.[1] Preparing a patient for discharge also requires a final clinical assessment to evaluate patient readiness. This assessment is necessary to determine if the patient has met the final discharge criteria. In most circumstances, discharge criteria are specific to the institution or facility and have been created in consultation with the anesthesia providers and approved by the anesthesia leadership. Box 17.4 clarifies requirements for having a responsible person who can provide transportation and care for the patient.[1]

Examples of discharge criteria, generally specific to the procedure and patient clinical presentation, may include, but not be limited to, the following:
- The patient is alert and oriented to person, time, and place or within the baseline preoperative status
- Vital signs are stable and/or within the preoperative baseline status
- Oxygen saturation is greater than 94% and/or within the baseline preoperative status

---

BOX 17.3 Risk Factors and Predictors for Unanticipated Hospital Admission

Surgical factors
- Pain
- Bleeding
- Extensive surgery; prolonged length > 3 hours
- Surgical complications and unanticipated operative events
- Abdominal surgery
- General and urologic surgery

Anesthesiologic factors
- ASA 2–4
- Mallampati score 2
- Nausea and vomiting
- Somnolence
- Aspiration

Social factors
- Discharge without escort

Medical factors
- Medical complications related to diabetes mellitus, ischemic heart disease, and sleep apnea
- Medication error
- Increased body mass index
- Advanced age > 80 years

ASA, American Society of Anesthesiologists.
Adapted from Shnaider I, Chung F. Outcomes in day surgery. *Curr Opin Anaesthesiol.* 2006;19:622–629; Whippey A, Kostandoff G, Paul J, et al. Predictors of unanticipated admission following ambulatory surgery: A retrospective case-control study. *Can J Anaesth.* 2013; 60(7):675–683; and Marley RA, Clapp TJ. Outpatient anesthesia. Table 42.11 in: Nagelhout JJ, Elisha S, (eds.). *Nurse Anesthesia.* 6th ed. Elsevier; 2018.

- No signs of respiratory distress (e.g., stridor, croupy cough) are present
- The circulation is intact, with a capillary refill of less than 3 seconds in any affected extremity
- Pain is controlled (e.g., patient describes the pain as "tolerable" and/or within baseline preoperative status)
- Patient can swallow and retain fluids with minimal or no nausea or vomiting
- Dressings are intact without excessive drainage or bleeding
- Patient can void if required due to surgical procedure or regional/spinal anesthetic
- Patients who are unable to void have been provided with appropriate instructions for follow-up if indicated
- Patient can ambulate consistent with preoperative abilities if not directly impacted by the procedure
- Written discharge instructions have been reviewed with the patient and patient's responsible individual
  - If possible, the teach-back method is used or a verbal understanding of the instructions is communicated
- Resources have been provided that the patient can contact if any problems should arise at home (e.g., emergency contact information for providers)
- If the patient is returning to a group home, nursing home, or other outside facility, a report has been called to the facility and a handoff given to that facility. A note should also be written in the electronic health record documenting this information.
- All patients, except those receiving strictly local anesthesia, must have safe transport home
- Patients should have a 24-hour caregiver identified prior to having the procedure.
  - In the event the patient absolutely has no way of arranging to return home with a responsible individual to provide care, the patient must remain in the unit/hospital until such time that a surgeon and anesthesiologist responsible for overseeing the case of the patient determines that the patient has returned to a presedation level of awareness and function and is able to manage themselves following discharge. A note in the electronic health record must document a decision to discharge in the absence of a responsible individual. In addition, the surgery/procedure should be scheduled as the first case of the day to allow for additional recovery time.
- Patient has accepted readiness for discharge
- If a female patient has received sugammadex as a neuromuscular blocking agent and is also taking hormonal contraceptives, the effectiveness of the contraceptives may be reduced. These include birth control pills, hormonal implants, skin patches, and certain intrauterine devices. The patient must be advised that a nonhormonal contraceptive alternative should be used for 7 days after the surgical procedure to prevent an unwanted pregnancy.[7]

The primary emphasis on the discharge process should be focused on criteria and not on time-based arrangements. In other words, mandatory minimum stays are usually not required by discharge policies unless specified by the surgeon. In some situations, a facility may incorporate a postanesthesia discharge scoring tool to determine the readiness for discharge. Box 17.5 shows an example of a discharge scoring tool.

BOX 17.5 Criteria for Determination of Discharge Score for Release Home to a Responsible Adult

Variable Evaluated	Score*
Vital Signs (Stable and Consistent with Age and Preanesthetic Baseline)	
Systemic blood pressure and heart rate within 20% of the preanesthetic level	2
Systemic blood pressure and heart rate 20% to 40% of the preanesthetic level	1
Systemic blood pressure and heart rate greater than 40% of the preanesthetic level	0
Activity Level (Able to Ambulate at Preoperative Level)	
Steady gait without dizziness or meets the preanesthetic level	2
Requires assistance	1
Unable to ambulate	0
Nausea and Vomiting	
None to minimal	2
Moderate	1
Severe (continues after repeated treatment)	0
Pain (Minimal to No Pain, Controllable with Oral Analgesics; Location, Type, and Intensity Consistent with Anticipated Postoperative Discomfort)	
Acceptability:	
Yes	2
No	1
Surgical Bleeding (Consistent With That Expected for the Surgical Procedure)	
Minimal (does not require dressing change)	2
Moderate (up to two dressing changes required)	1
Severe (more than three dressing changes required)	0

*Patients achieving a score of at least 9 are acceptable for discharge.

Modified from Marshall SI, Chang F. Discharge criteria and complications after ambulatory surgery. *Anesth Analg.* 1999;88:508–517; and Berg SM, Braehler MR. The postanesthesia care unit. Table 80.4 in: Gropper MA, ed. *Miller's Anesthesia.* Elsevier, 2020.

Evidence-Based Practice: Important Elements for Discharge Criteria

Jakobsson provides the following summary related to the assessment of patients following day surgery with regards to discharge readiness:

- A standardized tool should be used
- The objective user of the tool should be a skilled personnel
- Basic criteria include stable vital signs, adequate pain and nausea control, ability to stand and mobilize independently
- Factors that are patient- and procedure-dependent possibly requiring evaluation include oral intake of food and fluids as well as a requirement to void
- Determination of an escort and a companion for the first night at home should be assessed
- Consideration of a discharge checklist to confirm patient readiness

Source: Jakobsson JG. Recovery and discharge criteria after ambulatory anesthesia: can we improve them? *Curr Opin Anesthesiol.* 2019;32(6): 698-702. https://doi.org/10.1097/ACO.0000000000000784

POSTOPERATIVE FOLLOW-UP

Several regulatory bodies, including the Center for Medicare and Medicaid Services, as well as The Joint Commission, require post discharge evaluations within 72 hours of discharge. The original impetus for this evaluation was to reduce postoperative complications resulting in unplanned returns to emergency departments, unplanned returns to the operating room, and unplanned readmissions. These agencies have not provided guidelines on how these evaluations are to be conducted other than to require complete documentation of the evaluation exchange. Many practices have adopted a postoperative telephone call as the tool for this follow-up. The postoperative follow-up phone call is now standard and common practice. The postoperative discharge telephone call can serve a few purposes, including the collection of quality data. Most importantly, these calls allow for the clarification of patient or caregiver questions or concerns and the reinforcement of any pertinent patient education. Box 17.6 shows examples of the questions asked during the postoperative calls.

PATIENT AND FAMILY EDUCATION

"Patient education is a long-standing nursing tradition. Nursing has used patient education as a tool for providing safe, cost-effective, quality healthcare since the middle of the 19th century."[2] The predischarge period provides opportunities to educate both the patient and caregiver regarding anticipated discharge care needs. Topics may include wound care, safe medication practices, home safety assurance, dietary needs, mobility, and durable medical device utilization, to name a few. For more details regarding discharge challenges and patient teaching, see Chapter 18.

CHAPTER HIGHLIGHTS

- Phase II staffing recommendations, equipment needs, and clinical assessment parameters can be found in ASPAN's *2023–2024 Perianesthesia Nursing Standards, Practice Recommendations and Interpretive Statements.*
- Poorly managed pain and comfort control, as well as PONV, are among the potential issues delaying discharge to home.

BOX 17.6 Postdischarge Follow-Up

- How are you doing in general?
- How is your pain? (have the patient provide a pain score)
- If you are still having pain, are you taking your pain medication as directed?
- Are you able to eat and drink?
- Are you experiencing any nausea or vomiting?
- What does your surgical site look like? Is there any redness or bleeding?
- Do you have or have you had a fever?
- Is your circulation, motion, and sensation intact? (for extremity procedures)
- Are you having any difficulty voiding? (this question is especially important with certain procedures and anesthesia types)
- Are you able to get around in your house? Are there any limitations?
- Have you had to contact your physician for any reason or return to the emergency department?
- Did you have any issues while in our care?
- Have you made your follow-up appointment?
- Were your discharge instructions clear and helpful, or do you have additional questions?
- How was your overall satisfaction with your experience? Were there any areas of concern or feedback that would allow us to improve?
- Is there anything we could have done to make your stay better?
- Were there any particular employees you wanted to mention?
- Allow for any other comments/concerns that the patient wants to share.

Cook AE. Discharge criteria, education, and postprocedure care. Box 38.4 in: Schick L, Windle PE, eds. *Perianesthesia Nursing Core Curriculum: Preprocedure, Phase I and Phase II PACU Nursing.* Elsevier; 2021.

- Extended care is needed when a patient requires additional monitoring and interventions due to clinical or social barriers to discharge criteria.
- Many organizations providing ambulatory care services have implemented a postoperative phone call to conduct patient follow-up after discharge.

CASE STUDY

A 25-year-old male, Charley, has been discharged from PACU Phase I to Phase II. He had an inguinal hernia repair under general anesthesia, with local anesthesia to the incisional area. Charley has a history of opioid use disorder (OUD) and is concerned about the potential for relapse. The local anesthesia is starting to wear off. Charley begins to complain about the pain. He has received the maximum opioid and nonopioid medications. The surgical site is intact, with no observable swelling or bleeding. A soft gel ice pack is placed over the dressing. According to the electronic medical record, Charley has been on medication-assisted treatment (MAT) for his OUD, using daily methadone at a locally supervised clinic.

- What would you ask Charley concerning his MAT status for that day?
- How could you show a respectful, nonjudgmental attitude?
- What options can be provided to Charley for additional pain and comfort support?

REFERENCES

1. American Society of PeriAnesthesia Nurses. *2023-2024 Perianesthesia Nursing Standards, Practice Recommendations and Interpretive Statements.* ASPAN; 2022.
2. Smith S. Progressive postanesthesia care: phase II recovery. In: Burden N, Quinn DMD, O'Brien D, Dawes BSG, eds. *Ambulatory Surgical Nursing.* 2nd ed. WB Saunders; 2000:477-503.
3. Gan TJ, Belani KG, Bergese S, et al. Fourth Consensus Guidelines for the management of postoperative nausea and vomiting [published correction appears in *Anesth Analg.* 2020 Nov;131(5):e241]. *Anesth Analg.* 2020;131(2):411-448. Available at: https://doi.org/10.1213/ANE.0000000000004833.
4. Munsterman C, Strauss P. Early rehydration in surgical patients with prolonged fasting decreases postoperative nausea and vomiting. *J Perianesth Nurs.* 2018;33(5):626-631. Available at: https://doi.org/10.1016/j.jopan.2017.06.124.
5. Smith I, Skues MA, Philip BK. Ambulatory (outpatient) anesthesia. In: Gropper MA, ed. *Miller's Anesthesia.* 9th ed. Elsevier; 2020:2251-2283
6. Redmond MC. Extensions of care: phase III recovery. In: Burden N, Quinn DMD, O'Brien D, Dawes BSG, eds. *Ambulatory Surgical Nursing.* 2nd ed. WB Saunders; 2000:527-549.
7. McLaughlin MF. Postoperative/postprocedure assessment. In: Schick L, Windle P, eds. *PeriAnesthesia Nursing Care Curriculum: Preprocedure, Phase I and Phase II PACU Nursing.* 4th ed. Elsevier; 2021:859-894.

18 Patient Teaching and Discharge Challenges

Amy Berardinelli, DNP, RN, NE-BC, CPAN, FASPAN

LEARNING OBJECTIVES

A review of the content of this chapter will help the reader to:

1. Describe the impact of institutional policies and procedures on discharge education and practices at ambulatory surgical centers.
2. Describe the procedures for patient teaching in the ambulatory surgery setting.
3. Describe relevant postprocedural factors affecting the safe discharge home of patients after ambulatory surgery.
4. Describe the nursing care that is appropriate for patients being discharged after ambulatory surgical procedures.

Education is the passport to the future, for tomorrow belongs to those who prepare for it today.

–Malcolm X

OVERVIEW

Preparation for patient discharge after any surgical procedure begins in the surgeon's office at the time a determination is made that a patient is a candidate for a surgical procedure. This is when discharge planning and teaching commence. When patients are misled, misinformed, or ill-prepared for their course of recovery, discharge challenges occur.

More and more healthcare organizations are discharging patients home on the same day their surgical procedure takes place (same-day discharge). Free-standing ambulatory surgery centers (ASCs) are no longer the only facilities allowing same-day discharge, however. Large level I trauma centers perform surgeries for a mixture of patients, including inpatients, outpatients that are later admitted, and patients who are discharged on the same day as their surgery. Perianesthesia registered nurses, regardless of their work environment, require training in order to provide optimal patient education about discharge. Of course, safety is the number one priority. Surgical departments are constantly trying to achieve the greatest efficiency in the use of operating rooms, equipment, and time while also focusing on achieving the most positive outcomes. Comprehensive patient teaching is one factor that can increase efficiency. It begins preoperatively and is extremely important for patients who will be discharged home on the same day as surgery. Premature discharge may lead to poor outcomes, which may result in emergency department visits, as well as unplanned readmissions. A delayed discharge home causes inefficiencies in workflow and patient throughput and may lead to an unanticipated hospital admission or increased length of stay, both of which can result in increased costs for the healthcare organization and the patient.

Several factors are associated with a patient's surgical and anesthetic courses. The type and length of surgical procedures vary, as does the anesthetic plan. To safely discharge a patient home on the same day as surgery, the surgeon and anesthesiologist must develop a plan that best suits the patient's procedure and health status. Ideally, a multimodal anesthetic plan provides the quickest, safest recovery. A short-acting, rapid-onset and -offset, opioid-sparing anesthetic plan with minimal side effects provides patients with the pharmacokinetic traits required for a safe discharge to home. The perianesthesia nurse plays a large role in ensuring that the patient returns home safely and seamlessly. Institutional discharge policies and surgical and anesthesia order sets, as well as competency in perianesthesia nursing, including discharge teaching, are vital for successful patient and surgery center outcomes.

FACTS AND FIGURES

The Ambulatory Surgery Center Association offers patients, insurers, and providers access to an annual quality reporting program for ASCs. Of the more than 5400 ASCs in the United States, 96.9% of them collect data that are reported to the federal government. Two performance reporting programs allowing the public to compare ASCs online are the Centers for Medicare and Medicaid Services' Ambulatory Surgical Center Quality Reporting (ASCQR) program and the ASC Quality Collaboration (ASC QC) program. Both entities publish findings on ASCs, and they show that ASCs are extremely safe based on their low incidences of adverse events.[1] The ASCQR has been collecting ASC outcomes data since 2012, and as of 2018, it had reported on nine measures related to patient outcomes, safety, and satisfaction and facilities' quality and efficiency. The ASC QC focuses on developing processes to standardize ASC quality measures. Because reporting to it is voluntary, not all ASCs participate; however, as of 2017, 1484 ASCs from 49 states had supplied data for 11 distinct ASC performance measurements.[1]

FEDERAL AND INSTITUTIONAL DISCHARGE STANDARDS AND POLICIES

Successful patient discharge from an ASC is dependent on the patients' understanding of the discharge instructions and their commitment to compliance with them, as well as to the facility's discharge standards and policies. The federal government must approve all ASCs providing care for Medicare beneficiaries. In addition to federal requirements, state licensure is obtained through an onsite inspection process. The two most common accreditation organizations providing guidelines for ASCs are the American Association for Accreditation of Ambulatory Surgery Facilities and The Joint Commission.

Comprehensive protocols, guidelines, and policies developed by an interprofessional team at each ASC address the patient's readiness for discharge, as well as transportation home, and they assist the care team in making safe decisions. The patient's safety after receiving sedation or anesthesia is critical, which is why recommendations are made for a responsible individual to not only transport the patient home but to also remain with the patient for a predetermined period. Discharge criteria should be clearly specified in a facility's discharge policy. Objective markers lead to consistent practice decisions. These markers are easily audited to drive the practice to promote safe quality care based on evidence.

Discharge Scoring Tools

Although not required by regulatory agencies, discharge scoring tools provide a systematic scoring process for assessing whether a patient meets the appropriate criteria for discharge from each phase of recovery. The development and use of a discharge scoring tool avoids the need for nurses to make subjective decisions and ensures that patients meet the appropriate milestones based on evidence-based practice and research. Discharge scoring tools have been utilized since 1970 and include the Aldrete Score, Fast Track Pathway Tool, Post-anesthetic Discharge Scoring System, DASAIM Discharge Assessment Tool, and Modified Aldrete Score (Table 18.1). The American Society of PeriAnesthesia Nurses (ASPAN) recommends that perianesthesia nursing facilities utilize a postanesthesia scoring system when assessing patient readiness for discharge.[2]

Identifying a Responsible Individual Who Can Accompany the Patient Being Discharged

Definitions of a responsible individual, as well as professional society guidelines on this person, vary. Each institution is responsible for developing clearly defined guidelines as to the discharge requirements for patient escorts and care once patients are at home. The responsible individual should also be present during discharge teaching. Another variable is the amount of time a responsible adult should stay with a discharged ASC patient. The most common recommended time is 24 hours.

The U.S. population is aging . The elderly population having surgery has additional challenges related to multiple co-morbidities and complex medication regimes. ASC nurses have an obligation to assess not only the patient but the family and their socioeconomic status. Caring for a loved one postoperatively can be very stressful. Often, the caregiver is required to take time off from work and find alternative childcare, all of which may be emotionally and financially burdensome. Furthermore, older adults may not always have a loved one or responsible adult to care for them at home. These situations require alternative discharge planning. If

these situations are not properly identified in the surgeon's office prior to the day of surgery, they often lead to cancellations until a responsible adult and transportation are secured.

Discharge Instructions for Patient and Family

Discharge education and planning begin in the surgeon's office when a decision is agreed upon that surgery is going to be the choice of treatment. The education and planning continue during the preadmission testing visit, as well as during the preoperative phase on the day of surgery. The presence of a responsible adult in addition to the patient during discharge teaching and planning increases the success of the discharge process. Anxiety, stress, and anesthetic medications may cause patients to forget or ignore verbal instructions, and this is why giving instructions early to patients and families leads to improved outcomes.

The ASC nurse verbally reviews the written instructions prior to discharge with the patient and the responsible adult. The surgeon's orders, as well as information about new and continuing medications, are reviewed. Having a pharmacist available to provide medication education is ideal; however, this practice is more readily available in hospital-based surgery centers.

> **Evidence-Based Practice: Discharge Instructions**
> According to Strouse and Rosenberg, patients in the outpatient surgical setting are particularly vulnerable to postoperative complications unless they can demonstrate a strong understanding of the surgical process including self-care expectations. In addition, it is estimated that only 12% of individuals are proficient in health literacy and over one-third of ambulatory surgical patients have poor health literacy. Recommendations to maximize patient understanding include first and foremost, identifying barriers to learning. Fear? Pain? Feeling rushed? Drowsiness? Keeping educational content limited to only crucial information and providing the information using eye contact, common terminology, and active listening techniques. Always engage return demonstrations when appropriate.

Source: Strouse S, Rosenberg S. Health literacy and discharge education. *MedSurg Nursing*. 2022;31(6):402-404.

Enhanced Recovery After Surgery

Enhanced recovery after surgery (ERAS) programs have or should be part of all patients' surgical journeys. The key to

TABLE 18.1 Modified Aldrete Score

Category	Score = 0	Score = 1	Score = 2
Activity	Not moving extremities	Moves two extremities	Moves four extremities
Respiration	Apneic	Dyspnea or shallow breathing	Able to take a deep breath and cough freely
Circulation	Blood pressure 50 mm Hg of preanesthetic level	Blood pressure 20–50 mm Hg of preanesthetic level	Blood pressure 20 mm Hg of preanesthetic level
Consciousness	Not responding	Arousable on calling	Fully awake
O_2 saturation	O_2 Saturation less than 90% even with O_2 supplementation	Needs O_2 inhalation to maintain O_2 saturation greater than 90%	Able to maintain O_2 saturation greater than 92% on room air

The total score is 10, with patients scoring 9 or higher fit for discharge home.

From Chung F: Discharge criteria: A new trend. *Can J Anaesth*. 1995;42(11):1056–1058; and Schick L, Windle PE. *PeriAnesthesia Core Curriculum*. 4th ed. Elsevier, 2021. Table 14-5.

successful ERAS implementation is directly linked to leadership, as ERAS is a multidisciplinary approach to surgical patients' care. Audits, assessments, and continued education lead to a sustained and successful program. The ERAS protocols are based on evidence and research and are designed to standardize and streamline medical care. When followed appropriately, they expedite recovery, reduce confusion, improve perioperative pain, and reduce complications. Protocols are in place for the optimal use of parenteral analgesia, the best operative approach, the early planning for and implementation of an appropriate diet, the medically appropriate removal of lines and urinary catheters, and the planning for discharge. The earliest adopters of the ERAS protocol were the colorectal surgeons, with many other specialties following suit, including surgeons providing general surgical procedures, obstetrician–gynecologists, orthopedic surgeons, and neurospinal surgeons.[3] Chapter 19 provides more detail on ERAS principles.

PHASE I, PHASE II, AND THE EXTENDED CARE PHASE OF RECOVERY: BYPASSING OF PHASE I

Recovery stages in the postanesthesia care unit (PACU) coincide with the late phases of intraoperative care. Patients are emerging from the effects of anesthesia and are not considered fully recovered until they have returned to their baseline preoperative physiologic states. The overall process of returning to baseline may take several days and continue in the home. However, there are distinct phases of postanesthesia recovery in the ASC: Phase I, Phase II, and extended care. Some patients can bypass Phase I and go directly to Phase II from the operating room.

The nursing role in *Phase I postanesthesia care* is to provide basic life-sustaining care while patients emerge from anesthesia so they can transition to Phase II care.

The nursing role in *Phase II postanesthesia care* is to prepare and educate the patient and support person to make a safe transition home or to an extended care environment.

The nursing role in the *extended care phase* is to observe and provide interventions once the Phase I and Phase II discharge criteria are met. Patients often remain in extended care until the surgeon determines they are or are not safe to be discharged home. Sometimes the reason for extended care is to monitor postoperative pain or postoperative nausea and vomiting (PONV) to ensure that these issues are managed appropriately prior to discharge. ASCs have policies and procedures set up for determining the types of care required in this phase.

A common pathway to recovery in an ASC is the *bypassing of a patient*, not long ago referred to as the fast-tracking of a patient. A bypassed patient proceeds directly to Phase II from the operating room, thus bypassing Phase I. The clinical decision to bypass a patient is made as the patient emerges from anesthesia. If the patient meets the Phase I discharge criteria and is otherwise medically appropriate, the team (i.e., anesthesia provider, surgeon, operating room circulator, and perianesthesia registered nurse) may decide to have the patient bypass Phase I. The main benefits of this are a shorter patient recovery time, decreased costs, and increased productivity of the ASC.

CRITERIA FOR SAFE PATIENT DISCHARGE AND CLINICAL READINESS

As noted earlier, using discharge scoring tools and written discharge instructions can lead to a safe patient discharge from an ASC. According to the ASPAN, "a physician is responsible for the discharge of the patient from the postanesthesia care unit."[2] The facility's department of anesthesia and medical staff must generate and approve the discharge criteria utilized at each ASC. Ultimately, it is the responsibility of the physician, surgeon, and anesthesiologist to ensure that patients are sufficiently recovered to be safely discharged to go home. Therefore, sound, clear facility policies and procedures are needed to standardize care. If a patient is discharged prematurely, complications, readmissions, and possible legal ramifications may ensue.

Discharge criteria have historically included an assessment of the patient's vital signs and level of return to baseline mobility, how well pain is being controlled, and whether PONV is being managed. The patient's ability to tolerate oral liquids and to void are controversial criteria, and decisions about their importance depend on the individual physician. Once a patient meets the discharge criteria for a safe transfer to home, other benchmark goals must be reached for the patient to have a full recovery. The establishment of and education related to standardized discharge criteria are important. ASC nurses can give patients written and verbal instructions about their discharge plans. Some of the common factors in these plans are the signs and symptoms of which patients should be aware and the name and contact information of the person a patient should contact in case of an emergency.

Return to Baseline Vital Signs Following Surgery

Baseline vital signs are captured in several preprocedural areas, such as the surgeon's office, preadmission testing center, and patient's primary care office, and on the day of surgery in the preoperative area. Information on a patient's normal baseline vital signs is important when the nurse is evaluating the patient for discharge readiness. If the vital signs were obtained in the preoperative area on the day of surgery, the patient may have been anxious, and the signs recorded may not reflect the true baseline signs. Stable postanesthesia vital signs are often based on the systolic blood pressure and heart rate being within 20% of the patient's preanesthetic level. When evaluating the patient's readiness for discharge, the nurse needs to record the age-appropriateness of the patient's signs, the patient's co-morbidities, the type of anesthesia received, and the type of surgery completed, as well as the trends in vital signs recorded intraoperatively.

Vital sign assessments in both Phase I and Phase II are based on facility-specific guidelines and expert opinion. During Phase I, signs should be recorded every 5 to 15 minutes, and during Phase II, every 30 to 60 minutes. Expert recommendations are that signs be recorded, at a minimum, on arrival and at discharge from the ASC and also as clinically indicated during the patient's stay.[4] Clinical indications for additional monitoring may include signs of a rising temperature, persistently low oxygen saturation values, lingering hypotension, and other warnings of potential complications and decompensation.

Respiratory Status Following Surgery

In Phase I, the assessment of the airway patency, respiratory rate, and oxygen saturation is conducted with close attention to the monitoring of oxygenation and ventilation. Once patients meets Phase I discharge criteria, they are typically breathing room air. Patients with underlying pulmonary conditions who require supplemental oxygen at baseline meet discharge criteria when they are weaned back to their home oxygen requirements. Ultimately, a Phase II patient ready for discharge to home is no longer at risk for ventilatory depression.

Adults over 60 years of age who weigh over 100 kg are at an increased risk for oxygen desaturation. The most common airway emergency following anesthesia is related to the loss of pharyngeal muscle tone due to the effects of inhaled anesthetics, neuromuscular blockades, and opioid medications for treating pain. Perianesthesia nurses are trained to identify when a patient is attempting to breathe against an obstructed airway. Airway support treatments include a jaw thrust maneuver or continuous positive airway pressure. Once the airway obstruction has been treated and adequate ventilation ensured, the importance of identifying the cause is imperative. Other causes of upper airway obstruction following anesthesia are residual neuromuscular blockade, laryngospasm, airway edema, rising carbon dioxide levels, and obstructive sleep apnea syndrome. Patients who continue to exhibit a significant respiratory impairment should be evaluated for possible causes. These may include, but are not limited to, perioperative aspiration, pulmonary edema, pulmonary emboli, and intraoperative ventilation issues. Patients demonstrating respiratory failure no longer meet the criteria for discharge to home.

Baseline Mental Reorientation After Surgery

The patient's mental status, responsiveness, and orientation to surroundings are required elements of postanesthesia evaluations. To be ready for discharge, patients should have returned to the baseline orientation appropriate for their developmental and preoperative status. There are several circumstances that can prevent a patient from meeting these orientation milestones, such as postoperative delirium, postoperative cognitive dysfunction (POCD), emergence excitement, delayed awakening, and neurovascular injuries such as stroke. Older adult patients are at a higher risk of suffering from mental status alterations following anesthesia,[5] In addition, half of patients ages 65 and older have had at least one procedure in their lifetime requiring anesthesia.[5]

Postoperative delirium is not always an immediate finding during the postoperative assessment. Because it is an acute and fluctuating condition, it may not occur until patients have been home for a day or two. It is manifested by disorientation or a difficulty in remembering things. Symptoms can occur in Phase I or Phase II recovery and up until 5 days following a procedure. Any individual with ongoing memory loss or concentration concerns should relay those symptoms to the anesthesia provider prior to surgery. The anesthetic plan can be tailored to the specific needs of the patient to mediate postanesthesia mental status changes. Postoperative delirium has been linked to poor surgical outcomes, such as increased length of stay, functional decline, institutionalization, higher mortality rates, and increased costs.[6] Patient and family preparation related to the prevention of delirium includes information about orientation protocols, the benefits of early mobilization, the encouragement of a family presence, and the need to avoid polypharmacy.

Postoperative cognitive dysfunction (POCD) is a more serious condition and is also medically less understood. Long-term effects of POCD can include memory loss, difficulty retaining information, and a decreased ability to concentrate. Since these symptoms can often be present in elderly people prior to surgery, conducting a presurgical mental test is needed to determine if an underlying cognitive decline is present.

The American Society of Anesthesiologists organized a multidisciplinary group to address the special anesthetic needs and circumstances of those with or at risk of cognitive impairment, including those age 65 and older. The group's suggestions for limiting confusion in seniors following surgery are listed in Box 18.1.[6]

Emergence excitement is associated with a rapid wake up or emergence from inhaled anesthesia. It is more common in children than adults; however, emergence excitement occurs

---

BOX 18.1 Six Tips for Seniors to Help Limit Confusion After Surgery

1. Ask your physician to conduct a presurgery cognitive test, which is an assessment of your mental function. The physician can use the results as a baseline for comparison after surgery.
2. Be sure your caregiver, a family member, or a friend stays with you or can visit you as you recover, carefully observes your physical and mental activity after surgery, and reports anything troubling to your physician.
3. Check with your physician before taking medications after surgery that can affect your nervous system, such as those for anxiety, seizures, muscle spasms or those to aid with sleep.
4. If you wear hearing aids or glasses, ask that they be made available as soon as possible after the procedure.
5. Request a hospital room for recovery with a window, if possible, so you can tell whether it is day or night.
6. If you will be staying overnight in the hospital, pack a family photo, a clock, a calendar, or other familiar objects from home, to help you readjust.

American Society of Anesthesiologists. *Six Tips to Reduce Confusion in Older Patients After Surgery*. 2018, March. https://www.asahq.org/about-asa/newsroom/news-releases/2018/03/six-tips-to-reduce-confusion-in-older-patients-after-surgery

---

in approximately 3% of adults.[7] The occurrence is typically within the first 10 to 15 minutes of recovery. There are several sedation–agitation scales, such as the Riker Sedation–Agitation Scale (Table 18.2), Richmond Agitation–Sedation Scale, Motor Activity Assessment Scale, and New Sheffield Sedation Scale. Medical emergencies can arise during emergence excitement episodes because patients may attempt self-extubation or the removal of arterial and venous access devices or may injure themselves or others. Death is also a possibility. The most common risk factors have been identified as preoperative medication with benzodiazepines, breast procedures, abdominal surgeries, and long surgical procedures.[7]

Delayed awakening occurs when a patient lacks responsiveness after surgery. If after 60 to 90 minutes a patient is not responding to stimuli, determining an underlying cause is emergent. Common causes are residual drug effects, underlying disease, and metabolic disturbances, such as hypothermia, electrolyte imbalances, and hyperglycemia or hypoglycemia.[8] The airway, breathing, and circulation should be assessed, as well as the temperature. If a residual medication effect is suspected, appropriate reversal agents should be initiated. If none of the above causes is determined, ruling out a cerebrovascular accident is appropriate.

PHYSICAL CONSIDERATIONS FOLLOWING SURGERY
Bleeding and Drainage After Surgery

Each surgical procedure has a different level of acceptable drainage, whether it is of blood, serosanguineous fluid, urine, or another bodily fluid. The expertise of the Phase II nurse is important in dealing with drainage issues. Knowing how to evaluate the surgical site based on the type of surgery done and understanding the surgeon's expectations for patient recovery are crucial. Evaluation of the patient's surgical site prior to discharge is expected. The condition of the dressing, cast, or drain is documented by the nurse in the electronic medical record. Any condition other than what is expected for the type of surgery must be discussed with the surgeon and anesthesia provider so that the patient can be reevaluated prior to discharge home. Unintended surgical bleeding can lead to

TABLE 18.2 Riker Sedation–Agitation Scale

Score	Description	Definition
7	Dangerously agitated	Pulls at endotracheal tube; tries to remove catheters; climbs over bed rail; strikes at staff; thrashes side to side
6	Very agitated	Does not calm despite frequent verbal reminding of limits; requires physical restraints; bites endotracheal tube
5	Agitated	Anxious or mildly agitated; attempts to sit up; calms down to verbal instructions
4	Calm and cooperative	Calm; awakens easily; follows commands
3	Sedated	Difficult to arouse; awakens to verbal stimuli or gentle shaking but drifts off again; follows simple commands
2	Very sedated	Arouses to physical stimuli but does not communicate or follow commands; may move spontaneously
1	Unarousable	Minimal or no response to noxious stimuli; does not communicate or follow commands

Urden LD, Stacy KM, Lough ME. *Critical Care Nursing.* 7th ed. Elsevier, 2014. Page 171.

vascular compromise, hemodynamic instability, the formation of hematomas, and, potentially, wound dehiscence.

Circulation in the Extremities After Surgery

Surgical interventions that require a cast, an encircling dressing, or a splint postoperatively necessitate a thorough circulatory assessment to ensure the apparatus is not too tight and is preventing the appropriate circulation. Pulse checks, sensation evaluations, and mobility checks to investigate the neurovascular and skin integrity are done frequently throughout the discharge process and at discharge. Comparing the operative with the nonoperative extremity is valuable for identifying compromised circulation. The use of Doppler ultrasound when palpable pulses are difficult to assess is an alternative method for ascertaining the blood flow through the vessels. Using a skin marker to signify where the blood flow is detected is a good practice for reassessments during recovery. Extremities that required a tourniquet during surgery also need postoperative assessment to ensure proper blood flow has returned. Information related to tourniquet use should be relayed during handoff from the operating room team to the perianesthesia nurse. Preoperative teaching related to good glucose control, as well as smoking cessation, can be reinforced to support optimal circulation outcomes.

Pain After Surgery

A patient who has acute pain as a result of ambulatory surgery may have an extended recovery or even an unplanned hospital admission. Multimodal analgesia is both patient- and procedure-specific, with the goal of promoting pain management and making the patient comfortable. It utilizes a combination of medications from various drug classes, such as nonsteroidal antiinflammatory drugs (NSAIDs), local anesthetics, nonopioid analgesics, and alpha-2 antagonists. ASCs are transitioning to this multimodal approach to pain management in response to the opioid epidemic, to improve patient outcomes and satisfaction, as well as to achieve optimal pain control and comfort.[9]

Postoperative complications related to pain have been significantly reduced since the initiation of multimodal analgesia and ERAS protocols. However, pain management after surgery may still be problematic. Opioids continue to be prescribed and used regardless of their adverse effects (e.g., nausea, vomiting, sedation, constipation, respiratory depression, pruritis, opioid-induced hyperalgesia, misuse, and addiction).[9] The use of local and regional anesthesia in single-injection or extended-release formulations assists in reducing adverse opioid-related effects, as well as promotes improved pain control postoperatively.

Management of acute postoperative pain is most effective when open communications between surgeon and patient related to postoperative discomfort and expectations take place. These discussions begin in the surgeon's office and continue throughout the preadmission testing visit and on the day of surgery. Prior knowledge of the patient's pain tolerance assists the surgeon, anesthesia provider, and perianesthesia nurse in providing the best pain management. Use of a pain scale, such as a numerical rating scale, visual analog scale, or categorical scale, assist the provider in determining the patient's level and tolerance of pain.

Nausea and Vomiting After Surgery

Postoperative nausea and vomiting (PONV) and postdischarge nausea and vomiting continue to be common adverse effects of anesthetic agents. In ASCs, the rate of PONV has been reported to be between 30% and 50%.[10] The agents most likely to produce such side effects are the inhalational anesthetics, although other anesthetic and nonanesthetic factors are also contributors. Consequences of PONV may lead to delayed discharge, unexpected hospital admissions, pulmonary aspiration, and increased costs. The most effective way of preventing PONV is to identify risk factors for it preoperatively during the patient evaluation and to treat them prophylactically. The following factors should be considered during the preoperative evaluation as they are identified risk factors: female gender, history of PONV or motion sickness, nonsmoker, duration of anesthesia, use of opioids, and type of surgery (Table 18.3). Treatment for PONV may take place in all phases of the procedure, whether preoperative, intraoperative, or postoperative. Prophylactic treatment for PONV involves modifying the course of anesthesia with the addition of pharmacologic and nonpharmacologic interventions. The brain

TABLE 18.3 Likelihood of Developing PONV

Risk Factors	Percentage of Likelihood
No risk factors	10%
1 Risk factor	20%
2 Risk factors	40%
3 Risk factors	60%
4 Risk factors	80%

Adapted from Gan TJ, Belani KG, Bergese S, et al. Fourth consensus guidelines for the management of postoperative nausea and vomiting. *Anesth Analg.* 2020;131(2):411–448. Figure 5.

has several receptors associated with PONV, and when activated, these receptors cause nausea or emesis, or both (i.e., dopamine receptor type 2, serotonin type 3 receptor, histamine type 1 receptor, and muscarinic acetylcholine receptor type 1).[10] Pharmacologic agents that block these receptors include transdermal scopolamine, droperidol, promethazine, prochlorperazine, ondansetron, dolasetron, granisetron, and dexamethasone. Depending on the patient's risk factors, one or a combination of the agents may be used. Additional treatment for prophylaxis includes adequate hydration with IV fluids, the prevention of hypotension, and the ensuring of effective analgesia, similar to the ERAS anesthetic technique.[10]

Patients at risk of PONV are in jeopardy of pulmonary aspiration if emesis ensues, as well as potential wound dehiscence and increased pain and discomfort. Prophylactic treatment does not always prevent PONV. In these cases, a rescue treatment is initiated. An important fact to remember when treating patients for PONV in the postoperative area is that giving the patient more of the same class of drug when one drug in that class has not been effective does not help. For instance, if ondansetron 4 mg was given for PONV and proved to be ineffective, another dose of ondansetron or another drug in the same class will most likely not reap any benefits. Giving dosages from the same class within a 6-hour period is not recommended. The medications scopolamine, aprepitant, and dexamethasone should never be redosed.[11] It should be noted that aprepitant reduces the effectiveness of hormonal contraceptives and hormonal therapies for 28 days. Patients who receive aprepitant during their surgical course should be given verbal and written instructions from the Phase II nurse regarding alternative birth control methods prior to discharge from the facility.[12]

Oral Intake After Surgery

Discharging a patient to home who is actively vomiting is unacceptable; however, the necessity for a patient to tolerate oral intake postoperatively is controversial. Studies have determined no significant differences in the recovery of adults who were required to drink and tolerate fluids prior to discharge from an ASC and of adults who were not so required.[13] Therefore, it is not necessary to require that patients drink fluids at this time, although ensuring that patients are properly hydrated is imperative. In some ASCs, oral fluid intake is no longer mandated for adult patients. Mandated oral intake may be linked to PONV and lead to a longer postoperative stay. Another benefit of the ERAS protocols is a decrease in postoperative dehydration due to the preoperative allowance of oral fluids and the shortening of time in which patients are not allowed to ingest anything orally before surgery.

Voiding After Surgery

Voiding prior to discharge after surgery is another topic of controversy. Often, waiting for a patient to void leads to a delayed discharge. Current evidence supports a safe discharge to home without voiding for patients who do not have risk factors for postoperative urinary retention. A thorough preoperative evaluation should help identify risk factors for postoperative urinary retention, including a history of urinary retention, pelvic or urologic surgery, spinal or epidural anesthesia, and perioperative catheterization, either with a straight catheter or an indwelling catheter. When urinary retention is suspected, a bladder scan is performed by the perianesthesia nurse. Urinary retention is most commonly defined as the inability to void for 30 minutes or more and having a bladder volume of 600 mL or greater. Studies have indicated that male patients who are 50 years of age and older, patients with instillation of more

than 750 mL of intraoperative IV fluids, and a bladder volume of more than 270 mL when leaving the operating room have been significant risk factors for postoperative urinary retention.[14] High-risk patients may still be discharged home prior to voiding. This is most successful when at-home catheterization is taught and a follow-up visit is scheduled soon after discharge to home. Indwelling catheter care and straight catheter instruction are routinely delivered by the Phase II nurse via verbal and written instructions as well as teach-back methods.

Ambulation Following Surgery

Early ambulation postoperatively leads to improved patient outcomes. Not only is early ambulation cost-effective but mobilization also improves patient outcomes both physically and psychologically. ASC nurses are expected to educate patients about ambulation. The most appropriate and efficient approach is to work in collaboration with a physical therapist.

The return to baseline ambulation is dependent on the type of surgery, as some patients may be discharged home with assistive devices. ASC nurses have a responsibility to assess the patient's and family members' comprehension and ability to utilize the devices. This is done through teaching and demonstration. Ensuring the patients are able to safely use their assistive devices is imperative.

MANAGING PROBLEMATIC RESPONSES TO ANESTHESIA DURING AND AFTER SURGERY

Malignant Hyperthermia

Malignant hyperthermia (MH) is a genetic condition that predisposes individuals to a hypermetabolic reaction to volatile anesthetic agents or the depolarizing neuromuscular blocking agent succinylcholine. A patient in a fulminant MH crisis exhibits the following symptoms: increased end-tidal carbon dioxide, increased heart rate, muscle rigidity, and fever. These symptoms can lead to muscle breakdown, an altered body chemistry, and increased blood acid levels. Ultimately, cardiac arrest, brain damage, internal bleeding, organ failure, and death can result. Because MH is a potentially fatal condition, research on it is limited due to ethical considerations and because the disorder is so rare. Only 700 cases are reported in the United States annually.[15]

Individuals who might develop MH have either experienced a previous MH crisis, have a blood relative with a history of MH, or have had a positive result of the genetic test for MH or a muscle biopsy for a caffeine–halothane contracture test. Genetic testing determines if the patient is predisposed to MH, and the muscle biopsy determines the patient's susceptibility to it. Patients with a known susceptibility to MH can be safely scheduled for surgery at an ASC. An anesthesia assessment to review the patient's MH history and susceptibility is step one. On the day of surgery, the anesthesia workstation is prepared by replacing vaporizers and flushing circuits. Trigger-free anesthesia is planned. This may involve regional anesthesia and/or total IV anesthesia.

Problematic Responses to Regional Anesthesia

Regional anesthesia is a common anesthetic technique used in ASCs. Use of multimodal anesthesia includes regional anesthesia in conjunction with general anesthesia or procedural sedation. Regional anesthesia is similar to local anesthesia, which blocks sensation to small areas of the body, except that regional anesthesia numbs larger body areas. Types of regional anesthesia include spinal blocks, epidurals, and peripheral nerve blocks. Spinal blocks and epidurals provide numbness from the waist down. For a spinal block, the anesthetic agent is injected directly into the dural sac as a single injection, whereas in an epidural, the agent is injected into the epidural space and may be connected to an infusion pump. Spinal blocks are used for lower body surgeries to include genital, urinary tract, and lower extremity orthopedic cases. Epidurals are most commonly used during labor and delivery, although they may be used for continuous analgesia after lower body procedures such as hysterectomies. Both spinal and epidural anesthesia may reduce the need to intubate patients, as well as offer a recovery with fewer complications than general anesthesia and opioid use. Single-injection methods are more common in ASCs, as these patients are being discharged home and require a return of sensation for ambulation.

Peripheral nerve blocks involve a local anesthetic medication that is injected through a needle or catheter in either a single injection or via a catheter. A single-injection nerve block is a one-time injection of an anesthetic agent around the nerve bundle. These injections can have a numbing effect for 3 to 24 hours depending on the type of agent used. The effects of newer liposomal preparations of anesthetic agents can actually last up to 96 hours. For more involved surgeries needing longer periods of analgesia, a catheter is placed alongside the nerve. The catheter may be attached to an infusion pump that has a basal rate or self-dosing option, or both. Peripheral nerve blocks are most commonly used for the arms, legs, and abdomen, but they may also be used for breast, ophthalmologic, and oral surgeries. As a note, surgical oncologists have been advocating for regional anesthesia use because it is associated with a reduced recurrence of cancer. Both the adrenergic and inflammatory responses to surgery are diminished with the use of regional anesthesia, as opposed to general anesthesia. Postoperative oncology patients have displayed a preserved immunity in response to local anesthetics and the reduction of opioid use.[16]

Patients who receive a peripheral nerve block are always required to regain sensation prior to discharge home. Anesthetization of a body part means that postoperative pain is reduced; however, the area requires protection. For instance, an interscalene nerve block may be performed to treat postoperative pain for arthroscopic shoulder surgery. The patient is discharged home with a sling, and the ASC nurse gives verbal and written instructions on how to protect the limb. Patients may also be discharged home with devices that continuously infuse the numbing agent, often referred to as pain pumps. The ASC nurse instructs the patient and family member about the device's functionality and the side effects of the medication. Patients discharged home with a blocked body part should be given a contact phone number to report any concerns or for emergency needs.

Local anesthetic systemic toxicity (LAST) is extremely rare yet life-threatening. LAST occurs when the local anesthetic is inadvertently injected intravenously and circulates systemically. The prodromal signs and symptoms include perioral numbness, tinnitus, and agitation. The symptoms can progress to more extensive central nervous system effects, causing seizures or a coma. The treatment for LAST is seizure management, advanced cardiac lifesaving techniques, and IV 20% lipid emulsion. Nursing education, annual competencies, and mock codes to respond to a LAST situation are proven methods to ensure that perianesthesia nurses are able to identify symptoms and react accordingly.

THE DISCHARGE PLAN

The discharge plan for each patient is generated by the surgeon and staff at the surgeon's office, sometimes with the help of the primary care physician and staff, and by the ASC staff on the day of the procedure. It is based on their knowledge of the patient's physical and mental status, the procedure the patient will be having, any risks or specific needs of the patient, and any issues that arise on the day of surgery. Even a patient's socioeconomic and cultural factors might be part of the plan if they will affect the patient's discharge and recovery at home. Impairments in vision, hearing, and ambulation may need to be addressed. A written or digital copy of the plan should accompany the patient from physician's office to surgery center operating room to PACU to home. Adjustments made along the way should be clearly noted.

On the day of surgery, once the patient has been assessed by the perianesthesia nurse and the nurse has validated that the patient is hemodynamically stable and alert, has tolerable pain and nausea, and has sensory and motor controls that have returned to baseline, the plan for discharge can be implemented.

Planning for Transportation After Discharge

Identifying and ensuring that an ambulatory surgery patient has a reliable and safe mode of transportation home, as well as a support system and plan in place for postoperative care, are the responsibilities of the surgeon, anesthesia provider, preadmission testing nurse, perianesthesia nurse, and patient. Patients are unable to safely drive themselves or take public transportation alone due to the medications received and procedure performed. It is essential that the perianesthesia nurse ensure that the patient's responsible driver is sober and able to safely transport the patient to her or his home.

Preoperatively, failure to identify patient transportation needs when going both to and from the procedure may lead to a canceled or rescheduled procedure. Identifying the need postoperatively leads to added stress on the perianesthesia nurse, a delayed discharge, and added costs. If a responsible ride cannot be secured to take the patient home, an inpatient stay may be warranted. In these instances, the hospital incurs additional fees, and many of these costs are shifted to the patient. Various vendors across the nation are now offering transportation in which a healthcare professional accompanies patients being discharged home after surgery. Some even offer in-home care for assistance in recovery. Self-pay and insurance coverage are accepted.

DISCHARGE INSTRUCTIONS FOR THE PATIENT AND FAMILY

Preventing a hospital admission after discharge after surgery is a priority. The prevention success rate is dependent on the patient's and caregivers' understanding and ability to follow the discharge instructions. The perianesthesia nurse is responsible for assessing the patient and family to develop a patient- and family-centered plan for safe discharge to home. Assessing and preparing a 25-year-old for discharge to home may require a different approach than assessing and preparing an 85-year-old. Age-appropriate and patient-appropriate teaching promotes a successful discharge to home by identifying the learning style of, stimulating the interest of, considering the limitations and strengths of, and involving the family of the patient. Delivering the instructions in a quiet, stimulation-free area may lead to better concentration and retention. Research has shown that the more skilled the perianesthesia nurse is in providing postoperative instructions, the more confident patients are in caring for themselves after surgery.[17] Patients often bypass Phase I and therefore have a speedier recovery and discharge. However, the perianesthesia nurse is responsible for being aware of and instructing patients on potential problems, such as pain, nausea, and bleeding. Utilizing the teach-back method remains the most effective way of ensuring that the patient and family member understand the expectations associated with the postoperative recovery plan.[18] Open-ended questions and return demonstrations require the patient and family member to verify their understanding of the instructions and actions that were just explained to them. Ultimately, the goal is for a safe discharge to home with a safe journey to a full recovery.

Verbal, Written, and Digital Instructions

Patient teaching formats are changing as technology advances. Written and verbal instructions at the Phase II level of care are commonplace, but the use of technology may be implemented as a backup feature. Whether the online or multimedia video or audio instructions are created by the ASC staff or purchased from an outside vendor, they enhance direct interpersonal interactions. Patients may be sent videos via email or may receive a phone call with recorded instructions once they are home and recovering. Newer digital applications have been designed to provide patients with reminders of many important postoperative activities, such as moving about, doing deep breathing, taking medications, and attending postoperative appointments. Instructions, including charts and diagrams, may also be uploaded to the patient's electronic health record, allowing for access to these instructions whenever needed.

Documentation That Instructions Have Been Given

Once the Phase II perianesthesia nurse has provided the patient and family with discharge instructions, documentation is completed in the patient's electronic health record. The documentation includes the patient's and family's readiness and ability to comprehend the instructions, any barriers to learning, and how the barriers were addressed, as well as which documents and additional instruction forms were sent home with the patient.

The documentation includes the nurse's assessment of the patient's physical and mental status, a copy of the patient's discharge plan, and a copy of the discharge instructions. Aspects to document include who received the instructions, how the instructions were received, and how well the patient and family member understood the instructions. The identity of the responsible individual who transported the patient and will be caring for the patient at home is added. Copies of the medication reconciliation and any additional teaching forms are given to the patient and family member once they have been signed by the responsible adult. The signed original copies are retained for the electronic medical record. There are situations in which the person transporting the patient home is not the person responsible for assuming care for the patient at home. In these instances, the discharge instructions can be communicated over the phone by the nurse to the caregiver. Documentation of this in the electronic medical record is imperative.

Timing of Discharge Instructions

As was stated earlier in the chapter, "postoperative" teaching should begin in the surgeon's office, continue during the preadmission testing process, and go on throughout the day of surgery. The surgeon's office and office for preadmission testing are ideal settings for education because in these settings, the patient is relatively relaxed and has not yet been exposed to anesthetic agents that might cloud the memory. These appointments prior to the day of surgery give healthcare providers an opportunity to address any special needs. For example, the patient may need an interpreter, crutch training,

or arrangements for transportation home from the ASC, all of which can be prepared for preoperatively. Patients can be given written and verbal instructions about the procedure and recovery and allowed to ask open-ended questions. If the family member who will be the at-home caregiver during recovery can accompany the patient to the appointments, this is advantageous, as education is more successful when the patient and family member have received the same information before the procedure. On the day of surgery, the Phase II nurse should simply be reevaluating the knowledge and understanding of the patient and family member, not performing the initial teaching. When obstacles are initially identified on the day of surgery, the perianesthesia nurse absorbs the responsibility for them in terms of providing solutions, and this leads to decreased patient satisfaction, poor efficiency, increased costs, and a possible hospital admission.

Topics Covered in Discharge Instructions

Discharge instructions are provided to the patient and family member on how to continue postoperative care once in the home. General instructions are included relating to anesthesia precautions, and instructions related to the specific surgical procedure are also noted. Ways of identifying postoperative complications are described, contact information is given on whom to notify about complications, and steps for what to do in case of an emergency are outlined.

General Topics

A patient and family member can expect a similar discharge experience at ASCs across the nation. The physician is responsible for discharging the patient after surgery. The perianesthesia nurse utilizes discharge criteria developed by the facility, as well as nursing skills, to determine a patient's readiness for home. The ultimate goal is to discharge all patients safely with an understanding of their continued recovery once at home.

Activity, diet, medication, and hygiene are standard items for postoperative discharge instructions. *Activity levels* are specific for each patient and procedure. Early ambulation leads to improved patient outcomes. Stimulation of the cardiovascular system provides oxygen to cells to promote healing and circulation. Encouraging ambulation is an important component of postoperative teaching. Patients may experience discomfort, and perianesthesia nurses are competent in explaining the difference between excessive physical activity and a lack of physical activity. Patients should be encouraged to stand and walk every hour, sit at the table for meals, and intermittently change positions. These activities, along with deep breathing, encourage circulation and oxygenation throughout the body and reduce the incidence of deep vein thrombi. Some patients may have activity limitations preoperatively or postoperatively due to the surgical procedure. For example, patients who are discharged home and have a non–weight-bearing status are given detailed instructions by the physician as to the patient's limitations and expected course of recovery.

Patients may inquire about sexual activity. Unless contraindicated due to the surgical procedure, most patients can resume sexual activity. If the procedure was urologic or gynecologic, the physician may provide specific instructions related to sexual intercourse postoperatively. Ideally, the patient received this information from the surgeon when scheduling the surgery or during the preadmission testing visit.

Returning to a *normal diet* postoperatively is common. Guidance on what to eat and how to advance slowly is a conversation had with the patient prior to discharge home. Both the perianesthesia nurse and the anesthesia provider may engage in this conversation. Postoperative patients do best when they start by tolerating fluids and slowly advance to solids. Starting with a light meal is advisable. Eating heavy foods, such as fried or greasy foods, as well as dairy products, may lead to episodes of nausea and vomiting. Most importantly, adequate hydration enhances postoperative recovery.

A medication reconciliation is performed at the preadmission testing visit to determine which *medications* to continue and which to stop prior to surgery. During the day of the surgery preoperative assessment, the perianesthesia nurse reviews the patient's medication list, which includes each medication and its dosage, as well as the time when each medication was last taken. If certain medications, such as anticoagulants or beta blockers, were not taken correctly, the surgeon and anesthesiologist are informed by the preoperative nurse and a decision whether to perform surgery or to cancel is made. Challenges occur when the medication reconciliation is not properly completed throughout the continuum of care. Some ASCs utilize pharmacists to review the preoperative patient's medication list prior to surgery to ensure medications and dosages are correct and appropriate. This offers a safe, high-quality process for discharging ASC patients home, especially when new prescription medications are added to their regimen.[19]

During the postoperative phase, the perianesthesia nurse reviews the patient's medications once again, to include those the patient is already taking and those prescribed by the surgeon. If the patient is being discharged home with new medications, education on the use and side effects is reviewed with the patient and family member by the nurse or pharmacist. If the patient is being discharged home with an opioid prescription, the patient should be taught about the risk of constipation and how to prevent it, as well as how to dispose of the medication if any remains. Studies have indicated that due to ERAS protocols and multimodal anesthetic techniques, fewer opioids are being administered during operative procedures, as well as fewer being prescribed for home. Despite this, opioids remain the analgesic of choice for postoperative pain. Patients and their family members should be given information related to the opioid epidemic to include where the closest take-back or dropbox is for the safe disposal of unneeded opioids.[20]

Bathing and *hygiene* postoperatively can often be difficult for postoperative patients. Bandages, crutches, casts, and other apparatuses make showering and bathing challenging. Preoperatively, medical assistive devices may have been prescribed to aid in entering a shower or covering a cast. Patients do not always bring these devices with them the day of surgery. The perianesthesia nurse should inquire about durable medical equipment, as well as offer instruction on its use. Postoperatively, bacteria-proof dressings allow the patient to shower immediately because they provide a protective barrier. Perianesthesia nurses cannot always visually distinguish between waterproof and non-waterproof dressings. The type of dressing is communicated during handoff from the operating room team. Discharge orders related to bathing should be entered by the physician. Other surgical procedures that may pose bathing challenges are gynecologic procedures. Tub bathing is usually prohibited for a period of time. Sponge bathing may be safest for those being discharged home with splints and casts. The need to keep bandages dry is vital and can be challenging when attempting to balance on crutches or keep an upper extremity in a sling.

Topics for Specific Procedures

In addition to the general discharge instructions, each procedure has varying guidelines and potential complications. The guidelines may address incisional care, what to do about bleeding or drainage, how to position the patient, and which activities should be limited. Some incisions are covered with a dressing, and others may be adhered with surgical glue and remain open to air. Any surgical procedures may result in postoperative bleeding. Some patients may be discharged home with a drain that requires emptying and the recording of the discharge. Discomfort in orthopedic patients may be reduced and temporarily eased by sleeping in a recliner. Ophthalmology patients may be required to wear sunglasses and remain out of direct sunlight. Each procedure is unique, as is each patient. The skills and knowledge of the perianesthesia nurse, as well as a team approach to the patient's postoperative care, lead to improved patient satisfaction and outcomes. Reducing surgical site infections and other postoperative complications is dependent on the care team's ability to teach the patient and family member the proper care, as well as the patient's and family members' commitment to carrying out the instructions.

Precautions Related to Types of Anesthesia

Anesthesia techniques vary based on the surgical procedure, the patient, and the physician preference. The technique used may have postoperative effects that need to be addressed in the discharge instructions. Even multimodal anesthesia may require postoperative precautions. *General anesthesia* may cause side effects such as dizziness, memory loss, PONV, shivering, or sore throat. *Regional anesthesia* blocks sensation to a body part. Although the sensation is blocked for analgesia, the motor function may be impacted. Care must be taken to protect the limb from injury, such as keeping a blocked upper extremity protected in a sling. Patients who received spinal anesthesia are instructed to be aware of postdural puncture headache, as well as how and where to seek treatment for symptoms.

HOSPITAL ADMISSIONS OF AMBULATORY SURGERY CENTER PATIENTS
Unanticipated Hospital Admissions

An unanticipated hospital admission may occur if a patient exhibits uncontrolled pain, persistent PONV, or bleeding or drainage in excess, or if the surgeon requests admission for additional monitoring. To reduce the number of ASC-related unanticipated hospital admissions, the team makes efforts to ensure that patients are properly optimized for surgery. In addition, appropriate selection criteria for the outpatient setting should be applied, and confirmation that the patient has the appropriate caregivers to provide transport and support at home is crucial to the success of outpatient care.

Plans for Unplanned Hospital Admissions

In many states, each ASC is required to have a written transfer agreement with a receiving hospital. If the ASC does not have a written agreement, then the surgeon must have admitting privileges at an inpatient hospital in order to transfer an ASC patient to that hospital. Policies and procedures must be in place for the transfer of electronic and written medical records, as well as for patient transportation to the hospital. In emergency cases, the ASC should have emergency protocols in place that define the process of responding to critical events, including calling 9-1-1 and stabilizing the patient until help arrives.

DISCHARGE AGAINST MEDICAL ADVICE

An unfortunate and often dangerous occurrence is when a patient is discharged against medical advice (AMA). As much as healthcare providers want to provide proper treatment for all patients, sometimes a patient is unwilling to accept or comply with the policies and protocols regarding discharge postoperatively. The most common occurrence is related to a lack of a responsible individual to transport the patient home or to help care for the patient for a determined amount of time. When a patient leaves AMA, the care team may feel distress due to an inability to fully understand why the patient left and a concern for adverse outcomes due to care being abruptly stopped. Adult patients have a legal right to refuse medical care. Restraining or preventing a patient from leaving a facility may be and can be considered battery. Thorough and detailed documentation of the situation, including the risks of leaving AMA as discussed with the patient, must be recorded in the record.

CHAPTER HIGHLIGHTS

- Patient preparation for discharge following outpatient surgery is of the upmost importance.
- Ensuring that ambulatory surgical patients are discharged home to a safe environment with the appropriate instructions leads to the patient's full recovery.
- The perianesthesia nurse must have knowledge of the potential impact of anesthesia, as well as the actual surgery, to best prepare the patient and family for discharge to home.
- Protocols to address unplanned events and situations must be in place per facility oversight.

CASE 18.1

Harold is an 80-year-old widower who lives alone. His children live locally and check on him frequently, but Harold is stubborn and demands his independence. He is scheduled for a left cataract replacement in the local ASC. Due to a history of a traumatic brain injury, hypertension, and diabetes, his home care is complicated. His home medications include dilantin, phenobarbital, lisinopril, daily aspirin, and metformin. This case presents multiple challenges for the perianesthesia nurse who is preparing the patient's chart for surgery. The following questions have come to mind:

- What is the capacity of Harold to learn due to the nature of his brain injury? What is the best method for preoperative teaching?
- Despite cataract surgery being minimally invasive, due to Harold's age and living status, what resources does he need for immediate home care? Will his family be willing to intervene and provide home support? How is food preparation done now, and how will it be supplemented during his initial recovery?
- Given his current medication practice at home, are there any medications that Harold should be advised to stop?
- Would Harold benefit from a preoperative home study?
- Would Harold benefit from the services of a care navigator or a social worker?

REFERENCES

1. Ambulatory Surgery Center Association. *ASC Quality Reporting.* Available at: https://www.ascassociation.org/advancingsurgicalcare/safetyquality/ascqualityreporting. Accessed July 27, 2021.
2. American Society of PeriAnesthesia Nurses. *2021-2022 PeriAnesthesia Nursing Standards, Practice Recommendations and Interpretive Statements.* ASPAN; 2020.
3. Crosson JA. Enhanced recovery after surgery—the importance of the perianesthesia nurse on program success. *J Perianesth Nurs.* 2018;33(4):366-374. Available at: http://doi.org/10.1097/ALN.0b013e31823c1067.
4. Apfelbaum JL, Silverstein JH, Chung FF, et al. Practice guidelines for postanesthetic care: an updated report by the American Society of Anesthesiologists Task Force on Postanesthetic Care. *Anesthesiology.* 2013;118(2):291-307. Available at: https://doi.org/10.1097/ALN.0b013e31827773e9.
5. Janjua MS, Spurling BC, Arthur ME. Postoperative delirium. Updated May 15, 2022. In: *StatPearls.* StatPearls Publishing; 2021. Available at: https://www.ncbi.nlm.nih.gov/books/NBK534831/.
6. American Society of Anesthesiologists. *Six Tips to Reduce Confusion in Older Patients After Surgery.* March 18, 2018. Available at: https://www.asahq.org/about-asa/newsroom/news-releases/2018/03/six-tips-to-reduce-confusion-in-older-patients-after-surgery.
7. Lepousé C, Lautner CA, Liu L, Gomis P, Leon A. Emergence delirium in adults in the post-anaesthesia care unit. *Br J Anaesth.* 2006;96(6):747-753. Available at: https://doi.org/10.1093/bja/ael094.
8. Misal US, Joshi SA, Shaikh MM. Delayed recovery from anesthesia: a postgraduate education review. *Anesth Essays Res.* 2016;10(2):164-172. Available at: https://doi.org/10.4103/0259-1162.165506.
9. Barker JC, Joshi GP, Janis JE. Basics and best practices of multimodal pain management for the plastic surgeon. *Plast Reconstr Surg Glob Open.* 2020;8(5):e2833. Available at: https://doi.org/10.1097/gox.0000000000002833.
10. Golembiewski J, Chernin E, Chopra T. Prevention and treatment of postoperative nausea and vomiting. *Am J Health Syst Pharm.* 2005;62(12):1247-1260. Available at: https://doi.org/10.1093/ajhp/62.12.1247.
11. Gan TJ, Belani KG, Bergese S, et al. Fourth consensus guidelines for the management of postoperative nausea and vomiting. *Anesth Analg.* 2020;131(2):411-448. Available at: https://doi.org/10.1213/ane.0000000000004833.
12. Kanaparthi A, Kukura S, Slenkovich N, et al. Perioperative administration of Emend® (aprepitant) at a tertiary care children's hospital: a 12-month survey. *Clin Pharmacol.* 2019;11:155-160. Available at: https://doi.org/10.2147/cpaa.s221736.
13. Jin F, Norris A, Chung F, Ganeshram T. Should adult patients drink fluids before discharge from ambulatory surgery? *Anesth Analg.* 1998;87(2):306-311. Available at: https://doi.org/10.1097/00000539-199808000-00013.
14. Rosseland LA, Stubhaug A, Breivik H. Detecting postoperative urinary retention with an ultrasound scanner. *Acta Anaesthesiol Scand.* 2002;46(3):279-282. Available at: https://doi.org/10.1034/j.1399-6576.2002.t01-1-460309.x.
15. Rüffert H, Bastian B, Bendixen D, et al. Consensus guidelines on perioperative management of malignant hyperthermia suspected or susceptible patients from the European Malignant Hyperthermia Group. *Br J Anaesth.* 2021;126(1):120-130. Available at: https://doi.org/10.1016/j.bja.2020.09.029.
16. Wu Z, Wang Y. Development of guidance techniques for regional anesthesia: past, present and future. *J Pain Res.* 2021;14:1631-1641. Available at: https://doi.org/10.2147/jpr.s316743.
17. Berardinelli A, Bernhofer EI. Postsurgical follow-up phone calls: worth the investment? *J Perianesth Nurs.* 2020;35(6):665-670. Available at: https://doi.org/10.1016/j.jopan.2020.03.014.
18. Agency for Healthcare Research and Quality. *Health Literacy Universal Precautions Toolkit.* 2nd ed. Use the Teach-Back Method: Tool #5 | Agency for Healthcare Research and Quality (ahrq.gov); 2015. Accessed July 28, 2021.
19. Marotti SB, Kerridge RK, Grimer MD. A randomised controlled trial of pharmacist medication histories and supplementary prescribing on medication errors in postoperative medications. *Anaesth Intensive Care.* 2011;39(6):1064-1070. Available at: https://doi.org/10.1177/0310057x1103900613.
20. Merrill KC, Haslam VC, Luthy KEB, Nuttall C. Educating patients about opioid disposal: a key role for perianesthesia nurses. *J Perianesth Nurs.* 2019;34(5):1025-1031. Available at: https://doi.org/10.1016/j.jopan.2018.12.008.

ADDITIONAL READING

Albrecht E, Chin KJ. Advances in regional anaesthesia and acute pain management: a narrative review. *Anaesthesia*. 2020;75:e101-e110. Available at: http://dx.doi.org/10.1111/anae.14868.

Aldrete JA, Kroulik D. A postanesthetic recovery score. *Anesth Analg*. 1970;49(6):924-934.

Truong L, Moran JL, Blum P. Post anaesthesia care unit discharge: a clinical scoring system versus traditional time-based criteria. *Anaesth Intensive Care*. 2004;32(1):33-42. Available at: https://doi.org/10.1177/0310057x0403200106.

Brown DL. *Atlas of Regional Anesthesia*. Elsevier Health Sciences; 2010.

Brown I, Jellish WS, Kleinman B, et al. Use of postanesthesia discharge criteria to reduce discharge delays for inpatients in the postanesthesia care unit. *J Clin Anesth*. 2008;20(3):175-179. Available at: https://doi.org/10.1016/j.jclinane.2007.09.014.

Chung F, Chan V, Ong D. A post-anesthetic discharge scoring system for home readiness after ambulatory surgery. *J Clin Anesth*. 1995;7(6):500-506. Available at: https://doi.org/10.1016/0952-8180(95)00130-a.

Cronin J, Livhits M, Mercado C, et al. Quality improvement pilot program for vulnerable elderly surgical patients. *Am Surg*. 2011;77(10):1305-1308.

Martin DP, Warner ME, Johnson RL, et al. Outpatient dismissal with a responsible adult compared with structured solo dismissal: a retrospective case-control comparison of safety outcomes. *Mayo Clin Proc Innov Qual Outcomes*. 2018;2(3):234-240. Available at: https://doi.org/10.1016/j.mayocpiqo.2018.06.002.

Feliciano T, Montero J, McCarthy M, Priester M. A retrospective, descriptive, exploratory study evaluating incidence of postoperative urinary retention after spinal anesthesia and its effect on PACU discharge. *J Perianesth Nurs*. 2008;23(6):394-400. Available at: https://doi.org/10.1016/j.jopan.2008.09.006.

Gartner R, Callesen T, Kroman N, Kehlet H. Recovery at the post anaesthetic care unit after breast cancer surgery. *Dan Med Bull*. 2010;57(2):1-5.

Hooper VD. SAMBA consensus guidelines for the management of postoperative nausea and vomiting: an executive summary for perianesthesia nurses. *J Perianesth Nurs*. 2015;30(5):377-382. Available at: https://doi.org/10.1016/j.jopan.2015.08.009.

Horstman MJ, Mills WL, Herman LI, et al. Patient experience with discharge instructions in postdischarge recovery: a qualitative study. *BMJ Open*. 2017;7(2):e014842. Available at: https://doi.org/10.1136/bmjopen-2016-014842.

Jakobsson JG. Recovery and discharge criteria after ambulatory anesthesia: can we improve them? *Curr Opin Anaesthesiol*. 2019;32(6):698-702. Available at: https://doi.org/10.1097/aco.0000000000000784.

Lee JH. Anesthesia for ambulatory surgery. *Korean J Anesthesiol*. 2017;70(4):398-406. Available at: https://doi.org/10.4097/kjae.2017.70.4.398.

Morris BA, Benetti M, Marro H, Rosenthal C. Clinical practice guidelines for early mobilization hours after surgery. *Orthop Nurs*. 2010;29(5):290-316. Available at: https://doi.org/10.1097/nor.0b013e3181ef7a5d.

Persico M, Miller D, Way C, et al. Implementation of enhanced recovery after surgery in a community hospital: an evidence-based approach. *J Perianesth Nurs*. 2019;34(1):188-197. Available at: https://doi.org/10.1016/j.jopan.2018.02.005.

Song D, Chung F, Ronayne M, Ward B, Yogendran S, Sibbick C. Fast-tracking (bypassing the PACU) does not reduce nursing workload after ambulatory surgery. *Br J Anaesth*. 2004;93(6):768-774. Available at: https://doi.org/10.1093/bja/aeh265.

Stephenson ME. Discharge criteria in day surgery. *J Adv Nurs*. 1990;15(5):601-613. Available at: https://doi.org/10.1111/j.1365-2648.1990.tb01860.x.

Trevisani L, Cifalà V, Gilli G, Matarese V, Zelante A, Sartori S. Post-anaesthetic discharge scoring system to assess patient recovery and discharge after colonoscopy. *World J Gastrointest Endosc*. 2013;5(10):502-507. Available at: https://doi.org/10.4253/wjge.v5.i10.502.

Waddle JP, Evers AS, Piccirillo JF. Postanesthesia care unit length of stay: quantifying and assessing dependent factors. *Anesth Analg*. 1998;87(3):628-633. Available at: https://doi.org/10.1097/00000539-199809000-00026.

Willey J, Vargo JJ, Connor JT, Dumot JA, Conwell DL, Zuccaro G. Quantitative assessment of psychomotor recovery after sedation and analgesia for outpatient EGD. *Gastrointest Endosc*. 2002;56(6):810-816. Available at: https://doi.org/10.1067/mge.2002.129609.

19 Enhanced Recovery After Surgery: The Continuum of Care from Diagnosis and Surgery to Recovery

Jacque Crosson, DNP, RN, CPAN, FASPAN

LEARNING OBJECTIVES

A review of the content of this chapter will help the reader to:

1. Describe the importance of patient education in enhanced recovery protocols.
2. Explain the benefits of multimodal analgesia for patient recovery.
3. Describe the influence of nursing on the success of enhanced recovery programs and patient outcomes.

INTRODUCTION TO ENHANCED RECOVERY AFTER SURGERY

The enhanced recovery after surgery (ERAS) program consists of multimodal evidence-based protocols delivered by multidisciplinary care teams to enable patients to recover sooner with fewer postoperative complications and better outcomes. An important factor in its success is patient participation in the plan of care from the moment surgery is planned until recovery is complete.[1] Patient involvement includes preoperative education to fully understand the benefits of enhanced recovery protocols on surgical outcomes.[2,3] Pioneered by Professor Henrik Kehlet over 25 years ago and initially referred to as fast-track surgery, ERAS now benefits from the continued refinement of protocols based on new evidence and the development of new consensus guidelines. Multiple surgical specialties have embraced enhanced recovery, and implementation continues in medical centers across the world.

Patient education and active involvement in the process are the most important aspects of a successful ERAS program. Nursing education should parallel patient education so that the perianesthesia registered nurse understands the evidence supporting the patient's enhanced recovery and can serve as a cheerleader for the patient.

In the past, patients may not have played a key role in their care, whereas, with ERAS, this is now encouraged. With enhanced recovery protocols, it is an expectation that patients independently participate in the plan of care. Successful implementation of enhanced recovery protocols improves the following patient postoperative outcomes[4-6]:

- Decreased length of stay
- Decreased rates of morbidity without an increase in rates of postoperative complications or readmissions
- Early return of bowel function
- Superior pain management with a reduction in opioid utilization
- Sustained high levels of patient satisfaction

Evolution of ERAS in Europe and the United States

In the early 1990s, several European surgeons developed the concept of fast-track surgery. Inspired by Dr. Kehlet's positive results in colorectal surgery in 1995 and 1999 in terms of early patient discharge, an enhanced recovery work group was formed by European academic surgeons and scientists in 2001.[7-9] The group focused on developing evidence-based protocols with multimodal interventions that would minimize the surgical stress response.[8,9] The term *fast-track surgery* was replaced with *enhanced recovery after surgery*. Emphasis was placed on the optimization of patients preoperatively, patient education, keeping patients fed and euvolemic, implementing multimodal pain management, avoiding unnecessary tubes and drains, and encouraging early mobilization and early feeding.[8] This work produced the first publication by the group delineating the first consensus protocol for patients having colonic surgery based on an extensive review of the evidence.[9] Despite its efforts to outline the optimal standardized practice, the ERAS group found that perioperative care in some European countries continued to be variable and inconsistent with evidence-based practices.[7,9] In response, the ERAS study group created a nonprofit medical society in 2010 to promote research, refine protocols, expand perioperative education, and assist with the implementation and auditing of protocols.[7] The ERAS Society, based in Sweden, continues to host implementation programs around the world. The first implementation of enhanced recovery protocols in the United States occurred in 2016, when four Connecticut hospitals joined the Connecticut Surgical Quality Collaborative. Currently, there are three U.S. Centers of Excellence which include Brigham and Women's Hospital in Boston, Massachusetts, the Carolinas Medical Center in Charlotte, North Carolina, and Mayo Clinic Arizona in Phoenix, Arizona.

The American Society for Enhanced Recovery (ASER) was launched in 2014 at the Second U.S. Enhanced Recovery Congress[9] for the purpose of promoting patient optimization and recovery through education and research.[10] In October 2016, ERAS USA was founded to improve perioperative care and enhance postoperative recovery through implementation of "evidence-based practice, audit, education, and research"[11]; its founding was a recognition of the importance of multidisciplinary collaborative teams.[9,11]

Evidence-Based Practice: Ambulatory Surgery

Although most published data describing enhanced recovery programs have been established from inpatient surgical settings, the basic principles of these recommendations also apply to the ambulatory patient. These include methodologies to better manage pain and comfort, reduce opioid utilization, minimize postoperative nausea and vomiting, promote early ambulation which reduces complications related to stagnate circulation and oxygenation, and enhance the quality and speed of postoperative recoveries. These desirable outcomes can be assessed with a quality program intended to evaluate length of stay, postoperative opioid requirements, unplanned transfers to a higher level of care, and readmission or urgent care visits within 30 days. Patient reported outcomes related to the overall clinical experience should also be monitored for opportunities to improve these pathways.

Source: Afonso AM, Tokita HK, McCormick PJ, Twersky RS. Enhanced recovery programs in outpatient surgery. *Anesthesiol Clin.* 2019;37(2):225-238. https://doi.org/10.1016/j.anclin.2019.01.007

TABLE 19.1 ERAS Phases of Care

Preoperative Phase	Intraoperative Phase	Postoperative Phase
Patient education	Short-acting anesthetics	Early removal of drains and catheters
Patient optimization	Regional anesthesia	Maintenance of euvolemia
Cessation of smoking	Avoidance of tubes and drains	Minimized use of opioids
Cessation of alcohol	Minimized use of opioids	Multimodal nonpharmacologic comfort
Avoidance of fasting	Active warming	measures
Carbohydrate loading	Maintenance of euvolemia	Aggressive postoperative nausea and vomiting
Avoidance of bowel preps	Antiemetic medications	management
Prewarming	Minimally invasive surgery	Early oral nutrition
Preemptive analgesia		Early mobilization
Thromboprophylaxis		Discharge criteria
Antibiotic prophylaxis		
Early discharge planning		

OVERVIEW OF ERAS PROTOCOLS

Every enhanced recovery program includes specific elements to be implemented in each phase of perioperative care. Actions critical to its success are the abilities to audit the process and ensure that these elements are incorporated into the patient's plan of care. Also, it is necessary for each member of the care team to understand the importance of these elements, including the evidence supporting them and their impact on patient outcomes. Providers' standardized order sets ensure that all aspects of enhanced recovery protocols are implemented, and result in increased compliance. Table 19.1 shows the key interventions for each phase of the patient's plan of care.

Patient Optimization for Surgery

The need for surgery can be stressful and concerning for everyone. Learning that a surgical procedure is required to cure a condition or disease can be overwhelming. Providers are key in alleviating these fears through concise, factual, and easily understood explanations of what is needed and why.[12] Another key tenet of enhanced recovery is to ensure the patient appreciates the reasons for enhanced recovery protocols and understands how the protocols support swifter recoveries, better surgical outcomes, and fewer complications. Critical to the success of this entire process is the patient's participation in the plan of care.[13] Providers must discuss the importance of patient optimization prior to surgery. For patients with medical conditions such as diabetes, hypertension, or cardiac disease, the assessment should include the determination of the severity of disease and how well patients are complying with medications or treatments.[14] When patients participate in their overall healthcare, they are better stewards of enhanced recovery protocols since they want to recover faster and return home sooner. Noncompliant patients are challenging for providers, as are those unwilling to grasp the concepts offered through enhanced recovery principles. As with all disease processes, patients must be actively involved in their care and management to decrease their own morbidity and mortality rates. Patient mobility is important for successful recovery after surgery. If necessary, the patient may require physical therapy prior to surgery (e.g., prehabilitation) to be prepared for early mobilization postoperatively. The nutritional status will be evaluated, and for some patients, protein supplementation may be recommended. Cessation of alcohol use and smoking will be recommended, and counseling offered.

Patient education and steps for physiologic optimization begin with the provider. Educational programs prior to surgery explain why active participation is key and why optimized health is important. The fasting guidelines and recommendations for carbohydrate intake should be explained so that the patient understands that clear liquids can be continued until two hours prior to surgery. Each section of this chapter reveals how patient education and re-education can motivate patients to be excellent participants in their care and have the best outcomes possible.

Preoperative Patient Education

Prior to any surgical procedure, patient and family education is necessary so that all understand what to expect and how to prepare for surgery. Utilizing ERAS evidence-based protocols and preoperative education and counseling is even more critical. For patients to fully participate in their plan of care, they must first understand the importance of physiologic optimization prior to surgery and the expectations for postsurgical participation in their care.[13] Cessation of smoking and alcohol intake should begin a minimum of 4 weeks prior to the procedure.[5,12,14] Improvement in mobility status is encouraged and prepares the patient for postoperative early mobilization.[4] For patients with impaired mobility, prehabilitation (e.g., proactive programs designed for preoperative preparation) is recommended.[4] Cardiac function, blood pressure, and glucose control should be optimized prior to surgery. Patient education must include the importance these steps have in recovery. In one randomized controlled study, findings suggested that when patients received perioperative counseling, the overall length of hospitalization was reduced.[3]

Physiology of the Surgical Stress Response

The perioperative goal for patients requiring surgery is to alleviate the surgical stress response. Regional anesthesia techniques inhibit inflammatory responses and mitigate the endocrine-metabolic response, which causes a rise in cortisol, catecholamines, and glucagon; hyperglycemia; and reduced insulin resistance.[4,5,8,14,15] Surgical stress propels the body into a catabolic state, intensifying cardiac demands and tissue hypoxia, reducing coagulation responses, and altering pulmonary and gastrointestinal functions.[4,5,8] The body's response to surgical stress can precipitate organ dysfunction, increase rates of morbidity and mortality, and extend the period of postoperative recovery.[5] Enhanced recovery programs aim to preserve normal physiology by means of perioperative interventions intended to decrease the surgical stress response.

NPO Status

A 12-hour period of fasting puts the body into starvation mode. This results in a depletion of liver glycogen stores. When this happens, the body has no available energy source to fuel metabolic demands during the immediate postoperative period.[5] Historically, fasting after midnight was thought to decrease the risk of aspiration or regurgitation during anesthesia.[5] Fasting guidelines from the American Society of Anesthesiologists now allow for a light meal six hours prior to the induction of anesthesia and clear liquids two hours prior to the induction of anesthesia.[16] A key element of patient education is telling patients they can consume clear liquids, such as a clear, high-energy drink, up until two hours prior to surgery.[8,12,17] This improves the hydration status, decreases thirst and fatigue, and improves patient satisfaction.[8] The addition of carbohydrates improves glucose tolerance and decreases the impact of catabolism (wasting) on muscles.[5,12] Optimizing the patient nutritional status prior to surgery positively impacts the physiologic status and surgical outcomes.

Carbohydrate Loading

Allowing preoperative carbohydrate beverages has a positive impact on the preoperative patient. From the time the last light meal is consumed, six hours prior to surgery, ERAS patients are instructed to ingest carbohydrate-loading drinks up to two hours prior to surgery or, if ordered by their surgeon, a commercial carbohydrate beverage that may include immune system boosters. Preloading with carbohydrates prior to surgery decreases the need for the human body to rely on muscle tissue (catabolism) for energy.[12] Additionally, insulin resistance is decreased, keeping glucose control within normal limits during the perioperative and postoperative periods. Increased glucose levels may lead to decreased wound healing, directly impacting surgical outcomes.[12]

Mechanical Bowel Preparation

Patients may or may not be prescribed a mechanical bowel preparation, also known as a bowel prep (e.g., oral ingestion of gut cleansing medications). Historically, patients scheduled for a bowel resection were prescribed a bowel prep to decrease the risk of an anastomotic leak and decrease the risk of infection.[5] The negative effects of this bowel purge included dehydration, electrolyte imbalances, extended fasting, and patient dissatisfaction.[5] Currently, practices may vary between surgeons. If a bowel prep was ordered, patient compliance should be ascertained during the preoperative assessment.

Prevention of Postoperative Nausea and Vomiting

Risk factors for postoperative nausea and vomiting (PONV) include laparoscopic surgery, female gender, nonsmoker, and a history of motion sickness.[18] In many cases, the utilization of minimally invasive surgical procedures such as laparoscopy can lead to a higher prevalence of PONV in patients. PONV can lead to patient dissatisfaction, prolonged hospitalization, and increased costs of care and an increased length of stay.[5] Aggressive multimodal approaches to prevent PONV should be part of the patient's plan of care. Two agents from two different classes of antiemetics should be considered. Classes of antiemetic medications include 5-HT3 antagonists, NK-1 antagonists, corticosteroids, antihistamines, anticholinergics, butyrophenones, and phenothiazines.[5,12,18,19]

Cessation of Smoking

Smoking has deleterious effects on the physiologic optimization of patients prior to surgery. At the time of diagnosis and when the need for a surgical intervention is determined, cessation of smoking counseling should begin.[17] This allows for a four-week respite that can support improved postoperative respiratory functioning.[12,14,15,17]

Cessation of Alcohol

Consumption of alcohol impacts liver function, bleeding, and wound and cardiopulmonary complications.[15] For those patients consuming alcohol daily, cessation reduces the risk of withdrawal symptoms during hospitalization and decreases the postoperative rates of morbidity.[12,15] ERAS protocols recommend a minimum of four weeks of abstinence for optimal benefits.

Multimodal Analgesia

Multimodal analgesia utilizing one or more analgesic agents, each with different mechanisms of action, is standard perioperative patient care.[12,20] The importance of this approach for patient education is that it tackles pain transmission through several mechanisms and can also reduce overall opioid requirements. Pain signals from the surgical site to the brain are carried by peripheral nerves. These afferent signals are blocked with the use of local or regional anesthesia. Preemptive analgesia is prescribed preoperatively and generally given during the preoperative preparation process. Analgesic medications are given prior to surgical incision to decrease the intensity and extent of postoperative pain.[21] Classes of medications given preoperatively include nonsteroidal anti-inflammatory drugs (NSAIDS), acetaminophen, and gabapentinoids. When local and regional anesthesia techniques are utilized with minimally invasive incisions and the patient receives preemptive analgesia, it is possible to minimize opioid utilization. Patient preoperative education should focus on the concepts of multimodal analgesia and how it improves pain management postoperatively without relying specifically on opioids.

Understanding the importance of how different medication classifications improve postoperative pain management and why they must be taken as ordered is important in ERAS protocols:

- NSAIDS are anti-inflammatory medications that inhibit cyclooxygenase and prostaglandin production.[17,19]
- Acetaminophen is a centrally acting pain medication and the one most used.[17,19]
- Gabapentinoids block the transmission of nerve pain; their side effects of sedation and dizziness should be monitored.[19]

Patients are instructed to take both NSAIDS and acetaminophen every six hours, staggered, around the clock for their baseline analgesia postoperatively. When their pain level becomes intolerable, an opioid is recommended. Utilizing the synergistic effects of more than one type of non-narcotic analgesia provides better pain relief for patients without the side effects of opioids (e.g., nausea, hypotension, dizziness, constipation).[17] This is an important educational point for the patient to understand prior to surgery.

Early Ambulation

One of the most important tenets of ERAS is patient mobilization.[22] Multimodal pain management techniques allow patients' pain to be well controlled. This makes ambulation easier on the day of surgery and can facilitate sitting in a recliner rather than spending time in bed. When patients are up and moving, they feel more normal, their bowel function returns sooner, and they meet discharge criteria for going home sooner. Patient education must include the reason for mobility so patients can participate in the plan of care. Ambulation also decreases the potential for thromboembolism, pneumonia, and atelectasis.[22]

Implementation of Nursing Education

Nursing education should mirror information the patient has received from the surgeon. In order for perianesthesia nurses to reinforce education on the day of surgery, they must know what the patient understands; this helps them continue to advocate on behalf of the patient and family, addressing any misconceptions or misunderstandings.[6,13] Reinforcing expectations and clarifying the patient understanding of ERAS protocols ensures that patients have better outcomes from their surgical experience. It is also important for nurses to give preemptive analgesia at the appropriate time and verify the ingestion of carbohydrate drinks and NPO status. Prewarming patients, applying sequential compression devices, administering chemical thromboembolism prophylaxis, and ensuring that the appropriate preoperative antibiotics were ordered are important interventions leading to the best surgical outcomes. In a Delphi study by one research group, the following elements were identified as important for ERAS implementation:

- A multidisciplinary team working and learning together[23]
- An effective feedback system[23,24]
- Strong leadership and vision[23]
- Regularly scheduled meetings[23,24]
- Senior management engagement[24]
- A dedicated ERAS nurse or nurse coordinator[23,24]
- Regular audits and data collection[23,24]

Perianesthesia nursing involvement is key to the success of any ERAS program. Nurses' demonstrated knowledge of protocols is necessary to support patient compliance and optimization. When necessary, the perianesthesia registered nurse may need to alert the care team if deviations to the plan of care have been discovered.

Education on the Day of Surgery

By the time enhanced recovery patients present on the day of surgery, they should have received education from their surgeon relating to the procedure and the protocol of the plan of care.[12] Verifying patients' perspectives and what they have learned prior to surgery allows the perianesthesia registered nurse to reinforce what is known and fill in gaps in information.[13] When the preoperative expectations of the patient and family differ significantly from the known protocols, it is imperative to engage the surgeon so that expectations are discussed and the patient can ask questions. Patient participation in the plan of care is imperative to enhanced recovery success and the patient's positive surgical outcomes.

Order Sets of the Surgeon and Anesthesiologist

Successful ERAS programs include standardized order sets that can be customized for each patient. Provider compliance improves when providers can select from preexisting orders that follow protocols. This is essential when auditing processes to determine protocol compliance. Currently, there are multiple surgical specialties that have protocol pathways for enhanced recovery (Box 19.1). In 2010, the ERAS Society was registered as a not-for-profit medical society.[11] Its guidelines have been published, and, in many cases, they have been combined with guidelines from other medical societies.[11] Specialty guidelines are available for bariatric, breast, cardiac, cesarean, colorectal, gynecologic, head and neck, liver, orthopedic, pancreatic, thoracic, and urologic procedures. Each guideline provides both a summary of and recommendations based on the best evidence for perioperative care.

BOX 19.1 ERAS Guidelines

Guidelines for many types of procedures are available on the ERAS Society website at no charge: https://erassociety.org/guidelines/list-of-guidelines/
   Examples include:

- Consensus Statement for Perioperative Care in Total Hip Replacement and Total Knee Replacement Surgery
- Guidelines for Vulvar and Vaginal Surgery
- Consensus Review of Optimal Perioperative Care in Breast Reconstruction
- Guidelines for Perioperative Care in Bariatric Surgery

Verification of Ingestion of a Carbohydrate Drink and NPO Status

Fasting after midnight on the day of surgery has been standard practice to reduce the risk of pulmonary aspiration during surgery. As reported in the colorectal guidelines, a meta-analysis of random controlled trials demonstrated that patients who fasted after midnight had neither decreased gastric contents nor an increased pH of gastric fluid compared with patients who were allowed to ingest clear liquids until two hours prior to surgery.[15] For patients with a history of delayed gastric emptying, the guidelines recommend a minimum fast of eight hours.[25] Consumption of a minimum of 50 g of an oral carbohydrate two to three hours prior to the induction of anesthesia decreases muscle breakdown, increases the patient's sense of well-being, reduces postoperative insulin resistance,[25] and eases thirst, hunger, and anxiety.[15] Once the perianesthesia registered nurse ascertains that the patient has consumed liquids up until two hours prior to surgery, the nurse knows that the patient's fluid status is euvolemic and that preoperative fluids should be kept at a to-keep-open (TKO) rate.

Multimodal Preemptive Analgesia

Celecoxib 400 mg orally, acetaminophen 1000 mg orally, and gabapentin 600 mg orally are examples of multimodal medications given preoperatively for preemptive analgesia.[26] Pain management begins with the administration of these medications in the preoperative area.[5] The goal of preemptive analgesia is to block the activation of pain receptors before the incision has been made.[5] Utilization of preemptive analgesia has been correlated with a reduced use of opioids postoperatively.[5]

Prewarming

Upon induction of anesthesia, redistribution hypothermia can decrease a patient's core temperature up to 1.6°C.[27] Hypothermia can cause intraoperative and postoperative complications such as coagulopathies, increased blood loss, decreased wound healing, immune suppression, cardiovascular challenges, and an increased length of stay in the hospital.[5,12,27] Prewarming prior to anesthesia induction helps to prevent inadvertent hypothermia. The use of forced-air prewarming devices is highly encouraged for all patients at least 30 minutes before they enter the operating room.

Bowel Preparation

Patients may or may not have been ordered a bowel prep prior to surgery. Verification is important to determine the patient's potential fluid status preoperatively. Some surgeons continue to utilize bowel preps as part of a preoperative surgical protocol.

Whether prepped or not, this information is important to the overall management of the patient's fluid balance.

Antimicrobial Prophylaxis

Antimicrobial prophylaxis 30–60 minutes prior to incision decreases the risk of a surgical site infection.[5,12] Additional dosing during prolonged procedures should also occur.[15,25] Patients should be instructed to shower at home with chlorhexidine antimicrobial soap or a similar product, and the skin prep in the operating room should ideally consist of chlorhexidine- and alcohol-based solutions when not contraindicated.[25]

Thromboembolism Chemoprophylaxis

Patients who are having surgery for a diagnosis of cancer are at a higher risk for deep vein thrombosis. The administration of pharmacologic thromboprophylaxis is recommended in many enhanced recovery protocols and includes the application and use of sequential compression devices during surgery.[15] Mobilization, along with antithrombotic prophylaxis, decreases the risk for deep vein thrombosis postoperatively.[17]

Reinforcement of Patient Education

The most important part of patient preparation on the day of surgery is the reinforcement of education along the continuum of care. Ask clarifying questions to ascertain what the patient understands, and supplement this knowledge as indicated. Some patients are ready and understand all the events that will occur throughout their hospitalization, and some are not. Setting the patient up for success is still possible in the preoperative arena. Summon providers as needed to ensure that all questions are answered and that all patients can state verbally what will happen in the enhanced recovery process. This is the optimal opportunity to clarify and set expectations for the patient's experience. Any questions or concerns should be managed preoperatively so that the plan of care is understood by the patient, family, and all members of the healthcare team.

INTRAOPERATIVE ERAS CARE

With the advances that have been made in surgical technology, most surgical procedures can be done with minimally invasive techniques. Regional anesthesia options allow for exceptional pain management, and this decreases the need for opioids during and after surgery. The ability to make smaller incisions and provide better pain management allows the patient to become mobile earlier without the side effects of opioids. Understanding the anesthesia plan is important for perianesthesia registered nurses. Liposomal bupivacaine utilized in regional anesthesia provides pain relief for up to 72 hours postoperatively.[5] Use of low doses of ketamine for pain control during surgery in lieu of opioids often allows the patient to arrive in the postanesthesia care unit (PACU) more awake and alert with fewer side effects than in the past. When narcotics are minimized, nausea, hypotension, pruritis, and dizziness occur less frequently, and this enables the patient to be ready for oral hydration sooner. The volume of intravenous (IV) fluids administered during surgery should be noted in the handoff from the anesthesia provider to the perianesthesia nurse. Many enhanced recovery protocols encourage goal-directed fluid therapy throughout the perioperative period, using vasopressors as needed to maintain the mean arterial pressures once normovolemia is achieved.[5,12,15] Active warming should have occurred so that the patient remained normothermic. Mechanical deep vein thrombosis prophylaxis with the use of sequential compression devices should be instituted throughout the surgical course. Tubes, drains, and catheters should be minimized. The absence of medical equipment or devices (e.g., tubes, drains, catheters) that can impede the ability to ambulate improves patient mobility postoperatively. When they have been used, their timely removal is important. During handoff between the perioperative nurse and the anesthesia provider, the procedure, approach, medications, anesthetic plan, and any medical devices utilized should be included in the patient's report so that the perianesthesia nurse can continue the plan of care.

Minimally Invasive Incisions

Laparoscopic approaches to surgery are common. Utilization of robotics for surgery allows for greater visualization of the surgical field through smaller incisions. A key to patient recovery is the ability to perform large complex surgical procedures through small incisions. Less invasive surgeries allow the patient to become mobilized quickly with less pain. Even though minimally invasive approaches are utilized, regional anesthesia techniques provide superior pain control for the patient. If it is necessary for the patient to have an open incision or laparotomy, regional anesthesia techniques can still provide adequate pain relief so that the patient is able to become mobilized on the day of surgery. Timing of the regional anesthesia is crucial; it is generally done at the beginning of the procedure. Many surgeons are now performing their own regional blocks at the beginning of surgery, utilizing the benefit of the laparoscope to identify landmarks prior to infiltration of the local anesthetic. This allows for the local anesthesia to have the maximum effect by the time the surgery is completed. Often, liposomal bupivacaine is infiltrated during regional blocks, providing patients with up to 72 hours of pain control. Examples of regional anesthesia for abdominal procedures include transversus abdominis plane blocks and quadratus lumborum blocks. Chest wall blocks for breast surgery include paravertebral and fascial blocks, such as pectoralis, serratus, or erector spinae blocks.[19]

Decreased Use of Drains and Catheters

Enhanced recovery protocols avoid the need for tubes, drains, and catheters. Nasogastric tubes are deemed unnecessary as they obstruct early feeding. There may be times when one is necessary because of the procedure performed, but routine use is no longer supported by the evidence.[5] Foley catheters, if utilized, should be removed within 24 hours of surgery.[5] This reduces the potential for infection and, more importantly, facilitates better mobility for the patient. Any additional tubes should only be used if necessary. Anything foreign to the body can be a source of infection and should be removed when no longer necessary.

Euvolemia

Current fasting guidelines allow patients to consume fluids until two hours prior to surgery. On the day of surgery, the patient should be in a state of euvolemia. In the past, fasting restrictions had patients stop eating and drinking at midnight. By the time they arrived for the procedure, it could have been more than eight hours since fluids had been ingested. If a bowel prep had been ordered, patients would have been more dehydrated due to fluid losses with no replacement. Prior to enhanced recovery protocols, these patients received generous amounts of fluids during their surgical procedures to manage any hemodynamic instability. This led to the potential for fluid overload in the postoperative period, often causing a shift in intracellular fluids. Third spacing of fluid can lead to abdominal distention and slowing down of bowel function,[5] impeding the patient's ability to consume a regular diet. Bloating can also cause nausea and the potential for vomiting, keeping patients from becoming mobile. When the goal is for patients to remain euvolemic, the recovery progresses, patients can resume eating an appropriate diet, ambulation occurs, and patients are more satisfied since they feel they are making progress toward discharge.

Regional Anesthesia

Local anesthetics have been utilized for surgical wound infiltration and are an effective method for postoperative pain management.[5] The ability to anesthetize the nociceptors on the skin prior to surgical incision was a key factor in decreasing the surgical stress response. As anesthesia techniques have advanced, more advanced regional blocks have evolved. It is now widespread practice for regional anesthesia to be utilized in almost every type of surgical procedure. Whether the patient is having a total hip replacement or an inguinal hernia repair, regional anesthesia is a common component of postoperative pain management. Discussions prior to surgery between members of the healthcare team and the patient include options for postoperative pain management. As active participants in their care, patients should always be involved in the decision. Since some regional anesthesia occurs in the preoperative area for orthopedic procedures, patients need to understand what is involved and what to expect. Another huge advancement in the utilization of regional anesthesia is the ability for surgeons to perform these procedures. Abdominal and chest wall blocks have become part of the armamentarium for a surgeon to ensure adequate pain control for their patients. Regional anesthesia techniques have become part of a surgeon's routine during surgery and can be done effortlessly. The type of regional anesthesia and medication utilized need to be reported when the patient's record is handed off to the perianesthesia registered nurse. There are now many types of regional anesthesia used during surgical procedures. A key component of continuing education for the patient is reinforcement of the pain management plan of care.

Opioid Sparing

Opioids have many deleterious side effects, such as sedation, hypotension, nausea, dizziness, and pruritis, to name a few. These side effects cause the patient to feel miserable and unable to participate in their care. When patients have received opioids only for pain management during surgery, an entire day of recovery can be lost due to adverse effects. Opioids are an important part of pain management but should not be the only agents provided. In addition to regional anesthesia, IV acetaminophen, ketorolac, ketamine, and dexmedetomidine are all important components of a balanced multimodal anesthetic plan of care. The ability to block multiple pain receptor sites is important in controlling postoperative pain and setting the patient up for success. Successful patient recovery depends on the patient's ability to participate in the plan of care.

POSTOPERATIVE ERAS CARE

Postoperative care is a continuation of the enhanced recovery protocol that began when it was determined that the patient required surgery. Perianesthesia registered nurses should be prepared to manage the patient with an understanding of the patient is on the enhanced recovery continuum. Critical

information received during handoff from the anesthesia provider and the perioperative registered nurse assists the perianesthesia registered nurse in planning interventions along the enhanced recovery protocol. The amount and timing of opioids given is important, as additional dosing may not be necessary. When regional anesthesia techniques have been utilized, opioids may be spared. Timing for the next dose of an anti-inflammatory or acetaminophen is necessary so that the patient has around-the-clock coverage. Non-narcotic medications and nonpharmacologic measures should be the first-line interventions for pain control. The perianesthesia registered nurse can anticipate aggressive management of PONV. The dosage and class of antiemetic used is important in getting the patient ready for fluids. Patients should be kept normothermic and IV fluids should be administered according to orders. Every intervention provided should follow enhanced recovery protocols, with patient education provided. Perianesthesia registered nurses should be cheerleaders for the patient, providing encouragement and reinforcing milestones accomplished.

Order Sets of the Surgeon and Anesthesiologist

Standardized order sets enable all members of the healthcare team to follow enhanced protocols. Orders that include around-the-clock non-narcotic analgesia, opioids for breakthrough pain, level of activity, type of diet, and use of antiemetics give nurses the knowledge to manage patient symptoms quickly so that there is no interruption in care. Knowing the protocol and having the appropriate orders to initiate interventions allow patient progression through the recovery process. Order sets are also beneficial when patients may be cared for in other units in the other institutions in which the staff is not familiar with enhanced recovery protocols. There is a clear plan of care when orders are standardized.

Nonpharmacologic Interventions

Prior to any pharmacologic intervention, nonpharmacologic interventions should be implemented. When patients undergo surgery on a hard, flat table, they may awaken feeling discomfort in parts of the body not impacted by the surgery. Positioning during surgical procedures allows the surgeon to have good visualization of the surgical field. Upon awakening from anesthesia, patients may not be able to articulate the source of pain and may assume it is from the surgical site. Prior to administration of any pain medication, it may be helpful to reposition the patient for comfort, utilizing heat packs, ice packs, or pillows. This may be the only intervention necessary until the patients awakens further and can better describe if and how they are experiencing pain.

Multimodal Analgesia

Managing the patient's pain should include all classes of pain medication. If acute pain is present upon arrival in the PACU, the nurse may find it appropriate to partner with anesthesia colleagues for ketamine dosing. Continuation of all non-narcotic medications as ordered should be the baseline strategy for postoperative discomfort. If opioids are necessary, smaller dosages can be provided when all modalities of medications have been given. Whether the patient is being discharged home or transferred to a hospital unit, the handoff report must include next dosages needed of NSAIDs and acetaminophen.

Euvolemia

Maintaining euvolemia in the postoperative patient follows enhanced recovery protocols. Applying a heparin or saline lock to an IV catheter once patients are tolerating fluids gives patients greater freedom to ambulate and improves their sense of well-being and accomplishment because they are recovering as planned. If during the postoperative course the patient becomes hypotensive, small 250-mL fluid boluses may be ordered until the patient's blood pressure returns to baseline. Blood pressure parameters and interventions should be included in the standard postoperative order sets handed of from the anesthesiologist. It is important to know that urine output of 20 mL/h is a normal response to surgical stress and may not require any intervention.[5]

Early Ambulation and Mobilization

Patients confined to bedrest have increased postoperative complications, including atelectasis, deep vein thrombosis, muscle wasting, and decreased bowel function. Mobilization of the patient decreases the risk for postoperative complications. The sooner patients ambulate and the longer they are sitting up in a chair out of bed, the quicker they recover and can be discharged to home.[5] Enhanced recovery protocols provide superior pain management with reduced opioid requirements, improved patient satisfaction, a decreased length of stay, and decreased postoperative complications.[26]

SUCCESSFUL RECOVERY

Functional recovery is considered complete when patients can tolerate a general diet, independently ambulate, and have their postoperative pain controlled with oral analgesics.[5] As patients move along the continuum of enhanced recovery, their involvement is necessary: They are the *key* participants in the process. Collaboration by an all-inclusive multidisciplinary team creates an environment that supports patient success from diagnosis to full recovery.

CHAPTER HIGHLIGHTS

- Enhanced recovery after surgery (ERAS) programs are based on evidence-based protocols that allow patients to recover rapidly.
- ERAS protocols mitigate the surgical stress response by modulating both inflammatory and neurohumoral responses.
- Patient participation in the plan of care is necessary for the success of ERAS programs.
- ERAS protocols have been utilized in Europe for over 20 years.
- Physiologic optimization of patient medical conditions impacts surgical outcomes.

- Multidisciplinary healthcare teams are necessary for the successful implementation of ERAS programs.
- Perianesthesia registered nurses are critical actors in the implementation and success of ERAS programs.

CASE STUDY

Carol is a 63-year-old Caucasian female with a history of hypertension, type II diabetes, anxiety disorder, and smoking. She was recently diagnosed with ovarian cancer. Her preoperative counseling and education were completed 4 weeks ago. She was escorted to the appointment by her husband. Carol was shown a video in the surgeon's office describing the benefits of enhanced recovery after surgery and was allowed to ask questions until she verbalized her understanding of the process. Written information on enhanced recovery was also provided. At the time of her consultation, she was given information on smoking cessation and resources for relaxation and meditation to control her anxiety. Carol verbalized her desire to be compliant with smoking cessation and diabetic management.

Carol presents to your institution on the day of her surgery. Upon entering the preoperative room, she immediately turns to you and says, "I could not stop smoking; I was too anxious. I need something for this anxiety before I can do anything else!" As her preoperative registered nurse, how can you assist Carol with her preoperative anxiety? What nonpharmacologic interventions may be needed at this time? As her preoperative registered nurse, are you concerned about the information provided that she could not stop smoking?

During the preoperative interview, when she was asked if she had any questions regarding her surgical procedure, Carol said, "Dr. Jones did not tell me anything about what she is going to do today. I only remember her telling me that I would be able to go home today." As her preoperative registered nurse, what is your next step? Are Carol's expectations regarding her hospitalization realistic? How do you ensure that Carol's expectations are addressed?

Dr. Jones and the anesthesia team have visited Carol in her preoperative room and answered all her questions and concerns. She has signed her consent for surgery. As you complete your documentation, Carol states, "I hope that anesthesia doctor has a lot of drugs to give me. I want to be unconscious throughout my hospitalization." As Carol's preoperative registered nurse, what concerns do you have regarding her desire to be rendered unconscious? Are you concerned about whether Carol plans to participate in her plan of care? What additional education regarding pain management strategies needs to be offered?

REFERENCES

1. Conn LG, Rotstein OD, Greco E, Tricco AC, et al. Enhanced recovery after vascular surgery: protocol for a systematic review. *Syst Rev.* 2012;1(52):1-7. Available at: https://doi.org/10.1186/2046-4053-1-52.
2. Gillis C, Gill M, Marlett N, et al. Patients as partners in enhanced recovery after surgery: a qualitative patient-led study. *BMJ Open.* 2017;7:e017002. Available at: https://doi.org/10.1136/bmjopen-2017-017002.
3. Forsmo H, Erichsen C, Rasdal A, Tvinnereim J, Korner H, Pfeffer F. Randomized controlled trial of extended perioperative counseling in enhanced recovery after colorectal surgery. *Dis Colon Rectum.* 2018;61(6):724-732. Available at: https://doi.org/10.1097/DCR.0000000000001007.
4. Carli F. Physiologic considerations of enhanced recovery after surgery (ERAS) programs: implications of the stress response. *Can J Anaesth.* 2015;62(2):110-119. Available at: https://doi.org/10.1007/s12630-014-0264-0.
5. Kalogera E, Dowdy SC. Enhanced recovery pathway in gynecologic surgery: improving outcomes through evidence-based medicine. *Obstet Gynecol Clin North Am.* 2016;43:551-573. Available at: https://doi.org/10.1016/j.ogc.2016.04.006.

6. Brown D, Xhaja A. Nursing perspectives on enhanced recovery after surgery. *Surg Clin North Am.* 2018;98(6):1211-1221. Available at: https://doi.org/10.1016/j.suc.2018.07.008.
7. Ljungqvist O, Young-Fadok T, Demartines N. The history of enhanced recovery after surgery and the ERAS society. *J Laparoendosc Adv Surg Tech A.* 2017;27(9):860-862. Available at: https://doi.org/10.1089/lap.2017.0350.
8. Powell AC, Stopfkuchen-Evans M, Urman RD, Bleday R. Decreasing the surgical stress response and an initial experience from the enhanced recovery after surgery colorectal surgery program at an academic institution. *Int Anesthesiol Clin.* 2017;55(4):163-178. Available at: https://doi.org/10.1097/aia.0000000000000162.
9. Tanious MK, Ljungqvist O, Urman RD. Enhanced recovery after surgery: history, evolution, guidelines, and future directions. *Int Anesthesiol Clin.* 2017;55(4):1-11. Available at: https://doi.org/10.1097/aia.0000000000000167.
10. American Society of Enhanced Recovery (ASER). *About Us.* American Society for Enhanced Recovery. Available at: aserhq.org.
11. ERAS® Society. *History.* Available at: https://erassociety.org/about/history.

12. Temple-Oberle C, Shea-Budgell MA, Tan M, et al. Consensus review of optimal perioperative care in breast reconstruction: enhanced recovery after surgery (ERAS) society recommendations. *Plast Reconstr Surg.* 2017;139(5):1056e-1071e. Available at: https://doi.org/10.1097/prs.0000000000003242.

13. Mendes DIA, Ferrito CRAC, Gonçalves MIR. Nursing interventions in the enhanced recovery after surgery®: scoping review. *Rev Bras Enferm.* 2018;71(suppl 6):2824-2832. Available at: https://dx.doi.org/10.1590/0034-7167-2018-0436.

14. Kehlet H, Wilmore DW. Multimodal strategies to improve surgical outcome. *Am J Surg.* 2002;183(6):630-641. Available at: https://doi.org/10.1016/s0002-9610(02)00866-8.

15. Gustafsson UO, Scott MJ, Schwenk W, et al. Guidelines for perioperative care in elective colonic surgery: Enhanced Recovery After Surgery (ERAS®) Society recommendations. *Clin Nutr.* 2012;31(2012):783-800. Available at: https://doi.org/10.1016/j.clnu.2012.08.013.

16. American Society of Anesthesiologists (ASA). Practice guidelines for preoperative fasting and the use of pharmacologic agents to reduce the risk of pulmonary aspiration: application to healthy patients undergoing elective procedures: An updated report by the American Society of Anesthesiologists task force on preoperative fasting and the use of pharmacologic agents to reduce the risk of pulmonary aspiration. *Anesthesiology.* 2017;126(3):376-393. Available at: https://doi.org/10.1097/ALN.0000000000001452.

17. Wainwright TW, Gill M, McDonald DA, et al. Consensus statement for perioperative care in total hip replacement and total knee replacement surgery: enhanced recovery after surgery (ERAS®) society recommendations. *Acta Orthop.* 2020;91(1):3-19. Available at: https://doi.org/10.1080/17453674.2019.1683790.

18. Gan TJ, Belani KG, Bergese S, et al. Fourth consensus guidelines for the management of postoperative nausea and vomiting. *Anesth Analg.* 2020;131(2):411-448. Available at: https://doi.org/10.1213/ane.0000000000004833.

19. Charipova K, Gress KL, Urits I, Viswanath O, Kaye AD. Maximization of non-opioid multimodal analgesia in ambulatory surgery centers. *Cureus.* 2020;12(9):e10407 Available at: https://doi.org/10.7759/cureus.10407.

20. Mariano ER, Schatman ME. A commonsense patient-centered approach to multimodal analgesia within enhanced recovery protocols. *J Pain Res.* 2019;12:3461-3466. Available at: https://doi.org/10.2147/jpr.s238772.

21. Carli F. Henrik Kehlet, M.D., Ph.D., recipient of the 2014 excellence in research award. *Anesthesiology.* 2014;121(4):690-691. Available at: https://doi.org/10.1097/ALN.0000000000000396.

22. Batchelor TJP, Ljungqvist O. A surgical perspective of ERAS guidelines in thoracic surgery. *Curr Opin Anaesthesiol.* 2019;32(1):17-22. Available at: https://doi.org/10.1097/aco.0000000000000685.

23. Francis NK, Walker T, Carter F, et al. Consensus on training and implementation of enhanced recovery after surgery: a Delphi study. *World J Surg.* 2018;42:1919-1928. Available at: https://doi.org/10.1007/s00268-017-4436-2.

24. Watson DJ. The role of the nurse coordinator in the enhanced recovery after surgery program. *Nursing.* 2017;47(9):13-17. Available at: https://doi.org/10.1097/01.NURSE.0000522018.00182.c7.

25. Nelson G, Bakkum-Gamez J, Kalogera E, et al. Guidelines for perioperative care in gynecologic/oncology: enhanced recovery after surgery (ERAS) society recommendations—2019 update. *Int J Gynecol Cancer.* 2019;29(4):651-668. Available at: https://doi.org/10.1136/ijgc-2019-000356.

26. Kalogera E, Bakkum-Gamez J, Jankowski CJ, et al. Enhanced recovery in gynecologic surgery. *Obstet Gynecol.* 2013;122(2):319-328. Available at: https://doi.org/10.1097/aog.0b013e31829aa780.

27. American Society of PeriAnesthesia Nurses. *2021-2022 Perianesthesia Nursing Standards, Practice Recommendations and Interpretive Statements.* ASPAN; 2020.

20 Principles of Intraoperative Care

Valerie A. Pfander, DNP, APRN, ACCNS-AG, CPAN, FASPAN

LEARNING OBJECTIVES

A review of the content of this chapter will help the reader to:

1. Describe the components of the surgical environment.
2. Identify the roles and responsibilities of the surgical team.
3. Discuss the steps of preparing a patient for surgery.
4. Explain the handling and labeling considerations of specimen management.
5. Examine intraoperative safety concerns and mitigation strategies.
6. Describe the components of a standardized handover process.

OVERVIEW

Intraoperative care is provided by nurses, anesthesiologists, nurse anesthetists, surgical technologists, surgeons, and surgical assistants working together as a team. The intraoperative phase of care includes delivery of safe and effective care by monitoring patient homeostasis during the procedure, maintaining sterile techniques to decrease the risk of surgical site infection, and providing ongoing patient assessment to ensure patient safety and comfort.

Perioperative nursing is a unique, highly specialized area of nursing practice that takes place in the surgical environment. During this phase of care, patients are at their most vulnerable. Safety and advocacy of the patient are the primary concerns of the circulating perioperative nurse. Although the intraoperative period is defined as beginning when the patient enters the operating room, the role of the circulating nurse begins with patient interactions in the preoperative area. The circulating nurse traditionally introduces herself or himself to the patient before the patient is transported to the operating room. During this time, a review of the preprocedural safety checklist is completed and a handover of relevant information occurs between the preoperative nurse and the circulating nurse.

Ambulatory surgery centers (ASCs) are healthcare facilities providing outpatient or same-day surgeries and diagnostic procedures. According to a report from the Centers for Disease Control and Prevention, in 2010 there were 25.7 million ambulatory procedures (or 53% of all ambulatory procedures) performed in hospital settings and an additional 22.5 million (47%) performed in ASCs.[1] Contemporary trends indicated a steady increase in the volume and types of surgeries being performed over the past decade, and this was due in part to advances in technology and best practices. Patients in an ambulatory setting tend to have fewer co-morbidities and less critical needs than those having surgery in a hospital-based setting. However, same-day surgery centers often have a rapid turnover of patients, and this means that the staff must work in a fast-paced, rapidly changing environment.

The Association of Operating Room Nurses has established evidence-based nationally recognized guidelines for perioperative practice. Recommendations from these guidelines should be used to guide safe care for patients undergoing surgical and other invasive procedures.[2] These guidelines include ambulatory supplements that are reviewed and vetted for their applicability to ASCs.[2]

THE SURGICAL ENVIRONMENT

The surgical suite is divided into three designated zones, unrestricted, semi-restricted, and restricted.[3] The unrestricted zones are areas in which traffic is not limited, such as the surgical waiting room. This area is often accessible from the exterior of the building and does not require surgical attire to be worn. The semi-restricted zones are often designated by a red line on the floor. These areas are restricted to employees and patients and include surgical supply rooms, scrub areas, and corridors leading to an operating room. Surgical scrubs and head coverings should be worn in the semi-restricted areas. Restricted zones are the insides of operating rooms or areas in which sterile processes are in progress (Figure 20.1). Restricted areas are limited to employees and patients. Surgical scrubs, face masks, and head and facial hair coverings are required.

Sterility of the Surgical Environment

The purpose of a clean and safe surgical environment is to prevent contaminants from entering the operative site of the patient and causing a surgical site infection. All individuals involved in an invasive procedure have the responsibility to ensure the environment is safe for the patient.[4] Actions taken by the perioperative team to ensure sterility include handwashing, surgical scrubbing, wearing of surgical attire, and the preservation of a sterile field for instruments and supplies. Additional measures to control contamination of a surgical

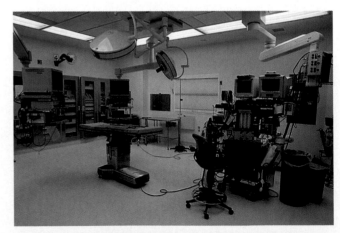

Fig. 20.1 The operating room suite and instrumentation. Falcone T, Walters MD. Figure 111.1 in: Baggish MS, Karram MM, eds. *Atlas of Pelvic Anatomy and Gynecologic Surgery*. Elsevier: 2021.

site include preoperative patient bathing, surgical site skin preparation, prophylactic antibiotic administration within one hour of incision, adequate glycemic control, and maintenance of perioperative normothermia.[4]

Hybrid Operating Room

A hybrid operating room combines a traditional operating room with a procedural space equipped with guided imaging devices to allow for minimally invasive, often catheter-based, highly complex procedures. Hybrid rooms are often used for vascular surgery, cardiac procedures, neurosurgery, and trauma cases.[5] Advantages to using a hybrid operating room include higher procedural accuracy, less operative time, and less risk of complications due to the transfer of patients between radiology or catheterization laboratory suites and the operating room (Figure 20.2).[6]

ROLES AND RESPONSIBILITIES OF THE SURGICAL TEAM

The intraoperative surgical team may vary based on the workplace setting, but it consists of a circulating registered nurse, an anesthesia provider (physician or certified registered nurse anesthetist), a surgeon, and a surgical technologist. Other team members that may be included based on surgical specialty include a certified surgical assistant, a registered nurse first assistant, and an advanced practice provider.

Circulating Registered Nurse

The circulating nurse functions outside of the sterile field and is responsible for managing the care provided in the operating room. The registered nurse circulator completes the nursing documentation, prepares and positions the patient for surgery, monitors the imaging equipment, performs counts of surgical items, and acts as a patient advocate to ensure safe patient care is being provided. As a nonsterile member of the surgical team, the circulator also assists the surgeon, anesthesia provider, and other operating room team members when necessary.

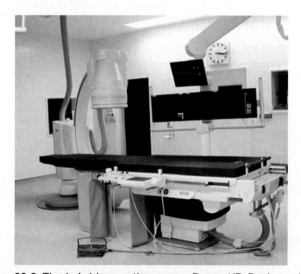

Fig. 20.2 The hybrid operating room. Donas KP, De Azevedo FM. Logistics in the hybrid operating room for complex endovascular aneurysm repair. Figure 5.1 in: Donas KP, Torsello G, Ouriel K, eds. *Endovascular Treatment of Aortic Aneurysms*. Elsevier; 2018.

Scrub Person

The scrub role is most often performed by a surgical technologist but can be performed by a registered nurse. The scrub person establishes and maintains a sterile field and assists the surgeon with passing instrumentation and other sterile items onto the surgical field.[2] The scrub person often anticipates the surgical plan and communicates closely with the surgeon throughout the procedure.

Anesthesia Provider

Anesthesiologists are physicians who evaluate, monitor, and supervise the delivery of anesthesia during a clinical procedure.[7] During the course of the operation, an anesthesiologist or other anesthesia provider such as a certified registered nurse anesthetist and certified anesthesiologist assistant monitor vital signs, perform patient assessments, administer medications, and oversee the patient's physical well-being.

Surgeon

The surgeon is responsible for the preoperative diagnosis of the patient, for performing the operation, and for overseeing postoperative care and treatment.[8] Typically, the surgeon leads the team to ensure that cooperation and collaboration are optimal in caring for the patient and that safe practices are implemented.

First Assistant

The first assistant role can be filled by a registered nurse first assistant, an advance practice provider (e.g., nurse practitioner, physician assistant, or clinical nurse specialist), or a certified surgical assistant. The role requires knowledge of surgical physiology and tissue handling and manipulation. The first assistant works under the direct supervision of the surgeon and performs technical tasks such as holding open incisions, controlling bleeding, and closing incisions. In addition to collaborating with the surgeon in the operating room, the duly credentialed first assistant also actively participates in preoperative and postoperative care.

PREPARING FOR A PROCEDURE
Informed Consent

Informed consent is gained through a process of communication between a provider and a patient, not through a signature on a form.[9] The informed consent establishes a mutual understanding between the patient and the provider about the risks and benefits of and the alternative options to a proposed procedure.[9] To enhance patient safety, the following efforts are recommended by The Joint Commission[9]:

- Encourage active patient participation in obtaining the consent, ask open-ended questions, and encourage the patient to ask questions.
- Ensure that the patient comprehends the event to which the patient is consenting.
- Use everyday language; do not assume the patient understands the medical terminology on the consent form.
- A signature on a consent form alone is not sufficient for informed consent.
- Give the patient time to consider the information provided.

Patient Skin Antisepsis

Removing soil and microorganisms from the patient's skin prior to surgery reduces the risk of the patient developing a surgical site infection.[2] This is accomplished using several methods, including preoperative bathing, proper hair removal by clipping, not shaving, the hair; and the application of an antiseptic product to the skin around the surgical site. The most commonly used skin antisepsis products are povidone–iodine (Betadine), iodine-based alcohol (Dura-prep), chlorhexidine gluconate, and chlorhexidine gluconate in 70% isopropyl alcohol (ChloraPrep). In some cases, the type of antiseptic product is chosen based on the procedure type and the surgeon's preference.[2]

A non-scrubbed perioperative team member applies the skin antiseptic using sterile technique in the operating room. It is important to allow the antiseptic to dry for the full time recommended in the manufacturer's instructions for use before sterile drapes are applied.[2] Allowing for the full drying time improves the efficacy of the product, protects the patient's skin, and decreases the risk for a surgical fire.[2]

Patient Positioning

The circulating nurse guides the efforts for proper patient positioning to provide exposure of the surgical site, maintain the patient's comfort and privacy, provide access to venous access lines and monitoring equipment, allow for airway maintenance, maintain circulation, and prevent undue stress on pressure points.[2] The surgeon and anesthesia provider may have additional positioning requirements based on the location of the surgery and the need for safe access to the patient's airway. Failure to properly position a patient can result in serious injuries from compression or stretching, leading to nerve damage and ischemic changes from reduced blood flow.[2]

The perioperative team is familiar with proper positioning for a variety of surgical positions, including supine, Trendelenburg, reverse Trendelenburg, lithotomy, jackknife, semi-Fowler, high Fowler, Sims, lateral, and prone. Select examples can be found in Figures 20.3 and 20.4. Additionally, the perioperative team is familiar with a variety of positioning devices to aid in achieving or maintaining the required position and ensuring patient safety, such as foam or gel positioners and positioning straps.

The circulating nurse can ensure patient privacy during positioning by keeping doors closed, limiting traffic into the room, and exposing only the area of the patient's body that is necessary to provide care. Patients who are obese or have disabilities may present additional challenges during positioning. The circulating nurse can advocate for the patient by creating an environment of respect and sensitivity.[2]

Special considerations are taken for pregnant patients to displace the uterus to the left to prevent supine hypotensive

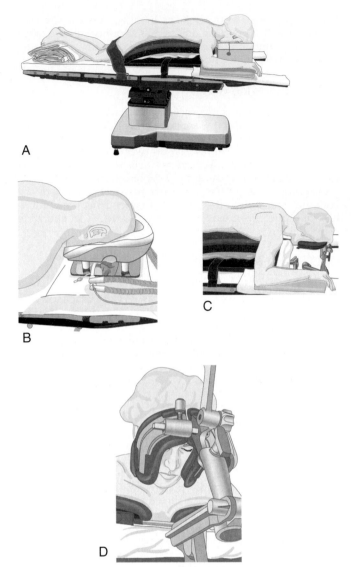

Fig. 20.4 Prone position with Wilson frame. Thompson JL. Positioning for anesthesia and surgery. Figure 23.6 in: Nagelhout JJ, Elisha S, eds. *Nurse Anesthesia*. Elsevier, 2018.

syndrome.[2] In addition, patients with risk factors for pressure injuries should be appropriately protected from undue pressure.[10]

> **Evidence-Based Practice: What is the best intraoperative position for obese patients?**
> When possible, place obese patients in a 30-degree reverse Trendelenburg position to improve lung volume and pulmonary compliance. A ramped position with the head elevated facilitates mask ventilation and increases chances for correct placement of an endotracheal tube.[10]

SPECIMEN MANAGEMENT

There are a variety of laboratory studies used for intraoperative specimens, such as histologic (tissues), microbiologic (cultures), cytologic (cells), hematologic (blood), and immunohematologic (transfusion or /antibody–antigen) tests. There are also a variety of specimen classifications, such as fresh, frozen, biopsy, culture, forensic, and gross examinations.

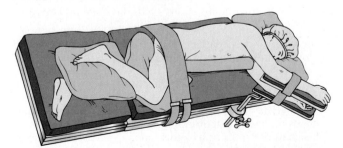

Fig. 20.3 Lateral decubitus position. Thompson JL. Positioning for anesthesia and surgery. Figure 23.9 in: Nagelhout JJ, Elisha S, eds. *Nurse Anesthesia*. Elsevier, 2018.

It is critical for surgical specimens to be handled appropriately. Mishandling of specimens can result in a patient not getting a timely or accurate diagnosis. Lost or improperly collected specimens can lead to additional surgeries being performed. Potential errors can arise when specimens are improperly collected, incorrectly labeled, or incorrectly preserved (e.g., in the wrong preservative or solution) or when there is a delay in transporting them to the laboratory. To mitigate potential specimen errors, follow the five rights of specimen handling:[2]

- Right patient
- Right laboratory test or preservative
- Right time and date of collection
- Right surgeon
- Right specimen

Specimen containers must be labeled with two patient identifiers, the specimen's name, the specimen site, the date of excision, and a biohazard label.[2] A standardized process should be developed for preserving various specimen types. Staff in the ambulatory setting collaborate with a pathologist and the surgeon to create a facility policy. The policy should include directions for when to use preservatives or chemical additives such as formalin to preserve the specimen tissue.

SURGICAL COUNTS

Surgical counts are necessary to ensure patient safety and prevent unintentional retention of an item such as a soft goods item (sponges, towels), instrument, sharp (suture needles, Bovie tips, blades), or small miscellaneous items. The most frequently retained surgical item is the cotton gauze surgical sponge.[11] The most common sites of retention are the abdomen or pelvis, the vagina, and the chest.[11] Some surgical supplies are extremely small, such as micro sutures which are as fine as a human hair and about the size of an eyelash. Given the small size of this suture in a surgical field that also contains blood and irrigation fluids, it may get overlooked, and one can see why performing a surgical count of such items is essential.

Surgical counts should be visibly observed and audibly counted concurrently by two members of the perioperative team, often the circulating nurse and the scrub person. Additional safety considerations during the count include the recording of each category counted (e.g., sponges, sutures) before moving on to the next category of items, the prohibiting of nonessential conversation during the count, and the need to restart the count if an interruption occurs.[2,12] Counts of sponges, sharps, and instruments should be documented in the intraoperative record.[12] Factors contributing to sentinel events involving retained items usually include the failure to follow institutional policy or industry guidelines, poor communication, a fast-paced environment, and the competence of the surgical team.[11,13]

INTRAOPERATIVE SAFETY CONCERNS
Universal Protocol

The Universal Protocol is a method of preventing surgery on the wrong site, the wrong procedure from being performed, and the wrong person having surgery.[14] The Universal Protocol consists of three steps: a preprocedural verification process, the marking of the procedure site, and the performing of a timeout.[14] A standardized process should be used to ensure this protocol is followed for every patient for every procedure. In addition to the steps of the Universal Protocol for preventing surgical errors, many facilities employ a presurgical safety checklist. The checklist often reviews crucial safety elements such as the removal of jewelry, the presence of dentures, the compliance of a preoperative history and physical examination, and the documentation that a responsible individual can be contacted on the patient's behalf postoperatively, to name a few (Figure 20.5).

The preprocedural verification process helps to address any discrepancies before starting the procedure and is often performed in the preoperative area. This process should involve the patient and verify the correct procedure, for the correct patient, at the correct site.[14]

Marking the procedure site is essential when there is the potential for more than one possible location. Ideally the site should be marked by the person performing the procedure, and this practice is driven by facility policies.[14] The site should be marked before the procedure is performed and include the patient's verification when possible. The mark should not be ambiguous and the protocol for marking should be used consistently throughout the organization.[14] The site mark needs to remain visible after the application of the skin preparation and draping.[14]

A timeout should be conducted immediately before the incision is made or the start of the procedure with all members of the surgical team present. During the timeout, all team members should agree, at a minimum, on the correct patient identity, the correct surgical site, and the correct procedure to be done.[14] This can be verified by including the actual surgical consent that describes the planned procedure. The procedure should not be started until all questions or concerns are resolved. Many facilities also utilize a postoperative debriefing process before the patient leaves the operating room. This tool verifies the consensus of the team that the correct procedure on the correct site was done on the correct patient.

Surgical Fire

A surgical fire can occur on a patient's skin or hair, surgical drapes, an airway, or a piece of equipment. The incidence of a surgical fire is low, but the injury to a patient could be severe.[15] All members of the surgical team should be aware of the causes and implications of a surgical fire.

Surgical fires occur when an oxidizer (e.g., oxygen, nitrous oxide), a fuel source (e.g., skin prep, surgical drapes), and an ignition source (e.g., electrosurgery unit, laser, fiberoptic lights) are present.[15] These three components are known as the *fire triangle* or *fire triad*. Strategies to prevent and extinguish fires are based on controlling the three elements of the fire triangle.[15]

A fire risk assessment should be performed for each patient. All of the surgical team members need to discuss the potential fire risk and the plans to manage the risk. In many facilities, this communication occurs as part of The Universal Protocol.

Strategies to control ignition sources include[2]:

- Storing the electrosurgery unit in a holder
- Placing light sources on a rubber mat
- Keeping drapes and linens away from activated electrosurgery units, lasers, or light sources.

Strategies to control fuels include[2]:

- Preventing the skin prep from pooling
- Ensuring that the drying time recommended by the manufacturers' instructions for use has been met
- Removing any prep-soaked materials
- Using water-soluble gel to cover facial hair.
  Strategies to control oxidizers include[2]:
- Checking anesthesia circuits for leaks prior to the start of the procedure

Surgical Safety Checklist

World Health Organization | Patient Safety
A World Alliance for Safer Health Care

Before induction of anaesthesia	Before skin incision	Before patient leaves operating room
(with at least nurse and anaesthetist)	(with nurse, anaesthetist and surgeon)	(with nurse, anaesthetist and surgeon)
Has the patient confirmed his/her identity, site, procedure, and consent? ☐ Yes	☐ **Confirm all team members have introduced themselves by name and role.** ☐ **Confirm the patient's name, procedure, and where the incision will be made.**	**Nurse verbally confirms:** ☐ The name of the procedure ☐ Completion of instrument, sponge and needle counts
Is the site marked? ☐ Yes ☐ Not applicable	**Has antibiotic prophylaxis been given within the last 60 minutes?** ☐ Yes ☐ Not applicable	☐ Specimen labelling (read specimen labels aloud, including patient name) ☐ Whether there are any equipment problems to be addressed
Is the anaesthesia machine and medication check complete? ☐ Yes	**Anticipated critical events**	**To surgeon, anaesthetist and nurse:** ☐ What are the key concerns for recovery and management of this patient?
Is the pulse oximeter on the patient and functioning? ☐ Yes	**To surgeon:** ☐ What are the critical or non-routine steps? ☐ How long will the case take? ☐ What is the anticipated blood loss?	
Does the patient have a:	**To anaesthetist:** ☐ Are there any patient-specific concerns?	
Known allergy? ☐ No ☐ Yes	**To nursing team:** ☐ Has sterility (including indicator results) been confirmed? ☐ Are there equipment issues or any concerns?	
Difficult airway or aspiration risk? ☐ No ☐ Yes, and equipment/assistance available	**Is essential imaging displayed?** ☐ Yes ☐ Not applicable	
Risk of >500 ml blood loss (7 ml/kg in children)? ☐ No ☐ Yes, and two IVs/central access and fluids planned		

This checklist is not intended to be comprehensive. Additions and modifications to fit local practice are encouraged.   Revised 1 / 2009   © WHO, 2009

Fig. 20.5 Surgical safety checklist. From the World Health Organization (WHO): WHO surgical safety checklist (website), 2009. http://apps. who.int/iris/bitstream/handle/10665/44186/9789241598590_eng_Checklist.pdf;jsessionid=4314C271516C1924525DA0A6BD661033?seque nce=52. (Accessed 19 October 2022).

- Tenting the surgical drapes to allow air flow
- Keeping the oxygen percentage as low as possible for non-intubated patients
- Informing the surgeon when an open oxygen source is being used (e.g., mask, nasal cannula)

Staff should be aware of the location of fire alarm pulls, medical gas shut-offs, and fire extinguishers. Fires should be extinguished as soon as possible to prevent injury to the patient. If it can be done safely, a fire on the patient can be extinguished by using a nonflammable liquid such as saline or water, or by smothering with a towel.[2] Staff in the ambulatory surgery environment, as in any surgical environment, should incorporate regular drills for the prevention of surgical fires, as well as for managing a fire in the event it should occur.

HANDOFF PROCESS

Handoff or handover is an opportunity to exchange critical information when the responsibility for the well-being of the patient is transferred between healthcare providers. Well-conducted, standardized handoff processes can increase communication between perioperative team members and promote patient safety.[2,16] A handoff should occur between the inpatient unit or emergency room staff and the preoperative staff, the preoperative staff and the operating room staff, the operating room staff and the postoperative staff, and any time a healthcare provider switch-out occurs, such as when

one leaves for a break or at the end of the shift. The crucial element of any handoff process includes the opportunity to ask questions and receive answers.

Poor handoffs can result in patient care errors and adverse patient outcomes.[16] Actions contributing to poor handoffs include distractions, interruptions, inadequate preparation, lack of a structured report, production pressure, incomplete exchange of information, and poor interpersonal interactions.[16]

Strategies to ensure a safe and thorough handoff include limiting the discussion to patient-specific information, allowing one person to speak at a time, and keeping distractions and interruptions to a minimum.[2] Use of an evidence-based communication tool can aid in having a standardized process, such as:

- SBAR: situation, background, assessment, recommendation[2]
- I PASS THE BATON: introduction, patient assessment, situation, safety concerns, the background, actions, timing, ownership, next[2]
- SWITCH: surgical procedure, wet, instruments, tissue, counts, have you any questions[2]
- Surgical Patient Safety System (SURPASS) checklist
- World Health Organization (WHO) Surgical Safety checklist

CHAPTER HIGHLIGHTS

- The surgical environment is divided into three primary zones, the unrestricted, semi-restricted, and restricted access areas.

- The perioperative team is intraprofessional and includes, but is not limited to, physicians, registered nurses, surgical technicians, advanced practice providers, and unlicensed assistive personnel.
- The role of the perioperative nurse includes participating in surgical preparation and providing for patient safety using a presurgery safety checklist.
- The role of the perioperative nurse includes maintaining safety and advocacy during the surgery.
- The role of the perioperative nurse includes the safe transfer of care using the principles of patient handoff for communication.

CASE STUDY

James is a 42-year-old white male who came today for surgery. He is wheeled into the surgical suite and prepped for a laparoscopic procedure. The anesthesia provider intubates the patient and begins administering anesthetic gases. The presurgical skin preparation is completed using a standard antiseptic solution. The surgeon is anxious to begin and refuses to wait the full amount of time required for the solution to dry. The procedure begins and the lights inside the operating room are dimmed for better viewing with the scope. During the procedure, the scrub tech announces an issue with an instrument. The surgeon sets the laparoscopic cautery hook down on the surgical drape covering the patient's chest and turns to address the instrument issue. While turning toward the back table, the surgeon inadvertently steps on the cautery pedal. Suddenly, the anesthesia provider announces that she sees smoke coming from the patient's chest area. A small flame is discovered coming from the drape.

- What were the risk factors leading to this event?
- What should be done next?
- Should the surgery be aborted?
- How should the fire be extinguished?
- What are the risks of the fire spreading to the patient's airway or other parts of the body?
- What should be done to contain the fire?
- What are other potential causes of a surgical fire?

REFERENCES

1. U.S. Department of Health and Human Services, Centers for Disease Control and Prevention. Ambulatory surgery data from hospitals and ambulatory surgery centers: United States, 2010. *Natl Health Stat Report*. 2017;102. Available at: https://www.cdc.gov/nchs/data/nhsr/nhsr102.pdf.
2. Association of PeriOperative Registered Nurses (AORN). *Guidelines for Perioperative Practice*. AORN; 2021.
3. Association of PeriOperative Registered Nurses (AORN). *Periop 101: A Core Curriculum. The Perioperative Environment*. AORN; 2022.
4. Berrios-Torres SI, Umscheid CA, Bratzler DW, et al. Centers for Disease Control and Prevention Guideline for the prevention of surgical site infection, 2017. *JAMA Surg*. 2017;152(8):784-791. Available at: https://doi.org/10.1001/jamasurg.2017.0904.
5. Fuchs-Buder T, Settembre N, Schmartz D. Hybrid operating theater. *Anaesthesist*. 2018;67(7):480-487. Available at: https://doi.org/10.1007/s00101-018-0464-z.
6. Jin H, Liu J. Application of the hybrid operating room in surgery: a systematic review. *J Invest Surg*. 2020;35(2):378-389. Available at: https://doi.org/10.1080/08941939.2020.1838004.
7. American Society of Anesthesiologists. *Role of Anesthesiologist*. 2022. Available at: https://www.asahq.org/madeforthismoment/anesthesia-101/role-of-physician-anesthesiologist/.
8. American College of Surgeons. *What is the job description for surgeons?* n.d. Available at: https://www.facs.org/education/resources/medical-students/faq/job-description.
9. The Joint Commission. *Quick Safety 21: Informed consent: More than getting a signature*. 2022. Available at: https://www.jointcommission.org/-/media/tjc/newsletters/quick-safety-21-update-4-4-22.pdf.
10. Carron M, Fakhr BS, Ieppariello G, Foletto M. Perioperative care of the obese patient. *Br J Surg*. 2020;107(2):e39-e55. Available at: https://doi.org/10.1002/bjs.11447.
11. Gibbs VC, Coakley FD, Reines HD. Preventable errors in the operating room: retained foreign bodies after surgery—Part I. *Curr Probl Surg*. 2007;44(5):281-337. Available at: https://doi.org/10.1067/j.cpsurg.2007.03.002.
12. Association of Surgical Technologists (AST). *Recommended Standard of Practice for Counts*. 2014. Available at: https://www.ast.org/uploadedFiles/Main_Site/Content/About_Us/Standard Counts.pdf.
13. Warwick VR, Gillespie BM, McMurray AM, Clark-Burg KG. The patient, case, individual and environmental factors that impact on the surgical count process: an integrative review. *J Perioper Nurs*. 2019;32(3):9-19. Available at: http://dx.doi.org/10.26550/2209-1092.1057.
14. The Joint Commission. *The Universal Protocol*. 2022. Available at: https://www.jointcommission.org/standards/universal-protocol/.
15. Ehrenwerth J, Wahr JA, Nussmeier NA. *Fire Safety in the Operating Room*. UptoDate. 2021. Available at: https://www.uptodate.com/contents/fire-safety-in-the-operating-room#!.
16. Lorinc A, Henson C. All handoffs are not the same: What perioperative handoffs do we participate in and how are they different? *APSF Newsletter*. 2017;32(2):29-33. Available at: https://www.apsf.org/article/all-handoffs-are-not-the-same-what-perioperative-handoffs-do-we-participate-in-and-how-are-they-different/.

21 Diverse Care Considerations in the Perianesthesia Patient

Rachel Moses, MSN, RN, CPAN

LEARNING OBJECTIVES

A review of the content of this chapter will help the reader to:

1. Describe cultural competence.
2. Identify opportunities to improve care delivery for patients with diverse religious or gender backgrounds.
3. Discuss mental health issues impacting the safe planning of care.
4. Identify nursing care for specific diverse clinical presentations.

OVERVIEW

Every patient who enters through the doors of a surgery center has a particular set of needs. Each one has an individual set of circumstances affecting their outlook, their concerns, and even their medical diagnoses. These needs can be based on a patient's cultural upbringing, location in the social hierarchy, experiences with personal relationships, and any number of circumstances they have experienced throughout their lives.

This chapter delves into a few of the specific considerations that can affect how a patient progresses through the perioperative experience. This text should be understood as the briefest of overviews and should not be taken as a comprehensive assessment. It is the obligation of each perianesthesia registered nurse to maintain cultural and social competencies and to continue educating themselves to ensure that they are always giving the most sensitive care to their patients. Each institution should have yearly competencies directed at updating staff on institutional and best practice policies as they relate to diversity.

CULTURAL CONSIDERATIONS

Healthcare is practiced in an increasingly diverse and exponentially expanding sphere. Over the last century, the world has become an incredibly interconnected place in which healthcare workers are expected to give culturally sensitive care to every patient with whom they interact. This can be challenging given that caregivers are as diverse as their patient populations, and no clinician can possibly have been previously exposed to each and every culture that they will care for over their careers.

Over the past few decades, schools and care organizations have begun to recognize the importance of *cultural competency*.[1] Culture is an incredibly nebulous concept that includes the beliefs, behaviors, customs, arts, and history of a population of people. It encompasses all manner of social constructs that

ultimately influence how children are raised, the societal values they are taught to uphold, and how they care for each other. Cultures may be bound by geography, as in American Appalachia; limited to specific religious groups, such as Hasidic Jews; or informed by social commonalities, as in the lesbian, gay, bisexual, transgender, or queer (LGBTQ+) community. Regardless of its origins or demographics, each culture is unique in its combination of beliefs, attitudes, and values.

To best understand how a caregiver is affected by culture, it is important to recognize the multiple layers that exist within a society. Each patient has a defined culture in which they were raised, and each medical professional does as well. The race, religion, and socioeconomic status of the home in which an individual is raised has an impact on every belief system formed as an adult. The medical field itself is made up of a myriad of microcultures. Each job delineation (doctor, nurse, phlebotomist) creates an overarching culture, and each specialization within that designation creates its own microcosm of expectations, behaviors, and norms.[1] A nurse in the intensive care unit often has a different demeanor and outlook on patient care than a labor and delivery nurse, and both have different ways of treating patients than a neurosurgeon.

Cultural Competencies

Cultural competence is a complex idea. It would be easy to think that cultural competence is simply having knowledge of different cultures. In healthcare, however, this idea encompasses not only the knowledge one must have of another culture, but also one's ability to give a patient care that is congruent with their cultural beliefs.[1] Cultural competence requires that a caregiver possess cultural knowledge, awareness, sensitivity, and respect. Cultural knowledge is simply an acquired knowledge base about other cultures. Cultural awareness is the caregiver's ability to recognize outward signs of cultural affiliations. Cultural sensitivity involves the altering of the caregiver's approach to patient care depending on the patient's cultural beliefs or practices.[1] Above all, cultural competence requires a willingness to respect different cultural values and practices, whether or not they are shared by the caregiver.

It is the responsibility of medical professionals to question their own beliefs, perceptions, and prejudices. Caregivers should actively practice introspection, identifying biases that might affect how they perceive patients of different cultures. In an ideal world, once a bias is identified it should be removed. This is not so simple in practice. Many beliefs are deeply ingrained and sometimes even integral to a person's identity. The goal of introspection is to identify these biases and consider their impact and influence on patient care. The most that any caregiver can do is to strive to be better and to learn more each day. That drive for self-improvement is necessary to provide culturally competent care, and it is a quality that patients recognize. Maintaining that drive is a constant process. Biases must be constantly revisited and reevaluated to ensure that awareness is maintained.

Cultural Healthcare Disparities

It is important to recognize that healthcare disparities are prevalent in societies around the world, including in the United States. Typically, healthcare disparities point to an individual's inability to access or receive appropriate healthcare attributable to a specific feature or characteristic of each individual. Researchers have described the problem succinctly: "Race or ethnicity, sex, sexual identity, age, disability, socioeconomic status, and geographic location all contribute to an individual's ability to achieve good health."[1] Healthcare disparities are linked to poor patient outcomes. Healthy People 2020 specifically targeted the goal of reducing health disparities, recognizing the alarming health inequities caused by them. Some studies show a continued lack of progress toward this goal, with wide gaps noted in immigrant/refugee and ethnic minority healthcare goals.[2,3]

The Joint Commission (TJC) is a healthcare regulatory body from which healthcare organizations must seek accreditation for certain reimbursement structures. It is the expectation of TJC that healthcare organizations respect patient rights, including reasonable accommodations for cultural or religious beliefs.[4] This expectation aligns with the Healthy People 2020 goal of decreasing health disparities related to race. Healthcare organizations are expected to educate their staff in providing culturally competent care to meet TJC standards.[4]

RELIGIOUS DIVERSITY

Religion can be a characteristic of a larger population or it can be the basis of a culture in and of itself. Culturally competent care must include religious sensitivity. This is a complex concept, as several religions have various restrictions on how and what type of care can be given by medical providers. Providers sometimes dismiss a patient's religious beliefs, yet religion and spirituality factor heavily into the decisions many patients make about the medical care they receive. Different religions may have different expectations of dietary choices, clothing choices, and medication use. Some may prohibit certain medical procedures. Providers must address religious concerns with sensitivity and caution if they are to have any chance of forming a strong relationship with patients and improving their outcomes.[4] Healthcare providers should use the same sensitivity in addressing religious concerns related to healthcare as they would cultural or social concerns. Patients should still be given all the medical information necessary to their care even when it conflicts with their religious beliefs, but the choices they make based on their religious convictions should be respected by all members of the health care team.

Medical Considerations Related to Religion

Clinical concerns and interventions can be broken down by specific religion. One of the more common religious clinical concerns encountered by medical providers is the refusal of blood and blood products, a practice often observed by Jehovah's Witnesses. In such a case, patients' requests that they not be administered blood products should be readily identified on their charts. Some facilities have even begun labeling patient identification bands with this information to further prevent errors. Additionally, these patients should be offered blood refusal declination forms listing all forms of blood products or derivatives that might be necessary, and patients should be allowed to choose any that are acceptable to them. A blood derivative such as albumin might be acceptable to a patient, even if red blood cells are not. To further accommodate these patients, providers can give preoperative support with use of medications such as epoetin alfa vials to stimulate red blood cells or iron supplements to effectively prepare for surgery. Some surgeries can utilize blood-saving techniques in which the patient's own blood can be preserved and returned to the patient at the conclusion of surgery. Such options should be discussed with patients in full so that they may decide if they wish to utilize them. It should be noted that this is only an example, and not all Jehovah's Witness patients find these alternatives acceptable.[5]

Certain religious adherents have clothing requirements, including Muslims and Sikhs. If this clothing is required to be removed, caregivers should ensure that it is replaced at the earliest opportunity that does not impede medical care. For example, a Hijab removed before thyroid surgery because it could easily be displaced when surgical site assessments take place, may be replaced after the surgery is complete. This respects the cultural tradition while maintaining safe patient care. Religious adherents with dietary restrictions include Hindus (typically vegetarian), Seventh Day Adventists (vegetarian, alcohol, and caffeine prohibited), Jewish people (pork and shellfish prohibited, Kosher-certified foods required), and Muslims (pork, alcohol, and shellfish prohibited). Some religions, including Islam, Hinduism, and Seventh Day Adventist, may observe periods of fasting. Religion can also affect pregnancy and birth control beliefs and the acceptance of organ transplantation, as well as death and dying practices.

COMMUNICATION AND LANGUAGE CONSIDERATIONS

Effective communication is critical at every stage of the perioperative period. Healthcare providers must be able to effectively communicate with their patients if they hope to facilitate good patient outcomes. Poor communication has been shown to lead to poor health outcomes, including an increased risk of hospitalization.[6] It is important to remember that communication involves not only the spoken or written word; it also involves the ability to understand the information given. Multiple factors contribute to a patient's ability to understand instructions. The following section presents a few instances where simple adjustments on the part of the provider ensure effective patient communication.

Hearing, Vision, and Speech

Some patients present with physical impediments to communication, such as vision or hearing loss. Patients with vision impairments can be given instructions in ways that accommodate their degree of sight. If patients can see well enough to read, ensure that all written instructions are in large print and that patients have their glasses nearby when instructions are given. If the person is blind, instructions can be read out loud. Additional important information given them at discharge can be in written form and given to a family member or friend, but this limits the patient's autonomy and ability to carry out self-care. A better option is to send instructions electronically, so that patients can access them with their own e-reading devices and refer to their own plan of care whenever they wish.

Patients with hearing loss also require interventions based on their level of hearing. Hard-of-hearing individuals should be given instructions in a quiet place with low environmental noise. Ensure that their hearing aids, if they use them, are in place and working. Some patients who do not have hearing-enhancing devices might visualize the speaker's mouth to enable lip reading. Deaf patients, just like non-English-speaking patients, should be offered a qualified medical sign language interpreter. These interpreters must either be present in person or through video conferencing to effectively translate speech. It is important to note that although someone is deaf, it does not necessarily mean that sign language is that person's preferred communication method. The person may use sign language to communicate, lip reading to understand what others are saying, and speech to communicate back. Each person is different, and the caregiver should ask and be sensitive to the communication preferences.

Communication is the ability to both receive and express information. Communication requires both input and output. Some patients have difficulty expressing ideas through speech. This can be due to aphasia in patients with residual stroke symptoms; surgical changes to the throat and larynx; new tracheostomies or postsurgical jaw banding or wiring; and a myriad of other causes. Patients who have long-standing reasons might come with an assistive device of their own, such as a cell phone or computer with a text-to-talk feature. Others whose conditions are more temporary should be given a pen and paper so that they can communicate their wishes and needs to the caregiver. Make sure that the patient's literary status is known. If a patient is unable to read or write, giving them a pen and paper to write will likely cause stress and inhibit rather than help communication.

Literacy and Health Literacy

An alarming 40% of adults are illiterate, with limited ability to understand written materials.[1] While overall literacy rates in the United States have improved over recent years, some patients still have a limited ability to read and write. Patients who have a high verbal fluency can in fact mask a limited literacy.[6] Even patients who can read and write might be stymied if the reading level is above their own level. Manuscripts or documents that use a great deal of medical jargon can impede understanding. This leads to poor adherence to instructions and can lead to poor patient outcomes.

It is critically important that caregivers not only assess a patient's understanding of written documents and forms to be signed, but also that the information is understood by the patient and family.[1] Proficiency in health literacy, the ability of an individual to understand and access materials related to healthcare, is less than sufficient in 88% of adults.[1] Many vulnerable patients are at risk for low health literacy. Older adults, minorities, individuals with a low socioeconomic status, and those who are medically underserved are more likely to struggle to understand medical instructions. Healthcare is a complex world, and patients' abilities to navigate it affect the care they receive. People with limited health literacy have been shown to use emergency services more often and to return within two weeks more frequently than those with high health literacy. Low health literacy of parents or guardians has also been proven to impact children's health adversely.[6] Caregivers must ensure not only that their teaching is understood but also that the materials provided are at an appropriate reading level that is accessible to those with a limited health literacy.

Improving health communication—and health literacy—was a goal of Healthy People 2020.[7] When the goals of Healthy People 2020 were evaluated, no improvement was found. Healthy People 2030 has reinstated the goal of increasing health communication. The recommendation is that providers use teach-back methods when educating patients; doing so engages patients and ensures that they understand the instructions given. It is also recommended that providers engage in shared decision making with their patients. These recommendations have the aim of improving health communication and thereby improving patient outcomes.[7]

Primary and Secondary Language Considerations

Language plays a critical role in all patient interactions in the healthcare system. It is one of the most important tools for ensuring that patients understand instructions about their care. While English is the most prominent language in the United States, Americans speak and sign hundreds of languages. It is essential that competent interpreters be used for all verbal instructions and that written materials be available in the patient's primary language.[1] Family members and caregivers should not be excluded from patient education. It is just as important for them to understand the steps in care as it is for the patient, particularly if they will be involved in the patient's recovery process, and interpreters should be used if the family is not fluent in English. It is a rule in most healthcare organizations that licensed medical interpreters be used. Family and friends are not acceptable alternatives unless they have signed an appropriate declination. Be sure to understand the expectations of the healthcare organization before utilizing a family member as an interpreter.

CONSIDERATIONS ABOUT GENDER AND SEXUALITY

Clinicians are now beginning to understand that they are caring for patients with a diverse set of personal identities. Education on gender expression and sexuality is becoming widely recognized by physician and nursing training centers around the world as a critical patient care competency.[8] Unfortunately, most nurses and physicians who completed formal education more than a few years ago missed this crucial education.[8] Regardless of the healthcare practice's size, all caregivers will eventually end up treating a patient with an identity with which they are unfamiliar. A knowledge gap in this area can create barriers to care, result in harmful or ineffective treatment regimes, and further jeopardize a medically vulnerable population.

Although cultural competency and sensitivity were referred to earlier in this chapter, it is important here to touch specifically on cultural humility. *Cultural humility* is the concept that no matter how much information a caregiver may learn about a culture, every individual within that culture experiences it in a personal way.[8] Caregivers must continue to be self-reflective of their own bias and must avoid making assumptions about individuals.[8] The focus should always be on providing patient- and family-centered care by meeting the unique needs of the individual patient. While cultural competency can support meeting those needs, each patient has an individual identity and experiences their culture in ways that affect the care they need.[8]

Definitions of Gendered Terms

There are several definitions that might be unfamiliar to clinicians when caring for persons within this population. Definitions can change or mean different things to different people within this community. Caregivers who are unfamiliar with its verbiage should check with patients to clarify the meaning of terms and ensure they understand what patients mean. Table 21.1 gives a brief overview of some of the more common definitions used by this population.

The Importance of Gender and Sexuality Competencies

Estimates vary for the number of people living in the United States who are in the LGBTQ+ community. The Williams

TABLE 21.1 LGBTQ+ Definitions

Gender identity	A person's inner sense of who they are, be it male, female, nonbinary, or having no gender
Gender binary	The concept that there are only two genders (male and female) and that every person must be either one or the other
Sex	Termed "sex assigned at birth," this is the sex an infant is assigned based on physical or biologic characteristics seen at birth
LGBTQ+	Acronym used to describe the community of lesbian, gay, bisexual, transgender, and queer or questioning; additionally encompassing any other form of gender or sexuality expression not explicitly mentioned outside of the binary structure
Lesbian	A sexual orientation that describes a woman who is primarily emotionally or physically attracted to people of the same gender
Gay	Someone who is emotionally or physically attracted to someone within the same gender; often used to describe men who are attracted to men, although the term is more widely encompassing
Transgender	A person whose birth-assigned sex is incongruent with their gender identity; while often this is associated with a binary gender (transgender male, transgender female), it can encompass gender fluid or nonbinary persons, as well
Queer	Can be a term encompassing multiple different gender expressions and sexualities; additionally seen in "gender queer," which describes those whose gender identity falls outside of traditional gender binaries; has been used as a slur against gender-nonconforming persons, but in recent history has begun to be reclaimed by members of the LGBTQ+ community
Asexual	A person who feels little or no sexual attraction to another person regardless of gender
Nonbinary	Gender identity that allows individual expression of gender outside of traditional or "binary" expression
Assigned female/male at birth	Indicates birth sex, typically assigned based on anatomic or biologic features; abbreviated AFAB (assigned female at birth) or AMAB (assigned male at birth)
Intersex	A varied group of medical congenital conditions in which sexual anatomy develops outside of the expected female/male development patterns
Gender-affirming chest surgery	In the slang, described as "top surgery"; this is a gender-affirming surgery that involves bilateral mastectomies for those AFAB who do not identify as female
Gender-affirming genital surgery	Any surgery that helps to align a person's genitals or internal reproductive organs to their gender identity (can include removal or creation of different structures); in slang, described as "bottom surgery"
Misgender	Referring to someone by a gender (or using gendered language terms such as "Sir" or "Ms.") that indicates a gender different than the person's identity

National LGBTGIA+ Health Education Center. LGBTQIA+ glossary of terms for health care teams. https://www.lgbtqiahealtheducation.org/publication/lgbtqia-glossary-of-terms-for-health-care-teams/. Published February 3, 2020. Accessed July12, 2021. Derived from https://www.lgbtqiahealtheducation.org/wp-content/uploads/2020/10/Glossary-2020.08.30.pdf

Institute estimates that 0.6% of the population, or around 1.6 million people, identify as LGBTQ+.[9] Population estimates of gender-nonconforming (GNC) adults are difficult to accurately calculate. Few surveys of demographics, including those done by the U.S. government, contain questions related to sexuality and gender expression. In recent years, 27 states and Guam have added survey questions on the Behavioral Risk Factor Surveillance System (BRFSS) related to gender expression and sexuality.[10] These states have also agreed to publicize data through the Centers for Disease Control and Prevention (CDC), but even these estimates are lacking.[10] The BRFSS survey is only given to noninstitutionalized adults who have phone access and agree to answer survey questions over the phone.[10] This not only misses information from the other 23 states that do not participate, but it also excludes those experiencing a housing crisis, those without phone access, and anyone who is not comfortable sharing information about their sexuality over the phone.[10]

There are a variety of reasons that persons who are GNC tend to be hesitant with regard to sharing information about sexuality and gender. This population is vulnerable to violence, which occurs at alarmingly high rates. In a study of transgender individuals, as many as 10% reported physical violence from family members and 8% had become homeless after disclosing their sexuality.[11] In addition, 30% of transgender respondents had experienced homelessness at some point

in their lives. In the workplace, 19% reported employment discrimination (e.g., not being hired for jobs, being fired from jobs, or being denied promotions) based on their gender identity. Sexual assault was reported by 47%. Of those who sought public services (e.g., transportation, drug/alcohol treatment centers, restaurants, gyms), 31% reported discrimination or poor treatment. Nearly 20% avoided accessing public services altogether for fear of discrimination. An astounding 59% avoided use of public restrooms because of previous negative experiences.[11]

These barriers extend to medical care for LGBTQ+ individuals. Sexual minorities experience higher rates of being uninsured, are less likely to have regular medical caregivers, and are more likely to avoid or put off necessary medical procedures than their gender-conforming counterparts.[12] They often have poorer access to care, with these gaps in care widening if they also belong to a racial minority.[12] LGBTQ+ persons have increased rates of morbidity and mortality, higher risks of certain illnesses, higher rates of tobacco and illegal substance use, and almost double the rate of suicide as compared their heterosexual counterparts.[8]

When that population is narrowed to only those who identify as transgender, 40% state that they have attempted suicide in their life; in the general population that rate is only 4.6%.[10] Transgender persons experience profound medical discrimination, with 33% reporting negative healthcare interactions (including treatment refusal, harassment, assault, and needing to teach their providers about transgender care), and these negative reports increase for disabled people and persons of color.[11] These statistics are alarming. Clinicians should actively strive to mitigate these barriers, educating themselves on both best practices and cultural sensitivity. By conscientiously identifying personal bias, caregivers can avoid having another negative medical experience for this marginalized population.

Care Considerations

When caring for someone in the LGBTQ+ community, the first question that should be asked is "How would you like me to address you?" While it is common practice to ask patients what they prefer to be called, it is particularly important in these interactions. A GNC person's given name can be associated with a gender with which they no longer affiliate. They may have chosen a name that more closely matches their identity than their legal name does. As with any other patient, patient satisfaction is increased when caregivers refer to them according to their preference.[13] Across all care environments and with every patient population, the appropriate way to refer to a patient is to use what the patient chooses.

Along with naming considerations, asking a patient what pronouns they prefer is particularly important. As discussed, patients in the LGBTQ+ community can feel alienated and unwelcome in medical settings. By asking patients what their pronouns are and then using those pronouns, the caregiver shows patients that they are in a safe, inclusive environment where they can feel comfortable receiving care.[13] A patient who is nonbinary may request to be referred to as "they, them," while a transgender woman might prefer "she, her." There is not a specific guide to say what pronouns a patient will use. The only important rule to remember is that the patient's pronouns are whatever the patient says. Asking for a patient's pronouns during the check-in process and charting those preferences in the medical record or reporting them during a verbal handoff is important.[8,13]

Most people are taught pronoun usage from a young age. Variations in how they are used can feel cumbersome to speakers unfamiliar with this community. While it seems inevitable that mistakes will be made, the caregiver should make every attempt to name and gender the patient appropriately and have a plan in place for what to do when mistakes are made. Apologizing for errors is an automatic response—and, indeed, a respectful one—but it is not always the most helpful in this setting. Apologizing for misgendering patients can make patients feel uncomfortable, as if they are inconveniencing the provider, or can force them to minimize something that is critical to their identity. A better response is to say, "Thank you for correcting me" or "Thank you, <insert corrected gender and name>." This allows the patient to be recognized and validated while not drawing undue attention to the error. Clinicians who wish to become more comfortable should practice with a friend or family member, using different pronouns in regular conversation to make it feel more natural. When possible, it is better to practice with someone who does not personally have diverse pronouns. It is the caregiver's responsibility to gain comfort with a population, not that population's responsibility to help the caregiver to feel comfortable.

In general, gendered language remains a common part of the English vernacular. Caregivers would be well served to begin adopting gender-neutral expressions across their practice. Additionally, when discussing chosen names and which pronouns to use, avoid use of the word *preferred*. Stating that a patient has "preferred" pronouns can indicate that the patient made a choice in their gender or sexuality instead of simply using the name or pronouns that most identify with their gender. This is a nuanced difference, but it is important when showing an otherwise vulnerable population that they are accepted and welcome in the medical care setting.[8] Caregivers should also hold each other responsible and create accountable work environments. If colleagues misgender a patient or use hurtful language, they should be respectfully corrected. Whether it is misgendering a patient, telling insensitive jokes, or using outdated language, an accountable workplace keeps the space comfortable for both patients and co-workers of diverse gender identities.

MENTAL HEALTH CONSIDERATIONS

Mental health conditions also impact perioperative patient care. In most perianesthesia situations, these patients require individualized interventions based on their diagnoses. If patients are unable to meaningfully express their emotional or mental health needs, caregivers should look to family members or guardians for guidance. If neither the patient nor family can offer clinicians any insight, some knowledge can be gleaned from the diagnosis itself. The following sections include some brief insights into the more common mental health diagnoses and guidance for the caregiver on accommodating patients with these experiences.

Mental Health Diagnoses That Affect Care

Mood Disorders

Mental health diagnoses can be categorized into overarching groupings. Mood disorders, for instance, affect a person's ability to regulate both mood and emotions. These disorders can be further divided into three distinct categories: depression, anxiety, and bipolar disorder. Each of these conditions is characterized by distinct symptoms. Management in the perioperative period typically includes completing a thorough health history and managing symptoms. A more in-depth discussion of these disorders follows.

The term *depressive disorder* covers multiple diagnoses, with *major depressive disorder* representing the common presentations. Symptoms must be present for prolonged periods (at least 2 weeks). Characteristic symptoms of this condition include regular and recurrent depressed mood and anhedonia, or loss of interest or pleasure in activities. One of these must be present, along with any five of the following: unintentional weight or appetite loss, sleep dysregulation, fatigue or loss of energy, feelings of excessive guilt or worthlessness, psychomotor agitation or retardation, inability to concentrate or make decisions, suicidal ideations, or passive recurrent thoughts of death.[14]

Anxiety disorders are characterized by fear (a response to a real or perceived threat) and anxiety (the anticipation of a potential or future threat). While the disorders appear to regularly overlap, the diagnosis is typically made based on certain situations or triggers causing a response and the type of response. For example, agoraphobia is the marked fear or anxiety triggered by leaving one's home environment, using public transport, or being in enclosed or wide-open spaces; the environment causes the trigger. In panic disorders, the response is the diagnostic criterion. Panic responses are physical reactions to fear, including but not limited to, racing heartbeats, shaking, sweating, shortness of breath, and chest pain.[14]

Bipolar disorder covers a few conditions, but the most well-known is *bipolar I disorder*, which is demonstrated by cyclical periods of mania followed by periods of hypomania, major depression, and euthymia. Manic episodes last at least 1 week and entail elevated energy or activity levels, mood changes (elevated mood, increased irritability), and an increase in goal-directed activities. Heightened distractibility, an increased display of high-risk behaviors, flights of ideas, grandiosity, and a decreased need for sleep may also be present. Manic episodes are interspersed with periods of hypomania (like mania but of shorter duration), major depressive disorder episodes, and normal or euthymic periods.

The preoperative care and workup of a patient with a mood disorder should include a review of any medications used to treat the illness and asking whether the patient is currently taking the medications, when the last dose was taken, and when the next dose is due. If patients are regularly using benzodiazepines, this should be discussed with the anesthesiologist to allow for bridging medications as necessary. Patients with depression or bipolar disorders may not have acute manifestations in the perioperative period, but those with an anxiety disorder may react strongly and require the use of rescue medications. Surgery and anesthesia are stressful for most people but can be triggering for those with anxiety. Discuss with the patient in the preoperative period how they typically manage anxiety at home. This should be passed on in each handoff report through the continuation of the perioperative period. Guiding patients through breathing exercises and using nonpharmacologic therapeutic techniques should be top interventions for nurses. In severe cases, the anesthesiologist may prescribe medications to decrease anxiety. The patient should be observed carefully, as some of these medications have very long half-lives.

> **Evidence-Based Practice: Suicidality**
> *Multiple mental health disorders have an increased risk of suicide. Certain departments, such as emergency or primary care medicine, regularly screen their patients on arrival for suicidal ideations. Does your facility screen for suicidal ideations? Do you have a policy to follow? What should you do if someone's screen is positive?*

Psychotic Disorders

Psychotic disorders are categorized by variances in one of five categories: delusions, hallucinations, disorganized motor behaviors or thinking, and negative symptoms (e.g., diminished emotional expression, anhedonia, avolition).[14] One of the more familiar psychotic disorders for medical providers is schizophrenia. Schizophrenia typically presents between the late teenage years and the mid-thirties. While mood disturbances may be present, hallucinations, delusions, or disorganized speech must be present for the diagnosis to be made.[14] Globally schizophrenia ranks as one of the top 20 causes of disability.[14] People with schizophrenia have mortality rates two to four times higher than the general population. It is important to address suicidality with all patients, and certainly with schizophrenic patients. Five to six percent of patients who have schizophrenia complete suicide, and almost 20% attempt it over the course of their lives. Psychiatric co-morbidities include substance use disorders, high rates of tobacco use, and an increased prevalence of anxiety and panic disorders, as well as schizotypal or paranoid personality disorders. Medical comorbidities include metabolic, cardiac, and pulmonary disease, as well as obesity and diabetes. This population does not regularly participate in health maintenance, and this can be attributed to some of the aforementioned conditions.[14]

Caring for a patient with a psychotic disorder is complex. Patients are likely taking an antipsychotic medication, and this should be addressed in the comprehensive history prior to proceeding; the last dose taken and next dose due should be noted. The perianesthesia nurse should be aware of co-morbid conditions that could complicate the medical picture. Typically, the most difficult aspect of caring for these patients is accompanying them as they progress through the perioperative period. Increased rates of paranoia, aggression, and, particularly, delusions can render establishing a trusting relationship with these patients difficult. The nurse must persevere to ensure that the information given is accurate, honest, transparent, and calming. Therapeutic communication should be used to attempt to establish a bond of trust between patient and caregiver, which allows the patient to feel safer while progressing through the postoperative period. Avoid prolonged eye contact if the patient is experiencing high levels of paranoia. If a support person is present to whom the patient responds well, consider allowing the person to stay with the patient through the awake periods of the perioperative experience.

Developmental Delay/Syndromes

Autism spectrum disorder is a diagnosis characterized by social deficits related to communication and interaction with repetitive behavioral or thought patterns. It is typically diagnosed early in the developmental period of childhood, though symptoms can be unintentionally masked into adulthood and cause a definable impairment in important areas of independent functioning in the absence of a better-defined intellectual disability. Severity is based on a rating of level 1 to 3, with level 1 "requiring support and level 3 "requiring very substantial support." Communication deficits include verbal and nonverbal deficits. Clinicians might notice limited eye contact, a lack of tonality in speech, or a lack of gestures to accompany speech in patients who are more verbal, but patients span the spectrum from verbal to completely nonverbal patients. These patients may have concurrent sensory sensitivities to light, sound, and touch. Ordinary experiences may provide overwhelming input for patients with these co-morbidities.[14]

Before caring for autism spectrum patients, a perianesthesia nurse should discuss with caregivers the progression of the disorder for the individual patient. Caregivers should be able to inform the nurse of sensory sensitivities to avoid and soothing techniques that the patient utilizes, as well as any problems with communication and how the patient can best communicate. Patients at a high level of functionality may be able to have these conversations with the nursing staff themselves. In cases of severe sensory sensitivities, ensure that the entire team is aware of the plan of care. For example, all should know whether the lights should be lowered; whether the patient should be touched on awakening and, if so, whether a single person should be designated to do so; or whether a quiet area can be found for preoperative care and recovery. Having parents or a guardian present can be helpful in this scenario.

> **Evidence-Based Practice: Experience of Children with Autism**
> Benich et al, conducted a qualitative study to explore the experience of children with autism in the perioperative environment with a goal of identifying opportunities to optimize the experience. Several common challenges were identified including discovery of behavioral triggers, the need for comfort objects, and communication barriers. Interventions that families identified as helpful involved the inclusion of immediate and familiar people around the child as well as recommendation to minimize preoperative waiting times to help keep the child calm. Comfort objects may include specific clothing, toys from home, or digital devices for distraction or communication.

Source: Benich S, Thakur S, Schubart JR, Carr MM. Parental perception of the perioperative experience for children with autism. *AORN J.* 2018;108(1): 34-43. https://doi.org/10.1002/aorn.12274

Intellectually disabled patients, also known as having *intellectual development disorder*, typically have disorders of development that cause deficits in multiple domains. In the conceptual domain, reasoning, problem solving, and abstract thinking may be affected; in the social domain, the ability to interact with peers, produce language, and demonstrate communication skills may be affected; and in the practical domain, developmental milestones may be missed and there may be limitations of functions of daily living. Intellectual disability is not measured by intelligence quotient (IQ) scores; it is measured by the level of adaptive functioning loss described as mild, moderate, severe, or profound. Mild impairments may mean that a patient with a good support network can be fairly independent and make their own decisions, while profound impairments typically mean that the patient is completely physically dependent on other people.[14]

These patients often come in with a family member or caregiver. It is important to know that these patients may appear more independent than they actually are. The nurse should verify if they have a legal guardian who is making their decisions. Appropriate guardianship paperwork must be filed in the medical chart and should be passed on in handoff. These patients might respond better to care with a familiar caregiver at the bedside. Depending on intellectual abilities, some pediatric interventions, such as play therapy and distraction, can be effective in this population. Teaching should be geared to the patient's level unless the patient is unable to effectively learn, in which case teaching should be geared to the caregiver, parent, or guardian.

Delirium: Neuropsychiatric Syndrome

Delirium is a unique diagnosis in that it crosses specialties. Psychiatrists often refer these patients but consider delirium to be a medical diagnosis. Internal medicine doctors, surgeons, hospitalists, and even sometimes anesthesiologists can feel ill-equipped to manage this diagnosis. Delirium is an acute state of confusion, manifesting as disorientation, inattention, hallucinations, and/or delusions.[14] A common complication of anesthesia is emergence or postoperative delirium. Risks for *emergence delirium* include extremes of age, that is, children and elderly persons, who are at high risk; a history of psychiatric disorders; and a history of long-term substance abuse. Additionally, certain medications used during anesthesia can increase the risk of emergence delirium. These medications include benzodiazepines, ketamine, haloperidol, opioids, atropine, metoclopramide, and scopolamine.[15]

Treatment of delirium is dependent on finding and treating the underlying cause. Before doing anything else, the perianesthesia nurse must assess the physical status of the patient for signs of hypoxemia, pain, or bladder distention, which can all cause increased agitation or restlessness in the emergence period. Once physical causes are ruled out, treatment focuses on preventing harm to the patient and those around them. Multiple staff members may be required to help redirect the patient and prevent the patient from dislodging medical equipment. If necessary for patient or staff safety, restraints or anxiolytics might be used. If these are ineffective, sedatives may be required. In this case, the nurse should monitor for hemodynamic, respiratory, and airway stability.[15] Delirium should abate with time, but in some cases, it can last for an extended period. While delirium is uncommon, surgery centers should have a plan in place for how to proceed if a patient has prolonged delirium.

SOCIOECONOMIC CONSIDERATIONS

Each individual's socioeconomic status (SES) affects their health and the healthcare they receive. An individual's SES includes income, housing, employment, insurance, all of the social settings experienced over the course of their lives, and other lifestyle factors. SES has a profound impact on health. Studies completed over the last half century show growing health inequities between those with high and low SESs. People with a low SES have increased rates of morbidity and disability, a higher disease burden, and a higher incidence of co-morbidities than their more economically advantaged counterparts.[16] Some researchers believe SES to be the greatest determinant of health and life expectancy.[17]

Caregivers should consider each individual's SES when preparing patients for surgery and carefully assess social determinants such as food or housing or financial insecurity. The United States is one of the few countries in the world that does not offer universal health care coverage. An estimated 41.3 million people were uninsured in 2013, with an additional 23% of insured adults considered underinsured.[15] A lack of insurance affects a person's health in a number of ways. Both the uninsured and underinsured report struggling to pay medical bills and skipping or delaying necessary medical care (including prescription medications) because of their cost.[15] Nurses involved in surgery planning and intake should be aware of the social services offered by the facility to assist in these situations. Nurses should assess the ability of patients to complete follow-up care as necessary and to reinforce low- or no-cost follow-up options. If the facility includes a social services team, nurses should help initiate a referral for patients and families.

Being unhoused (experiencing homelessness) is a social condition that has a myriad of implications in the perioperative period. Living without shelter is itself a risk factor for injury, illness, and higher mortality rates.[18] Being unhoused is also a condition associated with a great deal of stigma within the medical community, causing patients from this population to feel unwelcome in healthcare settings. This stigma is exacerbated by the prejudices of many medical professionals about medical conditions for which this group is more at risk, such as chronic pain, mental illness, and addiction.[18] Perianesthesia nursing staff should be careful to assess their own biases, evaluating the care they provide with a critical eye and constant questioning of their own practices. They must ask themselves, "Am I being appropriately attentive to patient complaints of pain regardless of the patient's demographics? Am I helping the patient access social services as part of the care I administer?" Though the unhoused population is usually a small percentage of the patients served at an ambulatory surgery center, nurses must remain aware of the special needs of this population and strive to meet those needs in every interaction.

CHAPTER HIGHLIGHTS

- Nurses in an ambulatory surgical setting care for a wide array of patients with a variety of cultural, physical, emotional, and social needs.
- Nurses in an ambulatory surgical setting should be prepared to address these needs in order to effectively care for their patients.
- Nurses must remain committed to exploring and learning about the wide variety of circumstances surrounding best care for patients.

CASE STUDY

A male-presenting patient checks in for surgery under the legal name Molly for a hysterectomy. While completing the check-in, the receptionist asks what the patient's preferred name is, and the patient says it is Jared. The receptionist brings the patient into the preoperative area and tells the nurse, "This is Molly. She's here for a hysterectomy."

How should the nurse respond?

After assuming care of the patient, the nurse asks for the patient's preferred pronouns. The patient uses the pronouns "he/him." The nurse acknowledges these pronouns and conscientiously tries to use them consistently.

When the anesthesiologist comes in, how can the nurse facilitate introducing the patient to ensure that the anesthesiologist is able to verify the patient's identity but also use the patient's chosen name and appropriate pronouns?

Before the patient is taken to surgery, the nurse misgenders the patient when giving the report to the operating room nurse.

What is the most appropriate way to correct the mistake?

If this surgery is part of a transition surgery, what might another term for it be?

REFERENCES

1. Purnell LD, Fenkl EA. *Transcultural Healthcare: A Population Approach.* 5th ed. Springer; 2021.
2. Berge JM, Fertig A, Tate A, Trofholz A, Neumark-Sztainer D. Who is meeting the Healthy People 2020 objectives? Comparisons between racially/ethnically diverse and immigrant children and adults. *Fam Syst Health.* 2018;36(4):451-470. Available at: https://doi.org/10.1037/fsh0000376.
3. Yearby R. Structural racism and health disparities: reconfiguring the social determinants of health framework to include the root cause. *J Law Med Ethics.* 2020;48(3):518-526. Available at: https://doi.org/10.1177/1073110520958876.
4. Swihart DL, Yarrarapu SNS, Martin RL. Cultural religious competence in clinical practice. In: *StatPearls* [Internet]. StatPearls Publishing; 2021. Available at: https://www.ncbi.nlm.nih.gov/books/NBK493216/.
5. Scharman CD, Burger D, Shatzel JJ, Kim E, DeLoughrey TG. Treatment of individuals who cannot receive blood products for religious or other reasons. *Am J Hematol.* 2017;92. 1370-1381. Available at: https://doi.org/10.1002/ajh.24889.
6. Healthy People 2020. *Health Literacy.* Available at: https://www.healthypeople.gov/2020/topics-objectives/topic/social-determinants-health/interventions-resources/health-literacy. Accessed August 01, 2021.
7. Office of Disease Prevention and Health Promotion. *Health Communication.* Available at: https://health.gov/healthypeople/objectives-and-data/browse-objectives/health-communication. Accessed August 01, 2021.
8. Kuzma EK, Graziano C, Shea E, Schaller FV, Pardee M, Darling-Fisher CS. Improving lesbian, gay, bisexual, transgender, and queer/questioning health: using a standardized patient experience to educate advanced practice nursing students. *J Am Assoc Nurse Pract.* 2019;31(12):714-722. Available at: https://doi.org/10.1097/JXX.0000000000000224.
9. UCLA Williams Institute. *How Many Adults and Youth Identify as Transgender in the United States?* 2022. Available at: https://williamsinstitute.law.ucla.edu/publications/trans-adults-united-states/. Accessed September 14, 2022.
10. Gonzales G, Henning-Smith C. Barriers to care among transgender and gender non-conforming adults. *Millbank Q.* 2017;95(4): 726-748. Available at: https://doi.org/10.1111/1468-0009.12297.
11. McDonagh D, Skubish S. Transgender patient care principles in radiation oncology. *Radiation Therapist.* 2019;28(2): 159-177.
12. Hsieh N, Ruther M. Despite increased insurance coverage, non-white sexual minorities still experience disparities in access to care. *Health Aff.* 2017;36(10):1786-1794. Available at: https://doi.org/10.1377/hlthaff.2017.0455.
13. Bernstein SM. The world was not built for us: improving access to care for transgender youths. *Pediatrics.* 2018;142(6):e20182781. Available at: https://doi.org/10.1542/peds.2018-2781.
14. American Psychiatric Association. *Diagnostic and Statistical Manual of Mental Disorders.* 5th ed. 2013.
15. Odom-Forren J. *Drain's Perianesthesia Nursing: A Critical Care Approach.* 7th ed. Elsevier; 2018.
16. Kivimäki M, Batty GD, Pentti J, et al. Association between socio-economic status and the development of mental and physical health conditions in adulthood: a multi-cohort study. *Lancet Public Health.* 2020;5(3):e140-e149. Available at: https://doi.org/10.1016/S2468-2667(19)30248-8.
17. Wang J, Geng L. Effects of socioeconomic status on physical and psychological health: Lifestyle as a mediator. *Int J Environ Res Public Health.* 2019;16(2):281. Available at: https://doi.org/10.3390/ijerph16020281.
18. Gilmer C, Buccieri K. Homeless patients associate clinician bias with suboptimal care for mental illness, addictions, and chronic pain. *J Prim Care Community Health.* 2020;11:2150132720910289. Available at: https://doi.org/10.1177/2150132720910289.

22 Special Needs of Pediatric Patients

Myrna Eileen Mamaril, DNP, RN, NEA-BC, CPAN, CAPA, FAAN, FASPAN

LEARNING OBJECTIVES

A review of the content of this chapter will help the reader to:

1. Describe the relationship of pediatric patients and their families during ambulatory surgery.

2. Summarize important considerations about the pediatric environment of care in ambulatory surgery centers.

3. Compare and contrast the anatomy and physiology of pediatric patients with those of adult patients.

4. Review critical pediatric preoperative risk assessment factors associated with PACU respiratory complications and adverse events.

5. Identify key pediatric patient and family educational strategies for successful ambulatory surgery outcomes.

6. Discuss four pediatric PACU emergencies using the pediatric advanced life support resuscitation interventions.

OVERVIEW

Same-day pediatric surgery has become increasingly popular with patients and families. This practice now extends not only to hospital-based outpatient surgery and free-standing surgery centers, but also to physician–owned, office-based surgery facilities. Ambulatory surgery has clear benefits for hospitals and healthcare providers, but patients and their families also often prefer outpatient surgery for a variety of reasons. Today, there have been tremendous technical advances in surgical procedures and improvements in anesthetic agents and regional techniques for treating pain. The majority of the children undergoing surgery in these facilities are healthy and have few co-morbidities, and usually the surgery involves relatively simple procedures associated with prompt recovery.

In 2015, in an important initiative for ensuring the safety of children, the American Academy of Pediatrics (AAP) generated a policy statement identifying the *Critical Elements for the Pediatric Perioperative Anesthesia Environment*. The goal was to advocate for the quality health care of children undergoing anesthesia for surgical procedures.[1] The AAP identified important requirements of ambulatory surgery centers (ASCs) for the surgical and anesthetic care of infants and children that addressed the administrative, clinical (medical providers and nurses), and operational competencies.

One of the most essential goals for perianesthesia nurses working in ASCs is to foster a therapeutic family-centered relationship. The family-centered care philosophy recognizes that the family is the most important constant in the child's life. Consequently, when the child is having surgery, the entire family is also affected. Perhaps the most outstanding opportunity for these specialized pediatric ambulatory surgery nurses is the holistic involvement they have in every aspect of the young patient's and family's surgical experience from admission to discharge. Minimizing parental separation from their pediatric patients, especially children younger than five years of age, promotes feelings of normalcy and well-being.[2] By continuing to demonstrate respectful nursing communication, perianesthesia nurses genuinely support patients' and their families' cultural, ethnic, spiritual, and socioeconomic strengths along the entire perioperative care continuum, including during the preparations for discharge.

This chapter presents the essential elements needed for providing a safe, competent patient- and family-centered ambulatory surgery care environment. Epidemiologic, physical, cognitive, and psychosocial developmental trends are reviewed, along with the pediatric anatomic and physiologic differences. Multimodal pharmacologic and complementary techniques are explored for the management of pain in this vulnerable population. Most importantly, critical preoperative risk factors in the preparation and assessment of perioperative pediatric patients, as well as complications and adverse events that can occur in the postanesthesia care unit (PACU), are examined. Finally, PACU emergency situations are reviewed by highlighting the 2020 American Heart Association's (AHA) pediatric advanced life support (PALS) guidelines.

CREATING A SAFE PEDIATRIC ASC ENVIRONMENT

Safe Physical ASC Environment

The perianesthesia care environment in which pediatric patients are provided care should have the equipment appropriate for the population being served. The following list of general items should be available for the routine care of pediatric patients: scales showing weights in kilograms for all age groups (e.g., infants, small children, older children, adolescents, and young adults); chair scales that can accommodate wheelchairs; patient lift scales for immobile patients; a bariatric floor scale if indicated; axillary, tympanic, oral, and temporal artery thermometers; various-sized stethoscopes (e.g., infant to adult size); assorted sizes of blood pressure cuffs (e.g., premature infant to large adult sizes); pediatric electrocardiogram (ECG) leads that are easy to attach and remove; a variety of pulse oximeter probes; end-tidal carbon dioxide monitoring equipment if indicated; a readily available anesthesia nerve block cart; emergency medications (e.g., dantrolene sodium and a dosage chart for malignant hyperthermia); malignant hyperthermia cart and pediatric code cart; pediatric medication dosage charts; appropriately sized pediatric pajamas or gowns; assorted diaper sizes and scales for weighing urine output; gowns, gloves, and masks for children for whom isolation precautions have been implemented (e.g., consider disposable thermometers and/or designated stethoscopes for these children); items for distraction, such as televisions, books, games, and toys (e.g., age-appropriate toys without small pieces) that are nonallergenic and washable; rocking chairs, pillows, and footstools for caregivers who are holding children; safe seating for family members; access to a breast pump and related supplies for nursing mothers; and changing

---

BOX 22.1 Equipment Suggested for Pediatric Patients

Blood pressure cuffs
Electrocardiogram leads
Infant and baby bottles and pacifiers
Medication dosing charts
Padded side rails
Pediatric code cart
Pediatric emergency medications
Pediatric gowns
Pediatric isolation equipment
Pulse oximeter probes
Scales
Stethoscopes
Thermometers
Vascular access equipment

Adapted from Mamaril ME, Schnur M. Pediatric patients. In Stannard D and Krenzischek DA, eds. *Perianesthesia Nursing Care: A Bedside Guide for Safe Recovery.* 2nd ed. Jones and Bartlett Learning; 2018.

BOX 22.2 United Nations Declaration of the Rights of the Child

All Children Need:
To be free of discrimination
To develop physically and mentally in freedom and dignity
To have a name and nationality
To have adequate nutrition, housing, recreation, and medical services
To receive special treatment if handicapped
To receive love, understanding, and material security
To receive an education and develop their abilities
To be the first to receive protection in disaster
To be protected from neglect, cruelty, and exploitation

Permission from: Barrera P, Hockenberry MJ. Perspectives of pediatric nursing. In Hockenberry MJ, Wilson D, eds. *Wong's Nursing Care of Infants and Children.* 10th ed. Mosby Elsevier; 2020.

---

tables.[3] Box 22.1 has a summary of the recommended primary equipment. Additional pediatric supplies and equipment include approved protective devices to protect surgical sites, tubes, and intravenous (IV) lines; multiple sizes of IV catheters; arm restraints for self-protection; measuring tapes to determine sizes (e.g., height, reddened areas, abdominal girth); assorted cribs for infants and toddlers; stretchers with appropriate side rail pads; and baby bottles, glucose water, assorted formulas, and pacifiers.[3] Finally, all equipment should be in various sizes to accommodate all ages and size ranges of patients seen in the facility.

If children are allowed to move about in a preoperative play area, there should be child-sized furniture available and nonslippery floor surfaces. Care should be taken to have rounded edges on all counters and furniture so as not to injure children. Electrical outlets should be covered with plastic protectors or placed out of reach. If children change into surgical pajamas in such an area, their feet should be covered with slippers that have nonskid bottoms. Preoperative and PACU areas should be separated so those children who are NPO (nothing by mouth) do not come in contact with food or drinks.

Pediatric patients' and their families' coping methods during this stressful surgical period should be supported through educational programs that focus on developmental and emotional needs. Engage in therapeutic play and offer referrals to child life therapists if available. Patient and family advocacy requires that perianesthesia nurses not only recognize the rights of the child but also understand their duty to protect children in their care (Box 22.2).[4,5] The United Nations Convention on the Rights of the Child (UNCRC) was first introduced in 1989 and subsequently established fundamental principles to improve the well-being of children and to ensure their basic rights so that better healthcare can be provided for all children (see Box 22.2).[4,5] ASC nurses should uphold the UNCRC's aims of respecting every child's dignity and basic human rights by demonstrating caring, compassion, and empathy to their vulnerable patients. Gender issues and the patient's preferred name, as well as pronouns that address self-identification of the child, are essential and must be communicated to the healthcare team.

Safe Psychosocial ASC Environment

The establishment of a professional, therapeutic relationship is foundational for providing high-quality perianesthesia nursing care.[3,4] After welcoming the patient and family to the ASC, the preoperative nurse should establish from the patient and/or parent the name with which the child prefers to be addressed. This name should then be documented in the child's electronic record to ensure all healthcare team members are aware of the child's wishes. Attention to the emotional needs of the young patient is central to the perianesthesia nurse's perioperative plan of care. It is important that the nurse first reassures the child that no one will hurt them and encourages both the parent and the child to participate in the nursing assessment process. For example, when taking the temperature, have the parent take the temperature first on themselves and then have the parent take the temperature on their child. Creating a safe psychosocial care environment involves effective communication skills. Ethically, the perianesthesia nurse uses an advocacy framework for the child and family by actively listening to and showing interest, concern, and sensitivity to the child's and family's needs.

LEGAL CONSENT

One of the first priorities of perianesthesia nursing care is to ensure the parent or accompanying caregiver is the legal guardian. The documentation in the medical record should include signatures from the legal guardian for consents for surgery or procedures and anesthesia, as well as responsibility for the patient upon discharge to home. If the parent or legal guardian is not with the child, it may be permissible in certain situations to obtain consent by telephone when two healthcare providers, such as the surgeon and/or anesthesiologist and the nurse, are listening simultaneously and the physician is informing the parent or legal guardian about the procedure and its risks and benefits, and the parent or legal guardian then gives verbal consent. The time, date, method, and type of consent, along with the name of the parent or legal guardian, should be documented in the medical record per facility policy. There may be times when children become emancipated through marriage, pregnancy, high school graduation, military service, and/or living independently.[3] These emancipated minors may be recognized as adults and can consent to surgery and invasive procedures according to each state's legal statutes.

EPIDEMIOLOGIC TRENDS IN PEDIATRIC ANESTHESIA
General Anesthesia

More than 3.9 million pediatric surgeries are performed each year.[6] In December 2016, the U.S. Food and Drug Administration

(FDA) issued a warning regarding general anesthesia and sedation drugs used in children under the age of three years who are undergoing anesthesia for more than three hours or who are having repeated use of anesthetics. This warning suggested that anesthesia may affect the neurodevelopment of children's brains.[7] The FDA also listed 11 common general anesthetics and sedative drugs that bind to the GABA and NMDA receptors.[7] When reviewing this evidence, researchers found confounding variables, such as the inclusion of some children who had previously had possible neurologic co-morbidities.[7-10] According to Sun et al. and Davidson et al., children and infants who had less than one hour of anesthesia for their surgeries did not have poorer neurodevelopmental outcomes.[8,9] However, Andropoulos and Greene did recommend that an extensive preoperative discussion take place with parents whose young children were having multiple procedures to inform the parents of the risks and benefits of multiple exposures.[10] They recommended considering the possibility of delaying the surgery until after three years of age.[10] Since this warning was issued, there have been rigorous studies exploring the use of general anesthetics and sedatives for same-day surgeries lasting less than one hour. All have demonstrated no association with a poorer neurodevelopmental outcome in randomized controlled trials for infants of less than 60 weeks' gestation.[8-10]

Evidence-Based Practice: Pediatric Anesthesia

According to the Practice Recommendations for Pediatric Anesthesia produced by the American Society of Anesthesiologists, care of the pediatric patient in the postanesthesia care unit should be supervised by a pediatric anesthesiologist or anesthesia provider trained and experienced in the care of pediatric patients. Additionally, staff providing direct clinical care to the pediatric patient should be trained in pediatric advanced life support or similar training. The clinical unit where the postoperative care of pediatric patients occurs must also be equipped with appropriated pediatric-sized equipment as well as medications and supplies. Ambulatory care centers should also produce a clinical protocol for the transfer of children to a higher level of care in the event that complications arise.

Source: American Society of Anesthesiologists. Statement on Practice Recommendations for Pediatric Anesthesia. Amended October 13, 2021. https://www.asahq.org/standards-and-guidelines/statement-on-practice-recommendations-for-pediatric-anesthesia

Postoperative, Postanesthetic Maladaptive Behavioral Changes

It has been reported by some parents that their children displayed maladaptive behavioral changes in the late postoperative period, sometimes days, weeks, or even months after anesthesia and surgery.[11-13] These maladaptive behaviors have been described as regressive bed wetting, sleep disturbances, temper tantrums, and even unusual attention-seeking behaviors.[11-13] A research study by Fortier et al. reported that preoperative anxiety, sevoflurane anesthesia agents, younger ages, the occurrence of emergence delirium, and lower birth weights were associated with the development of postoperative maladaptive behavior.[12] Studies have also found that postoperative pain in pediatric patients was an influencing factor following ambulatory surgery discharge.[12,13]

PEDIATRIC PHYSICAL, COGNITIVE, AND PSYCHOSOCIAL STAGES OF DEVELOPMENT

The pediatric stages of development are the physical, psychosocial, and cognitive changes that begin in infancy and continue through adolescence (Tables 22.1 to 22.5). According to Wilson, all "body systems undergo a progressive maturation" in which they continue to develop, change, and mature through adolescence.[14] The infancy period is characterized by the most rapid physical growth, and the adolescent period also encompasses many physical changes (Box 22.3). An infant beginning to acquire motor skills in a cephalocaudal sequence and growing and maturing in a proximodistal sequence is going through physical changes.[14] These physical developmental changes are correlated with other pediatric cognitive and social stages of development.

Erikson's Stages of Development

Erikson's stages of psychosocial development begin with the infant acquiring a sense of trust while "overcoming a sense of mistrust."[14] The infant attains this sense of trust when needs are met through feeding, comfort, caring, and love from others, especially the parents. Trust is fundamental to successfully attaining all other stages of Erikson's developmental model. Autonomy versus shame and doubt is the next developmental stage for children 1–3 years of age. Preschool children 3–5 years of age are in the initiative versus guilt stage. School-age children 5–10 years of age are in the industry versus inferiority stage, and the last pediatric developmental stage is adolescence, from 10–18 years of age, which is the identity versus role confusion stage.

Piaget's Stages of Learning

The cognitive theory of development was developed by Piaget. It describes his sensorimotor phase of development, in which children learn about the world through different senses or learning constructs.[3,14] Infants from birth to 24 months are in the sensorimotor stage of development and are learning about their world through their senses. Infants progress through reflexive behaviors to repetitive and imitative acts and learn to separate from objects and persons, thus beginning to understand time and space concepts.[3,14] The next stage of development is the preoperational stage (3–5 years), in which the child learns about the world through their experiences in developing a sense of time, which include playtimes, naptimes, and mealtimes. The concrete operational stage (5–10 or 12 years) is a period in which the child learns there are rules and uses logical thinking to understand others' viewpoints.[3] Piaget's last pediatric stage of development is the formal operations stage (adolescence to adulthood), in which teenagers learn to use abstract thinking, gain improved verbal communication, and acquire technologic skills.

Common Fears at Different Developmental Stages

Many infants and children experience and exhibit common fears at different ages and stages of development from infancy to adolescence (see Tables 22.1 to 22.5).[3] Separation anxiety begins between the ages of 4 and 8 months, when the infant realizes the parent is absent (see Table 22.1).[3] By 12 months of age, the infant anticipates the departure of the parent by watching their behaviors.[14] Stranger anxiety is exhibited between the ages of 6 and 8 months, when infants begin to discriminate between familiar and unfamiliar people.[14]

Toddlers also experience the fear of separation from parents, as well as the fear of interacting with strangers. Loss of control, getting hurt, and dealing with intrusive procedures are other fears for this age group (see Table 22.2).[3] Preschoolers are afraid of the unknown or being left alone or abandoned. They too, are afraid of separation from parents, bodily injury, or loss of function (see Table 22.3).[3] School-age children are

TABLE 22.1 Physical, Cognitive, and Social Stages of Development in Infants

Physical Development	Cognitive Development	Social Development	Common Fears	Nursing Implications
At birth, infants have weak and immature musculature and immature nervous systems Their neck muscles are unable to support their head in an upright position As the months pass, the infant's muscles strengthen and the nervous system matures The infant gains control of the head and is soon sitting upright Infants move by crawling, reaching, and eventually standing The infant does experience physical pain	The neonate interacts largely by reflex, such as the sucking reflex Over the course of the first year, the infant shows an increasing response to sounds and sights, exhibiting interest in toys such as rattles and developing the ability to distinguish strangers The infant begins to demonstrate an understanding of cause and effect and may begin to vocalize	The infant is very social, often cooing or squealing in delight, smiling at anyone who smiles back at the infant Infants are curious At 6 months of age or older, infants experience separation anxiety from parents that may last until 30 months of age The infant's personality is developing	Fear of separation from parent or caregiver Stranger anxiety	Observe infant before making contact Speak softly and smile Observe for signs and symptoms of hunger, such as crying Keep infant on parent or primary caregiver's lap Handle infant gently but firmly, always supporting the head and neck Perform least invasive procedures first Keep infant warm Ensure that hands and equipment (e.g., stethoscope) are warm before touching Provide comfort measures, such as a pacifier Use distraction techniques with various items such as music, keys, toys, or penlight Persistent crying, irritability, or inability to console or arouse infant may indicate physiologic distress

Used with permission from Mamaril ME, Schnur M. Pediatric patients. In Stannard D, Krenzischek DA, eds. *Perianesthesia Nursing Care: A Bedside Guide for Safe Recovery.* 2nd ed. Jones and Bartlett Learning, 2018.

TABLE 22.2 Physical, Cognitive, and Social Stages of Development in Toddlers

Physical Development	Cognitive Development	Social Development	Emotional Responses	Common Fears	Nursing Implications
Toddler's gross motor skills continue to improve Walking is mastered, and running, jumping, and climbing are tried The toddler is very curious and lacks an understanding of dangerous situations The household needs to be childproofed The toddler's fine gross motor skills are revealed through activities such as coloring and playing with blocks or dolls	Toddlers are learning to speak and imitate words, identify body parts, know colors, and understand simple commands	Toddlers are very energetic and enjoy exploring, playing simple games, and engaging in parallel play Temper tantrums may be developing The child at this age believes the world revolves around them Crying loudly, biting, kicking, and hitting may be normal expressions of frustration	Children in this age group that undergo urologic procedures often react with anger, and postoperative crying and arching may not be indicative of pain, but may indicate anger as they react to invasion of their genitals; This is especially evident in boys Distraction and discussion about going home often helps, and getting them dressed in their own clothing postoperatively as soon as possible may assist them as a positive diversionary measure Breath holding can occur in this age group, leading to sudden oxygen desaturation Children that engage in breath holding in the PACU often have a history of breath holding when they are angry or crying; it is important to ask parents about this preoperatively so that the nurse and staff can be prepared for it postoperatively	Being left alone Separation from parents Interacting with strangers Interruptions in usual routine Loss of control Getting hurt/ fear of injury Intrusive procedures Fear of the toilet Fear of going down the drain Fear of the dark	Gain trust of child and parent or caregiver Physically position nurse at the child's eye level to be less intimidating Avoid separating the child from the parent or caregiver if possible Address child by name Smile and speak in a calm, quiet tone Encourage child to participate in care Respect modesty Promote holding a familiar or transitional object in times of stress Be truthful; avoid words and phrases that may be frightening, such as "put to sleep" or "stick needle" Provide safe limits for expression of negative feelings Expect and accept regressive behavior Offer choices to enhance child's feeling of control Prepare immediately before surgery or procedure

Used with permission from:
Mamaril ME, Schnur M. Pediatric patients. In Stannard D, Krenzischek DA, eds. *Perianesthesia Nursing Care: A Bedside Guide for Safe Recovery.* 2nd ed. Jones and Bartlett Learning, 2018.

TABLE 22.3 Physical, Cognitive, and Social Stages of Development in Preschool Children

Physical Development	Cognitive Development	Social Development	Emotional Responses	Common Fears	Nursing Implications
Preschooler's gross motor skills and hand-to-eye coordination continue to improve They have much energy and love to move, run, jump, hop, skip, and dance to music	Preschoolers are developing initiative and like to pretend and imitate others They like to color "inside the lines," play "make believe," and talk a lot They love to tell stories and may have a difficult time distinguishing between reality and fiction; Piaget calls this pre-concrete thinking They are just beginning to understand time Preschoolers may regress to the toddler stage under stress	Preschoolers may be loud as they are still learning what is the appropriate volume of speech They may believe they have superhuman powers Preschoolers love to learn and enjoy playing games and working on large puzzles Preschoolers are beginning to think by the rules	Children in this age group have some understanding of what is going to occur Preoperative tours are often helpful and also prepare families for what to expect on the day of surgery Encouraging children to make choices at this age is also important The light of the pulse oximeter can become a fascinating toy, as opposed to a scary clip Storytelling by nurses and anesthesia care providers is a great distraction	Fear of the unknown and the dark Fear of being left alone Fear of being lost or abandoned Fear of separation from parents or caregiver Fear of injury, pain, mutilation, loss of function Fear of pain as a punishment Fear of loss of control Fear of adults that look or act "mean"	Speak quietly in clear, simple language; avoid baby talk; avoid scary terms such as "cut," "shot," "germs," or "put to sleep" Physically position nurse at the child's eye level as it is less intimidating Encourage the child to hold transitional objects, such as favorite toys Encourage hands-on practice with equipment Provide distraction techniques such as guided imagery Offer child treatment choices Respect the child's modesty Keep the child warm Prepare the child for uncomfortable procedures and make a plan for distraction, a position of comfort, availability of a favorite toy, or other intervention that will lessen anxiety Optimize parental visitation

With permission from: Mamaril ME, Schnur M. Pediatric patients. In Stannard D, Krenzischek DA, eds. *Perianesthesia Nursing Care: A Bedside Guide for Safe Recovery*. 2nd ed. Jones and Bartlett Learning; 2018.

TABLE 22.4 Physical, Cognitive, and Social Stages of Development in School-age Children

Physical Development	Psychological Development	Cognitive Development	Social Development	Emotional Responses	Common Fears	Nursing Implications
School-age children continue to improve their large muscle and fine muscle skills They demonstrate industry and participate in gymnastics, dancing, and team sports that reflect the increasing growth and development of their muscles and nervous systems They draw, paint, and play musical instruments	Children of this age group are generally happy and excited about life School-age children have a need to develop a sense of achievement and competence, such as engaging in team activities such as sports, scouting, or church events They are usually eager, enthusiastic, and willing to cooperate It is important for children to master skills and develop self-confidence and self-esteem	Children during this period learn through concrete operational thought Children are constantly learning new concepts, such as letters, colors, words, and numbers They are gaining knowledge and are able to make abstract associations	Children enjoy same-sex peer groups They like activities such as games, parties, and team sports During this period, children develop close friendships and best friends Children understand what is acceptable behavior in public School-age children know the difference between right and wrong	School-age children may have shared stories of surgical experiences with siblings or friends Preconceived ideas may affect their emotions and fears Preoperative tours are a benefit to this age group Asking questions may promote a better understanding of worries and concerns	Fear of the unknown Fear of separation from parent or caregiver Fear of loss of control Fear of pain, loss of body function Fear of body injury, mutilation Fear of rejection of peers Failure to live up to others' expectations Anger over dependence Fear of physical disability, disfigurement, or not being able to participate in sports Fear of procedures involving genitals Guilt about illness	Listen attentively Acknowledge fears Respect dignity and need for increasing privacy Provide honest, factual information Offer optimized parental visitation Help establish coping skills and distraction techniques

Used with permission from: Mamaril ME, Schnur M. Pediatric patients. In Stannard D, Krenzischek DA, eds. *Perianesthesia Nursing Care: A Bedside Guide for Safe Recovery*. 2nd ed. Jones and Bartlett Learning; 2018.

TABLE 22.5 Physical, Cognitive, and Social Stages of Development in Adolescents

Physical Development	Psychological Development	Cognitive Development	Social Development	Emotional Responses	Common Fears	Nursing Implications
Adolescents continue to develop, increasing strength and coordination in their large muscles and fine motor movement	Adolescent years are a time of emotional struggle for independence as the teenager searches for his or her personal identity	Adolescent is able to synthesize information and draw a conclusion	Adolescent is rapidly maturing into adulthood	Teenagers often stay up late into the night; postoperatively, they may appear to be slow to arouse from anesthesia because of sleeping very little the night before surgery	Fear of being left out or socially isolated	Speak in a respectful, friendly manner as one would to an adult
Adolescent is still developing	Adolescents feel a sense of invincibility	They continue to master academic subjects and engage and think abstractly	Friendships continue, and adolescents may begin to date		Fear of inheriting parent's problems (e.g., alcoholism, mental illness)	Obtain history from patient if possible
The sexual development process takes approximately 4 years	Emotions are labile and may be volatile		The peer group is very important, and experimentation may occur	Since teens also like to feel in control, respect their growing independence and include them in determining the best time for the parents to rejoin them at the bedside	Fear of infection	Be sensitive and interview privately when questioning about tobacco, drug, or alcohol use
Adolescents adjust to their ever-changing bodies			At this age, many enter the workforce		Fear of loss of control	Consider pregnancy testing for menstruating females or per facility policy
Height and weight increase with muscle mass				The various levels of maturity in the teen population result in a wide spectrum of needs and responses	Fear of loss of privacy	Assess for body piercings
					Fear of altered body image, disfigurement	Respect independence
					Fear of separation from peer group	Allow parent or caregiver to be involved if patient wishes
					Fear of pain	Explain things clearly and honestly; allow time for questions
						Respect patient's modesty
						Address patient's concerns of body integrity or disfigurement
						Provide discharge instructions to the patient and parent or caregiver
						Implement interventions aimed at gaining control, increased coping measures, and learning distraction techniques

Used with permission from: Mamaril ME, Schnur M. Pediatric patients. In Stannard D, Krenzischek DA, eds. *Perianesthesia Nursing Care: A Bedside Guide for Safe Recovery*. 2nd ed. Jones and Bartlett Learning; 2018.

afraid of the unknown, pain, bodily injury, and rejection by peers (see Table 22.4).[3] They may experience anger over the need to be dependent, or fear procedures involving genitals. Finally, the adolescent's common fears are a fear of being left out or socially isolated, infection, loss of privacy, and altered body image (see Table 20.5).[3]

INSTRUCTIONS FOR PATIENTS AND FAMILIES IN THE PREOPERATIVE PHASE

As parents prepare for a child's surgery, it is important for them to receive good preoperative information, which includes directions to the ASC and the time at which they should arrive for surgery. In addition, parents can be advised that the child should be bathed the night before surgery and may wear comfy loose-fitting clothes. Encourage the parent to bring an extra pair of underwear in case of accidents to help make the child feel secure and less ashamed should an accident occur.

During the preoperative phase, it is important to inquire about the child's health history, including current medications being taken; birth history (e.g., prematurity or post conceptual age, need for oxygen, stay in a neonatal intensive care unit, apnea, monitoring at home); allergies; recent upper respiratory infections, cough (productive), fever, or flu-like symptoms; and any recent exposure to communicable diseases.

The American Society of Anesthesiologists (ASA) has provided the following guidelines for preventing the risk of pulmonary aspiration during surgery: pediatric patients can drink clear liquids up to a minimum of two hours before anesthesia; can ingest breast milk up to four hours before, infant formula

up to six hours before, and nonhuman milk up to six hours before; and can eat a light meal up to six hours before (Box 22.4).

Although ambulatory surgery is a stressful time for children and their families, it also is an opportunity for strengthening family coping strategies and learning new information about managing recovery care. This is often the first time children have experienced surgery and anesthesia. The child's exposure to an ASC may have lasting effects, whether the experience was positive or negative. Important communication skills include:

- Accepting each family's uniqueness
- Respecting traditional and nontraditional family units
- Conveying open-minded, friendly, nonthreatening mannerisms
- Promoting autonomy, and
- Optimizing the child's and parents' privacy.

Finally, the many perianesthesia nursing implications for each unique developmental stage can be found in Tables 22.1 to 22.5.

PEDIATRIC ANATOMY AND PHYSIOLOGY
Anesthesia and Pediatric Anatomy and Physiology

The administration of anesthesia via a pediatric airway may have significant anatomic and physiologic effects in preterm infants, infants, and older children (see Table 22.1 and Figure 22.1).[3,15] Preterm infants and infants recovering from general anesthesia have the greatest risk of developing airway edema from intubation and subsequent oxygenation; their tracheal tissues are fragile

BOX 22.3 Pediatric Developmental Anatomic and Physiologic Characteristics

Neonate

Head accounts for 25% of the body's length and 33% of weight

Ribs composed mainly of cartilage and project at right angles from vertebral column (more circular)

Increased oxygen and metabolic demand; susceptible to hypoxia; obligate nose breathers

Limited glycogen stores

Immature respiratory center in the brain

Predisposed to hypothermia due to small muscle mass and inability to shiver

Fully developed parasympathetic nervous system, underdeveloped sympathetic nervous system

Large body surface area

Infant

Growth and development progresses at a rapid rate during the first 12 months of age

Body weight doubles at 5 months and triples at 12 months

Increased oxygen and metabolic demand; susceptible to hypoxia; obligate nose breathers

Vocal cords more cartilaginous

Limited glycogen stores

Immature respiratory center (pons and medulla) in the brain

Large body surface area; predisposed to hypothermia (small muscle mass and inability to shiver)

Fully developed parasympathetic nervous system, underdeveloped sympathetic nervous system

Chest wall is thin, rib cage is soft and pliable, breathing is predominantly diaphragmatic

Higher circulating blood volume (75 mL/kg)

Underdeveloped cervical ligaments; weak neck muscles (prone to hyperextension of neck)

Toddler

Trachea is short in length, increasing the potential for intubating the right mainstem bronchus

Rib cage is very pliable; chest wall is thin, breath sounds transmitted throughout chest

Underdeveloped bronchial tree and alveolar-capillary gas exchange units

Prone to temperature extremes

Larger body surface area; prone to temperature extremes, increased heat loss with anesthetic gases

Preschooler

Oxygen consumption requirements are about twice those of adults (6–8 mL/kg versus 3–4 mL/kg)

Cannot sustain rapid respiratory rates for a long time due to immature intercostal muscles

Smaller functional residual capacity with smaller oxygen reserves; consequently, rapid hypoxia

Liver and spleen in lower abdomen are less protected by rib cage and more prone to injury

Lower volume of cerebrospinal fluid/smaller subarachnoid space; less protection for infant's brain; injury to spinal cord occurs without fracture owing to cartilaginous nature of vertebral bones

School age

Bones begin to lose flexibility at 6 years of age (bone cortex thickens and become hardened)

Tracheal shape changes from funnel shape to cylindrical shape

Lung volume increases to 200 mL by 8 years of age

Bronchial tree has attained 16 divisions as in an adult

By 10 years of age, size and flexibility of airway match those of adults

Adolescents

Faster growth rate than any other period except infancy

By age 15 years, cardiac output is equal to an adult

By age 15 years, the body's response to shock is similar to that of an adult

Sebaceous glands increase production

Secondary sex characteristics: Breast tissue in females develops between 9 and 13 years of age

Adapted from Mamaril ME, Schnur M. Pediatric patients. In Stannard D, Krenzischek DA, eds. *Perianesthesia Nursing Care: A Bedside Guide for Safe Recovery.* 2nd ed. Jones and Bartlett Learning; 2018.

and their bronchi and alveolar-capillary gas exchange units are underdeveloped.[1,3,15] According to the AAP, infants under one year of age have a "four times higher risk of anesthesia-related cardiac arrest" than do children of 1–18 years.[1] If premature infants require 24-hour monitoring following anesthesia because of apnea, they may not be appropriate for surgery in an ASC.

BOX 22.4 Fasting Guidelines for Pediatric Patients

Ingested Material	NPO Time (Hours)
Clear liquids	2
Breast milk	4
Infant formula	6
Nonhuman milk	6
Light meal	6
Heavy meal (fried or fatty food)	6

Cladis FP, Davis PJ. Preoperative preparation. Table 16.13 in: Davis PJ, Cladis FP, eds. *Smith's Anesthesia for Infants and Children.* 10th ed. Elsevier; 2022.

Definitions of Developmental Ages

According to Hesselgrave, pediatric patients are classified according to the following developmental ages[16]:

- Neonate is the first 28 days of life
- Infant is 1–12 months of age
- Toddler is 1–3 years of age
- Preschooler is 3–6 years of age
- School age is 6–12 years of age
- Adolescence is 13–18 years of age.

IDENTIFYING PREOPERATIVE RISK FACTORS IN CHILDREN

Physiologic and Anatomic Risk Factors

There are unique pediatric risk factors associated with postanesthesia respiratory complications and/or adverse events.[3,15] The predictor risk factor variables include age (e.g., premature infant, post conceptual age < 40 weeks, child three years of age or less), sex (male), ASA physical status II or III) type of anesthesia (general), type of surgery (minor, airway, major), morbid obesity, congenital anomalies or syndromes (e.g., Down syndrome, skeletal dysplasia), airway co-morbidities (e.g., reactive airway, difficult airway, breath holding, tracheomalacia), preexisting

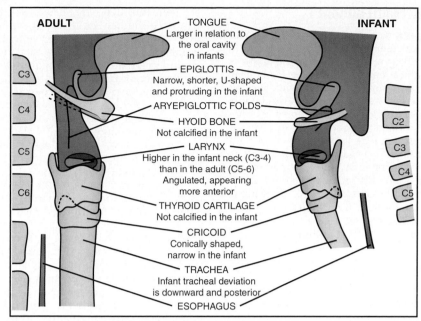

Fig. 22.1 Comparison of the anatomy of the adult and infant airways. Modified from Ellinas H. Difficult pediatric airway. Figure 188.2 in: Fleisher LA, Rosenbaum MA, eds. *Complications in Anesthesia.* 3rd ed. Elsevier, 2018.

pulmonary disorders (e.g., asthma, upper respiratory infection, exposure to passive or second-hand smoking, obstructive sleep apnea or disordered breathing), preexisting neuromuscular disorders, preexisting cardiac disorders, and African American ethnicity.[3,15,17] Nine pediatric risk factor categories were validated as independent risk factors for PACU complications on emergence from anesthesia. These risk factors include age, airway co-morbidities (syndromes or congenital anomalies), pulmonary comorbidities, neurologic co-morbidities, cardiac co-morbidities, tobacco smoke exposure, obesity, obstructive sleep apnea, and African American ethnicity. Perianesthesia nurses need to identify in their preanesthesia nursing assessment all pediatric preoperative risk factors that are linked to PACU respiratory complications.[15]

Environmental Risk Factors

Exposure to second-hand tobacco smoke and or environmental allergens such as mold or dust mites may predispose infants and children to pulmonary preoperative co-morbidities such as reactive airway disease or asthma and may cause postoperative respiratory complications on emergence from anesthesia.[3,15,17] Passive or second-hand smoke exposure in older children also has also been linked to laryngospasm in the PACU.[3,15,17] Children who have been exposed to environmental allergens at home may suffer from an asthma reactive airway, especially African American infants and children.[3,15,18]

IDENTIFYING SITUATIONS THAT PUT CHILDREN AT RISK IN DAILY LIFE
Pediatric Suicide

During the preanesthesia phase of care, the nurse should include in the preoperative screening assessment factors that identify pediatric patients at risk for suicide or self-harm. Pediatric suicide is the second leading cause of death for children, adolescents, and young adults ages 15–24 years.[19] Furthermore, it is the ninth leading cause of death for children

ages 5–11 years.[20] Tragically, suicide rates have doubled over the past 10 years.[21] Interestingly, pediatric suicide occurs more commonly after puberty.[21] While suicide ideation and attempted suicide are more common in females, actual death by suicide is more common in males. Teenage boys commit suicide three times more often than girls.[22] Finally, research studies reveal it is more common in children with gender identity issues than in heterosexuals.[21] Some of the suicide methods include firearms, suffocation/hanging, poisoning (e.g., carbon monoxide, overdose), and other methods, including cutting and drowning.[22]

Perianesthesia nurses should also note certain behavioral risk factors. These include aggressive or disruptive behavior, changes in behavior or performance, depression, drug or alcohol abuse, personality disorders, previous suicide attempts, history of psychiatric illness, and the use of antidepressant drugs and/or self-injury.[21] Patients reporting traumatic events, such as bullying, disappointments, loss or rejection (such as family or parental death or divorce), physical or sexual abuse or trauma, and/or pressure to succeed are also at high risk for suicide.[20]

It is important when assessing pediatric patients for potential suicide ideations to interview teens separately from parents. Ask the patients the following nonthreatening questions: "I know that a lot of people your age have a lot going on. What has been going on in your mind?" or "How have things been going with school? Friends? Parents?" or "Have you felt threatened?" The AAP recommends the following teen screening questions[19]:

- Have you ever thought about killing yourself or that you would rather be dead?
- Have you ever done something with the purpose of doing yourself harm or killing yourself?

Once the perianesthesia nurse has identified suicide risk factors, the nurse has an ethical duty to inform the parents and validate any concerns and observations. The anesthesia provider and surgeon should also be consulted to determine if the surgical procedure should be performed. Finally, the nurse should provide access to pediatric behavioral health services for appropriate and timely follow-up.[20]

Child Abuse and Child Maltreatment

Another important preoperative risk factor to look for is suspected intentional physical, emotional, or sexual abuse or neglect of children.[23] The four major types of child abuse or maltreatment include physical harm by inflicting injury from hitting, kicking, beating, burning, or shaking; child neglect from failing to provide basic needs; sexual abuse demonstrated by fondling genitalia, intercourse, incest, rape, sodomy, or prostitution; and emotional abuse revealed through rejection, isolating, terrorizing, ignoring, corrupting, or verbally assaulting. Any form of abuse may also be combined with another form of abuse. According to Wilson, the most critical responsibility for nurses when child maltreatment is identified is to document in detail the assessment data of the injury and physical examination, protect the child from further abuse, and report suspected child abuse to the nurse manager, social protective child services, and local authorities.[23]

Child Trafficking

Preoperative screening for child trafficking can be challenging. Traffickers are often well-spoken, well-dressed, and well-rehearsed.[3] They often pose as a family member or a friend who does not allow the child to answer questions. Typically, the trafficker is a noncustodial adult who provides vague or misleading answers about the child's health. The child or adolescent may seem reluctant to answer questions or have vague or inconsistent explanations of the illness or injury. The perianesthesia nurse should become suspicious if children are not able to provide their address, identification cards, or documents. They also may appear depressed and anxious, avoid eye contact, or have a flat affect. A common tactic for traffickers is to threaten their victim's loved ones. In the United States, runaway or homeless children are the most vulnerable. Children at risk present to healthcare providers by disclosing a high number of sexual partners, unwanted pregnancies, and even abortions.[24] When screening pediatric patients, the nurse should not be judgmental but may ask, "Have you ever been forced to do something that you didn't want to do?" Additional screening questions include:

- Can you come and go from home whenever you please?
- Has anyone at home or work ever physically harmed you?
- Have you ever been threatened for trying to leave your job?
- Is anyone forcing you to do things you do not want to do?
- Do you have to ask permission to eat, sleep, or use the bathroom?
- Are there locks on your doors and windows that keep you from leaving?
- Have you ever been denied food, water, sleep, or medical care?

The most important nursing action is to protect the child from further trafficking. Report suspected child trafficking to the nurse manager, social protective child services, local authorities, and the National Human Trafficking Resource Center Hotline (1-888-373-7888). Screening questions to identify trafficking should be asked when the patient is alone. Never ask them if a noncustodial adult is present as the adult may be the person who is trafficking the patient. Asking screening questions with the trafficker present places the child's safety at risk.

INNOVATIVE MULTIMODAL TREATMENT FOR PAIN IN PEDIATRIC PATIENTS

The assessment and management of pediatric pain in infants and children is challenging for the perianesthesia nurse. In fact, there is evidence that pain is poorly managed by parents, even once children are recovering at home after their surgeries.[25] Pain is generally subjective, and children have varied responses to pain and distress that should be interpreted according to the individual's cognitive and emotional development at specific ages. Multimodal therapies are the standard of care for perioperative pain management.[25] Combining the traditional opioids and oral analgesics with local, regional, and peripheral nerve blocks has proved to be a successful pharmacologic intervention.[25] Finally, effective perioperative pain management is critical for good patient comfort, the prevention of postoperative complications, and the satisfaction of the patient and parents.

Ambulatory surgery multimodal pain management uses many pharmacologic and nonpharmacologic treatment modalities.[26] The pharmacologic medications include regional and local anesthesia, dissociative anesthesia, and IV sedation (both deep and conscious).[26] When managing postoperative or postprocedural pain in children, the perianesthesia nurse takes into account the preoperative medications, the type of surgery or invasive procedure and its complexity, and the intraoperative medications that were administered. The intraoperative interventions for pain may include IV opioids, nonopioids, local anesthetics, wound instillations or tissue infiltrations, nerve blocks, and topical anesthetics.[3,25] A multimodal approach including non-narcotic analgesics and nonpharmacologic methods in addition to opioids when necessary is recommended to optimize safe and effective pain management in children.[3]

Preoperative Pain Medications

Preoperative pain considerations begin with a multidisciplinary approach involving the anesthesia provider, surgeon, perianesthesia nurse, patient, and patient's family. This interdisciplinary approach considers the specific surgical procedure, expected severity of pain, and duration of the procedure, as well as the duration of expected postoperative pain.[3,26,27] Preoperatively, the perianesthesia nurse introduces different age and developmentally appropriate pain assessment tools to the patient, as well as to the parents. Pain scales that may be used include the FLACC (face, legs, activity, cry, consolability) scale for infants and nonverbal patients, the Wong–Baker Faces scale for toddlers and preschool children, the Oucher scale (a variant of the faces scale), the visual analog scale for school-age and adolescent children, and the numerical rating scale for school-age and adolescent children.[3] There are a number of other options for pediatric pain assessment tools, and the choice may be driven by facility protocols.

Preoperative premedication is known to reduce anxiety, lessen the stress of separation from parents before being transported into the operating room, and enhance the induction of anesthesia.[3,26,27] Midazolam is a short-acting benzodiazepine with a fast-acting onset of administration and is the most commonly prescribed premedication. Oral midazolam 0.25-0.5 mg/kg is frequently administered 15–20 minutes before the start of the scheduled operating room case or induction.[26] Although midazolam has antianxiety benefits, it may have untoward effects such as amnesia, restlessness, agitation, and excessive sedation in some children.[3,26,28]

Postoperative Pain Medications

Postoperative pediatric pain is a result of physiologic injury or tissue damage from a surgical procedure. This tissue insult activates the inflammatory response, as well as the nerve conduction from the site of injury. Sources of physical discomfort are incisional pain, invasive tubes, IV lines, and even blood pressure cuffs and pulse oximeter probes. Emotional components of pain may result from the absence of parents, fear of abandonment, lack of security objects, and unfamiliar surroundings.

Perianesthesia nurses effectively treat pediatric pain in several ways. The ongoing presence of the nurse and the nurse's frequent observations of the child's verbal and nonverbal responses are crucial, as is the anticipation of the patient's predictable surgical pain and astute nursing interpretations of the complexity of the child's pain. Some of the developmental responses for pediatric pain may include the following[3]:

- Infants may cry, flail arms and legs, and grimace
- Toddlers may scream, cling, total body resistance
- Preschoolers may cry, hit, kick, cling, or withdraw
- School-age children may have passive coping mechanisms
- Adolescents may have increased body control and may even be more embarrassed about their lack of privacy than the surgical pain.

All children need to be monitored closely for adequacy of pain control and for the potential of adverse side effects. Neonates, infants under 55–60 weeks' postgestational age, and children with specific preexisting diseases such as obstructive sleep apnea are at increased risk for respiratory depression due to decreased clearance and elimination of opioids.[26]

Children's medication dosages are calculated by weight and may be based on total body weight, ideal body weight, or lean body mass.[3,26] Age is taken into consideration in neonates and infants. Dosages may be decreased and intervals increased to account for immature organ development.[28] Initial dosages are titrated depending on the response of the patient. Children as young as 4 years of age may be cognitively and physically capable of using a patient-controlled device.[28,29] A wide variety of interventions, including the presence of family, comfort measures, complementary therapies such as reiki, behavioral distraction techniques, guided imagery, and pharmacologic choices, are typically available to the nurse for a multimodal approach to minimizing pain.[3] Other nonpharmacologic techniques include cognitive behavioral methods, music therapy, television cartoons, interactive videos, animated applications on electronic tablets, and cell phones.[27,29]

Complementary Distraction Techniques

Nonpharmacologic considerations include distraction and relaxation techniques. These methods can involve playing with toys, coloring books, motorized cars, and lava lamps, to name a few. Child life therapists may be available at many facilities to provide therapeutic play interventions, such as music and educational pediatric mannequins that demonstrate surgical body parts. Flavored anesthetic masks used with inhalation induction agents can help to increase the child's comfort level in the operating room. Another very effective consideration is to allow parents to be present in the operating room to support their child during induction based on the facility's guidelines.[27] According to Kain, children older than four years of age, parents with low anxiety levels, and children with a low baseline level of activity benefit from a parental presence during induction.[27]

The Society for Pediatric Anesthesia has issued evidence-based recommendations for the use of opioids in children during the perioperative period.[25] The goal was to address the most important issues of opioid administration for children after surgery. These goals include the following statements[25]:

- Regular pain assessments should be part of the perioperative care and treatment of pediatric patients who are receiving opioid medications, and assessment should consider the unique circumstances of the child's psychological state and the extent of surgery
- Expert consensus is to use an as-needed strategy for opioid dosing until further evidence is available.
- Opioid pain medications should not be prescribed with benzodiazepines except for children for whom there is a specific indication and alternative treatment options are inadequate. Doses should be limited to the lowest effective level, and parents should be warned about the potential for excessive sedation and respiratory depression.
- For pediatric patients with chronic pain who are maintained on opioids, continue established preoperative dosing during the perioperative period as a baseline. Acute postsurgical analgesia should be provided over and above the baseline opioids. Use of nonopioid analgesia is encouraged, including regional analgesia techniques, alpha-2 agonists, ketamine, acetaminophen, nonsteroidal anti-inflammatory drugs, and neuropathic pain medications such as gabapentinoids or antidepressants.
- Patients with obstructive sleep apnea, obesity of over the 95th percentile of the body mass index, and recurrent nighttime oxygen desaturations are at higher risk for opioid-induced respiratory depression. Opioid dosing should be based on the ideal or lean body weight, and the dose of opioid should be reduced by 50% to 67% for obstructive sleep apnea patients. Additionally, extended respiratory monitoring is required when opioids are being administered to this population in the perioperative period.
- Educational resources must be provided to inform parents of the appropriate indications for pain medications and strategies for the safe use of opioids, nonopioids, and other measures to manage their child's postoperative pain. Parents should receive both verbal and written detailed discharge instructions regarding home pain management, with instructions regarding safe storage and disposal of leftover medications.

POSTANESTHESIA CONSIDERATIONS AND COMPLICATIONS

Postanesthesia Agitation (Emergence Agitation; Emergence Delirium)

Postanesthesia agitation (PAA) is also known as emergence delirium, emergence agitation, and postanesthetic excitement. PAA includes disorientation, nonpurposeful movements, lack of focused eye contact, incoherence, inconsolability, restlessness, and agitation.[3] Scientific evidence suggests that general anesthetic agents such as sevoflurane and/or hypoxemia or hypercarbia contribute to the physiologic causes.[3] Other causes may be pain, fear, anxiety, or a full bladder. During the admission of the child in the Phase I recovery unit, the nurse should auscultate the patient's bilateral breath sounds and monitor the pulse oximetry for adequate oxygenation and ventilation. The next nursing intervention is to protect the patient from injury and determine the need for other interventions. After ruling out possible physiologic causes, the nurse assesses for pain, fear, and anxiety. Since the agitated child is not capable of self-reporting, pain may be assessed based on the likelihood of pain associated with the patient's procedure in the context of the analgesia and anesthesia received.[3,30] Although PAA can last up to 45 minutes, it is typically self-limiting. However, undesirable outcomes of the delirium may include surgical site bleeding or patient injury, loss of venous access or surgical drains, increased pain, and potential injury to members of the healthcare team.[3,30]

Additional clinical resources should be alerted to assist if needed.

Neurologic Complications

Failure to awaken from anesthesia in the Phase I unit has several possible causes and needs to be identified and reported to the anesthesia provider, as well as to the charge nurse or nurse manager. Residual effects from anesthetics and agents such as opioids or benzodiazepines, as well as the presence of hepatic or renal dysfunction, hypothermia, and hypoxia, may lead to prolonged sedation. Metabolic and/or electrolyte abnormalities from hyperglycemia, hypoglycemia, hypomagnesemia, and hyponatremia may also delay arousal from anesthesia. Children who have a ventriculoperitoneal shunt procedure as an outpatient may have a neurologic event, such as a bleed or stroke in the ASC. Furthermore, children who have a pseudocholinesterase deficiency or neuromuscular disease may also have delayed awakening from anesthesia. Finally, successful management is dependent on the differential diagnosis and appropriate treatment interventions, such as effective ventilation with a bag-valve mask, administration of appropriate reversal drugs, active warming of the hypothermic patient, evaluation of the electrolyte status, and consultation with a neurologic provider.

Upper Airway Obstruction

Pediatric airway obstructions present significant challenges that perianesthesia nurses frequently encounter when infants and children are emerging from anesthesia. Infants recovering from general anesthesia pose the greatest threat because they may develop airway edema from intubation, causing their fragile airway tissues to become occluded. The foremost metabolic demand for oxygen and glucose further puts them at greater risk for hypoxia.[15] Edema with narrowing of the trachea, as well as the underdevelopment of their bronchi and alveolar-capillary gas exchange units, increases the possibility of oxygen desaturation and respiratory adverse events in the Phase I unit.[15,31] Patients age 1–4 years who have a history of croup are at greatest risk of developing upper airway edema. Laryngospasm, bronchospasm, and acute airway anaphylaxis are potentially life-threatening conditions that children may experience during emergence from anesthesia or sedation. Laryngospasm is a reflexive closure of the upper airway as a result of a glottic musculature spasm; the spasm acts as a protective mechanism to prevent foreign material from entering the tracheobronchial tree.[32] Partial upper airway obstruction and mild respiratory distress may be easily resolved by repositioning the head and neck using a shoulder roll followed by using a jaw thrust.[31,32] Another effective intervention may be using the "laryngospasm notch" technique first used on adults; fingertip pressure is applied in front to the retro auricular depression at the tragus of the ears, and this causes the vocal cords to open, subsequently relieving the laryngospasm.[15,31] On the other end of the continuum, laryngospasm can cause total airway obstruction, and no inspiratory or expiratory breath sounds are heard. Likewise, apneic respirations and severe substernal chest retractions may quickly lead to oxygen desaturation, symptomatic bradycardia, or even pulseless electrical activity.[33] This respiratory arrest requires maintaining oxygenation and ventilation via high-flow oxygen (15 L) with a bag-valve mask, cardiac compressions if the heart rate drops below 60 beats per minute, and reintubation, along with pharmacologic paralytics, epinephrine, and judicious IV fluid resuscitation.[33] The perianesthesia nurse should be prepared to administer oxygen, nebulized racemic epinephrine, examethasone, lidocaine, atropine, or muscle relaxants and assist the anesthesiologist with reintubation if necessary.[31] When anaphylaxis-induced bronchospasm or acute airway anaphylaxis is suspected, epinephrine is the first-line treatment, along with oxygen and ensuring a patent airway.[33]

Lower Airway or Respiratory Obstruction

Another concerning pediatric airway condition is bronchospasm, which is a lower airway obstruction. Causes of bronchospasm may include asthma, anaphylaxis, histamine release, aspiration, mucous plug, or foreign body. Signs and symptoms may include expiratory wheezing, shallow noisy respirations, retractions, dyspnea, tachypnea, and oxygen desaturation.[31,33] Treatment of bronchospasm may vary due to different pathophysiologies. The most important first action is removing the irritant; then, high-flow oxygen is administered via a nonrebreather mask and physician-ordered bronchodilators are given, such as nebulized albuterol, levalbuterol, terbutaline, epinephrine, systemic steroids, inhaled steroids, or even magnesium sulfate infusions.[31,33] When anaphylaxis-induced bronchospasm or acute airway anaphylaxis is suspected, epinephrine is the first-line treatment, along with oxygen and ensuring a patent airway.[31,33] Additionally, the patient may require albuterol, antihistamines, and steroids to further treat the bronchospasm and fluid boluses to treat hypotension.[31,33] The perianesthesia nurse should be prepared to quickly identify the clinical symptoms of upper airway obstruction and preoperative risk factors and effectively manage laryngospasms, bronchospasms, noncardiac pulmonary edema, or acute airway anaphylaxis.[31] Finally, one of the most important perianesthesia nursing assessments is to frequently auscultate the child's bilateral breath sounds to identify not only the quality of inspiratory and expiratory adventitious sounds but also a complete versus partial spasm and the need to contact the anesthesia provider immediately.

Cardiovascular Complications

There are several cardiovascular complications that the perianesthesia nurse may identify during the recovery period. Tachycardia is a normal response in which the body attempts to increase the cardiac output resulting from dehydration or a prolonged NPO status. Other causes of tachycardia may be a full bladder, bowel, or stomach; an increased body temperature; and early respiratory distress. Bradycardia is usually the classic and ominous hallmark sign of respiratory distress (late sign), but also could be due to a vagal response from suctioning. However, it is important for the perianesthesia nurse to refer to the patient's preoperative baseline heart rate because children as young as 10 years may be athletes with a slow resting heart rate. Untreated hypertension in teenage African Americans may occur and is usually mediated with hydralazine or beta blockers. All inhalation gases depress the myocardium, causing hypotension. Hypotension may be reflected with fluid and blood losses, causing poor capillary refill in distal extremities. When the perianesthesia nurse palpates the distal pulses and central pulses, compares the findings, and notes a significant difference in the volume of the weak distal pulses compared with the strong central pulses, this may be a serious concern that should be reported to the anesthesia provider, as well as the surgeon, to be evaluated. If the child becomes bradycardic, consider assisting respirations with a bag-valve mask while another nurse provides high-quality compressions at a rate of 100–120 chest compressions per minute for heart rates less than 60 beats per minute. The 2020 pediatric advanced life support (PALS) guidelines recommend that early epinephrine 0.01 mg/kg (1:10,000 concentration) be administered intravenously for symptomatic bradycardia to prevent the child's cardiac rhythm from deteriorating into asystole.[33] High-quality compressions are required to cause the epinephrine to circulate systemically.

EMERGENCY RESUSCITATION OF PEDIATRIC PATIENTS IN THE PACU

Perianesthesia nurses must be prepared to manage the various forms of airway emergencies, as respiratory compromise can quickly lead to cardiac compromise. According to Christensen et al., hypoxia remains a leading cause of perioperative morbidity and mortality in children.[34] Although pediatric cardiopulmonary arrests in the perioperative period are rare, nearly 20% of such arrests occur during emergence or recovery from anesthesia.[34] According to Christensen et al., training the perianesthesia staff in the recognition, prevention, and early management of respiratory arrests presents opportunities to decrease mortality rates.[34] Likewise, the AAP's 2015 position statement recommended that perianesthesia nurses be competent in PALS.[1] PALS education and competency training provide cognitive knowledge and psychomotor skills in the managing of cardiopulmonary arrest in infants and children. Perianesthesia nurses must astutely identify and competently respond by effectively managing life-threatening postanesthesia pediatric emergencies with the implementation of the AHA's PALS guidelines.[33]

DISCHARGE EDUCATION FOR PEDIATRIC PATIENTS AND FAMILIES

Postanesthesia Phase II care focuses on discharge educational strategies to prepare the child and parents for home care and is one of the most important care activities of the child's perioperative course. When the perianesthesia nurse is reviewing discharge instructions with the parent, it is essential to determine that the caregiver understands and can use the teach-back method in a return demonstration.[3] This technique validates the learning and understanding of the written discharge instructions, ensures compliance, and shows that the parents or caregivers know how to properly care for the child once they return home. The perianesthesia nurse needs to optimize the timing of postoperative teaching so that the caregiver is able to pay attention and is not distracted by the child's crying or irritability. According to American Society of PeriAnesthesia Nurses standards, safe discharge is the responsibility of the perianesthesia nurse. Therefore, the healthcare provider should emphasize that one parent sit in the back seat with the child during the ride home.[35] If the child vomits or starts to cry, the second adult can immediately attend to the child while the other parent is driving. The nurse needs to reinforce that the patient should not lie down in the car but should sit upright and the parent should be sure to use the safety belt to prevent injury to the child.[3] Also, the nurse should state to the parent that the infant's head in the car seat should be supported to keep the head from flopping over and thus occluding the airway.

Provide instructions regarding the effects of anesthesia and medications, as well as pain assessment and management strategies, cautions about the risk of falling, ways of caring for the operative site (e.g., dressing, cast, brace), the resumption of the diet, and the possibility of nausea and/or vomiting.[3] For teenagers, it is important to stress any limitations on physical activity and restrictions on driving, especially when they are taking pain medications. When discussing postoperative care during the follow-up call after the patient is discharged to the home, it is important to review the discharge instructions and allow time for all the parent's questions and concerns to be addressed (Box 22.5).

CHAPTER HIGHLIGHTS

- When a child has ambulatory surgery, safe, high-quality perianesthesia nursing care is critical; it emphasizes that the child is an integral part of the family unit.
- Current evidence shows the epidemiologic trends of pediatric anesthesia and postoperative maladaptive behavior.
- Pediatric physical, cognitive, and social stages of development include a review of Erikson's and Piaget's conceptual frameworks.
- Important preoperative risk factors to identify in pediatric patients are physiologic or anatomic risk factors; environmental risk factors; pediatric suicide risk factors; child abuse risk factors, and child trafficking risk factors.
- Perianesthesia nurses advocate for multimodal pediatric pain management using pharmacologic and nonpharmacologic medications and methods.
- Postanesthesia considerations and complications highlight the critical PACU nursing interventions for emergence agitation/emergence delirium, upper airway obstruction, lower airway or respiratory obstruction, cardiovascular complications, neurologic complications, and obstructive sleep apnea.
- Key perianesthesia ASC education includes critical preoperative as well as PACU Phase II discharge instructions.
- PACU resuscitation of pediatric emergencies is demonstrated in the new 2020 PALS guidelines.

BOX 22.5 PACU Phase II Discharge Teaching

Monitor the child with close observation, which may include staying in the same room with the child during the night.

Keep the child quiet on a sofa or bed while watching TV or playing hand-held electronic games.

Do not let the child participate in contact sports or ride bicycles.

Provide a safe environment at home to prevent injury to the surgical site.

Discuss advancing the diet as tolerated and ordered, beginning with liquids and then trying soft food that is easily digested.

Instruct parents about the signs and symptoms of infection and how to maintain the surgical site dressing. For extremity surgery, ask the parents to demonstrate back the assessment of distal circulation and what to look for when there are signs of deteriorating perfusion to the fingers or toes. Ensure that they understand the importance of elevation in preventing and/or alleviating congestion in the operative extremity if indicated.

Foremost, ensure that the parents know who, when, and where to call in an emergency or if they are concerned about their child's recovery, including the contact numbers in the written instructions.

Discharge instruction tips

For younger children, it is best to go over discharge teaching with the family, if possible, while the child is still sleeping. The family will need to focus on the patient once he or she awakens, and it is more challenging for them once the patient is awake to listen attentively to instructions.

For adolescents, wait to give instructions until the patient is able to listen. Review any restrictions, such as those on driving, if applicable.

Adapted from Mamaril ME, Schnur M. Pediatric patients. In Stannard D, Krenzischek DA, eds. *Perianesthesia Nursing Care: A Bedside Guide for Safe Recovery.* 2nd ed. Jones and Bartlett Learning; 2018.

CASE STUDY

Preoperative assessment of a 3-month-old African American female undergoing general anesthesia for bilateral pressure and equalization tubes revealed the following: a full-term uncomplicated birth; a weight of 7.9 kg; vital signs of blood pressure 87/61, pulse 118, respiratory rate 22, oxygen saturation 96% (room air), temperature 36.9°C; no allergies; no medications; bilateral lungs auscultated clear; heart sounds S1 and S2, regular rate, no bruits; no recent upper respiratory infection or flu, except some clear mucus from both nostrils; healthy status, takes breast milk; NPO since 4 hours ago; disposition cooperative and playful. When questioning Mom about exposure to second-hand smoke, she denied any, stating that she rarely smoked cigarettes since having the baby.

- The anesthesia provider reviewed the preoperative nursing assessment and vital signs, as well as discussed the baby's health history. Then, the anesthesia provider assigned an ASA I physical health status to this patient.
- The intraoperative course went without incident with mask induction of sevoflurane. The anesthesia provider extubated the infant deep, placed an oral airway, and applied 6 L of oxygen via face mask to the patient, and her oxygen saturation was 97% in the operating room. When the patient was being transported to the PACU, she suddenly began emitting intermittent high-pitched crowing sounds.
- Vital signs on admission to the PACU: physiologic monitor revealed oxygen saturation 90% on 6 L of oxygen via face mask; heart rate 68; respiratory rate unresponsive; oral airway in place; mild inspiratory stridor; bilateral rise and fall of chest/diminished breath sounds bilaterally; mild sternal retractions.
- Vital signs 10 minutes later: oxygen saturation 66% on 6 L of oxygen via face mask; heart rate 38; respiratory rate no rise or fall of chest/no audible breath sounds

bilaterally; sternal retractions; lips and mucus membranes cyanotic.

The anesthesia provider quickly began providing positive end-expiratory pressure (PEEP) via Mapleson bag-valve mask with high-flow oxygen at 15 L. The perianesthesia nurse hit the code button, called for the code cart, and began chest compressions. The laryngospasm quickly resolved, and the infant started to cry. Her mucus membranes were pink, and her vital signs were 100% oxygen saturation with non-rebreather high-flow oxygen; heart rate 122; respiratory rate 28. The mom was escorted into the PACU to be with her baby. Once Mom was holding baby in the PACU, the perianesthesia nurse explained the respiratory complications that had occurred and gently questioned her again about the pulmonary risk of second-hand smoke to young infants. It was then that the mother shared that the only time the baby was exposed to secondary smoke was during the night hours when breast feeding. The perianesthesia nurse educated the mom regarding the importance of letting the healthcare team, especially the preoperative nurse and the anesthesia provider, know about passive smoke exposure before anesthesia.

Passive Smoke Exposure as a Risk Factor for Airway Complications During Outpatient Procedures

- Research study reviewed 405 children having outpatient procedures with general anesthesia by mask.
- Double-blinded outcomes were studied with respect to adverse airway events.
- Of the children, 168 experienced adverse airway events (breath holding, laryngospasms, and airway obstructions) in the PACU.
- Children who had had passive smoke exposure were 4.9 more likely to have laryngospasms and 2.8 times more likely to have airway obstructions.

Jones DT, Bhattachart N. Passive smoke exposure as a risk factor for airway complications during outpatient procedures. *Otolaryngol Head Neck Surg.* 2006;135:12–16.

REFERENCES

1. American Academy of Pediatrics. Critical elements for the pediatric perioperative anesthesia environment. *Pediatrics.* 2015;136(6):1200-1205. Available at: https://doi.org/10.1542/peds.2015-3595.
2. Algren CL. Family-centered care of the child during illness and hospitalization. In: Hockenberry MJ, Wilson D. *Wong's Nursing Care of Infants and Children.* 10th ed. Mosby Elsevier; 2020.
3. Mamaril ME, Schnur M. Pediatric patients. In: Stannard D, Krenzischek DA, eds. *Perianesthesia Nursing Care: A Bedside Guide for Safe Recovery.* 2nd ed. Jones and Bartlett Learning; 2018.
4. Barrera P, Hockenberry MJ. Perspectives of pediatric nursing. In: Hockenberry MJ, Wilson D. *Wong's Nursing Care of Infants and Children.* 10th ed. Mosby Elsevier; 2020.
5. Streuli JC, Michel M, Vayena E. Children's rights in pediatrics. *Eur J Pediatr.* 2011;170(1):9-14. Available at: https://doi.org/10.1007/s00431-010-1205-8.
6. Rabbits JA, Groenewald CB. Epidemiology of pediatric surgery in the United States. *Paediatr Anaesth.* 2020;30(10):1083-1090. Available at: https://doi.org/10.1111/pan.13993.
7. U.S. Food and Drug Administration. *FDA Drug Safety Communication: FDA Review Results in New Warnings About Using General Anesthetics and Sedation Drugs in Young Children and Pregnant Women. Drug Safety Availability.* 2016. https://www.fda.gov/media/101937/download.
8. Sun LS, Li G, Miller TL, et al. Association between a single general anesthesia exposure before the age of 36 months and neurocognitive outcomes in later childhood. *JAMA.* 2016;315(21):2312-20. Available at: https://doi.org/10.1001/jama.2016.6967.
9. Davidson AJ, Disma N, de Graaff JC, et al. Neurodevelopmental outcome at 2 years of age, after general anaesthesia and awake-regional anaesthesia in infancy (GAS): an international multi-centre, randomized controlled trial. *Lancet.* 2016;387(10015):239-250. Available at: https://doi.org/10.1016/s0140-6736(15)00608-x.
10. Andropoulos DB, Greene MF. Anesthesia and developing brains: implications of the FDA warning. *N Engl J Med.* 2017;376(10):905-907. Available at: https://doi.org/10.1056/nejmp1700196.
11. Sadhasivam S, Cohen LL, Hosu L, et al. Real-time assessment of perioperative behaviors in children and parents: development and validation of the perioperative adult child behavioral interaction scale. *Anesth Analg.* 2010;110(4):1109-1115. Available at: https://doi.org/10.1213/ane.0b013e3181d2a509.
12. Fortier MA, Del Rosario AM, Rosenbaum A, Kain ZN. Beyond pain: predictors of postoperative maladaptive behavior change of children. *Paediatr Anaesth.* 2010;20(5):445-453. Available at: https://doi.org/10.1111/j.1460-9592.2010.03281.x.
13. Abidin HZ, Omar SC, Mazalan MZ, et al. Postoperative maladaptive behavior, preoperative anxiety and emergence delirium in children undergoing general anesthesia: a narrative review. *Glob Pediatr Health.* 2021;8;2333794X211007975. Available at: https://doi.org/10.1177/2333794x211007975.
14. Wilson D. Promoting optimum growth and development. In: Hockenberry MJ, Wilson D, eds. *Wong's Nursing Care of Infants and Children.* 10th ed. Mosby Elsevier; 2020.
15. Mamaril ME. Preoperative risk factors associated with PACU pediatric respiratory complications: an integrative review. *J Perianesth*

Nurs. 2020;35(2):125-134. Available at: https://doi.org/10.1016/j.jopan.2019.09.002.

16. Hesselgrave J. Developmental influences on child health promotions. In: Hockenberry MJ, Wilson D, eds. *Wong's Nursing Care of Infants and Children.* 10th ed. Mosby Elsevier; 2020.
17. Chiswell C, Akram Y. Impact of environmental tobacco smoke exposure on anaesthetic and surgical outcomes in children: a systematic review and meta-analysis. *Arch Dis Child.* 2017;102(2):123-130. Available at: https://doi.org/10.1136/archdischild-2016-310687.
18. Hui JW, Ong J, Herdegen JJ, et al. Risk of obstructive sleep apnea in African American patients with chronic rhinosinusitis. *Ann Allergy Asthma Immunol.* 2017;118(6):685-688. Available at: https://doi.org/10.1016/j.anai.2017.03.009.
19. American Academy of Child & Adolescent Psychiatry. *Suicide in Children and Teens.* 2021. Available at: https://www.aacap.org/AACAP/Families_and_Youth/Facts_for_Families/FFF-Guide/Teen-Suicide-010.aspx.
20. Rufino KA, Patriquin MA. Child and adolescent suicide: contributing risk factors and new evidence-based interventions. *Children's Health Care.* 2019;48(4):345-350. Available at: https://doi.org/10.1080/02739615.2019.1666009.
21. Shain B, Committee on Adolescence. Suicide and suicide attempts in adolescents. *Pediatrics.* 2016;138(1):e1-e12. Available at: https://doi.org/10.1542/peds.2016-1420.
22. Nierengarten MB. Suicide attempts and ideation among teens are on the rise. *Contemp Pediatr.* 2018;35(8):32-34. Available at: https://cdn.sanity.io/files/0vv8moc6/contpeds/244809d86bb287d1b7fb31e000e185c548659360.pdf/cntped0818_ezineR2.pdf.
23. Wilson D. Health promotion of the toddler and family. In: Hockenberry MJ, Wilson D, eds. *Wong's Nursing Care of Infants and Children.* 10th ed. Mosby Elsevier; 2020.
24. Costa CB, McCoy KT, Early GJ, Deckers CM. Evidence-based care of the human trafficking patient. *Nurs Clin North Am.* 2019;54(4):569-584. Available at: https://doi.org/10.1016/j.cnur.2019.08.007.
25. Cravero JP, Agarwal R, Berde C, et al. The Society for Pediatric Anesthesia recommendations for the use of opioids in children during the perioperative period. *Paediatr Anaesth.* 2019;29(6):547-571. Available at: https://doi.org/10.1111/pan.13639.
26. Frizzell KH, Cavanaugh PK, Herman MJ. Pediatric perioperative pain management. *Orthop Clin North Am.* 2017;48(4):467-480. Available at: https://doi.org/10.1016/j.ocl.2017.06.007.
27. Kain ZN, Mayes LC, Caramico LA, et al. Parental presence during induction of anesthesia: a randomized controlled trial. *Anesthesiology.* 1996;84(5):1060-1067. Available at: https://doi.org/10.1097/00000542-199605000-00007.
28. Lauder G, Emmott A. Confronting the challenges of effective pain management in children following tonsillectomy. *Int J Pediatr Otorhinolaryngol.* 2014;78(11):1813-827. Available at: https://doi.org/10.1016/j.ijporl.2014.08.011.
29. Chidambaran V, Sadhasivam S, Mahmoud M. Codeine and opioid metabolism: Implications and alternatives for pediatric pain management. *Curr Opin Anaesthesiol.* 2017;30(3):349-356. Available at: https://doi.org/10.1097/aco.0000000000000455.
30. Aker JG. Pediatric anesthesia. In: Elisha S, Nagelhout JJ, eds. *Nurse Anesthesia.* 6th ed. Elsevier; 2017.
31. Hsu G, von Ungern-Sternberg BS, Engelhardt T. Pediatric airway management. *Curr Opin Anaesthesiol.* 2021;34(3):276-283. Available at: https://doi.org/10.1097/aco.0000000000000993.
32. Chattopadhyay S, Rudra A, Sengupta S. Laryngospasm in pediatric anesthesia: a review. *Int J Anes Res.* 2013;1(1):97-104.
33. American Heart Association. *Pediatric Advanced Life Support Provider Manual.* American Heart Association; 2020.
34. Christensen R, Voepel-Lewis T, Lewis I, et al. Pediatric cardiopulmonary arrest in the postanesthesia care unit: analysis of data from the American heart association gets with the guidelines—Resuscitation registry. *Paediatr Anaesth.* 2013;23(6):517-523. Available at: https://doi.org/10.1111/pan.12154.
35. American Society of PeriAnesthesia Nurses. *2023-2024 Perianesthesia Nursing Standards, Practice Recommendations and Interpretive Statements.* ASPAN; 2022.

23 Special Needs of the Older Patient

Myrna Eileen Mamaril, DNP, RN, NEA-BC, CPAN, CAPA, FAAN, FASPAN

LEARNING OBJECTIVES

A review of the content of this chapter will help the reader to:

1. Describe the demographic and statistical trends of older adults living in the United States.
2. Discuss the influence of cultural and ethnic attributes of geriatric patients.
3. Summarize important environment of care considerations in ambulatory surgery centers.
4. Compare and contrast the pathophysiology of aging and polypharmacy outcomes.
5. Review critical perianesthesia nursing assessments, interventions, and coordination of care implications.
6. Identify key older adult patient and family education strategies for successful ambulatory surgery outcomes.

OVERVIEW

Older adults are living longer with chronic, complex illnesses that affect all aspects of their lives. Many are faced with the need for surgery, invasive diagnostic procedures, and/or therapeutic interventions to improve their quality of life. Maintaining the health of an aging population focuses on developing a high level of wellness to address the mind–body–spirit approach to holistic perianesthesia nursing care. Ambulatory surgery centers (ASCs) embrace the wellness philosophy, which creates an ideal, patient-centered environment of care for these older adults. However, nurses realize that this vulnerable elderly population is at increased risk when undergoing anesthesia for surgery or invasive procedures due to significant co-morbidities and, in some cases, difficulties in gaining access to healthcare. More importantly, geriatric patients require an interdisciplinary approach to comprehensively evaluate preoperative co-morbidities, anesthesia risk factors, cognitive abilities, and frailty status to appropriately optimize their functional reserve for uneventful and positive postsurgical outcomes. Perianesthesia nurses must understand the importance of providing compassionate, high-quality care to older adults.

The chapter begins by defining the term *aging*, along with describing the demographic, historical, and statistical trends for geriatric surgical patients. Ethnic and cultural attributes of the elderly are described in terms of how they significantly affect health outcomes. The epidemiology of frailty, along with the pathophysiology of aging and other geriatric information such as screening and preoperative risk identification, is discussed. This information focuses on the assessment of the patient's physiologic functional reserves and cognitive status, issues of polypharmacy, and psychosocial and spiritual matters. Finally, an overview of patient and family education, including important preoperative preparations and safe postanesthesia discharge instructions for home care, is presented.

THE AGING POPULATION

The population of the United States is now composed of more elderly people than ever before. Redburn first used the term *population aging* to describe a demographic characteristic of adults age 65 years and older.[1] The growth in the size of aging populations is a result of improvements in health and increased longevity.[2] Miller describes how many images of aging are often associated with being "old" or "elderly" and reflect disease, deterioration, disability, or even dying.[3] According to Miller, the contrary is true, and older adults actually function well independently with a high quality of life and stable health conditions.[3]

Gerontologists, healthcare personnel, and even the American public define aging from many different perspectives.[3] A common definition is that aging is simply a physiologic process of chronologic growth and development, which begins at birth and continues into older adulthood. Another definition is that aging is a subjective or perceived state in which a person's estimated age is based on the appearance of good or frail health.[3] *Chronologic age* refers to the length of time that has passed since a person's birth. It has also been used to describe different stages of life; for elderly people, there are young elderly, of 65–75 years of age; old elderly, of 75–85 years of age; super elderly, of 85–99 years of age; and centurions, of 100 years of age and older. Other terms for age identity are subjective age, perceived age, cognitive age, stereotypical age, comparative age, and "how one actually feels" age. Today's geriatric scientists agree that aging is too complex a phenomenon to be based only on the year of birth.[3] Furthermore, it may be difficult to distinguish between the effects of normal aging and the disease processes that are common, but by no means inevitable, in the older population.

The term *elderly,* generally defined as anyone age 65 years or older, is a useful measure for making decisions about a person's financial status, future volunteer or job opportunities, and/or retirement.[3,4] People must be assessed medically to determine their functional or physiologic age in relation to their chronologic age. Many 70-year-olds are vigorous and healthy and maintain a physiologic age years younger than the age indicated by their birth certificates. Conversely, a chronically ill man of 55 years of age may function like a person of a significantly older age. When a healthcare team is assessing a person's age, caution is advised, because basing assumptions on appearances may be lead to poor decisions (e.g., the team may be overconfident about administering drugs or anesthetic agents to an older adult who appears to be in good health but is not). Researchers generally agree that the aging process alters the body's ability to respond or adapt to stress.[4] The apparently well-controlled elderly diabetic patient who is admitted for cataract surgery and interrupts his or her normal dietary schedule may have a higher likelihood of a glycemic reaction than the young teenager whose ability to adapt to interruptions or stressors is much greater.

Functional age is another important term that gerontologists use to describe physiologic health, psychological well-being, and the ability to function and participate in quality-of-life activities.[4] Miller suggests that an advantage of functional definitions of age over chronologic definitions is that functional age is associated with "higher levels of well-being."[3] The author also reports that the concept of functional status is associated with a more rational basis of care and the engagement of older adults in healthy, holistic lifestyles.

Aging is a natural process that gradually begins in early adulthood, continues throughout the life cycle, and leads to many noticeable changes in many organ systems. Consequently, a substantial proportion of older people report having at least one chronic condition or disease, including arthritis, osteoporosis, hypertension, anemia, heart disease, hearing impairments, visual impairments (especially cataracts), orthopedic problems, and diabetes.[4] These body system changes may decrease elderly persons' abilities to adapt physically, emotionally, and psychologically, especially when they learn they need surgery. Therefore, as the proportion of frail elders increases, so does the number of chronically ill, debilitated, or mildly cognitively impaired patients in outpatient surgery settings.

Older adults with well-controlled preexisting diseases who are having surgery make up a large number of the patients in an outpatient or ambulatory surgical setting. These older adults are physically healthy, self-sufficient, and mentally astute well into their nineties, with active lifestyles, close family relationships, and much participation in community or religious activities.

DEMOGRAPHIC AND STATISTICAL TRENDS IN AGING POPULATIONS

There were over 48.3 million ambulatory surgical and interventional procedures performed in hospital outpatient surgery centers and free-standing same-day surgery centers in 2010.[5] Over one third of those outpatient surgeries were performed on older adults.[5] One important driver of the growth in numbers of ASCs was a shift in the regulations of the Center of Medicare and Medicaid Services in 2019 on the facilities in which certain procedures could take place for Medicare patients: the shift was from hospital-based surgical settings to outpatient surgery center settings.[6] Total hip and total knee arthroplasties are now outpatient procedures.[6,7] Other types of surgery have also been approved for ASC settings, and this has meant that higher numbers of elderly patients are having elective procedures in ASCs.[6,7] These numbers will continue to grow due to advances in anesthesia agents and techniques, minimally invasive surgical techniques, technology for safety monitoring devices, and noninvasive technologies such as laser therapy.[6,7] White and colleagues report that the population between the ages of 65 and 75 years is increasing by more than 2% per year and the population over 80 years of age is increasing by more than 3% per year.[6] Interestingly, over 30% of the total geriatric outpatient surgeries done took place at free-standing ambulatory centers in the 2010s.[5,6]

The National Health Statistics Reports noted that the most common operations on the digestive system were endoscopy of the large intestine (colonoscopy) at over 2.2 million and endoscopic polypectomy of the large intestine at 1.1 million, or a total of 3.3 million.[5] The second most common operation was cataract extraction with insertion of an intraocular lens at 2.6 million and operations on the eyelids at 1 million.[5] Outpatient musculoskeletal procedures totaled over 1.3 million, and procedures involving the nervous system, including injections into the spinal canal as nerve blocks for pain management, totaled 2.9 million.[5] Even the duration of same-day surgery has decreased, with endoscopic procedures taking an average of 14 minutes, cataract surgeries with lens insertion approximately 10 minutes, and arthroscopies of the knee approximately 32 minutes.[5]

The U.S. Census Bureau estimates that by 2030, there will be 72 million older adults, and this will result in a dramatic increase in the surgical and nonsurgical outpatient procedures performed.[7] Even more significant is the proportion of those who will be 85 years and older, often referred as the "old-old" age group. This age group is expected to grow rapidly compared with the "old" age group of 65–84 years.[7]

CULTURAL AND ETHNIC CONSIDERATIONS OF OLDER ADULTS

Cultural and ethnic backgrounds of older adults significantly influence their values, behaviors, communication, health beliefs, and perceptions of outpatient surgery.[2] In the United States there has been a gradual shift in the size of certain groups; African Americans have been the largest minority, but Hispanics will soon become the largest minority group.[3] Warshaw et al. report that dramatic shifts in elderly cultural and ethnic minority populations should be expected during the twenty-first century because of immigration.[2] Currently, Asians have the longest life expectancy of all ethnic populations.[2] Although White Americans live longer than African Americans, until 75 years of age on average, African Americans who surpass 75 years are believed to have greater "hardiness" as survivors.[2] As the population ages and ethnic diversity increases, several important nursing considerations should be contemplated when interacting with these patients. Language and communications challenges may be significant when healthcare workers screen for and identify preoperative health risks. Multiple chronic co-morbidities of older frail adults are often complex. Understanding them thoroughly may be complicated by difficulties in communication when eliciting patient histories, and helping the patient to understand them may also be difficult for the same reason.[2] Older persons from different cultures may refuse surgeries that are too expensive or difficult to accept because of their cultural beliefs.[2] Some elderly patients may no longer have the mental capacity to participate in providing informed consent for surgery or anesthesia. Older adults from different cultures or ethnic backgrounds may be reluctant to seek medical care or have outpatient surgery because they view illnesses or disease processes as the "will of God" and an inevitable consequence of the aging process.[2] Perianesthesia nurses need to be aware of these feelings and assess their own cultural and ethnic beliefs in order to effectively care for this vulnerable older population.

CREATING A CARING AMBULATORY SURGERY ENVIRONMENT

Older adults have been productive and vital members of their families, the workforce, and society, and as such, they deserve respectful and considerate treatment. Ideally, those working and talking with elderly people should incorporate topics that older adults value, such as the type of work they did (or do) and the sports or hobbies they enjoy. When the psychological and emotional pressures of growing older are identified during a stressful preoperative interview, perianesthesia nurses should convey kindness, empathy, and respectfulness in their verbal and nonverbal communications.

Besides offering expert physical care, the perianesthesia nurse should provide an atmosphere that encourages elderly patients to maintain their self-esteem and independence through retaining as much control over the environment and situation as possible. Older adults should participate as fully as they are able in their care and in setting goals for that care. Competent patients must be permitted to make their own decisions, including the right to refuse care, a situation that the family and nurses may occasionally find difficult to accept.

If it is determined that a patient is incompetent to make his or her own decisions, it is important to follow the federal, state, and ambulatory surgery guidelines. Issues of individual rights and autonomy have been the subjects of much discussion. These issues are likely to become more and more contentious as the population ages and increasing numbers of seniors choose to question, rather than passively accept, decisions made about their health.

Aging does not mean loss of intelligence. Older people should not be treated like children or as though they are incapable of comprehension. Although measures of abstract intelligence such as solving mathematical problems or puzzles or assembling objects may decline in elderly persons, measures related to vocabulary, comprehension, and acquired information remain essentially unchanged. It is likely that any intellectual changes noted may be attributed to declining sensory function, a lessened ability to assimilate new information, and the need for increased time for processing that information. The nurse must allow sufficient time for the patient to respond to questions and process the information being provided. It must also be remembered that the motivation to learn or to follow directions may be impacted by depression, a very common and treatable condition in the elderly population.[2,3]

Time is a precious commodity in a busy ambulatory surgical unit. Perianesthesia nurses must be particularly creative, efficient, and resourceful so they can provide as much time as possible for interactions with their older patients. Elderly people can become confused or disoriented by hasty instructions or rapid activity. For nurses, presenting an unhurried demeanor in the face of constant pressures to perform numerous functions can be challenging. Sitting down, even briefly, for an interchange using a friendly smile, direct eye contact, and a caring voice with patients may neutralize the appearance of haste and impatience. Further, this communication style enhances mutual responsibility for care rather than an authoritarian relationship. Perianesthesia nurses have an ethical obligation to advocate for safe, quality, and compassionate elder care.

There is evidence to suggest that the memory of recent events declines with advancing years, whereas long-term memory remains essentially intact. This is an issue of particular importance to the nurse providing preoperative or discharge instructions to older patients. Elders appear to learn more efficiently when they are allowed to set their own pace. Sensory losses (especially of hearing), noisy environments, and distractions can reduce the ability or desire to remember instructions.[3]

Many older adults who have outlived family and friends are chronically deprived of the warmth of human touch, a gift that can readily be given in any nursing setting. Sometimes, the nurse is the only person, or one of a few, who may show genuine concern for an elderly person who is living alone. Thus, the most effective show of concern the nurse can offer is patience, a gentle touch, and the ability to actively listen, not just hear.

Some elderly patients may complain about a multitude of minor or perceived problems. The compassionate and astute nurse considers the patient's history or reference point for possible loneliness as one of several bases for such complaints. From that perspective, a caring approach, rather than one tinged with impatience or curtness, is more likely to establish a trusting relationship. Still, it is vitally important not to ignore or avoid the patient who is complaining. A real medical problem may be overlooked or missed when the behavior is seen outside of the context of the individual's ordinary daily behavior. It is a challenge to detect a subtle change in behavior and then try to determine whether it is related to a true medical problem. The perianesthesia nurse must understand the many effects of aging, as well as the symptoms of chronic diseases, and be able to differentiate between them. After careful assessment, a same-day-surgery nursing plan of care can be formulated to assist each older adult through a safe surgical and recovery course.

Specific Environmental Concerns in ASCs

Providing a safe and comfortable setting for older patients requires meticulous attention to numerous environmental issues. Floors must be free of obstruction and not slippery. The elderly patient is generally more sensitive to extremes in room temperature, particularly cold air conditioning or nearby fans, so a moderate room temperature should be maintained. Rooms should be well lit with nonglare lights. The choice of wall and door colorings is important; a darker color around door frames in contrast with walls helps older people identify exits. Colors brighter than pastels are detected better by the aging eye. Handrails provided in bathrooms and hallways help patients ambulate more safely. Nearby wheelchair-accessible bathrooms are appreciated.

Furniture should be selected for comfort, including the appropriate height for older people, who may have limited motion or strength. Ease of cleaning is an important consideration in furniture selection. Stretchers that lower for easy access without the use of a stepstool are ideal. When stepstools are used for access to higher surfaces, nontipping stools with attached handrails provide steadier assistance. Covered entrances and exits should be available to protect patients from weather conditions. This is particularly important for older adults, who could easily fall in rainy, snowy, or icy conditions.

ADVANTAGES AND DISADVANTAGES OF AMBULATORY SURGERY FOR OLDER ADULTS

The ambulatory approach offers the elderly person certain advantages. The decreased risk of nosocomial infections, particularly wound and respiratory infections, is one of the greatest advantages because the ability to combat infection may be altered in the aging immune system. There is less likelihood of mental confusion related to environmental changes and less disruption and loss of control over the older person's personal habits, eating schedules, and medication routines. Reduction in the time spent away from home, family, and friends is also an advantage that most elderly patients appreciate.

There may also be significant disadvantages for the older adult having same-day surgery. Frail elderly persons with complex co-morbidities and/or cognitive deficits may not be candidates for elective surgeries in free-standing surgery settings. Forgetful older patients may not follow NPO guidelines or changes to their preoperative medication schedules. They may not be aware of the need to discuss these issues with the nurse. After surgery, they may not follow directions or take medications as prescribed. At home alone, they may fall, contaminate the wound site by mishandling the dressing, or suffer from complications of a chronic systemic illness, all without the knowledge of their families or physicians. Being alone after surgery, fearing complications, and not coping with changes in daily routines necessitated by new medication protocols or care related to the surgery can be unsettling.

Transportation issues can be a financial and logistical burden, particularly when numerous trips to various care sites are required before and after surgery. Perianesthesia nurses may be able to assist in coordinating the necessary tests, such as laboratory and radiologic studies, so that they can be done in a single visit but at the same time not be tiring to patients, so as to conserve patients' resources, including their energy.

Safe discharge to go home is the responsibility of the perianesthesia nurse. This includes ensuring that the patient fully meets the discharge criteria and has the ability to be safe after discharge. A lack of appropriate home support creates another difficult situation for many older adults. Some patients may actually be the support or caregiver for a spouse or family member who requires daily care. If the patient is the only automobile driver in the home, transportation needs will have to be filled by someone else. The older adult may refuse to have friends or neighbors help for various reasons, ranging from privacy to pride. Regardless of the reason given, the nurse must persist until a plan has been mutually agreed upon that ensures the appropriate home support.

Financial concerns can also be a problem for older adults, particularly those with a fixed income. One reason for financial hardship might be the inability to purchase prescription drugs and/or nutritious food. Another problem might be the cost of transportation to and from medical appointments. A social services representative can be consulted to consider appropriate alternatives. In a free-standing surgery center or another facility without specialized resources, the physician should be contacted and asked to intercede appropriately. Writing prescriptions for lower-cost generic drugs is also a way the physician can financially assist vulnerable older adults.

EPIDEMIOLOGY OF FRAILTY

Frailty is an overarching public health crisis of population aging; however, as a concept and condition, frailty is poorly understood and underrecognized in clinical settings.[8] *Frailty* is most commonly found in older adults and is often described as a state of increased vulnerability resulting from a decline in physiologic reserves and functions across multiple organ systems.[8,9] Maxwell and Wang define frailty as a recognizable state of increasing vulnerability for the impairment to withstand stressors, such as surgery and anesthesia.[8] This places the frail elderly at a higher risk for negative health outcomes.[8-12] Physiologic dysregulation which contributes to

the trajectory of frailty, often begins in midlife before clinical manifestations are apparent. In fact, the intermediate stage known as *prefrailty* is related to early functional decline. This state of health can be detected and addressed to delay the development of advanced frailty and subsequent disability.[8-12]

Multiple studies have shown a strong association between frailty and adverse perioperative outcomes.[8-12] Frailty is now recognized as a "stronger indicator than chronologic aging that is frequently characterized by the gradual loss of energy, strength, endurance, and motor control."[8] Seib et al. found that frailty is predictive of postoperative morbidity in common ambulatory general surgeries and is independent of age, the type of anesthesia, and other co-morbidities.[12] These researchers conducted a retrospective cohort study that reviewed over 140,828 ambulatory general surgery patients and found that a high frailty score was associated with serious complications. Interestingly, they also found that the monitoring of anesthesia care and local anesthesia was the only modifiable co-variate associated with decreased odds.[12] Frailty was associated with worse perioperative outcomes for patients undergoing outpatient surgery for hernias, thyroid disorders, and parathyroid disorders.[12] In fact, frailty in older adults is considered the most important risk factor of the postoperative course.[12]

Perianesthesia nurses play an important role in screening for and identifying frailty and the unique risks in anesthesia and surgery associated with it. One of a number of frailty assessment tools can be used to identify frailty during preoperative screening The perianesthesia nurse should incorporate, document, and report the findings according to facility protocols (Figure 23.1).

PATHOPHYSIOLOGY OF AGING

Many changes occur in virtually every system of the body as part of the normal aging process. These changes may vary from patient to patient. It is critical to differentiate the normal changes related to aging from the pathologic changes of disease. The perianesthesia nurse should be aware of the relatively common physiologic and psychological characteristics of elderly persons.

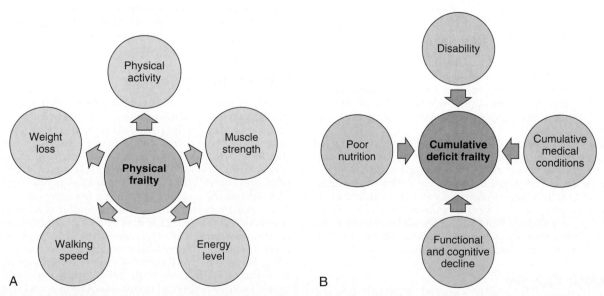

Fig. 23.1 The aging patient. Previll LA, Heflin MT, Cohen HJ. The aging patient. Figure 126.5 in: Wing EJ, Schiffman FJ, eds. *Cecil Essentials of Medicine.* 10th edition. Elsevier; 2021.

General Physiologic Changes of Aging

Physiologic decline with aging is a universal occurrence among body systems. Certain physiologic changes affect the body as a whole. There is an overall reduction in the body's ability to respond to stress of any type, such as changes in blood pressure, decreased oxygen levels, and decreased airway secretions. The older adult's tissues become less elastic and resilient and their reflexes become slower. There is a general decrease in the neuromuscular response and the efficiency of the immune system. Table 23.1 lists the physiologic changes in the aging patient and their implications for nursing.

An overall decrease in the number of cells in the body diminishes the effectiveness of virtually all organs and affects functions such as drug elimination via the liver and kidneys and cognitive skills such as remembering instructions. The elasticity of tissues is reduced, resulting in decreased lung compliance, artery rigidity, and wrinkling of the skin. Wound healing is slower because of a diminished response to inflammatory stimuli, slower rate of wound contraction, the effects of cellular aging, and inadequate amounts of proteins and vitamins as a result of poor nutrition.[2,3] Aging also leads to a decrease in fibroblasts, the cells that are responsible for the synthesis of protein and collagen.[2] Other factors that can lead to delayed wound healing include circulatory changes and a decreased resistance to infection.[2,3]

Circulatory Changes

In the cardiovascular system, disease, rather than normal aging, appears to be the most prevalent reason for most cardiac dysfunctions.[2] Blood pressure trends in older adults tend to increase with age, intrinsic cardiac contractile function declines, and cardiac reserve diminishes slowly in healthy elderly persons.[2] Multiple physiologic changes impact the oxygenation of blood, as well as the delivery of oxygen to tissues. The net effect of these physiologic changes, in addition to the impact of anesthesia, may promote hypoxia and confusion in surgical patients. They may also be due to anemia, which causes a decreased ability of the blood to transport oxygen and is a frequent finding in elderly people. The situation is further complicated by sclerosis of the vessels, which mechanically limits the blood flow to the periphery. Coronary artery disease is very common in older adults and remains the most common cause of death in adults 65 years and older.[2]

Respiratory and Pulmonary Changes

According to Warshaw et al., as the older adult ages, a mild decline in pulmonary function is observed.[2] Lung function declines in the areas of tidal volume, forced vital capacity, total lung volume, forced respiratory volume, forced inspiratory volume, aveolar-capillary diffusing capacity, and arterial oxygen pressure.

Changes in the pulmonary physiologic reserves in aging adults rarely result in significant impairments on their own.[2] Pulmonary disease must always be ruled out when an elderly patient becomes symptomatic.[2] Miller emphasizes that cumulative effects from external environmental exposures, such as the inhalation of tobacco smoke, aerosolized chemicals, or toxic fumes, throughout life place older adults at greater risk for diminished immune responses, chronic obstructive pulmonary disease, heart disease, or even cancer.[3]

Neurologic Changes

Nervous system function tends to decline with age, leading to impairments in cognition and motor, sensory, and autonomic nerve function. However, there may be an individual variability in the degree to which these changes occur in older adults. According to Warshaw et al., alterations in neurologic function may be profound, especially beyond age 75 years.[2] Warshaw et al. also report that studies of the brain (e.g., neuronal loss, dendrite changes, pigment accumulation, decreasing neurotransmitters, modest decreases in brain mass) are ongoing and focused on the clinical management of older adults.[2] Geriatric patients undergoing surgery are at risk for delirium (Box 23.1). Postoperative delirium is associated with an increased risk for mortality. An increased sensitivity to changes in oxygenation may lead to hypoxia and postoperative cognitive dysfunction in the older patient.

Renal and Urinary Changes

As one ages, changes occur in the kidneys, urethra, and bladder, and the physiologic mechanisms for controlling urination may also change.[3] Peak bladder capacity decreases, and residual urine moderately increases. These changes may cause symptoms of frequency. Renal blood flow decreases, and creatinine clearance also decreases with age. Changes in renal blood flow impact the delivery of anesthetic agents to the kidney and the rate of drug elimination. Older women develop pelvic floor muscle dysfunction that can lead to frequency and incontinence. In men, the prostate becomes enlarged and may develop hyperplasia, causing voiding problems; this is a common occurrence. The increased prevalence of prostate cancer is likely a reflection of more frequent surveillance and sophisticated diagnostic tests than an actual increase in numbers of cases.

Musculoskeletal Changes

Many older adults experience an increased incidence of osteoarthritis, rheumatoid arthritis, and problems with back and cervical spine mobility. These musculoskeletal changes present challenges for airway management throughout the anesthesia experience. Elderly patients frequently have intervertebral disc degeneration of the spinal column with disc herniation that may lead to nerve root impingement and symptoms of spinal stenosis. Regional anesthesia may be more difficult in elders. Osteoporosis is a common cause of traumatic injuries in elders, including hip fractures. Routine surgical positioning may contribute to postoperative pain in the older patient. Treatment of positioning discomfort with heat, ice, or repositioning may reduce the need for analgesics.

External Physical Changes

Elderly people tend to have changes in their physical appearance. A gradual loss of height may begin at 50–80 years of age and may result in the loss of as much as 2 inches in height. The loss of connective tissue results in changes in the body contours. Despite an overall increase in body fat content, the amount of subcutaneous fat actually decreases with age, and this decrease promotes the loss of body heat and reduces the amount of padding for bony prominences. The overall increase in body fat promotes absorption and provides increased storage depots for fat-soluble anesthetic drugs and agents. Both the tissues that store water and the total amount of intracellular water decrease proportionately. Because of this lessened fluid volume, the older adult is at increased risk for both dehydration and fluid overload. Typically, drier mucous membranes and wrinkled skin may complicate the assessment of dehydration in the elderly.

TABLE 23.1 Physiologic Characteristics of Aging and Their Implications for Nursing

Physiologic Changes	Effects	Nursing Implications
CENTRAL NERVOUS SYSTEM		
↓ Weight of brain, ↓ number of neurons	↑ Potential for central nervous system side effects of drugs	Observe for prolonged or toxic effects; encourage reduced drug dosages Enforce safety measures, siderails, observation; increase family involvement in home care; involve social services, home support services, caregiver support group for spouse or other caregiver Allow adequate time for instructions, no distractions; ↓ noise Provide verbal and written instructions; include family Provide supportive postanesthesia care for longer period Prepare for possible ↑ in length of stay in ASC Provide respectful, adult treatment
↓ Cerebral blood flow and CNS activity	May exhibit signs of Alzheimer disease or other organic dementias	
↓ Cognition and learning speed	↓ Understanding and memory	
↓ Minimum alveolar concentration requirements	Prolonged emergence from general anesthesia	
No change in intelligence		
PERIPHERAL NERVOUS SYSTEM		
↓ Number of neuromuscular connections ↓ Number of axons supplying peripheral muscles	↓ Dosage needs for regional anesthesia	Observe for prolonged or toxic effects of regional anesthetics Implement slower position changes Monitor fluid maintenance Provide appropriate analgesia based on patient assessment data Support multimodality approach to pain management and supplemental therapies (e.g., positioning, relaxation)
↓ Autonomic reflexes	↓ Response to stress and blood pressure changes	
Normal or lowered pain perception	Requires same amount of or less analgesia, depending on assessment of pain	
CARDIOVASCULAR SYSTEM		
↓ Contractility and ↓ cardiac reserve ↓ Cardiac output, atrophy of myocardial fibers	↓ Response to stress and blood pressure changes	Ascertain cardioactive medications taken preoperatively Use caution with fluid replacement Expect slower metabolism of drugs (↓ blood to organs) Assess heart and lung sounds for signs of overload or heart failure Allow adequate time for response to medications before redosing Be aware of possible ↓ workload of heart Provide adequate oxygenation, monitoring Use cardiac monitor in early recovery period Have medications and oxygen available Encourage deep breathing Avoid fluid overload Assess cardiovascular status Early ambulation Avoid extremes of blood pressure Provide oxygen support for adequate tissue oxygenation Use slow position changes and instruct for same at home Be gentle with venipunctures; may need to avoid tourniquets and vacuum-style equipment Apply adequate pressure to site after venipuncture or catheter has been removed Provide care instructions to patient
↑ Circulating time	Prolonged onset for drug action	
Sclerosis of coronary arteries	Potential for myocardial ischemia	
Sclerosis of cardiac conduction system	Conduction delays ↑ susceptibility to dysrhythmias	
Peripheral sclerosis and diffuse arterial disease	Potential for cerebrovascular accident, thrombosis, and embolism ↑ Peripheral vascular resistance	

Continued

TABLE 23.1 Physiologic Characteristics of Aging and Their Implications for Nursing—cont'd

Physiologic Changes	Effects	Nursing Implications
↓ Elasticity of vessels and heart valves	↓ Response to stress and blood pressure changes Potential for orthostatic hypotension	
Fragility of vessels	Bruising, difficult venipunctures	
RESPIRATORY SYSTEM		
Edentia and ↓ bone mass of jaw	Difficult intubation and airway maintenance	Provide appropriate airways, masks, laryngeal masks, and so on Provide dentures as applicable Ascertain NPO status preoperatively Ensure reflexes before oral fluids are given Position with head elevated after awake Protect unconscious airway Position for ease of chest expansion Elevate head when possible Provide oxygen support as needed Teach deep breathing and coughing Reduce anxiety, stress, pain
Depressed reflexes in upper respiratory tract and ↑ secretions	Increased potential for aspiration, regurgitation	
↓ Elasticity and recoil of lungs Calcification of costal cartilages Arthritic changes of ribs, sternum, and vertebrae Muscle strength of diaphragm and intercostal muscles	↓ Vital capacity, ↓ forced expiratory volume, ↓ residual capacity ↓ Functional residual capacity ↓ Chest expansion, stiffened chest wall ↓ Total lung capacity	
MUSCULOSKELETAL SYSTEM		
Atrophy of muscle mass	Decreased strength, less regional anesthesia required	Support for walking or exercise Observe for prolonged or toxic effects of regional anesthetic agent Provide skid-resistant slippers, handrails, other safety measures Encourage gentle exercise Administer analgesics Position for comfort Provide careful positioning, home safety instructions Use special positioning for procedure, support for back
Joint stiffness, arthritis	↓ Flexibility, pain, difficult ambulation Potential for accidental falls	
Osteoporosis	Potential for pathologic fractures	
Degenerative vertebral changes, ossification of spinal ligaments	Kyphoscoliosis, ↓ body height Difficulty for spinal, epidural injections	
SENSORY SYSTEM		
↓ Visual acuity, cataracts, glaucoma	Potential for confusion related to decreased sensory input	Provide large-print instructions, make magnifying glass available Provide constant reassurance and discussion about what you are doing Ascertain home support for care Allow patient to wear hearing aid when possible Provide microphone-style device Increase voice volume but not pitch, speak slowly, face patient Provide written instructions Allow adequate time for feedback to verify understanding Use safety precautions, especially after general anesthesia; handrails; stools; help with ambulation
↓ Hearing acuity, difficulty hearing high tones		
Vestibular changes	Dizziness, loss of balance Vertigo	
↓ Perception in small and taste		
INTEGUMENTARY SYSTEM		
Thinner layer of subcutaneous fat	Potential for hypothermia Potential for pressure sores	Provide warm blankets, ↑ room temperature when possible, cover head to prevent heat loss Pad and protect bony prominences, change position frequently Pad bony prominences, use paper tape or similar, avoid pressure to or abrasion of skin Be aware that it may mimic dehydration Be prepared for difficult venipuncture with "rolling veins"
↓ Elasticity and turgor and thinner skin	Potential for injury	
↓ Sebum secretion ↓ Collagen	Dryness of skin ↓ Subcutaneous support of blood vessels	

TABLE 23.1 Physiologic Characteristics of Aging and Their Implications for Nursing—cont'd

Physiologic Changes	Effects	Nursing Implications
RENAL/GENITOURINARY SYSTEM		
↓ Renal blood flow	↑ Excretion time for drugs ↓ Metabolism of drugs dependent on kidneys for excretion	Observe for prolonged drug effects Encourage drug doses Encourage oral fluids postoperatively Monitor IV infusions and urinary output Consider hyponatremia (Na$^+$ < 135 mmol/L) as one cause of confusion Observe for cardiac dysrhythmias, electrocardiographic changes (K$^+$ level > 4.5 mEq/L) Offer urinal frequently, assist to bathroom, monitor output Provide protection for bedding and clothing Reassure and support emotionally to decrease embarassment
↓ Glomerular filtration rate	Potential for fluid overload Potential for altered drug doses related to ↓ excretion, reabsorption	
↓ Ability to adapt to electrolyte and fluid changes	↓ Ability to conserve sodium ↓ Ability to excrete potassium	
Prostate enlargement in males ↓ Bladder capacity	Obstruction of urethra, dribbling	
Relaxation of pelvic musculature in females ↓ Bladder capacity	Stress incontinence	
GASTROINTESTINAL SYSTEM		
↓ Hepatic blood flow ↓ Function of hepatic microsomal enzymes	↓ Metabolism of drugs dependent on liver for excretion	Observe for toxic or prolonged drug effects Encourage lowered drug doses dependent on assessment data Use caution with oral fluids, food Position head up if appropriate
↓ Esophageal musculature	Changes in swallowing patterns May lead to reflux, spasms	

From Eliopolis C: A Guide to Nursing the Aging. Clinical Nursing Diagnosis Series. Williams & Wilkins; 1987. Pp 42–43; and Koehle MM. Special needs of the older adult. Table 27.4 in: Burden N, Quinn DMD, O'Brien D, Dawes BSG, eds. *Ambulatory Surgery Nursing*. 2nd ed. Elsevier; 2000.

Changes Resulting from Dietary Deficiencies

Chronic malnutrition leading to dietary deficiencies may be a problem for some older adults. Several physiologic changes may combine to affect the way in which medications are absorbed, metabolized, and excreted. The protein binding capacity is affected as the body ages. The effectiveness of many drugs and anesthetic agents is dependent on the amount of drug that remains unbound to serum proteins in the bloodstream. The unbound drugs are those that are pharmacologically active. The older adult who has less serum protein is at greater risk for developing toxic levels of drugs that are circulating unbound to protein molecules. This is particularly true of a drug such as digoxin that has a narrow therapeutic window and the ability to produce toxicity in older adults very quickly. Decreased cardiac output in the elderly results in a decrease in renal and hepatic blood flow, an overall decrease in the number of neurons and neuromuscular connections, and a slower circulating blood flow. These factors and many others may contribute to the clinical consequence of medications producing stronger and more lasting effects in elderly patients than in younger patients with higher serum protein levels.

Physiologic Changes and Anesthesia

Perianesthesia nurses must be knowledgeable about the effects of anesthesia and surgery in relation to the physiology of aging (Box 23.2). Ambulatory surgery nurses must also anticipate immediate and potential long-range effects that may continue once older adults have been discharged to go home. Perianesthesia

---

BOX 23.1 Risk Factors for Postoperative Delirium in Elders That Can Be Detected Preoperatively

Predisposing Factors

Age 80 years or older and male gender
Malnutrition or dehydration
Impairment of cognition or function
Sensory impairment (hearing and vision)
Co-morbidities and health problems
Drug interaction or more than three prescribed drugs

Precipitating Factors

Depression
Laboratory abnormalities such as anemia
Hyponatremia or hypernatremia
Drug use (opioids and anticholinergics)
High risk: Emergent or urgent surgical procedures (hip fractures); vascular or thoracic procedures; longer procedures or excessive blood loss
Moderate risk: Nonvalvular cardiac surgery, elective orthopedic surgery
Uncontrolled pain

Allen SL. Geriatric surgery. Page 1077 in: Rothrock J, ed. *Alexander's Care of the Patient in Surgery*. 16th ed. Elsevier; 2019.

BOX 23.2 Characteristics of Aging That May Affect Anesthesia

Increased pain threshold
Reduced requirement for anesthetic agents
Frequency of coexisting diseases (e.g., diabetes, hypertension, COPD, arteriosclerosis, anemia)
Delayed drug clearance
Reduced renal and hepatic function
Diminished autonomic tone
Altered responses to stress and environmental changes
Reduced thermoregulation
Edentia
Diminished protective airway reflexes
Reduced blood volume
Osteoporosis and arthritis
Decreased muscle mass
Malnutrition and anemia

Adapted from: Windle PE, Mamaril ME. The geriatric patient. In: Schick L, Windle PE. *PeriAnesthesia Nursing Core Curriculum: Preprocedure, Phase I and Phase II PACU Nursing.* Elsevier; 2021.

BOX 23.3 Polypharmacy

Masnoon et al. conducted a systematic review and found that the most common definition of polypharmacy was the ingesting of five or more medications daily.[13]
Other definitions of polypharmacy were:
   Persistent polypharmacy of more than five prescribed medications for 181 days
   Chronic polypharmacy of more than five prescribed medications in 1 month for 6 months (whether consecutive months or not)
   Major polypharmacy of more than 10 prescribed medications on 1 day
   Hyperpolypharmacy of more than 10 prescribed medications for more than 90 days[13]

---

nurses must inquire about and assess the home environment for safe discharge preparation so that both patients and their families know how to follow physicians' and facilities' discharge instructions. It is very important that the responsible individual or companion who will be staying with the patient be instructed to watch for cognitive issues such as confusion or forgetfulness for an appropriate time period. An older adult with particularly fragile veins and tissues should be instructed to protect the venipuncture site after removal of an intravenous (IV) catheter and to remove the tape (preferably paper tape or another nontraumatic type) from the skin carefully. Skin damage or discomfort related to the venipuncture site or other taped area can be bothersome and dangerous to the older patient with a compromised immune system.

Table 23.1 outlines some of these many physiologic changes that affect different body systems and the related nursing implications. Their interrelationships can complicate assessment and affect the progress of the older surgical patient who has been given an anesthetic. The perianesthesia nursing implications are important in a same-day-surgery setting.

RISKS OF POLYPHARMACY IN OLDER PATIENTS

The use of multiple medicines is commonly referred to as *polypharmacy* (from the Greek *polus,* for "many," and *pharmakeia,* for "the use of drugs").[13-15] Polypharmacy may be due to the overprescription of multiple drugs and is considered a significant risk factor for poor postoperative outcomes in the elderly population.[2,13-15] It may be associated with adverse outcomes such as geriatric syndromes, mental confusion, falls, adverse drug reactions, increased hospitalizations, and mortality.[13-15] Perianesthesia nurses should anticipate that a geriatric patient is taking several medications and may respond differently to medications, especially anesthesia, than younger patients. Box 23.3 lists aspects of polypharmacy in geriatric patients.

Pharmacokinetics is the study of the absorption, distribution, metabolism, and elimination of medications.[15] According to Kim and Parish, pharmacokinetics in older adults is influenced by the normal physiologic changes of aging and also by disease processes. An example is the metabolism of drugs in the liver, which may be reduced, as well as the elimination of drugs by the kidneys, which may take longer due to renal compromise. Older adults may respond differently and more sensitively to medication changes.[15]

Pharmacodynamics is defined as the way in which the body responds to medications. When the older adult's body loses some of its cell function, the resulting pharmacodynamics include a greater sensitivity to certain medications. For example, anticholinergics may have adverse effects on the central nervous system, such as confusion and mental status changes.[15] Examples of anticholinergic drugs used during anesthesia include atropine, scopolamine, and glycopyrrolate.

Shaw and Hajjar[14] estimate that chronic diseases are prevalent in older adults, with 80% having at least one chronic health condition and 40% having at least two chronic conditions,[14] such as arthritis, hypertension, diabetes, heart disease, lung disease, and cancer.[14-16] Consequently, multiple medications are often required for optimal management.[15] It is important to note that researchers found that outpatients taking five or more medications had an 88% increase in adverse drug events compared with those taking fewer medications.[15]

Adverse drug events are injuries that result from the administration of medications given certain factors.[16] Older adults who are engaging in polypharmacy are at an increased risk of experiencing adverse drug events. Often, older patients are uncertain about which medications they take and the reasons for taking them. This increases the risks for both drug-to-drug interactions and drug-disease interactions.[16] The addition of anesthesia agents adds a further risk of adverse drug events for older patients.

One important mechanism in drug interactions is the cytochrome P-450 enzyme system.[3] The P-450 system is composed of many specific enzymes responsible for the metabolism of, as well as the clearance of, many medications by the liver. They include herbal medications and some nutrients, as well as nicotine.[3] In elderly and frail elderly patients, this is especially a concern, as the P-450 system interacts with age-related changes and can modulate adverse reactions of prescribed medications.[3] Many medications administered during anesthesia care are metabolized via this enzyme system. Because multiple drugs use this enzymatic pathway, their metabolism may be slowed and the patient's recovery from anesthesia delayed.

Olotu et al. revealed that since polypharmacy is a relevant risk factor in older adults that is associated with poor postoperative outcomes, nonessential medications, including prescription drugs, should be discontinued during the perioperative period.[16] However, long-term cardiac medications, as well as preoperative analgesics, should be continued to avoid rebound complications.

Herbal Medicines

Herbal medications are derived from plant-based, bioactive products that are metabolized by the liver, and they can cause problems for older adults taking other medications.[2] Since many older adults take a disproportionately greater number of medications and herbal supplements than younger people, they become more susceptible to these adverse and altered effects (Table 23.2).

Many older adults may not disclose the fact that they are taking herbal medications for several reasons. They may perceive that over-the-counter herbals are harmless and as easily purchased as vitamins. Cultural and or ethnic reasons may factor into the disclosure because their use is part of a personal belief system. Other older adults may be secretive because of anticipated disapproval from the perioperative team. Widespread use of herbal medications may have negative outcomes for older adults who are undergoing anesthesia and surgery.[2,17,18]

When Lee, Moss, and Yuan conducted an integrative review of herbal medicines, they found that eight herbs had the greatest impact on surgical patients: echinacea, ephedra, garlic, ginkgo, ginseng, kava, St. John's Wort, and valerian.[18] Nonherbal supplements, such as vitamins, minerals, amino acids, and hormones, may also cause undesirable effects.[18]

TABLE 23.2 Potential Adverse Effects of Herbal Medicines in Elderly Patients Receiving Anesthesia

Herbal Medication	Adverse Effects
Black cohosh	Bradycardia, hypotension, joint pains
Bloodroot	Bradycardia, arrhythmia, dizziness, impaired vision, intense thirst
Boneset	Liver toxicity, mental changes, respiratory problems
Coltsfoot	Fever, liver toxicity
Dandelion	Interacts with diuretics, increased concentration of lithium or potassium
Ephedra	Anxiety, dizziness, insomnia, tachycardia, hypertension
Feverfew	Interference with blood clotting mechanisms
Garlic	Hypotension, inhibition of blood clotting, potentiation of antidiabetic drugs
Ginkgo biloba	Increased anticoagulation
Ginseng	Anxiety, insomnia, hypertension tachycardia, asthma attacks, postmenopausal bleed
Goldenseal	Vasoconstriction
Guar gum	Hypoglycemia
Hawthorn	Hypotension
Hops skullcap	Drowsiness, potentiation of antianxiety sedative
Kava	Damage to eyes, skin, liver, and spinal cord from long-term use
Licorice	Hypokalemia, hypernatremia
Lobelia	Hearing and vision problems
Mistletoe	Fever, liver toxicity (can be corrected)
Motherwort	Increased anticoagulation
Nettle	Hypokalemia
Senna	Potentiation of digoxin
Valerian	Sedative
Yohimbe	Anxiety, tachycardia, hypertension, mental changes

Adapted from: Miller CA. *Nursing for Wellness in Older Adults.* 8th ed, Wolters Kluwer/Lippincott Williams & Wilkins; 2020.

The risk of drug-to-drug and drug-disease interactions increases with the number of prescribed medications and is even greater with herbal medications.[2,8,18,19] Complications such as bleeding, stroke, myocardial infarction, coagulopathies, and prolonged or inadequate anesthesia during the intraoperative or postanesthesia phase of care increase the rates of morbidity and mortality in older adults taking herbal medications (Table 23.3).

Medication use generally appears to increase with age, suggesting that frail elderly patients may experience the double jeopardy of a diminished ability to absorb, metabolize, distribute, and excrete drugs and yet also have an increased need for their benefit as a result of their declining physiologic functions, such as decreased cardiovascular function. Maintaining the patient's usual medication protocol is important. Departments of anesthesia generally have policies regarding the use of antihypertensives, antiarrhythmics, mood elevators, aspirin, and anticoagulants before surgery and anesthesia. Diuretics are commonly omitted until after surgery to avoid a full bladder intraoperatively.

It is essential for perianesthesia nurses to know departmental policies regarding home medication usage. These policies are essential for safe preoperative screening, home medication instructions, avoiding case cancellations, and post discharge teaching. The nurse should reinforce these instructions and, on the day of surgery, verify and document that the instructions were followed.

Obtaining a complete medication history from an older adult can be a challenge. Some patients may have no idea as to the names of the medications they take, so it may be prudent to instruct elderly patients to bring the medications with them if they seem unsure. The ASC nurse is well advised to learn to recognize some of the more common medications by color and markings. Many elderly patients forget to mention certain medications or do not consider them important enough to list on medication histories. Eye drops, inhalants, topicals, supplemental oxygen, alcohol, cough medicine, antacids, laxatives, or over-the-counter medications such as analgesics and antihistamines are some common examples.

The nurse must anticipate which untoward interactions might occur between the patient's usual medications and those being given in the perianesthesia period.

Anti-inflammatory Agents

Aspirin and other anti-inflammatory agents that can interfere with blood coagulation are often taken for arthritis, bursitis, and other types of inflammatory processes. Most physicians recommend that patients discontinue such medications before the day of surgery. Although 7–10 days of abstinence from aspirin is suggested for effective platelet regeneration, many physicians do not recommend discontinuation of the drug long before surgery because exacerbation of the patient's chronic inflammatory disease may be more debilitating than the adverse consequences of continuation of the therapy.

Anticoagulant Agents

Many elderly patients take dipyridamole, warfarin, heparin, or other medications to prevent thrombosis or thromboembolism, particularly in the pulmonary and cerebral circulation. The surgeon or anesthesiologist often directs the patient to discontinue these types of drugs before surgery. For high-risk patients with complex medical histories, the primary physician may be consulted about preoperative discontinuation of these medications or use of an anticoagulation bridge protocol. Bleeding and clotting studies are often required just before surgery after the drug has been stopped to ensure adequacy of

TABLE 23.3 Selected Herbal Medicines, Their Uses and Actions, and Precautions About Using Them in Elderly Surgical Patients

Herbal Medicine	Uses	Actions and Precautions
Bilberry	Nonspecific acute diarrhea	High doses may inhibit platelet aggregation; monitor anticoagulation
Black cohosh	Menopausal symptoms (hot flashes, night sweats, insomnia)	Monitor liver function every 6 months for hepatotoxicity
Cat's claw	Osteoarthritis (knee); rheumatoid arthritis	Avoid organ transplant/autoimmune suppression
Chamomile	Inflammation of gastrointestinal tract	Avoid if allergy to chamomile
Echinacea	Respiratory infection (colds); urinary infection	Avoid in systemic diseases: HIV, TB, multiple sclerosis, leukocytosis; transplant patients
Evening primrose	Atopic dermatitis and eczema	Interaction with antipsychotic drugs; inhibits anticonvulsant drugs
Garlic	Lower cholesterol; minor respiratory issues	Inhibit platelet aggregation; risk for bleeding; monitor anticoagulation
Ginger	Prevention of motion sickness; PONV; anti-inflammatory	Avoid if active gallbladder disease
Ginkgo Biloba	Degenerative and vascular dementia, vertigo	Avoid with MAO inhibitors; inhibit platelet aggregation; bleeding; monitor anticoagulation
Ginseng	Restorative agent for fatigue, stress, exhaustion	Hypoglycemia, hypertension, avoid with MAO inhibitors
Hawthorn	Treatment in congestive heart failure patient	Potentiates digitalis and beta-blockers
Horse chestnut	Treatment of chronic venous insufficiency, night cramps, itching	Monitor bleeding times in patients taking anticoagulants
Kava	Treatment for anxiety	Hepatotoxicity; high potential for drug interactions (potentiate barbiturates)
Licorice	Inflammation of upper respiratory tract, gastrointestinal tract, gastric ulcers	Avoid in liver disorders, congestive heart failure, edema; may increase blood pressure; interacts with diuretics, antihypertensives, corticosteroids
Saw palmetto	Benign prostatic hypertrophy	No reported drug interactions
St. John's Wort	Use in mild to moderate depression, anxiety, and nervousness	Avoid in patient taking multiple medications; may cause serious interactions with general anesthesia
Valerian	Mild sleep-promoting agent in nervous and restless patients; anxiety-related sleep disturbances	May have additive effect when taking central nervous system depressants

Adapted from: Miller CA. *Nursing for Wellness in Older Adults.* 8th ed, Wolters Kluwer/Lippincott Williams & Wilkins; 2020.

the clotting mechanism. Patients should be observed for bleeding and must receive adequate physician instructions about when to resume the medications at home. They need to know about the possible symptoms of bleeding that could occur after discharge and to report these to the physician who is in charge of their care.

Insulin

One of the great advantages of the ambulatory approach to surgical care for the elderly is the maintenance of a more "normal" life routine, including the taking of medications and a usual schedule of meals. Insulin-dependent diabetic patients need to be able to rely on a consistent and planned approach to their day to effectively manage their insulin requirements. All members of the healthcare team who communicate with the patient must be clear and consistent about the instructions regarding drug and food regimens on the day of surgery. Patients may be asked to bring their own insulin so that they can take it after they have eaten after surgery. This method is often preferred to using insulin supplied by the facility because most patients are used to a particular brand.

Maintaining both dietary and insulin schedules as close to normal as possible is beneficial for the patient both physically and emotionally. Before the day of surgery, it is helpful to tell diabetic patients which foods and beverages will be available at the surgery unit. They have the option of bringing their own food if they are have a particularly strict dietary regimen.

Beta-blocking Agents

Many elderly patients take beta-blocking agents, which are prescribed for everything from hypertension to glaucoma. The primary effects of the beta-blockade include reduced myocardial contractility, conductivity, automaticity, and excitability, resulting in less workload for the heart. Other effects of beta-blockers, both desirable and undesirable, are listed in Table 23.4.

The postural hypotension associated with beta-blockers may be more common in older people, resulting in dizziness, fainting, gait difficulties, and impaired vision, problems easily dismissed as the normal consequences of aging.[2,3,13] Beta-blockers place patients at risk for experiencing or exacerbating preexisting heart failure, along with lethargy and dyspnea, by depressing the contractility of the myocardium. Hypoglycemia, which can be exacerbated by beta-blockers, may be poorly detected because the beta-blocker also masks the onset of the tachycardia that is a frequent danger signal of impending hypoglycemia. The astute ambulatory surgery nurse may be able to assess difficulties with beta-blockers through accurate history taking and thoughtful, probing questioning.

Some practitioners feel that the long-term or intermittent use of beta-blocking agents can place the patient at risk if epinephrine is administered concurrently, although controversy exists about the extent of interaction and the degree of associated risk.[2,20] Normally, the cardiovascular response to

TABLE 23.4 Physiologic Effects of Beta-blocking Drugs

Organ	Effect
Eye	Constriction of the ciliary muscle, causing a decline in visual acuity
Salivary glands	Depressed secretion of saliva, leaving mouth dry
Lungs	Constriction of the bronchial muscle, aggravating asthma and COPD
Pancreas	Stimulation of secretion of beta cells, which enhances the hypoglycemic effects of insulin in an insulin dependent diabetic
Heart	Slowing of heart rate or prevention of rates rising in response to exercise, illness, or other stimulation; cardiac output falls
Stomach/intestines	Increased motility and heightened tone, leading to gastrointestinal problems such as diarrhea, nausea, and vomiting
Liver	Slowed liver perfusion; less drug available to target organs
Urinary bladder	Detrusor muscle constriction, leading to urinary retention
Arterioles	Relaxation of arterioles, causing lowered perfusion, slowing the onset of action of some drugs
Male sex organs	Potentiation of impotency in men

COPD, chronic obstructive pulmonary disease.
Koehle MM. Special needs of the older adult. Table 27.5 in: Burden N, Quinn DMD, O'Brien D, Dawes BSG, eds. *Ambulatory Surgery Nursing.* 2nd ed. Elsevier; 2000.

epinephrine results from the stimulation of both alpha-receptors and beta-receptors in the autonomic nervous system. Beta-stimulation, which produces vasodilation and an increased heart rate, is balanced by alpha-stimulation, which promotes vasoconstriction and an increased arterial resistance.

The patient taking propranolol or another beta-blocking agent may experience a marked hypertensive episode, followed quickly by reflex bradycardia following the administration of epinephrine.[2] Hypertension occurs when the beta-blocking drug blocks the peripheral beta effects of the epinephrine, which usually would be vasodilation and an increased heart rate. Vasoconstriction and increased arterial resistance, the alpha effects of epinephrine, are accentuated. This can be followed by a reflex bradycardia or other type of arrhythmia during which propranolol can prevent the cardiovascular system from responding appropriately to the alpha-induced peripheral resistance. The beta-blocked myocardium is unable to respond to those increased demands, and further reflex bradycardia ensues.

Treatment is initiated with direct-acting drugs. Intravenous nitroglycerin and nitroprusside are used to decrease blood pressure.[2,13] Atropine may be effective in treating associated bradycardia. Ultimately, cardiac arrest or hypertensive stroke can occur if symptoms are left untreated.

Although this occurrence is rare, it cannot be dismissed in the ASC for many reasons. These include the frequent use of local anesthetics that may contain epinephrine, the tendency to use local and regional anesthesia for elderly patients whenever possible, and the number of elderly patients who are taking long-term beta-blocking agents. Some facility or anesthesia department policies discourage the use of epinephrine in patients taking beta-blockers. Others are less restrictive and instead recommend monitoring patients closely when epinephrine is administered.

Antidepressants

Depression is a common and highly treatable illness in the elderly population. An estimated 1% to 25% of older people experience symptoms of depression, such as low mood, sadness, pessimism, self-criticism, and difficulty sleeping, concentrating, or eating.[2-4,13] Older people have the highest rate of suicide of all age groups, a rate that is two to three times higher than that of the general population. Those at greatest risk usually meet the following criteria: male, white, age 75 years or older, low income, association with alcohol or drug abuse, single (e.g., widowed, divorced), suffering from chronic disease, especially chronic pain, and prior suicide attempt.[3,4]

The treatment for depression can include medications or psychotherapy, or a combination of both. Less commonly employed, but equally effective in some instances, is the use of electroconvulsive therapy, usually reserved for depression that is unresponsive to medication or for cases in which the use of antidepressant medications is contraindicated. There are many antidepressant medications on the market. These drugs appear to work by altering how specific neurotransmitters, such as dopamine, serotonin, and norepinephrine, act on receptors in the brain. The main categories of antidepressants include tricyclic antidepressants (e.g., amitriptyline), serotonin reuptake inhibitors (e.g., fluoxetine, paroxetine), monoamine oxidase inhibitors (e.g., isocarboxazid, phenelzine, selegiline), and atypical antidepressants (e.g., lithium, trazodone).

All of these medications have a wide range of side effects that can be particularly serious in elderly patients (Table 23.5). The general rule of thumb in prescribing an antidepressant to a senior is to "start low and go slow."[3] This may help to minimize side effects such as hypotension, anticholinergic effects, sedation, and gastrointestinal symptoms.

Orthostatic hypotension may be a problem associated with the antidepressants that have a moderate to strong ability to decrease blood pressure. Treatment with these drugs has been associated with an increased number of falls and fractures in the elderly patient. Those at greatest risk for developing orthostatic hypotension while taking antidepressants include frail elderly persons, patients with cardiovascular disease or diabetes, and patients taking other medications that affect the blood pressure.[2,3] Symptoms that should alert the ASC nurse to a problem include dizziness on standing, light-headedness, vertigo, increased number of falls, and complaints of palpitations or racing or pounding heart. Blood pressure monitoring while the patient is standing up or lying down should be performed for patients known to be taking any of these medications.

Anticholinergic effects are similar to the effects of atropine, occurring because of the antidepressant drug's ability to block specific receptors in the brain and elsewhere in the body.[2,3] Common symptoms may include a dry mouth, dry eyes, blurred vision, constipation, and urinary retention. Less common are fatigue, memory loss, confusion, hallucinations, and delirium.

TABLE 23.5 Side Effects of Antidepressants

Generic Name	Blood Pressure Effects	Anticholinergic Effects	Sedative Effects	Gastrointestinal Effects	Other Effects
DESIRABLE ANTIDEPRESSANTS					
Tricyclics					
Desipramine	Mild to moderate	Mild	Mild	–	–
Nortriptyline	Mild	Moderate	Mild	–	–
Atypical					
Trazodone	Moderate	Very mild	Moderate	–	Priapism
SEROTONIN REUPTAKE INHIBITORS					
Fluvoxamine	Mild	Mild	Mild to moderate	Moderate	Insomnia/agitation
Paroxetine	Mild	Mild	Mild	Moderate	Insomnia/agitation
Sertraline	Mild	Mild	Mild	Moderate	Insomnia/agitation
Reversible monoamine oxidase inhibitors					
Moclobemide	Moderate	Mild to moderate	Mild	–	Agitation
UNDESIRABLE ANTIDEPRESSANTS					
Tricyclics					
Amitriptyline	Moderate	Very strong	Strong	–	–
Doxepin	Moderate	Strong	Strong	–	–
Imipramine	Moderate	Moderate to strong	Moderate	–	–
Trimipramine	Strong	Moderate	Strong	–	–
Atypical					
Maprotiline	Moderate	Moderate	Moderate to strong	–	Seizures
Serotonin reuptake inhibitors					
Fluoxetine	Mild	Mild	Mild	Moderate	Long half-life Agitation Akathisia

Koehle MM. Special needs of the older adult. Table 27.6 in: Burden N, Quinn DMD, O'Brien D, Dawes BSG, eds. *Ambulatory Surgery Nursing*. 2nd ed. Elsevier; 2000.

As with the other side effects, sedation can occur early in treatment or at each dosage increase and may be compounded by the addition of new medications or new illnesses. Combining drugs such as antianxiety medications, sleeping pills, antihistamines, and antipsychotic drugs with antidepressants can increase the sedative side effects. The mild sedative effects may actually be helpful in relieving the sleep disturbances that occur in some depressed patients. Mild daytime sedation may also help the agitated patient. However, sedation that significantly interferes with the patient's ability to eat and participate in activities is not desirable, and dosage adjustments may be necessary. Patients taking antidepressants who present to the ASC with fatigue, difficulty in rousing early in the morning, late morning wakening, slurred speech, confusion, daytime sleepiness, or night-time incontinence should be referred for further investigation of their antidepressant therapy.

The serotonin reuptake inhibitors have been reported to cause gastrointestinal upsets, including nausea, vomiting, stomach pain, or a bloated feeling, in 20% to 40% of patients.[2,3,13] The severity can range from self-limited to severe. These side effects are particularly significant in an environment such as the ASC, where it is likely that procedures and medications causing further gastrointestinal upset will be administered or performed.[21]

Patients receiving antidepressants of the monoamine oxidase inhibitor family must be evaluated particularly carefully with respect to general anesthesia. Meperidine (Demerol) is an opioid that is no longer recommended in same-day surgery settings, except for shivering.[2,12,21,22] Meperidine especially is contraindicated in any patient receiving monoamine oxidase

inhibitors. Reactions have been hyperexcitability, convulsions, tachycardia, hyperpyrexia, and hypertension.

In summary, the perianesthesia nurse should have a working knowledge of the various types of antidepressant medications commonly prescribed for the elderly population. The ability to recognize that one of these medications may influence the patient's ability to receive an anesthetic agent (as in the case of monoamine oxidase inhibitors) or may be causing a dangerous side effect, such as postural hypotension, will assist the perianesthesia nurse in providing optimum patient care.

Anticholinergic Syndrome

The anticholinergic effects of antidepressants may occur immediately—in fact, often before the therapeutic effects begin—or they may take some time to occur after a patient has begun taking the medication. It is possible that the ambulatory surgery nurse may be the first healthcare professional to recognize a patient who is experiencing these anticholinergic effects.[2,3] The side effects vary with each drug and can be significantly worsened if a drug is used in combination with other drugs with similar effects. Commonly used agents that also have anticholinergic effects include antihistamines found in many allergy and cold remedies (diphenhydramine), antipsychotics (chlorpromazine, thioridazine), antinauseants (dimenhydrinate, scopolamine), anti-Parkinson agents (benztropine, procyclidine), anti-vertigo agents (meclizine), and anticholinergic drugs (oxybutynin).[2,3,22]

The medication history is critical in this population. Patients who are taking one or a series of "anti" drugs may be at significant risk for developing anticholinergic syndrome. They should be warned to watch for anticholinergic side effects. These effects are often difficult to pinpoint because in some ways they are rather vague. It is possible for patients to assume that fatigue, memory loss, and confusion are simply signs of "old age." It is important for health professionals to identify this potential cause of these worrisome side effects and intervene appropriately by informing the patient's physician about them or instructing the patient to stop taking the drug immediately.

Alcohol and Substance Abuse

It is estimated that anywhere from 1% to 15% (even higher for institutionalized elderly people) of the elderly population have an undiagnosed alcohol problem.[3] Physicians and others are often unwilling to recognize alcohol abuse and dependence in elderly people, perhaps believing that elderly people deserve to enjoy this substance. The fact remains that proper treatment can lead to productive years as a senior citizen rather than an early alcohol-related death.

Diagnostic problems constitute one of the greatest barriers to treatment of elderly alcoholics. When the perianesthesia nurse or physician perceives frailty, unsteadiness of gait, or dementia as the result of old age, such signs may also be associated with a substance abuse problem. Table 23.6 illustrates the difficulty encountered in differentiating the various signs of aging, problem drinking, and adverse drug reactions.

Patients must be asked about their substance use in a clear, nonthreatening, nonjudgmental manner. The most widely evaluated instrument to assist in data collection is the Michigan Alcoholism Screening Test, consisting of 25 true or false items; it is reasonably accurate in distinguishing alcoholic from nonalcoholic persons.[24] The CAGE (for cut down, annoyed, guilty, and eye-opener) questionnaire, now commonly incorporated into the admission assessments of patients in both inpatient and outpatient settings, is a very simple screening tool or reference.[20,23] The four questions are

C: Have you ever felt a need to cut down on your drinking?
A: Do you ever get annoyed by criticism of your drinking?
G: Do you ever feel guilty about your alcohol consumption?
E: Do you ever feel the need for an eye opener to get started in the morning?

Generally, two of four answers in the positive indicate a problem with drinking, particularly if combined with any evidence of symptoms, such as anxiety, depression, mood swings, fragmented sleep, and personal relationship problems.

Psychoactive substance abuse and dependence often involve more than one substance and are more prevalent in women. In a practical sense, this points to the need for very thorough history taking from the elderly patient, including an inquiry as to the use of, for example, sleeping pills or antianxiety agents. These agents are often members of the benzodiazepine or hypnotic families and can potentiate the effects of alcohol. Depression, as was mentioned, may be treated with tricyclic antidepressants or selective serotonin reuptake inhibitors, and these medications may potentiate an alcohol abuse or dependence problem. Coexisting substance abuse in the elderly person is generally of legally prescribed medications (as opposed to recreational drugs), such as antidepressants, hypnotics, and antianxiety agents.

A history of the long-term use of benzodiazepines for the treatment of sleep disorders is important to elicit from the elderly patient in the ASC. Frequently, older patients do not consider sleeping pills "medication" or may be embarrassed to admit that they need something to help them sleep.[2] Gentle questioning, perhaps prefaced by a reminder that the information is important to providing them the best care possible, may help to lessen their concerns.

Alcoholism and the use of other drugs may go undetected because of the difficulty in differentiating the symptoms from those of other illnesses, their treatments, or simply aging itself. Early recognition and referral can significantly improve the quality of life and reduce the incidence of serious illness. Ambulatory surgical nurses, who see a large number of elderly patients in their practice, should be aware of this problem and should be prepared to recognize and refer, when appropriate. Accurate assessment of current substance use and abuse is critical to providing the most appropriate anesthetic and surgical experience for the patient. The National Institute on Alcohol Abuse and Alcoholism website provides helpful information (www.niaaa.nih.gov).[3]

TABLE 23.6 Differentiating the Effects of Alcoholism and Aging from Adverse Drug Effects

Alcoholism	Aging	Adverse Drug Reactions
Confusion	Confusion	Confusion
Clouded sensorium disorientation	Clouded sensorium disorientation	Clouded sensorium disorientation
Recent memory loss	Recent memory loss	Recent memory loss
Slowed thought process	Slowed thought process	Slowed thought process
Muscle incoordination	Muscle incoordination	Muscle incoordination
Tremors	Tremors	Tremors
Inflammation of joints	Inflammation of joints	Gastritis
Gastritis	Gastritis	Hypertension, depression
Hypertension	Hypertension	Cardiac dysrhythmias
Depression	Depression	Anorexia
Congestive heart failure	Congestive heart failure	Diminished stress response
Cardiac dysrhythmias	Cardiac dysrhythmias	Excess excretion of Mg^{2+} and K^+
Anorexia	Anorexia	Edema
Diminished stress response malnutrition	Diminished stress response malnutrition	
Excess excretion of Mg^{2+} and K^+		
Edema		

Koehle MM. Special needs of the older adult. Table 27.7 in: Burden N, Quinn DMD, O'Brien D, Dawes BSG, eds. *Ambulatory Surgery Nursing*. 2nd ed. Elsevier; 2000.

NURSING IMPLICATIONS FOR THE CARE OF ELDERLY PATIENTS AT AMBULATORY SURGERY CENTERS

Key perianesthesia nursing interventions for the care of elderly patients are outlined in Box 23.4. The special needs of the older population must be addressed with as much concern as those of pediatric patients before, during, and after surgery.

Preoperative Nursing Implications

A comprehensive preanesthesia workup of the patient, including a nursing assessment and history taking, diagnostic testing, and provision of patient and family instructions, is essential for elderly patients, who may present with multiple physical, sensory, and social changes.

BOX 23.4 Nursing Considerations Throughout the Perianesthesia Care Continuum

Nurse and Patient During All Meetings

Allow added time for care, instructions, and responses
Avoid confusion, loud conversations, and distractions near patient
Provide warmth with a comfortable room temperature, clothing as allowed, blankets, slippers, limited exposure, warm solutions
Communicate slowly, clearly, in low tones; face the patient when speaking
Use gentleness in care
Address the patient respectfully and use the patient's proper name
Observe for untoward or exaggerated effects of medications
Encourage and allow patient's independence
Include support person in care and instructions whenever appropriate

Nurse in Physician's Office and Patient

Provide written and verbal directions to surgery facility or map
Provide clear instructions for parking and for locating ambulatory surgery department
Provide brief explanation of reason for:
  Preadmission interview (if one is scheduled)
  Diagnostics
  Importance of NPO and adherence to preadmission instructions

Preadmission Meeting Between Nurse and Patient

Provide adequate time for interview and assessment*
Solicit thorough health history; include past surgeries, chronic diseases, medications taken, allergies, name of personal physician, recent diagnostics
Assess physical status; include baseline vital signs, sensory losses, limitations in mobility, prosthetic devices
Assess mental status
Secure appropriate diagnostic tests and results
Verify transportation and home support system and document
Provide verbal and written instructions in large print; include time of arrival, appropriate clothing, medications to be taken or omitted, NPO instructions

Preoperative Meeting Between Nurse and Patient on Admission to Surgical Center

Verify transportation, home support, and contact information on admission
Give instructions a few at a time; speak slowly and clearly
Ascertain adherence to NPO and requested medication protocol
Assess physical status; include lung sounds, vital signs, and morning blood glucose level as appropriate
Assist with ambulation, positioning, and belongings
Allow patient to keep sensory aids and dentures if possible
Reassure patient about location of belongings
Use gentleness in care, protect fragile skin and tissues
Use alternatives to reduce medication needs, such as relaxation, touch, family presence, comfort measures
Observe closely for untoward effects of preoperative medications, respiratory and cardiovascular status

Communicate special needs to operating room and anesthesia team

Intraoperative Nursing Considerations

Avoid disturbing noises caused by instruments, loud music, inappropriate laughter and talking
Remain in visual, tactile, or voice contact with awake patient
Maintain warmth
Allow patient to keep sensory aids and dentures if possible
Positioning: change positions slowly and gently; avoid extremes (e.g., lithotomy)
Protect from skin and tissue injury
Nurse-monitored local anesthesia: provide special attention to vital signs, cardiac rhythm, sedative effects of medications

Postoperative Phase I

Provide extra time as necessary for arousal; oxygen support, slower ambulation
Monitor vital signs, respiratory and cardiovascular status closely
Observe closely for untoward effects of medications and anesthetic agents
Avoid fluid overload
Avoid sedation when possible
Provide analgesia as appropriate
Reorient patient to surroundings frequently
Protect from skin and tissue injury

Postoperative Phase II

Ambulate carefully: edge of stretcher first, physical support for walking, eyeglasses first, stepstool
As soon as possible
  Dress in clothes (wellness concept, warmth, familiarity)
  Return belongings and sensory aids
  Reunite with support person
Include support person in instructions
Verify plans for home support
Avoid sedating drugs
Provide clear verbal and large-print written instructions
Instruct on resumption of usual medication routine
Ascertain patient's understanding of instructions and ability for self-care through demonstration of skills and repeating of instructions

After Discharge

Contact after 24 hours
Identify caller clearly and slowly
Telephone call:
  Express concern and interest
  Obtain data on physical condition, complications
  Affirm patient's understanding of and compliance with special instructions
Initiate quality improvement monitors, second telephone follow-up, physician involvement as necessary based on data collected

---

*If a personal visit is not possible, telephone contact should be made to confirm time of arrival, transportation and home support arrangements, patient's understanding of NPO and medication instructions, allergies, and to obtain a basic health history.
NPO, nothing by mouth.
Koehle MM. Special needs of the older adult. Table 27.8 in: Burden N, Quinn DMD, O'Brien D, Dawes BSG, eds. *Ambulatory Surgery Nursing*. 2nd ed. Elsevier; 2000.

Ideally, this preparation occurs at least 1 week before surgery. The preadmission interview provides a built-in period for compiling information about the patient's health and living situation, consulting with the patient's primary physician and surgeon if necessary, and identifying and solving any problems that might affect the surgery. Avoiding cancellations on the day of surgery as a result of inadequate patient selection or preparation is important. Older adults are not opposed to preadmission visits, particularly if the purposes and benefits of such visits are explained to them. While at the ASC for the interview, the patient can become familiar with the layout of the building and the nearest parking areas. Meeting members of the nursing and anesthesia departments before the day of surgery often helps allay anxieties by reducing the number of unknowns.

For patients who do not wish to make an extra trip to the ASC before the day of surgery, a structured telehealth visit or telephone call can achieve many of the goals of the preanesthesia visit. The nurse can reaffirm what the attending surgeon and staff have explained about the patient's responsibilities with respect to preoperative preparation. The nurse can also obtain the medical and social history and verify the plans for transportation on the day of surgery and home support. The physician's office should provide the patient with information containing clear directions and/or a map for locating the ASC, easily readable instructions about preparing for the procedure, and a contact telephone number for the ASC staff.

Preoperative Nursing Assessment and History

The preoperative nursing assessment helps identify problems that might delay or affect the procedure so that a plan for preventing those problems can be formulated and communicated to the other members of the ambulatory surgical team. The atmosphere in the interview area should be comfortable for elderly patients. This includes a comfortable temperature, seating that is easy to get in and out of, and adequate lighting. The room should be located close to the ASC entrance to ensure as short a walk as possible for arriving patients. The interviewer must be careful not to position himself or herself in front of a brightly lit window, because the glare from the window can easily compromise the older adult's already diminishing visual acuity. A magnifying glass is helpful for some people for reading instructions or consent forms. Large-print instructions should be available, and any handwritten information should be written legibly.

Sufficient time must be allowed for assessment because, as was suggested earlier, older people may have multiple physical or social handicaps or they may simply talk and move more slowly than younger patients. Attempts to speed them up because of a heavy workload often result in even more time being required because the patient may misunderstand something said in a hurry or may neglect to inform the interviewer of important information. Distractions should be kept to a minimum. The interviewer should face the patient and speak in a strong, low-pitched voice. Hearing deficits are common in elderly persons and may particularly impair the hearing of the high-pitched sounds often used in times of haste.

The history and physical assessment of the nurse focus on nursing issues and often take place before the anesthesiologist's examination. In some facilities, the nurse initiates referral to the anesthesiologist only if the information in the history points to the need for further evaluation. Otherwise, the anesthesiologist sees the patient on the day of surgery. The patient should have completed a health history before the interview. It is the nurse's responsibility to identify and further investigate details that can escalate into large problems later.

The physical assessment includes all the parameters essential to any person's care, but for the elderly person, it should focus specifically on the respiratory and cardiovascular status, functional mobility, skin integrity, and sensory losses. Additional attention can then address any special needs that are identified. Where appropriate, the cognitive function can be assessed with a Mini-Mental Status Examination.[21] Tools such as this examination may become even more important in the future, when more and more patients with mild to moderate dementias will be seen in ambulatory clinics (Figure 23.2).

The older adult's health history requires special attention. Ascertaining the extent of chronic diseases allows for necessary adjustments in the planning of care. Sometimes, contact with the patient's personal physician is needed regarding specific health questions, particularly if the patient is a poor historian. If older patients do not know the names of the medications they are taking, they should be asked to provide that information before the day of surgery, so that the physician can instruct the patient about continuing or stopping the drugs before the surgical procedure.

Preoperative Diagnostic Tests

The older adult generally needs a more extensive diagnostic workup than a younger counterpart because of the increased incidence of chronic diseases and multiple medications; however, testing should be determined on the basis of clinical need rather than age alone. A complete blood count, blood glucose and potassium levels, electrocardiogram, and possibly a chest film and/or pulmonary function test may be clinically indicated, with more or less testing required for specific situations.

Preoperative Instructions for the Patient and Family

All patients should have adequate information regarding their responsibilities to and expectations of the surgical facility. The instructions may have to take into account the sensory and cognitive losses that many older adults experience. By no means should older adults be treated as though they are incapable of hearing or understanding. If the nurse identifies such losses, however, adjustments in teaching methods should be made. Some patients may pretend to understand out of embarrassment over sensory or memory losses.

For the patient with severe physical limitations, sending pajamas or a patient gown (from the surgery center or hospital) home to wear on the morning of surgery (covered with a robe or coat) eliminates the need for the patient to dress twice that morning. It saves the energy of the patient and family, as well as the nurse's time during admission. This practice, of course, must be in compliance with the facility's infection control policies and should be the exception rather than the rule.

Having a Support Person Present During the Preoperative Interview

It is helpful to include a support person or caregiver during the interview. If the patient has hearing or cognitive impairments, instructions may have to be repeated more than once, and caregivers may be able to reword them for patients in terms that are familiar to them. The instructions should also be provided in writing for later reference, especially instructions about fasting or nothing by mouth (NPO) requirements, medication protocols, appropriate clothing, time of arrival, and special home preparations (e.g., obtaining a walker, hiring a home health aide, making arrangements for home nursing if it is provided by the community). Many facilities are now insisting that patients and/or their responsible individuals sign

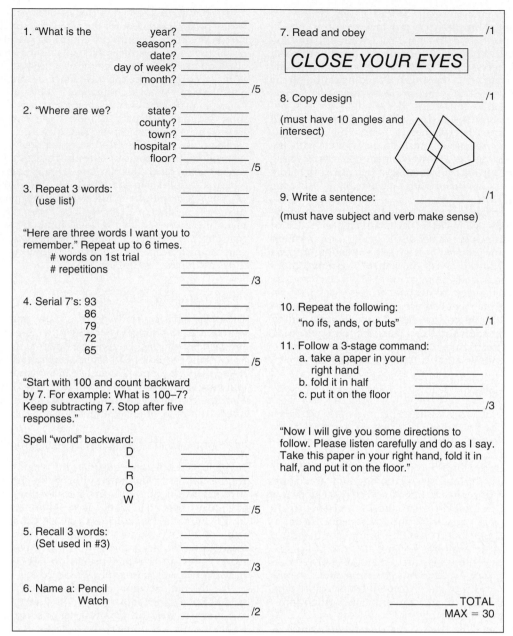

Fig. 23.2 Mini-Mental State Examination. Paulsen JS, Gehl C. Neuropsychology. Figure 44.3 in: Jankovic J, Mazziotta JC, Pomeroy SL, Newman NJ, eds. *Bradley and Daroff's Neurology in Clinical Practice*. 8th ed. Elsevier; 2021.

instruction sheets either as a paper copy or an electronic document attached to the patient's digital chart. This documentation affirms that the instructions were reviewed with patients and caregivers in instances when patients deny that they received any information. This can happen quite innocently when an older person is bombarded with information either in the preanesthesia clinic or on the day of surgery.

Older persons may be illiterate, and ASC nurses should be alerted to that possibility. This situation may become apparent when a patient is unsure about the written instructions or seems reluctant to, for example, sign the instruction sheet. A nonjudgmental approach to the illiterate patient is important for the maintenance of the therapeutic relationship. Together, the nurse, patient, and family member can determine the best way to ensure that the patient goes home with the appropriate information needed to facilitate recovery. If appropriate, the nurse may wish to use the opportunity to refer the patient to

community services available to assist the individual in learning to read and write.

Obtaining Consent for the Procedure

An elderly person who presents to an ambulatory surgical facility for surgical intervention is assumed by most staff to be legally competent and therefore able to complete the appropriate consent forms required by the facility for the surgery to proceed. Although physicians are legally obligated to obtain consent, they often enlist the assistance of the nurse in the task of documentation completion.

An individual is considered competent if, and only if, he or she can understand the nature of, consequences of, and alternatives to treatment, as explained by the physician.[3] The test of competency is the ability to repeat the diagnosis and proposed treatment in one's own words or manner. If the interviewing nurse believes that a patient is not legally competent in terms of understanding the surgery and its alternatives, it is important that the nurse follow the established institutional protocol for follow-up in these circumstances. Surgery should not go ahead without valid consent being provided. Several ways of proceeding are possible if it is determined that the patient is incompetent, but decisions on which to follow must be made in collaboration with other key players, such as physicians, social workers, family members, or those appointed to act on behalf of the incompetent adult. Once again, it is incumbent on the nurse to have a thorough understanding of the state or federal laws governing informed consent in acute care facilities.

Nursing Implications for the Day of Surgery, Discharge, and Follow-up

Before the patient is medicated and while the family or significant other is still in attendance, the individual who will be responsible for postoperative transportation and home support should be identified. The telephone number of this contact person should be verified. Special calling instructions for the postoperative nurses should be documented in the medical record.

The preoperative physical assessment on the day of surgery includes, but may not be limited to, the auscultation of breath sounds, evaluation of respiratory effort, and noting of the presence of peripheral edema and the regularity and rate of the apical pulse as an indicator of cardiac function. The fasting status should be confirmed and any medications taken that morning verified and documented. Preoperative medications should be used judiciously in elderly patients, particularly in those with preexisting cardiorespiratory illnesses. If preoperative medications are given, the patient must be monitored carefully for any untoward effects.

Some older people are very possessive of their belongings and may need to be reassured that the belongings will be secured. Promoting the concepts of autonomy and normalcy can be achieved by permitting the patients to retain their wigs, false teeth, hearing aids, and eyeglasses as long as possible. In many instances, there is no need for the patient to sacrifice these items.

Communication about the elderly patient's special needs to the operating room and anesthesia staff is important. A consistent location for documentation should be established for special information, such as "Do not place the blood pressure cuff on right (or left) arm," "Hearing aids out," "Patient is deaf in both ears," "Cane/walker in Phase II," and "Nitroglycerin tablets at foot of stretcher."

The elderly patient requires gentleness in care, both physical and emotional. The following are suggestions for addressing the elder patient's special needs in the operating room:

- Remain within the patient's sight as much as possible.
- Keep loud or disquieting noises to a minimum.
- Position patients carefully, avoiding extremes wherever possible.
- Place extra padding on beds and stretchers to protect fragile tissues.
- Keep the perioperative environment as warm as possible. Warm blankets, slippers, or socks and a covering for the head help prevent hypothermia and may also help the older patient feel less chilled.
- During local anesthesia with or without IV conscious sedation, monitor the older person's cardiovascular status, cardiac monitor rhythm, and respiratory function carefully.
- Titrate drug doses to produce intended effects while avoiding somnolence or other side effects.

- Allow sufficient time to evaluate the effects of IV medications before a second dose is given as a result of the reduced cardiac index and circulation time of some elderly individuals.
- Provide instructions slowly and clearly.

The postanesthesia care unit staff must take into account all of the factors related to the normal physiologic changes of aging, especially cardiovascular and respiratory parameters. Anesthetic drugs may linger, producing magnified effects and a slower arousal from general anesthesia. More time may be required before elderly patients can progress to a PACU Phase II (stepdown or discharge) level of care. Healthcare providers might ask whether there are programs that encourage spouses or friends of elderly persons to visit the postanesthesia care unit as one way of reducing the incidence of postoperative delirium. It is also important to verify that the optimum pain management has been achieved in the elderly population and that the patient is warm enough and has been given enough time for activities such as ambulation.

Because hypothermia is common in older adults, a temperature should be obtained on arrival in the PACU and periodically as appropriate. Rewarming may be necessary to promote recovery from general anesthesia and to provide comfort to the patient.

Constant reassurance that the procedure has been completed and that the patient is in the PACU Phase I or ambulatory surgical unit helps not only to reduce anxiety but also to prevent postoperative delirium or confusion. Acute confusion, also known as delirium and transient cognitive impairment, is a prevalent syndrome, occurring in 16% to 38% of elderly patients undergoing surgery.[21] Generally, reports of acute confusion following operative procedures are higher in older than in younger patients. Acute confusion is associated with an increased risk of morbidity and mortality among elderly patients and may unmask or exacerbate a chronic preexisting cognitive impairment. Common perioperative causes of acute confusion in the older patient include hemorrhage, hypothermia, hypotension, hypoxia, and the use of anticholinergic drugs such as atropine.[3] Uncontrolled postoperative pain, urine elimination problems, sensory disturbances, systemic infections (especially urinary tract infections), and limited physical mobility before surgery all contribute significantly to the development of postoperative delirium. Box 23.1 summarizes these causes.

The effective perianesthesia nursing preparation of vulnerable older adults may ensure an uneventful ambulatory surgical experience. The foremost concern is to provide education in a supportive and caring manner for these at-risk older adults, which may help decrease the risk of developing postoperative confusion. Nursing interventions for acute confusion should attempt to reestablish a normal physiologic status or assist patients in reorienting themselves to their same-day-surgery environment. PACU nurses should always consider different physiologic, anesthetic, or surgical causes of a patient's confused or agitated state first. Sedation or restraint for the hyperkinetic patient who is confused is a last resort reserved only for the patient who is at risk for harming self or others.

The health community generally believes that the practice of pain management ought to somehow differ for elderly patients as opposed to younger adults. Elderly patients are often given smaller amounts of analgesics than younger patients with the same magnitude of reported pain. Studies have shown, however, that older patients do not self-administer fewer analgesics than younger patients do.[16] There appears to be a lack of compelling evidence that older adults experience less pain than others. Clinical trials that have assessed the relationship between age and intensity of pain have failed to prove a significant link.[25]

Many healthcare providers and patients alike mistakenly consider pain to be a normal part of aging and something to simply be tolerated. Some elderly patients are reluctant to report their pain and stoically bear it.[25] The pain assessment process can be particularly difficult because of the patient's exhibiting concurrent physiologic, psychological, and cultural changes associated with aging, where the compounding factors are general or regional anesthesia.[25] The perianesthesia nurse must also be aware of the potential risk for drug-to-drug interactions or drug-disease interactions in patients with multiple chronic illnesses who may be taking numerous medications.[16]

Evidence-Based Practice: Managing Acute Pain for Older Adults

Physiological changes impact the experience of acute pain in the older adult. With aging comes a reduction of the A-delta fibers responsible for the sensation of sharp pain and a concurrent decrease in neurons responsible for the conduction of sensory and reactive nerves. These changes result in physiological, psychological, and social impairments related to pain such as functional limitations, sleep disturbances, depression, social isolation, and slower rehabilitation. In older adults, in addition to self-reports of pain, the incorporation of observational pain assessment tools can better determine pain levels.

Source: Hosseini F, Mullins S, Gibson W. Thake M. Acute pain management for older adults. *Clinical Medicine*. 2022;22(4):302-306. https://doi.org/10.7861%2Fclinmed.22.4.ac-p

---

The problem of overmedicating an older adult can be particularly worrisome when discharge to go home is the goal.[25] Choosing the appropriate analgesic dose can be a challenge. The literature does support early aggressive IV analgesia with narcotics, such as morphine and fentanyl or the fentanyl analogues, tapering off to the oral medications before discharge. Some hospitals and clinics are developing 23-hour surgery units, which allow patients to remain as "day patients" as long as they are officially discharged before they have been in the facility for 24 hours. This can be an especially helpful approach for the elderly patient whose pain would not be effectively controlled within a typical 8-hour time frame at most same-day surgery units. Many of these patients are offered the use of locally infused pain pumps or even IV patient-controlled analgesia pumps for the first 23 hours to get their pain under control and can be ready for home by the next day.

Additional adjuncts to pharmacologic remedies for pain should not be forgotten. Comfortable positioning, backrubs, soft music, transcutaneous electrical nerve stimulation devices, use of therapeutic touch if appropriate, and even a little "tender loving care" can be effective measures for easing pain and anxiety with minimal sedative or respiratory side effects.[26]

Fluid administration should be closely monitored to avoid circulatory overload. Sensory aids and dentures that may have been removed for surgery should be returned as soon as possible and preferably before the patient's reunion with family or friends. Movement and positioning should be accomplished slowly to avoid injury, dizziness, or fainting related to changes in blood pressure. Ambulation to a chair should be attempted in stages, with the attendance of a nurse. Stepstools, canes, and walkers are helpful for many older adults.

Reunions with family or friends are often comforting for the older adult, who may be unsettled by the disruption in the daily schedule. The support person should be included in the home care instructions because the patient may have trouble remembering them due to the effects of anesthesia or declining cognitive abilities.[26] Large print instructions are helpful for home reference. It is important that the patient understand instructions about resuming customary medications on the return to home.[26] It is often helpful to ask the patient to perform a return demonstration of the discharge instructions to the nurse to help identify any misunderstandings or difficulties the patient may be having with regard to the instructions.[26] Slowness in thought processes, movements, activities, and responses should be expected and accommodated. It may take a longer time for the older person to recover sufficiently for discharge to go home. Clearly, the elderly patient must be allowed sufficient time not only to be physically recovered before discharge from the facility but also to feel emotionally ready for discharge.

SCREENING FOR ELDER ABUSE

The National Research Council has defined *elder abuse* as intentional maltreatment imposing a significant risk of harm to vulnerable older adults by a caregiver or in a trusted relationship.[22,25] Pillemer et al. emphasized that these caregivers fail to provide basic human needs as well as to protect the elderly person from harm.[22] The National Center on Elder Abuse describes the following seven categories as domestic abuse, institutional abuse, and self-neglect/self-abuse[24]:

- Physical abuse
- Sexual abuse
- Emotional abuse/psychological abuse
- Neglect
- Abandonment
- Financial misappropriation, and
- Self-neglect.[27]

Neglect may include such other behaviors as denial of therapy, nursing services, clothing, therapeutic and equipment aids, and even visits from people who are important to the elderly individual. Elder neglect may be either intentional or unintentional on the part of the caregiver. Elder neglect is not necessarily always a consciously malicious act.

Elder Abuse Risk Profile

Although not restricted to any one economic, social, or cultural group, there are characteristics of both the abused and abusers that may be observed. These include, for the abused, being white, widowed, female, isolated, 75 years of age or older, physically or cognitively impaired, not financially self-sufficient, and living with relatives. The abuser, on the other hand, is generally a close relative or spouse of the abused, middle-aged or older, living with the abused elder, and often experiencing stress such as financial problems, medical problems, marital conflict, substance abuse, and unemployment. This individual may have been an abused child or may harbor some other form of low self-esteem or ineffective coping mechanisms.

Preoperative Screening for Elder Abuse

Elder abuse or neglect has become an increasing problem in contemporary society. Careful preoperative assessments are critical when observing and questioning older adults regarding their health history and home environment. Perianesthesia nurses working in same-day surgery settings are ideally situated to recognize the signs of neglect or abuse of elderly patients and then, most importantly, to take action on these findings based on the state and facility policies and procedures. Some signs and symptoms that may indicate abuse in elderly persons are listed in Box 23.5. The perianesthesia nurse, however, must not make false assumptions of abuse based totally on these observations, because many of the signs and symptoms listed may be due to the aging process. Accurate and comprehensive documentation must be maintained. The suspicion of abuse should be communicated with other healthcare team members in order to develop an individualized plan of care for each older adult patient.

Every case of suspected abuse or neglect is unique and requires an individualized approach. Nonetheless, the first step must always be to establish whether the patient is in any immediate danger, whether hospitalization for abuse is required, or whether it is safe for the patient to remain with the current caregiver. The patient's surgeon and primary physician should be notified as soon as possible. If overt physical abuse is evident, reporting the case to adult protective services and assisting in removing the patient from his or her current home situation may be necessary. The ASC nurse must be aware of the ethical, moral, and legal implications of elder abuse and must be knowledgeable about the facility's protocols and state regulations regarding reporting and intervening in cases of suspected abuse.

Under normal circumstances, one can assume that a patient who is having surgery at an ambulatory surgical facility is competent to make decisions for himself or herself. If, however, the ASC nurse finds that a patient may not be mentally competent and may be at risk for abuse by the accompanying caregiver, steps must be taken to establish a substitute decision maker or temporary guardian for the at-risk senior. Once again, the nurse should be aware of the resources available in the community. There may be other times when the nurse suspects abuse or neglect but the patient involved is assessed to be legally competent and capable of making rational decisions regarding care. The patient's autonomy and rights must be maintained under these circumstances, and the temptation to provide unsolicited help should be avoided.[3] Reassurance may be given, however, that help is available at any time it is requested. Should the competent patient choose not to accept the services or interventions offered, this decision must be accepted, while assurance is provided that help is available if needed.

BOX 23.5 Elder Abuse: Signs and Symptoms

Patterns of "health hopping" (e.g., relying on walk-in clinics, with no regular physician follow-up)
Previous unexplained injuries (e.g., hemorrhage beneath scalp, which may indicate repeated hair pulling)
Burns in unusual locations
Presence of old and new bruises, forming recognizable patterns or shapes
Multiple unexplained fractures of ribs or long bones
Sprains or dislocations
Genital/anal bruises or bleeding
Poor personal hygiene
Signs of sexually transmitted diseases
Extreme mood changes
Depression or oversedation
Lack of glasses, hearing aids, or dentures
Fearfulness
Complaints of sleep disorders
Feelings of guilt, hopelessness, or helplessness

Koehle MM. Special needs of the older adult. Table 27.1 in: Burden N, Quinn DMD, O'Brien D, Dawes BSG, eds. *Ambulatory Surgery Nursing.* 2nd ed. Elsevier; 2000.

Strategies for Interventions in Abusive Situations

Intervention strategies are directed toward the patient, the care provider, and the family of the patient. Primary prevention addresses the issue of elder abuse and neglect through education. Referrals to appropriate community resources, including the patient's family physician, caregiver associations, social services, and so on, may be helpful. The nurse should be aware of the other available resources that could assist the elderly person and caregivers, such as homemaker services, alternative housing services, respite care, adult day-care services, Meals on Wheels, financial counseling services, and legal assistance.

Interventions directed at abusers include legal proceedings (for intentional abuse), immediate relief from stress for caregivers through assistance in the care of the elder, counseling, education, and linking up with appropriate resources in the community. The pressure placed on all members of the healthcare team to reduce hospital admissions and hospital stays is making it increasingly difficult to justify hospitalization for social reasons. Perianesthesia nurses, then, must continually act as patient advocates and be watchful for suspected social or home circumstances that may place their elder patients at risk for abuse or neglect.

When perianesthesia nurses conduct a preoperative assessment, there should be a high degree of suspicion about elder abuse patients trying to hide maltreatment or self-neglect. It is important that the preoperative nurse question patients in privacy by asking if anyone has harmed them. The older adults' factual responses should be documented in their own descriptive words.

PERIANESTHESIA NURSING CARE DILEMMAS

Healthcare professionals may encounter specific care dilemmas when approaching the outpatient surgical care of elderly patients. First, preoperative planning is essential when ensuring appropriate resources are available to deal with the older adults' special needs, including adequate staffing for their more time-consuming comprehensive perianesthesia nursing care. Second, equipment, supplies, and medications for the short-term outpatient surgery needs of chronically ill patients must be available. Third, both assessment and instructional techniques must be altered if patients have psychological, cognitive, or physical limitations. Fourth, it is essential that the support personnel who are caring for these patients at home or in nursing homes are included in the older adults' plans of care.

Finally, as the U.S. population becomes increasingly more mobile and family units become more fragmented, many seniors are living far from their extended families, with no close relative living nearby who can be a responsible adult caregiver when they require same-day surgery. Giving elderly patients suggestions about social service organizations that can provide assistance and making sure that help is scheduled by the time patients leave for home may be necessary and welcome.

CHAPTER HIGHLIGHTS

- Geriatric patients face a myriad of health issues associated with the normal aging process.
- Cultural and ethnic values influence older adults' perspectives on their ambulatory surgery.
- Polypharmacy with prescribed medications or herbal medicines, or both, may cause serious adverse drug reactions in patients during anesthesia and surgery.

- Geriatric preoperative screening for significant risk factors is associated with postoperative outcomes.
- Perianesthesia nursing processes for the coordination of care for geriatric patients (e.g., preoperative care to the PACU Phase I level of care to the Phase II level of care to

discharge) are vital nursing assessments and interventions for this vulnerable population.
- Patient and family educational strategies are critical for older adults' understanding of and compliance with the healing process.

CASE STUDY

Mr. Ying is a 75-year-old Asian American undergoing a left hernia repair under general anesthesia. He weighs 120 kg and is 5 feet 10 inches tall. He has a history of obesity, obstructive sleep apnea, and hypertension. His ECG reveals premature atrial beats with sinus arrhythmias. He takes a beta-blocker, vitamin E, ginkgo, and garlic. Since his wife passed away from Covid-19 6 months ago, Mr. Ying has been depressed, and he is very nervous about having surgery. His sister is accompanying him to the surgery center and will be his caregiver once they return home.

It is important for the preoperative nurse to address the older Asian adult by his last name. In the Asian culture, older adults are perceived as wise elders to be respected. It is also important to ask the older adult how he prefers to be addressed to convey that the nurse is caring and creating a respectful, non-threatening environment.

Which risk factors should concern the perianesthesia nurse? The following are vitally important risk factors for the

preoperative nurse to identify and communicate to anesthesia providers, surgeons, and PACU nurses: obesity; obstructive sleep apnea, hypertension, and cardiac co-morbidities; polypharmacy that could lead to adverse drug reactions, including a side effect of bleeding caused by herbal medications; and psychosocial conditions.

What is the best approach for pain and comfort management for this patient? Multimodal pharmacologic pain management, along with complementary interventions, are important for the patient's postoperative recovery.

Finally, educational efforts preoperatively and at the time of discharge will help the patient understand why he needs to comply and follow his physicians' instructions. The psychosocial circumstances of this older Asian adult necessitate that his sister, the caregiver, also understand and follow his discharge instructions.

REFERENCES

1. Redburn DE. Graying of the world's population. In: Redburn DE, McNamara RP. *Social Gerontology.* Auburn House; 1998.
2. Warshaw GA, Potter JF, Flaherty E, McNabney MK, Heflin T, Ham R. *Ham's Primary Care Geriatrics: A Case-Based Approach.* 7th ed. Elsevier; 2021.
3. Miller CA. *Nursing for Wellness in Older Adults.* 8th ed. Williams & Wilkins; 2019.
4. Linton AD, Lach HW, eds. *Matteson & McConnell's Gerontological Nursing: Concepts and Practice.* 3rd ed. WB Saunders; 2007.
5. Hall MJ, Schwartzman A, Zhang J, Liu X. Ambulatory surgery data from hospitals and ambulatory surgery centers: United States, 2010. *Natl Health Stat Report.* 2017;102:1-15.
6. White PF, White LM, Monk T, et al. Perioperative care for the older adult outpatient undergoing ambulatory surgery. *Anesth Analg.* 2012;114(6):1190-1215. Available at: https://doi.org/10.1213/ane.0b013e31824f19b8.
7. United States Census Bureau. *The Nation's Older Population Is Still Growing. Census Bureau Reports.* 2017. Available at: www.census.gov/newsroom/press-releases/2017/cb17-100.html.
8. Maxwell CA, Wang J. Understanding frailty: a nurse's guide. *Nurs Clin North Am.* 2017;52(3):349-361. Available at: https://doi.org/10.1016/j.cnur.2017.04.003.
9. Richards SJG, Frizelle FA, Geddes JA, Eglinton TW, Hampton MB. Frailty in surgical patients. *Int J Colorectal Dis.* 2018;33(12):1657-1666. Available at: https://doi.org/10.1007/s00384-018-3163-y.
10. Axley MS, Schenning KJ. Preoperative cognitive and frailty screening in the geriatric patient: a narrative. *Clin Ther.* 2015;37(12):2666-2675. Available at: https://doi.org/10.1016/j.clinthera.2015.10.022.
11. Ko FC. Perioperative frailty evaluation: a promising risk-stratification tool in older adults undergoing general surgery. *Clin Ther.* 2019;41(3):387-399. Available at: https://doi.org/10.1016/j.clinthera.2019.01.014.
12. Seib CD, Rochefort H, Chomsky-Higgins K, et al. Association of patient frailty with increased morbidity after common ambulatory general surgery operations. *JAMA Surg.* 2018;153(2):160-168. Available at: https://doi.org/10.1001/jamasurg.2017.4007.
13. Masnoon N, Shakibs S, Kalisch-Ellett L, Caughey GE. What is polypharmacy? A systematic review. *BMC Geriatrics.* 2017;17(1):230-240. Available at: https://doi.org/10.1186/s12877-017-0621-2.
14. Shaw BM, Hajjar ER. Polypharmacy, adverse drug reactions, and geriatric syndromes. *Clin Geriatr Med.* 2012;28(2):173-186. Available at: https://doi.org/10.1016/j.cger.2012.01.002.
15. Kim J, Parish AL. Polypharmacy and medication management in older adults. *Nurs Clin N Am.* 2017;52(3):457-468. Available at: https://doi.org/10.1016/j.cnur.2017.04.007.
16. Olotu C, Weimann A, Bahrs C, Schwenk W, Scherer M, Kiefmann R. The perioperative care of the older adult: time for a new, interdisciplinary approach. *Dtsch Arztebl Int.* 2019;116:63-69. Available at: https://doi.org/10.3238/arztebl.2019.0063.
17. Izzo AA, Hoon-Kim S, Radhakrishnan R, Williamson EM. A critical approach to evaluating clinical efficacy, adverse events and drug interactions of herbal remedies. *Phytother Res.* 2016;30(5):691-700. Available at: https://doi.org/10.1002/ptr.5591.
18. Oresanya LB, Lyons WL, Finlayson E. Preoperative assessment of the older patient: a narrative review. *JAMA.* 2014;311(20):2110–20. Available at: https://doi.org/10.1001/jama.2014.4573.
19. Ang-Lee MK, Moss J, Yuan CS. Herbal medicines and perioperative care. *JAMA.* 2001;286(2):208-216. Available at: https://doi.org/10.1001/jama.286.2.208.
20. Mohanty S, Rosenthal RA, Russell MM, Neuman MD, Ko CY, Esnaola NF. Optimal perioperative management of the geriatric patient: a best practice guideline from the American College of Surgeons NSQIP and the American Geriatrics Society. *J Am Coll Surg.* 2016;222(5):930-947. Aailable at: https://doi.org/10.1016/j.jamcollsurg.2015.12.026.
21. Chow WB, Rosenthal RA, Merkow RP, et al. Optimal preoperative assessment of the geriatric surgical patient: a best practices guideline from the American College of Surgeons National Surgical Quality Improvement Program and the American Geriatrics Society. *J Am Coll Surg.* 2012;215(4):453-466. Available at: https://doi.org/10.1016/j.jamcollsurg.2012.06.017.
22. Pillemer K, Breckman R, Sweeney CD, et al. Practitioners' views on elder mistreatment research priorities: recommendations from

a research-to-practice consensus conference. *J Elder Abuse Negl.* 2003;23(2):115-126. Available at: https://doi.org/10.1080/08946 566.2011.558777.

23. Crawford FJ. The elderly patient. *AORN J.* 1985;41(2):356-359. Available at: https://doi.org/10.1016/s0001-2092(07)63270-0.

24. National Institute on Aging. *Elder Abuse.* July 21, 2023. https://www.nia.nih.gov/health/elder-abuse#types

25. Ardery G, Herr KA, Titler MG, Sorofman BA, Schmitt MB. Assessing and managing acute pain in older adults: a research base to guide practice. *Medsurg Nurs.* 2003;12(1):7-18.

26. Ead HM. Ensuring a smooth discharge home after ambulatory surgery. *J Perianesth Nurs.* 2016;31(3):254-256. Available at: https://doi.org/10.1016/j.jopan.2016.02.005.

27. Li M, Chang ES, Simon MA, Dong XQ. Elder mistreatment. In: Warshaw GA, Potter JF, Flaherty E, et al, eds. *Ham's Primary Care Geriatrics: A Case-Based Approach.* 7th ed. Elsevier; 2022:327-333.

23

24 Caring for the Family

Daphne Stannard, PhD, RN, CNS, NPD-BC, FCCM

LEARNING OBJECTIVES

A review of the content of this chapter will help the reader to:

1. Define *family*.
2. Differentiate between nursing-centered family interventions at the point of care: ensuring a family presence; providing the family with information and support; and encouraging family involvement in caregiving activities.
3. Describe how caring for patients and their families is a vital and required component of ambulatory surgical nursing practice.

OVERVIEW

Family can be defined in many ways. There are strict legal definitions of family that are purposefully narrow that are used for informed consents, other legal documents, and end-of-life decisions. However, the restrictive qualities of legal definitions exclude many of the types of families and family configurations seen in healthcare environments, making these limited definitions ill-suited for routine care issues. When the patient can communicate, the ideal definition of family is whomever the patient defines as family.[1] Typically, one's chosen family is a locus of meaning and connection. But, in the rapid-fire pace of an ambulatory surgical setting, it is difficult to assess the intention and quality of a particular family connection to a given patient. Thus, when the patient is unable to communicate, a practical definition of family is anyone who participates in the care and well-being of the patient.[2]

There is a reciprocal relationship between the patient and family. For example, the family is greatly affected by the patient's illness; likewise, a "sick" or dysfunctional family can greatly affect the patient.[1] Working with patients and their families allows ambulatory surgical nurses to support and strengthen meaningful relationships during times of great stress. But family-centered interventions at the point of care often differ from those that are offered away from a patient care area. Thus, family interventions can be understood on a continuum of proximity to the patient. Interventions at the patient's bedside or chairside are at one end of the continuum, while specialized programs occurring away from the patient are at the opposite end of the continuum (Figure 24.1). Nursing-centered interventions at the point of care are often unscripted and based on the responses of the patient and family and the particulars of the clinical situation. This stands in contrast to the more formalized interventions that are often offered away from the patient care area. Unit tours typically occur during quiet times and follow a predictable route. Post discharge phone calls commonly follow question prompts or a script, and many educational and support groups utilize a preplanned curriculum of sorts.

One type of intervention is not better than another, but nurses working in ambulatory surgical settings are uniquely situated to care for patients and their families at the point of care, and as such, the emphasis of this chapter will be on the nursing-centered family interventions that occur in patient care areas and their application to ambulatory surgical nursing practice.

FACTS AND FIGURES

In 2019, prior to the SARS-CoV-2 pandemic, nearly 20 million outpatient surgeries were performed in the United States.[3] This number represents a 6.4% increase in the number of surgeries performed in outpatient areas since 2015 and stands in contrast to a 1.5% decrease in the number of surgeries performed in inpatient settings during that same time period.[3] There are few regulations stipulating the provision of nursing care to patients and their families, but the Centers for Medicare and Medicaid Services acknowledges the importance of family representatives and defines them as "non-healthcare professionals supporting those who receive healthcare."[4]

In 1997, the American Association of Critical-Care Nurses (AACN) published a landmark evidence-based series entitled "Protocols for Practice: Creating a Healing Environment."[5] One of the white papers focused on the family needs and interventions in the acute care environment, and another focused on

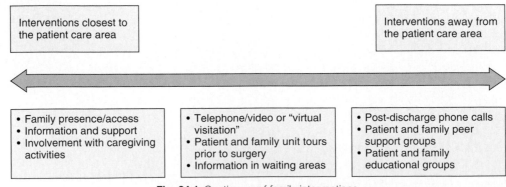

Fig. 24.1 Continuum of family interventions.

family visitation and partnership in the critical care unit. More recently, AACN published two practice alerts, one supporting unrestricted presence and participation of a support person[6] and the other supporting family presence during resuscitation and invasive procedures.[7] In 2016, the Society of Critical Care Medicine published guidelines for family-centered care in the neonatal, pediatric, and adult intensive care units (ICUs)[8], which was followed by a clinical practice guideline produced by the Emergency Nurses Association in 2017.[9] These evidence-based protocols, recommendations, and guidelines have a broad base of research literature as support, but the rigor and quality of some of the studies is weak. This is an important and evolving area of research, and more work is needed to inform nursing practice moving forward.

Evidence-Based Practice: Family Visitation

The American Association of Critical-Care Nurses published a practice alert in 2016 addressing family visitation in the adult intensive care unit. The recommendations for practice were based on leveled evidence from primarily peer-reviewed publications. In terms of situations in which the admission of families and/or visitors into the environment of care should be restricted, the practice alert identifies three primary reasons. These include:

- Family members who are known to be abusive, disruptive, or causing unsafe clinical situations.
- Family members wishing to participate in patient care should be free of communicable diseases and must follow infection control practices.
- Staff must consider ways of managing infectious disease situations in order to accommodate the safe presence of family to provide for the emotional support of patients.

Source: American Association of Critical-Care Nurses. Family visitation in the adult intensive care unit. *Crit Care Nurs.* 2016;36(1):e15-e19. https://doi.org/10.4037/ccn2016677

Many nurses know that caring for patients includes caring for families. For simple, logistical reasons alone, families are the ones who transport the recovered patient away from the facility. Families are the support people who distract and relax anxious patients in holding rooms before their procedures. Families are often the ones who pay the most attention to discharge instructions, as the patient may still be focused on the surgical procedure that was successfully completed. The American Society of PeriAnesthesia Nurses' (ASPAN) *PeriAnesthesia Nursing Core Curriculum: Preprocedure, Phase I and Phase II PACU Nursing* describes the necessity for a family-oriented environment in the preoperative phase and space for patients' families in Phase II recovery,[10] and the *Perianesthesia Nursing Standards, Practice Recommendations and Interpretive Statements*[11] published by ASPAN has a dedicated standard calling for family-centered care.

FAMILY-CENTERED CARE

Family-centered care is a philosophy of care delivery and way of caring for patients that includes and involves the family. Nurses who embrace family-centered care understand that caring for the family is an extension of caring for the patient. The goals for family-centered care are to transform the healthcare delivery system so that care settings will recognize and encourage patient and family strengths, choices, and independence.[12] Family-centered care is an approach to the planning and delivery of healthcare that is based on collaboration and partnership with patients, families, and clinicians. Three principal

nursing-centered interventions at the point of care that help to realize the goals of family-centered care are presented here.

Ensuring a Family Presence

The term *family presence* has been commonly associated with ensuring family access during resuscitation efforts and invasive procedures. However, the term can also be used in lieu of the term *family visitation*, which is falling out of favor because it does not imply active involvement with the patient and associated care.[1] Active involvement in care is emphasized by The Joint Commission[13] and is an intervention that will be discussed later in this chapter. Ensuring family presence is the cornerstone to all other family-centered interventions, as family access promotes family cohesion, connection, and involvement in care; fosters patient well-being; and provides the family with visual cues and other information.[2] While the other family-centered interventions are important and have been widely recognized as meeting the central needs of family members,[14] the primacy of family access cannot be overemphasized.

While family care in perianesthesia nursing areas is still an emerging field of research, when one draws on research that was conducted in similar areas (such as other acute and critical care areas), it has been demonstrated that family presence has the following effects on the patient:

- Reduces the incidence of delirium[15]
- Reduces the incidence of emergence delirium[16]
- Reduces cardiovascular complications[17-23]
- Improves pain management, lowers anxiety, and facilitates the use of positive postoperative coping strategies[24]
- Decreases intracranial pressure[25,26]
- Decreases negative behavior in children[27]
- Does not compromise patient safety[28]
- Increases patient satisfaction[29-31]
- Does not increase infection risk[18,32,33]

Additionally, family presence has the following effects on the family:

- Decreases family member anxiety[34-37]
- Increases family satisfaction and parental coping[37-39]
- Reduces the incidence of posttraumatic stress disorder in adolescents and adults[40,41]
- Assists with familial coping, especially with adverse outcomes and complications[42]

Finally, from the clinician's perspective, research has shown that family presence:

- Causes no delays in treatment or resuscitation[43,44]
- Causes no adverse effects on the technical performance of the staff[45]
- May decrease the risk of litigation[46-49]
- Enhances communication and facilitates family education[46-50]
- Humanizes the patient and supports patient dignity[46,48,49,51]

Caring for patients' families in ambulatory surgical settings is not usually as stressful as or associated with the high stakes of situations in critical care areas such as the emergency department and ICU during times of resuscitation or serious decompensation. However, given that patients in Phase I recovery are considered critically ill until they have a stabilized and patent airway and normalized hemodynamics (among other clinical characteristics), it is useful to review the benefits of family presence across the critical care continuum, as patients and families in ambulatory surgical settings can still experience anxiety, stress, emotional lability, and a desire to be close to loved ones.

Providing the Family with Information and Support

Another central aspect of family care is nurses' provision of information and support to patients' families.[2] Information has been identified as a crucial component in family coping and satisfaction. Support, in the form of nurses' caring behaviors and interactions, is enormously influential in shaping the care experience for both patients and families.[1] Taken together, these two nursing interventions are highly valued by families and are even more meaningful when family access is ensured.

Patients and families often have significant informational needs, which may become known during screening on the day of surgery in the preoperative holding area. Answering family questions has been reported in one study as being one of the causes for first case operating room delays.[52] Yet, ensuring that patients and families are well-informed in a language and manner that is understandable to them falls under the American Nurses Association (ANA) *Scope and Standards of Practice* as Standard 10 (Communication).[53] Other competencies under Standard 10 that are germane to providing information and support to patients and families include using communication styles and methods that demonstrate caring, respect, active listening, authenticity, and trust; conveying accurate information to patients, families, and members of the interprofessional team; maintaining communication with interprofessional team members and others to facilitate safe transitions and continuity in care delivery; and contributing the nursing perspective in interactions and discussions with the interprofessional team and other stakeholders.[53]

Providing information is often thought to be unidirectional, that is, it is the conveying of instructions or information from the clinician to the patient and family. However, per ANA Standard 10, communication should be bidirectional, and a nonrushed, nonjudgmental response will go far in conveying information in a caring manner.[53] Information imparted to family members can be instructional, such as, "Feel free to hold his hand on this side, so that you can avoid the IV," or can provide orienting information, which quite literally orients and familiarizes the family with the situation at hand and includes interpreting for the family the surrounding equipment, the patient's condition, and the anticipated trajectory or big picture.[2] A simple example of providing orienting information to a family member in language they can understand is, "The top line on this monitor tells us information about the heart."

Orienting information can share a blurry boundary with discharge instructions and teaching, but a crucial distinction between the two is that orienting information is typically provided in shorter segments, requiring less attention by the person receiving the information. This differs from discharge instructions, as the goals of discharge teaching are to ensure that the patient and family fully understand

- How to care for the surgical/procedural site once they are home
- Any dietary, medication, mobility, and functional restrictions related to the surgery/procedure
- Possible postsurgical/postprocedural complications that might arise and how to treat and when to report them, and
- Any follow up appointments or required care that is needed to maintain the surgical/procedural site until the postsurgical/postprocedural clinic visit

Ensuring that the family is ready to absorb discharge instructions is a form of clinical judgment and requires timing, active listening, and emotional engagement with the situation to ensure effective delivery of the education and facilitation of patient and family learning. Teaching anxious family members requires patience, understanding, and good communication skills on the part of the nurse, as well as a firm grasp of the content so that it can be simplified and re-stated in multiple ways to ensure family comprehension.[2]

Patients and families often recognize when the nurse is simply informing them as part of her or his job and when the nurse is informing them to provide them with an increased understanding of the situation. A nurse's rushed and unwelcoming behavior will often escalate family anxiety, so setting the tone by slowing the pace, frequently checking in for understanding, and listening and responding to a patient's and family's concerns become important strategies when providing crucial information.

Support is often demonstrated to patients and families through nonverbal caring actions on the part of the nurse. Support, thus, can be an intervention that is expressed alongside information giving and can also be conveyed through caring behaviors, such as an understanding nod, a squeeze of the hand, or a smile or hug. Being recognized as an important partner in care, being heard, and feeling cared for are all ways in which the nurse can support the patient and family and are vital advocacy roles that the ambulatory surgical nurse employs.

Nurses sometimes feel that specialized training or advanced degrees are necessary to help them prepare in caring for patients' families.[54] However, a family's interest is most typically aligned with the nurse's interest: to ensure that the best possible care is provided to the patient. In this way, nurses and family members are partners in care and are allies, of sorts; all are working together to ensure that the patient is fully informed, prepared, and ready for the surgery or procedure and is optimized for the best possible outcome following the surgery or procedure.

Encouraging Family Involvement in Caregiving Activities

Active family involvement is encouraged by The Joint Commission[13] and can range from minor involvement (such as asking a family member to pass the nurse a box of tissues on the other side of the gurney) to major involvement (such as inviting a family member to assist with the patient's oral care).[1] Nurses working in neonatal and pediatric areas have long involved families in the care of the patient to help prepare them for their caretaking duties once the patient is discharged. However, the same principles apply to adult patients, as family members often assist the patient in caring for a wound or help to manage mobility devices, among other therapies and assistive items, following a surgery or procedure.

There are many hurdles to fully involving family members in patient care, including facility policies (including restricting family access), inadequate staffing and lack of time, and hesitancy on the part of nurses and families (who may never have been invited to be involved in care before). As such, it is an understudied area in family research, but the few studies conducted in this area have shown that families desire increased involvement in the care of their loved ones and that involving them early in caregiving can help prepare them to better meet patient needs following discharge.[55] One strategy that has been suggested to increase family involvement during discharge teaching is to employ the teach-back method.[56,57] While this is an informational intervention, the method seeks active involvement in the teaching–learning activity. As such, this method may encourage patients and families to become more engaged in the discharge teaching process.

CHAPTER HIGHLIGHTS

- When the patient can communicate, the ideal definition of *family* is whoever the patient defines as family.[2] When the patient is unable to communicate, a practical definition of family is anyone who participates in the care and well-being of the patient.[3]
- Family interventions can be understood on a continuum of proximity to the patient. Interventions at the patient's gurney or chairside are at one end of the continuum, while specialized programs occurring away from the patient are at the opposite end (see Figure 24.1). Nursing-centered interventions at the point of care are often unscripted and based on the responses of the patient and family and the particulars of the clinical situation. This stands in contrast to the more formalized interventions that are often offered away from the patient care area. One type of intervention is not better than another, but nurses working in ambulatory surgical settings are uniquely situated to care for patients and their families at the point of care.
- Ensuring family presence is the cornerstone to all other family-centered interventions, as family access promotes family cohesion, connection, and closure; fosters patient well-being; and provides the family with visual cues and other information.[2] While the other family-centered interventions are important and have been widely recognized as meeting central needs of family members,[14] the primacy of family access cannot be overemphasized and has been shown in countless research studies to have many positive effects on the patient and the family.
- Information has been identified as a crucial component in family coping and satisfaction. Support, in the form of nurses' caring behaviors and interactions, is enormously influential in shaping the care experience for both patients and families.[1] Taken together, these two nursing interventions are highly valued by families and are even more meaningful when family access is ensured. Information imparted to family members can be instructional or orienting. Support can be an intervention that is expressed alongside information giving and can also be conveyed through caring behaviors.
- Active family involvement is encouraged by The Joint Commission[13] and can range from minor involvement (such as asking a family member to pass the nurse a box of tissues on the other side of the gurney) to major involvement (such as inviting a family member to assist with the patient's oral care).[1]

CASE STUDY

Mel Gonzales is a 68-year-old woman who is scheduled for a bilateral blepharoplasty. She has a significant cardiac history, with hypertension and a previous myocardial infarction at age 48. She is adherent with her exercise program, dietary restrictions, and medications, but as a precaution, she had her case scheduled in your ambulatory surgical facility. You are taking care of her postoperatively and have been in touch with the husband by phone during Phase I recovery, providing him with updates. Mel is now awake and asking for her husband, and you invite him to join his wife during Phase II recovery. Although the operative procedure Mel has had is not complex, there are a number of self-care interventions that the patient must employ to ensure uncomplicated healing. Mel considers herself to be independent but has a tight and loving relationship with her husband and wants him to help her with her postoperative care. As such, you involve both the patient and the family in your discharge teaching and employ the teach-back method to engage them and help to ensure that the discharge instructions are internalized and that Mel and her husband feel comfortable about carrying out the interventions at home.

REFERENCES

1. Stannard D, Cooper AS. Families of perianesthesia patients. In: Stannard D, Krenzischek D, eds. *Perianesthesia Nursing Care: A Bedside Guide for Safe Recovery.* 2nd ed. Jones & Bartlett; 2018: 187-195.
2. Stannard D. Caring for patients' families. In: Benner P, Hooper-Kyriakidis P, Stannard D, eds. *Clinical Wisdom and Interventions in Acute and Critical Care: A Thinking-In-Action Approach.* 2nd ed. Springer; 2011:267-300.
3. American Hospitals Association. *Total U.S.* Available at: https://guide.prod.iam.aha.org/stats/total-us. Accessed October 02, 2021.
4. Centers for Medicare and Medicaid Services. *Quality Measures and You: Persons and Family.* Available at: https://www.cms.gov/Medicare/Quality-Initiatives-Patient-Assessment-Instruments/MMS/QMY-Persons-and-Family. Accessed October 02, 2021.
5. American Association of Critical-Care Nurses. *Protocols for Practice: Creating a Healing Environment Series.* Author; 1997.
6. American Association of Critical-Care Nurses. Family visitation in the adult intensive care unit. *Crit Care Nurs.* 2016;36(1):e15-e19. Available at: https://doi.org/10.4037/ccn2016677.
7. American Association of Critical-Care Nurses. Family presence during resuscitation and invasive procedures. *Crit Care Nurs.* 2016;36(1): e11-e14. Available at: https://doi.org/10.4037/ccn2016980.
8. Davidson JE, Aslakson RA, Long AC, et al. Guidelines for family-centered care in the neonatal, pediatric, and adult ICU. *Crit Care Med.* 2017;45(1):103-128. Available at: https://doi.org/10.1097/ccm.0000000000002169.
9. Emergency Nurses Association. *Clinical Practice Guideline: Family Presence During Invasive Procedures and Resuscitation.* Author; 2017. Available at: https://media.emscimprovement.center/documents/familypresencecpg3eaabb7cf0414584ac2291feba3be481.pdf.
10. Schick L, Windle PE. *Perianesthesia Nursing Core Curriculum: Preprocedure, Phase I and Phase II PACU Nursing.* 4th ed. Elsevier; 2021.
11. American Society of PeriAnesthesia Nurses. *2021-2022 Perianesthesia Nursing Standards, Practice Recommendations and Interpretive Statements.* Author; 2020.
12. Institute for Patient- and Family-Centered Care. *Mission/Vision.* Available at: https://www.ipfcc.org/about/mission.html. Accessed October 02, 2021.
13. The Joint Commission. *Use an Advocate or Be an Advocate for Others.* Available at: https://www.jointcommission.org/resources/for-consumers/take-charge/use-an-advocate-or-be-an-advocate-for-others/. Accessed October 03, 2021.
14. Stannard D. It is time to balance the risks with notions of good. *J Perianesth Nurs.* 2021;36:441-442. Available at: https://doi.org/10.1016/j.jopan.2021.05.003.
15. Kandori K, Okada Y, Ishii W, Narumiya H, Maebayashi Y, Iizuka R. Association between visitation restriction during the Covid-19 pandemic and delirium incidence among emergency admission patients: a single-center retrospective observational cohort study in Japan. *J Int Care.* 2020;8:90. Available at: https://doi.org/10.1186/s40560-020-00511-x.
16. In WY, Kim YM, Kim HS, et al. The effect of a parental visitation program on emergence delirium among postoperative children in the PACU. *J Perianesth Nurs.* 2019;34(1):108-116. Available at: https://doi.org/10.1016/j.jopan.2018.04.003.
17. Fuller BF, Foster GM. The effects of family/friend visits vs. staff interaction on stress/arousal of surgical intensive care patients. *Heart Lung.* 1982;11(5):457-463.
18. Fumagalli S, Boniceinelli L, Lo Nostro A, et al. Reduced cardiocirculatory complications with unrestrictive visiting policy in an intensive care unit: results from a pilot, randomized trial. *Circulation.* 2006;113(7):946-952. Available at: https://doi.org/10.1161/circulationaha.105.572537.
19. Kleman M, Bickert A, Karpinski A, et al. Physiologic responses of coronary care patients to visiting. *J Cardiovasc Nurs.* 1993;7(3): 52-62. Available at: https://doi.org/10.1097/00005082-199304000-00006.
20. Happ MB, Swigart VA, Tate JA, Arnold RM, Sereika SM, Hoffman LA. Family presence and surveillance during weaning from prolonged mechanical ventilation. *Heart Lung.* 2007;36:47-57. Available at: https://doi.org/10.1016%2Fj.hrtlng.2006.07.002.
21. Lazure LL, Baun MM. Increasing patient control of family visiting in the coronary care unit. *Am J Crit Care.* 1995;4(2):157-164.

22. Schulte DA, Burrell LO, Gueldner SH, et al. Pilot study of the relationship between heart rate and ectopy and unrestricted vs. restricted visiting hours in the coronary care unit. *Am J Crit Care.* 1993;2(2):134-136.

23. Simpson T, Shaver J. Cardiovascular responses to family visits in coronary care patients. *Heart Lung.* 1990;19(4):344-351.

24. Grondin F, Bourgault P, Bolduc N. Intervention focused on the patient and family for better postoperative pain relief. *Pain Manag Nurs.* 2014;15(1):76-86. Available at: https://doi.org/10.1016/j.pmn.2012.06.006.

25. Hepworth JT, Hendrickson SG, Lopez J. Time series analysis of physiological response during ICU visitation. *West J Nurs Res.* 1994;16(6):704-717. Available at: https://doi.org/10.1177/019394599401600608.

26. Prins MM. The effect of family visits on intracranial pressure. *West J Nurs Res.* 1989;11(3):281-297. Available at: https://doi.org/10.1177/019394598901100303.

27. Lardner DR, Dick BD, Crawford S. The effects of parental presence in the postanesthetic care unit on children's postoperative behavior: a prospective, randomized, controlled study. *Anesth Analg.* 2010;110(4):1102-1108. Available at: https://doi.org/10.1213/ane.0b013e3181cccba8.

28. Fiorentini SE. Evaluation of a new program: pediatric parental visitation in the postanesthesia care unit. *J Post Anesth Nurs.* 1993;8(4):249-256.

29. Herd HA, Rieben MA. Establishing the surgical nurse liaison role to improve patient and family member communication. *AORN J.* 2014;99(5):594-599. Available at: https://doi.org/10.1016/j.aorn.2013.10.024.

30. Noonan AT, Anderson P, Newlon P, Patrin T, Ladue-Weber K, Winstead-Fry P. Family-centered nursing in the postanesthesia care unit: the evaluation of practice. *J Post Anesth Nurs.* 1991;6(1):13-16.

31. Tuller S, McCabe L, Cronenwett L, et al. Patient, visitor, and nurse evaluations of visitation for adult postanesthesia care unit patients. *J Perianesth Nurs.* 1997;12(6):402-412. Available at: https://doi.org/10.1016/s1089-9472(97)90003-4.

32. Adams S, Herrera A, Miller L, Soto R. Visitation in the intensive care unit: impact on infection prevention and control. *Crit Care Nurs Q.* 2011;34(1):3-10. Available at: https://doi.org/10.1097/cnq.0b013e31820480ef.

33. Tang CS, Chung FF, Lin MC, Wan GH. Impact of patient visiting activities on indoor climate in a medical intensive care unit: a 1-year longitudinal study. *Am J Infect Control.* 2009;37:183-188. Available at: https://doi.org/10.1016/j.ajic.2008.06.011.

34. Blum EP, Burns SM. Perioperative communication and family members' perceived level of anxiety and satisfaction. *ORNAC J.* 2013;31(3):14, 16-19, 34-36.

35. Carter AJ, Deselms J, Ruyle S, Morrissey-Lucas M, Kollar S, Cannon S, Schick L. Postanesthesia care unit visitation decreases family member anxiety. *J Perianesth Nurs.* 2012;27(1):3-9. Available at: https://doi.org/10.1016/j.jopan.2011.10.004.

36. Pagnard E, Sarver W. Family visitation in the PACU: an evidence-based practice project. *J Perianesth Nurs.* 2018;34(3):600-605. Available at: https://doi.org/10.1016/j.jopan.2018.09.007.

37. Wendler MC, Smith K, Ellenburg W, Gill R, Anderson L, Spiegel-Thayer K. "To see with my own eyes": experiences of family visits during phase 1 recovery. *J Perianesth Nurs.* 2016;32(1):45-57. Available at: https://doi.org/10.1016/j.jopan.2015.03.015.

38. Whitcomb JJ, Roy D, Blackman VS. Evidence-based practice in a military intensive care unit family visitation. *Nurs Res.* 2010;59(1S):S32-S39. Available at: https://doi.org/10.1097/nnr.0b013e3181c3c028.

39. McAlvin SS, Carew-Lyons A. Family presence during resuscitation and invasive procedures in pediatric critical care: a systematic review. *Am J Crit Care.* 2014;23(6):477-484. Available at: https://doi.org/10.4037/ajcc2014922.

40. Ferge JL, Banydeen R, Le Terrier C, et al. Mental health of adolescent relatives of intensive care patients: benefits of an open visitation policy. *Am J Crit Care.* 2021;30(1):72-76. Available at: https://doi.org/10.4037/ajcc2021799.

41. Jabre P, Belpomme V, Azoulay E, et al. Family presence during cardiopulmonary resuscitation. *N Engl J Med.* 2013;368(11):1008-1018. Available at: https://doi.org/10.1056/nejmoa1203366.

42. Tinsley C, Hill JB, Shah J, et al. Experience of families during cardiopulmonary resuscitation in a pediatric intensive care unit. *Pediatrics.* 2008;122(4):e799-e804. Available at: https://doi.org/10.1542/peds.2007-3650.

43. Dudley NC, Hansen KW, Furnival RA, Donaldson AE, van Wagene KL, Scaife ER. The effect of family presence on the efficiency of pediatric trauma resuscitations. *Ann Emerg Med.* 2009;53(6):777-784. Available at: https://doi.org/10.1016/j.annemergmed.2008.10.002.

44. O'Connell KJ, Farah MM, Spandorfer P, Zorc JJ. Family presence during pediatric trauma team activation: an assessment of a structured program. *Pediatrics.* 2007;120(3):e565-e574. Available at: https://doi.org/10.1542/peds.2006-2914.

45. Bjorshol CA, Mykelbust H, Nilsen KL, et al. Effect of socioemotional stress on the quality of cardiopulmonary resuscitation during advanced life support in a randomized manikin study. *Crit Care Med.* 2011;39(2):300-304. Available at: https://doi.org/10.1097/ccm.0b013e3181ffe100.

46. Basol R, Ohman K, Simones J, Skillings K. Using research to determine support for a policy on family presence during resuscitation. *Dimens Crit Care Nurs.* 2009;28(5):237-247. Available at: https://doi.org/10.1097/dcc.0b013e3181ac4bf4.

47. Dingeman RS, Mitchell EA, Meyer EC, Curley MAQ. Parent presence during complex invasive procedures and cardiopulmonary resuscitation: a systematic review of the literature. *Pediatrics.* 2007;120(4):842-854. Available at: https://doi.org/10.1542/peds.2006-3706.

48. McClement SE, Fallis WM, Pereira A. Family presence during resuscitation: Canadian critical care nurses' perspectives. *J Nurs Scholarsh.* 2009;41(3):233-240. Available at: https://doi.org/10.1111/j.1547-5069.2009.01288.x.

49. Pruitt LM, Johnson A, Elliott JC, Polley K. Parental presence during pediatric invasive procedures. *J Pediatr Health Care.* 2008;22(2):120-127. Available at: https://doi.org/10.1016/j.pedhc.2007.04.008.

50. Kuzin JK, Yborra JG, Taylor MD, et al. Family-member presence during interventions in the intensive care unit: perceptions of pediatric cardiac intensive care providers. *Pediatrics.* 2007;120(4):e895-e901. Available at: https://doi.org/10.1542/peds.2006-2943.

51. Demir F. Presence of patients' families during cardiopulmonary resuscitation: physicians' and nurses' opinions. *J Adv Nurs.* 2008;63(4):409-416. Available at: https://doi.org/10.1111/j.1365-2648.2008.04725.x.

52. Hicks KB, Glaser K, Scott C, Sparks D, McHenry CR. Enumerating the causes and burden of first case operating room delays. *Am J Surg.* 2020;219(3):486-489. Available at: https://doi.org/10.1016/j.amjsurg.2019.09.016.

53. American Nurses Association. *Nursing: Scope and Standards of Practice.* 4th ed. Author; 2021:94-95.

54. Chesla CA, Stannard D. Breakdown in the nursing care of families in the ICU. *Am J Crit Care.* 1997;6(1):64-71.

55. Al-Mutair AS, Plummer V, O'Brien A, Clerehan R. Family needs and involvement in the intensive care unit: a literature review. *J Clin Nurs.* 2013;22:1805-1817. Available at: https://doi.org/10.1111/jocn.12065.

56. Agency for Healthcare Research and Quality. *Use the Teach-Back Method.* Available at: https://www.ahrq.gov/health-literacy/improve/precautions/tool5.html. Accessed October 06, 2021.

57. Dinh TTH, Bonner A, Clark R, Ramsbotham J, Hines S. The effectiveness of the teach-back method on adherence and self-management in health education for people with chronic disease: a systematic review. *JBI Database System Rev Implement Rep.* 2016;14(1):210-247. Available at: https://doi.org/10.11124/jbisrir-2016-2296.

25 Substance Use Disorders

Valerie A. Pfander, DNP, APRN, ACCNS-AG, CPAN, FASPAN

LEARNING OBJECTIVES

A review of the content of this chapter will help the reader to:

1. Define *substance use disorder*.
2. Describe the impact of substance use on the body.
3. Describe the impact of substance use on surgical outcomes.
4. Identify nursing care specific to surgical patients with substance use issues.

OVERVIEW

Substance use disorder is a complex condition that affects the brain and leads to an inability to control the use of illicit drugs, alcohol, or other medications. Examples of subtances that are classified as having potential for abuse can be found in Table 25.1.[1] Substance use disorder can be broken down further into categories including, but not limited to, opioid use disorder and alcohol use disorder. The *Diagnostic and Statistical Manual of Mental Disorders* helps to define and differentiate criteria for substance-related disorders (Table 25.2).[2,3]

A person with substance use disorder has an intense focus on at least one substance to the point that it impairs normal day-to-day functioning.[4] People with substance use disorder are often aware they have a problem but are unable to stop using due to intense cravings for the substance. The craving or strong urge to use the substance leads to impaired control. Impaired control occurs when the strong urge to use the substance overcomes failed attempts to stop or cut down use.[4]

Substance use disorders cause physical and psychological problems and can lead to social problems with family, friends, and employers. Often those with substance use disorders are aware of the risks being taken by continuing to use but persist with this behavior despite knowing the problems it will cause in their home and work life.[4] Studies have shown that patients with substance use disorders experience higher rates of postoperative complications, including withdrawal and altered responses to typical pharmacology for anesthesia.[5] Given the growing incidence of drug and substance abuse in the general population, the probability of caring for an individual with a history of a current or previous substance use disorder in the ambulatory setting is high.

FACTS AND FIGURES

According to a national survey conducted by the Substance Abuse and Mental Health Services Administration (SAMHSA) in 2019, about 20 million people age 12 or older have experienced a substance use disorder in the past year.[6] In 2020, a national survey reported that 138.5 million Americans age 12 or older were alcohol users, 61.6 million people were binge drinkers, and 17.7 million were heavy drinkers.[6,7]

Substance use disorder is a leading cause of preventable illness and premature death. In 2020, there were nearly 92,000 deaths from drug overdoses in the United States.[8] The number of deaths from drug overdoses has increased 30%

TABLE 25.1 Substances of Abuse

Illicit Drugs
    Marijuana
    Cocaine/Crack
    Heroin
    Hallucinogens: LSD, PCP, Ecstasy
    Inhalants
    Methamphetamine
    Misuse of prescription psychotherapeutics: pain relievers, stimulants, tranquilizers, sedatives, benzodiazepines
    Opioids
Illicit drugs other than marijuana
Daily cigarette use
Smokeless tobacco: vaping
Cigars
Alcohol

Adapted from: Substance Abuse and Mental Health Services Administration. 2020 National Survey of Drug Use and Health (NDSUH) Releases. 2020. https://www.samhsa.gov/data/release/2020-national-survey-drug-use-and-health-nsduh-releases

TABLE 25.2 Criteria Differentiating Abuse, Dependence, and Substance Use Disorder

Criterion	Abuse	Dependence	Substance Use Disorder
Hazardous use	X		X
Social/interpersonal problems related to use	X		X
Neglected major roles to use	X		X
Legal problems	X		
Withdrawal		X	X
Tolerance		X	X
Use of larger amounts/longer		X	X
Repeated attempts to quit/control use		X	X
Much time spent using		X	X
Physical/psychological problems related to use		X	X
Activities given up to use		X	X
Craving			X

Source: Hasin D, Keyes K. The epidemiology of alcohol and drug disorders. Table 2.1 in: Johnson BA, ed. *Addiction Medicine: Science and Practice.* 2nd ed. Elsevier; 2020.

from 2019.[8] Given the growing incidence and high prevalence of drug and substance use, healthcare providers will likely be providing care to an individual impacted by the disorder. Further estimates suggest that one out of 10 patients admitted to the hospital has a concurrent substance use disorder.[9]

Ukaegbu and Tellioglu provide background and demographic data to define substance use disorders.[10] Often the term substance use disorder is used interchangeably with other terms such as drug abuse disorder, substance abuse disorder, and addiction disorder. Both genetic and environmental factors influence the potential spiral into substance use disorders. Substance use disorders are 1.3 times more common in males and often begin as young as 8–10 years of age.[10] Being a child of substance abusers increases the chances of any substance use disorder by twofold and increases the risk of alcohol and marijuana disordered use by threefold.[10] See Box 25.1 for additional risk factors.

THE MAJOR SUBSTANCES OF USE

Contemporary society is complex, and the factors that support the growing availability and access to substances of abuse change rapidly. Compounding the issues associated with substance use disorders is the stigma. According to Pulley, less than 1% of individuals sought treatment in 2013 even though nearly 9% identified as needing addiction therapy.[5] Additionally, many users abuse more than one substance. Many people with substance use disorder also fail to seek appropriate preventative healthcare and consequently have medical co-morbidities associated with the abuse that require medical optimization. In many cases, these individuals may not meet the criteria for surgery in an outpatient setting.

Alcohol

Alcohol is a drink that contains ethanol produced by the fermentation of grains, fruits, or other sources of sugar. In the United States, a standard drink contains 0.6 ounces of pure alcohol; this is found in a 12-ounce beer, 8-ounce drink of malt liquor, 5 ounces of wine, and 1.5 ounces of distilled spirits (gin, rum, vodka, whiskey).[7] According to the Centers for Disease Control and Prevention, the Dietary Guidelines for Americans recommends that to drink in moderation, men should have only 2 drinks or less per day and women only 1 drink or less per day.[7] As a substance of abuse, the drinking of alcohol falls into three categories. Binge drinking is the most common and is defined as drinking more than four (for women) and five (for men) drinks in a single setting.[7] Heavy drinking is defined as drinking more than 8 drinks in a week (for women) and 15 or more drinks in a week (for men.)[7] Alcohol is considered the third leading cause of deaths in the United States that are considered preventable.[9]

The last category of alcohol involves people who were formerly defined as alcoholic or alcohol dependent. The current terminology is alcohol use disorder. According to Moran et al., nearly 30% of patients presenting for any type of surgery (e.g., elective or emergent) have some degree of alcohol use disorder.[11] These individuals have developed both tolerance and physical dependency. The National Institute on Alcohol Abuse and Alcoholism (NIAAA) defines alcohol use disorder as a condition consisting of three or more of the following factors[12]:

- Drinking even though it causes trouble with family or work
- Drinking more than intended
- Having to drink more to get a desired effect
- Being unable to stop drinking after repeated attempts
- Continuing to drink even though it causes depression and anxiety.

Tobacco

Tobacco is one of the leading causes of preventable disease and death in the United States.[9] Individuals who are addicted to tobacco are actually dependent on the psychoactive characteristics of nicotine.[13] Over time, with chronic exposure, individuals become more tolerant of the nicotine and will experience extreme signs of withdrawal when the source is unavailable.[13] Tobacco exposure is best quantified using pack-years (number of packs of cigarettes smoked per day, multiplied by the number of years of smoking); as an example, an individual who smoked two packs of cigarettes daily for the prior 10 years is deemed to have a 20 pack-year history of tobacco use.

Risk factors for developing a tobacco use disorder can be found in Box 25.2. Aside from the long-term ill health effects of smoking, the pathophysiology of smoking impacts anesthesia care.[14] Smoking of cigarettes increases the likelihood of coronary heart disease, stroke, chronic obstructive pulmonary disease, and lung cancer and other cancers within the body, to name a few.[8] Smokers present with narrowed airways, ciliary action that is impaired, increased production of sputum, and airways that are more reactive than normal airways.[14] These impact the choice of anesthesia delivery, as well as the recovery from inhaled agents, including coughing, bronchospasms, and laryngospasms.

Marijuana

The term *medicinal marijuana* describes the utilization of parts of the marijuana plant for the purpose of alleviating symptoms of certain physical or emotional conditions. Most commonly, these products can be used for treating nausea, vomiting, anorexia, glaucoma, posttraumatic stress disorder, and pain.[15-17] Since the legalization of marijuana products across the United States, the access to and use of these products for recreation have also increased. While primarily inhaled, oral preparations

---

BOX 25.1 Common Risk Factors for Substance Use Disorders

Family history of substance use disorder
Male gender
Having another mental health disorder
Having a history of trauma
Peer pressure
Lack of family involvement
Taking a highly addictive drug

Ukaegbu R, Tellioglu T. Substance use disorder. In: Ferri FF, ed. *Ferri's Clinical Advisor 2023.* Elsevier; 2023.

BOX 25.2 Risk Factors for Tobacco Use

Peer pressure
Parental smokers
Poor school performance
Personality characteristics (e.g., rebellious, risk taker)
Desire to appear older
Easy access to e-cigarettes
Media and advertising

Adapted from: Brunetta PG, Kroon L. Smoking cessation. In: Broaddus VC, Ernst JD, King TE, et al., eds. *Murray & Nadel's Textbook of Respiratory Medicine.* 7th ed. Elsevier; 2022.

and salves are also available. The psychoactive component of cannabis is known as tetrahydrocannabinol, or THC. Patients admitting to smoking marijuana present with the same risk of pulmonary complications as patients who admittedly smoke tobacco.[9]

Opioids

Opioids can be classified as natural, semisynthetic, or synthetic compounds that bind with opioid receptors in the body and reduce feelings of pain (Table 25.3).[18] Used appropriately, opioids can be prescribed as a short-term treatment for moderate to severe pain that has not been responsive to nonpharmacologic and nonopioid measures. In addition to the analgesic effects of opioids, this class of drug can cause drowsiness, mental confusion, and euphoria, and at higher doses can depress respirations.[4]

Prescription opioids include oxycodone (Oxycontin), hydrocodone (Vicodin), morphine, methadone, and codeine. Synthetic opioids include fentanyl, methadone, tramadol, and carfentanil. There are also nonprescription opioids, also known as street drugs, such as heroin and fentanyl. Fentanyl is 50 times more potent than heroin and 100 times more potent than morphine. Overall, users often describe a sense of enhanced well-being or a state of euphoria when using opioids.[5,11] Abusers may inject, inhale, ingest, rectally insert, or snort these substances.

Methamphetamine

Methamphetamine (meth) is a highly addictive stimulant that affects the central nervous system. It is usually a white, bitter-tasting powder or pill.[19] Crystal methamphetamine is a form of the drug that looks like shiny bluish-white rocks. Methamphetamine can be smoked, snorted, injected, or swallowed. It is inexpensive to make this substance using over-the-counter cold medicine ingredients such as pseudoephedrine mixed with other dangerous chemicals.[19] There are currently no medications approved to treat methamphetamine addiction. Classified as a hallucinogenic, similar to lysergic acid diethylamide (LSD) and phencyclidine (PCP), users of methamphetamines experience disturbances in thought, mood, and perception.[5] This class of drugs is also referred to as: club drugs" or "designer drugs."[11] Patients with toxic levels of methamphetamines appear acutely psychotic, with hypertension and tachyarrhythmias.[20]

Cocaine

Cocaine is similar to methamphetamines in that individuals with dependence on cocaine seek the stimulant effects of ingestion. It is absorbed in a variety of ways, including orally, nasally, rectally, vaginally, through inhalation, or gastrointestinally through ingestion.[9] In addition to bringing a sense of euphoria, as well as a feeling of arousal and heightened self-confidence and well-being, cocaine increases cardiac work (e.g., elevates the heart rate and blood pressure) and raises the risk of myocardial events during anesthesia.[5,8]

PHYSIOLOGIC EFFECTS OF SUBSTANCE USE DISORDERS

Addiction is a complex disease that affects the brain in terms of physiology and behavior. Repeated use of an illicit substance and inappropriate use of prescribed medications can cause distorted thinking and behaviors, as well as changes in how the brain functions.[4] Brain imaging studies show that the areas of the brain that are impacted by substance use disorder include judgment, memory, decision making, learning, and behavioral control.[4] The changes in the brain structure and function caused by this disease, depending on the substance being used, can cause intense cravings, changes in personality, and abnormal behaviors.[4] Physiologic changes associated with chronic or acute substance abuse further complicate a medical presentation. For an overview of potential physiologic findings associated with common substance use disorder, see Table 25.4.

TABLE 25.3 Classifications of Opioids

Class of Opioid	Source	Drug Name
Natural opioids	Derived from the opium poppy plant	Codeine Morphine Opium
Semisynthetic opioids	Mixed with natural opioids	Oxymorphone Hydrocodone Oxycodone Hydromorphone
Synthetic opioids	Made in a lab with human-made materials	Dilaudid Demerol Oxycodone Vicodin Fentanyl Methadone Heroin

Adapted from: Schumacher M, Fukuda K. Opioids. In: Gropper MA, ed. *Miller's Anesthesia*. 9th ed. Elsevier; 2020.

TABLE 25.4 Physiologic and Psychological Effects of Common Substance Use Disorders

Substance	Potential Physiologic and Psychological Effects
Alcohol[5,11]	• Increased risk for pneumonia • Liver damage • Acute respiratory syndrome • Altered pain sensitivity • Withdrawal • Confusion • Electrolyte imbalances • Hypertension • Cardiomyopathy • Esophagitis • Pancreatitis • Malnutrition • Anemia
Tobacco[14]	• Impaired ciliary action • Increased production of sputum • Narrowing of airways • Reactive airway reflexes • Coughing • Bronchospasms • Laryngospasms
Marijuana[16]	• Elevated risk of myocardial infarction within one hour of use • Airway hyperactivity • Anxiety/paranoia • Psychosis • Tolerance to anesthesia agents • Stroke • Heightened pain perception • Withdrawal • Poor wound healing

Continued

TABLE 25.4 Physiologic and Psychological Effects of Common Substance Use Disorders—cont'd

Substance	Potential Physiologic and Psychological Effects
Opioids[5,11]	• Increased pain sensitivity • Withdrawal • Pulmonary hemorrhage • Unwanted sedation
Methamphet-amine[11]	• Arrhythmias • Aortic dissection • Coronary syndrome • Myocardial ischemia • Cardiomyopathy • Poor oral hygiene • Poor nutrition • Pulmonary hypertension
Cocaine[11]	• Psychosis • Dysphoria • Paranoia • Anxiety • Cerebral hemorrhage • Coronary vasoconstriction • Septal destruction • Soft palate necrosis • Interstitial fibrosis • Pulmonary hypertension

Adapted from: Moran S, Isa J, Steinemann S. Perioperative management in the patient with substance abuse. *Surg Clin North Am.* 2015;95(2):417–428. https://doi.org/10.1016/j.suc.2014.11.001; Pulley DD. Preoperative evaluation of the patient with substance use disorder and perioperative considerations; *Anesthesiol Clinics.* 2016;34(1):201–211. https://doi.org/10.1016/j.anclin.2015.10.015; Randles D, Dabner S. Applied respiratory physiology. *Anaesth Intensive Care.* 2021;22(6):364–368. https://doi.org/10.1016/j.mpaic.2021.04.009; and Sadighi T, Londahl-Ramsey V. Cannabis use: Change in screening for primary care preoperative clearance. *J Nurse Pract.* 2021;17(7):819–822. https://doi.org/10.1016/j.nurpra.2021.02.021

PREOPERATIVE ASSESSMENT OF PATIENTS WITH SUBSTANCE USE DISORDERS

Preoperative clinical assessments should include substance abuse screening to identify patients at risk for anesthesia and surgical complications. Many patients may be reluctant to disclose the history of past or current substance use. However, approaching the assessment in a nonjudgmental way can be reassuring. Current electronic documentation records have incorporated a variety of screening tools. For an example of a cannabis tool, see Figure 25.1. Improved access to treatment and a better understanding of the nature of substance use disorder have made advances in perioperative care safer; however, some individuals may be poorly optimized for surgery in the outpatient setting.[5]

Clearly, when a patient presents with acute intoxication, the surgical case must be cancelled.[20] When the decision to move forward with outpatient surgery is made, the perianesthesia nurse must keep several concepts in mind. Depending on the chosen substance and route of self-administration, some patients have extremely difficult venous access. These patients may also have covert or overt issues with nutrition and dental health. In preparation for the procedure, patients may have suspended use of the substance, and this increases the risk of presenting with or developing symptoms of withdrawal. As shown in Table 25.4, pain control will be challenging for many patients with substance use disorder. Lastly, many patients will physically demonstrate a need for higher anesthesia

requirements. A conversation regarding pain management expectations with the patient should be documented and the opportunity to provide realistic goals can be discussed.[9]

POSTOPERATIVE CARE OF PATIENTS WITH SUBSTANCE USE DISORDERS

Perioperative management of a patient with substance use disorder is complex and requires a multidisciplinary team, such as an anesthesiologist, surgeon, nurse, and pain management consultant.[21] Even though the number of patients with substance use disorder is increasing, nurses are often not trained on how to care for this population. The nursing care of patients with substance use disorder can be hampered by a lack of education and frustration with difficult patient interactions.[22] Education has been shown to improve healthcare workers' understanding of a patient with substance use disorder.[22]

Patients with substance use disorder having surgery may worry about receiving adequate pain relief, experiencing substance withdrawal symptoms, or the possibility of having a relapse.[21] Studies show that patients with opioid use disorders in particular have a lowered pain tolerance and increased sensitivity to pain, when compared with opioid-naïve control groups.[21] Additionally, patients with substance use disorder may have a co-morbid chronic pain condition that will continue to need management.[21] When a person has a substance use disorder, the probability of tolerance for that substance is high and may lead to the requirement of larger amounts of agents to feel any effects.[4] This tolerance may be different for each substance.

Before determining a course of care, it is important to ask whether the patient is in remission (no longer using), is receiving maintenance therapy such as methadone or buprenorphine, or has an untreated substance use disorder (potential withdrawal).[23] The clinical record should reflect documentation of a treatment provider's name and contact information during the preanesthesia interview. The anesthesia provider and the surgeon should be notified to coordinate a plan of care for the perioperative phase. This is an important aspect of nursing advocacy in an often-undermanaged population.

Evidence-Based Practice: Buprenorphine
Buprenorphine is a common treatment for individuals with substance use disorders. Original guidelines for management of the patient on buprenorphine products recommended that the product be suspended in anticipation of elective surgery and the patient placed on opioid therapy as a temporary bridge. Based on a systematic review, Quaye and Zhang recommend an individualized approach to determining the continuation or discontinuation of buprenorphine preoperatively suggesting that with the application of opioid-sparing methods, some patients may be maintained on baseline doses of buprenorphine. Patients on higher baseline doses (more than 16 mg daily) may need to titrate these doses to a lower daily dose to 8 mg daily. In addition to opioid-sparing techniques, a collaborative intraprofessional team approach should be incorporated when appropriate.

Source: Quaye AN-A, Zhang Y. Perioperative management of buprenorphine: Solving the conundrum. *Pain Medicine.* 2019;20(7):1395-1408. https://doi.org/10.1093/pm/pny217

Patients in Remission

Patients with substance use disorder who are in remission and have no signs or symptoms of substance dependence can continue to have triggers that lead to cravings.[24] The anxiety of

Have you used any cannabis over the past six months?   **YES/NO**

If **YES**, please answer the following questions about your cannabis use. Circle the response that is most correct for you in relation to your cannabis use over the past six months.

1.	**How often do you use cannabis?**				
	Never	Monthly or less	2 to 4 times a month	2 to 3 times a week	4 or more times a week
	0	1	2	3	4
2.	**How many hours were you "stoned" on a typical day when you had been using cannabis?**				
	Less than 1	1 or 2	3 or 4	5 or 6	7 or more
	0	1	2	3	4
3.	**How often during the past 6 months did you find that you were not able to stop using cannabis once you had started?**				
	Never	Less than monthly	Monthly	Weekly	Daily or almost daily
	0	1	2	3	4
4.	**How often during the past 6 months did you fail to do what was normally expected from you because of using cannabis?**				
	Never	Less than monthly	Monthly	Weekly	Daily or almost daily
	0	1	2	3	4
5.	**How often in the past 6 months have you devoted a great deal of your time to getting, using, or recovering from cannabis?**				
	Never	Less than monthly	Monthly	Weekly	Daily or almost daily
	0	1	2	3	4
6.	**How often in the past 6 months have you had a problem with your memory or concentration after using cannabis?**				
	Never	Less than monthly	Monthly	Weekly	Daily or almost daily
	0	1	2	3	4
7.	**How often do you use cannabis in situations that could be physically hazardous, such as driving, operating machinery, or caring for children?**				
	Never	Less than monthly	Monthly	Weekly	Daily or almost daily
	0	1	2	3	4
8.	**Have you ever thought about cutting down, or stopping, your use of cannabis?**				
	Never		Yes, but not in the past 6 months		Yes, during the past 6 months
	0		2		4

Fig. 25.1 Cannabis screening tool. Sazegar P. Cannabis essentials: Tools for clinical practice. *Am Fam Physician*. 2021;104(6): 598–608. Figure 5.

surgery and anticipated postoperative pain are stressors that could potentially elicit a trigger ultimately resulting in substance cravings. On the other hand, poorly controlled pain can also lead to cravings and relapse.[25] The anesthesia provider and surgeon should discuss the risks and benefits of a postoperative pain management plan. Regional anesthesia, principles of multimodal analgesia, and the use of nonpharmacologic interventions are highly encouraged as techniques to support opioid-sparing care.

These approaches can reduce the need for additional opioids postoperatively.[26] If opioids are needed postoperatively, administer the lowest effective dose and for a limited period.[21] Provide the patient education on cognitive behavioral approaches to manage anxiety and cravings.[21]

Discussion and coordination of a preoperative and postoperative handoff plan should be implemented prior to surgery with the patient's addiction treatment provider. Primary care coordination is critically important in this population. The perianesthesia nurse caring for the patient with a substance use disorder having surgery must be able to offer reassurance and the opportunity for the patient to verbalize anxiety related to the management of pain. Preoperative and postoperative nursing care should include an empathetic approach with listening, reassurance, advocacy, and transparency.[21]

Patients Receiving Maintenance Therapy

In addition to the considerations just discussed, patients with substance use disorder receiving maintenance therapy have special postoperative considerations. Medication-assisted treatment for opioid use disorders has been promoted to help reduce opioid misuse and to better support the health of the population in general.[9,21] Maintenance therapy often is with methadone, a full opioid agonist, or a compound with buprenorphine, a partial opioid agonist.[9,21] Buprenorphine is either prescribed alone (Subutex, Sixmo) or in combination with naloxone (Suboxone).[21]

Acute pain management for patients taking buprenorphine combined with naloxone is challenging due to the opioid reversal effects of naloxone. The provider and patient need to determine the benefits of discontinuing the buprenorphine product and resuming a bridge protocol of opioids to achieve pain management versus the risk of the patient having a relapse. If it is determined to not stop the buprenorphine product, a determination will need to be made of which type of analgesic regimen will be effective.[21] Some studies have shown that stopping buprenorphine products 5 days before surgery and switching the patient to buprenorphine only will ensure opioid receptor availability for effective pain management in the case of intermediate- or high-risk complex surgeries.[21] Newer studies suggest maintaining the therapeutic schedule of buprenorphine for simple, low-complexity outpatient procedures.[21]

DISCHARGE PLANNING FOR PATIENTS WITH SUBSTANCE USE DISORDERS

Patients with substance use disorders, whether in remission, receiving maintenance therapy, or untreated, require clear instructions on how to take any prescribed opioid analgesics and how to taper off of them appropriately.[21] This patient population has a high risk of medication side effects, adverse events, and relapse.[21] The perianesthesia nurse should encourage the patient to seek self-help groups and peer support and to collaborate with their mental health or substance use disorder clinician as soon as they are discharged.[21]

CHAPTER HIGHLIGHTS

- The most common substances frequently misused include opioids, methamphetamine, alcohol, nicotine, marijuana, and cocaine.
- Misuse of alcohol or illicit substances has substantial physiologic impacts.
- Many substances of abuse have known or suspected interactions with anesthetic agents.
- Postoperative care requires multidisciplinary planning for safe management of pain and discomfort using opioid-sparing techniques when possible.

CASE STUDY

A 45-year-old fisherman is being scheduled for a shoulder arthroscopy to repair a rotator cuff tear from repetitive motions on his fishing boat. He denied a history of smoking but failed to disclose that he smoked marijuana daily while fishing out at sea. On the day of surgery, his preoperative vital signs were normal. However, the preoperative nurse expressed concern to peers that his responses seemed delayed, "like he was stoned." Again, when questioned, the patient denied smoking or using substances. Following general anesthesia for an uneventful surgery, he arrived in the phase I PACU with a simple mask, oxygen at 6 L, and an oximetry reading of 94%. A short time after arriving in the PACU the patient began to develop stridor and dyspnea, with his oxygen saturations falling to 80%. The patient later admitted that he had smoked marijuana on the ride to the outpatient surgery center.

- What may have caused this patient's respiratory event?
- What interventions would have been prescribed to support the patient?

- What other potential complications can the perianesthesia nurse anticipate based on this new knowledge of recent marijuana inhalation?

REFERENCES

1. Substance Abuse and Mental Health Services Administration. *2020 National Survey of Drug Use and Health (NDSUH) Releases.* 2020. Available at: https:// www.samhsa.gov/data/release/2020-national-survey-drug-use-and-health-nsduh-releases.
2. American Psychiatric Association. *Diagnostic and Statistical Manual of Mental Disorders.* 5th ed. ASA; 2013.
3. Hasin D, Keyes K. The epidemiology of alcohol and drug disorders. In: Johnson BA, ed. *Addiction Medicine: Science and Practice.* 2nd ed. Elsevier; 2020.
4. American Psychiatric Association. *What Is a Substance Use Disorder?* December 2020. Available at: https://www.psychiatry.org/patients-families/addiction/what-is-addiction.
5. Pulley DD. Preoperative evaluation of the patient with substance use disorder and perioperative considerations. *Anesthesiol Clin.* 2016;34(1):201-211.
6. Substance Abuse and Mental Health Services Administration. *Mental Health and Substance Use Disorders.* 2020. Available at: https://www.samhsa.gov/find-help/disorders.
7. Centers for Disease Control and Prevention. *Alcohol Use and Your Health.* 2021. Available at: https://www.cdc.gov/alcohol/fact-sheets/alcohol-use.htm.
8. Centers for Disease Control and Prevention. *Death Rate Maps & Graphs.* 2022. Available at: https://www.cdc.gov/drugoverdose/deaths/index.html.
9. Weimer MB, Hines RL. Psychiatric disease, substance use disorders, and drug overdose. In: Hines RL, ed. *Stoelting's Anesthesia and Co-Existing Disease.* Elsevier; 2022:619-644.
10. Ukaegbu R, Tellioglu T. Substance use disorder. In: Ferri FF, ed. *Ferri's Clinical Advisor 2023.* Elsevier; 2023.
11. Moran S, Isa J, Steinemann S. Perioperative management in the patient with substance abuse. *Surg Clin North Am.* 2015;95(2):417-428. Available at: https://doi.org/10.1016/j.suc.2014.11.001.
12. National Institute on Alcohol Abuse and Alcoholism. *What Is Alcohol Use Disorder?* National Institute of Health; 2021. Available at: https://www.niaaa.nih.gov/short-takes-niaaa-what-alcohol-use-disorder-aud.
13. Brunetta PG, Kroon L. Smoking cessation. In: Broaddus VC, Ernst JD, King TE, et al., eds. *Murray & Nadel's Textbook of Respiratory Medicine.* 7th ed. Elsevier; 2022.
14. Randles D, Dabner S. Applied respiratory physiology. *Anaesth Intensive Care.* 2021;22(6):364-368. Available at: https://doi.org/10.1016/j.mpaic.2021.04.009.
15. Naguib M, Foss JF. Medical use of marijuana: truth in evidence. *Anesth Analg.* 2015;121(5):1124-1127. Available at: https://doi.org/10.1213/ANE.0000000000000928.
16. Sadighi T, Londahl-Ramsey V. Cannabis use: change in screening for primary care preoperative clearance. *J Nurse Pract.* 2021;17(7):819-822. Available at: https://doi.org/10.1016/j.nurpra.2021.02.021.
17. Ullrich S, Valdez AM. Rocky mountain high: preventing cannabis-related injuries. *J Emerg Nurs.* 2017;43(1):78-80. Available at: https://doi.org/10.1016/j.jen.2016.12.003.
18. Schumacher M, Fukuda K. Opioids. In: Gropper MA, ed. *Miller's Anesthesia.* 9th ed. Elsevier; 2020:680-741.
19. National Institute on Drug Abuse. *Methamphetamine Drug Facts.* 2019. Available at: https://www.drugabuse.gov/publications/drugfacts/methamphetamine.
20. Taylor JF, Dobyns JB. Perioperative considerations in patients using and abusing illicit substances. *Curr Rev Nurs Anesth.* 2021; 44(8):95-105. Available at: https://fdocuments.net/document/perioperative-considerations-in-patients-using-and-abusing-.html?page=1.
21. Ward EN, Quaye AN-A, Wilens TE. Opioid use disorders: perioperative management of a special population. *Anesth Analg.* 2018;127(2):539-547. Available at: https://doi.org/10.1213/ane.0000000000003477.
22. Russell R, Ojeda MM, Ames B. Increasing RN perceived competency with substance use disorder patients. *J Contin Educ Nurs.*

2017;48(4):175-183. Available at: https://doi.org/10.3928/00220124-20170321-08.

23. Anitescu M. The patient with substance use disorder. *Curr Opin Anaesthesiol.* 2019;32(3):427-437. Available at: https://doi.org/10.1097/aco.0000000000000738.

24. Volkow ND, Koob GF, McLellan A. Neurobiologic advances from the brain disease model of addiction. *N Engl J Med.* 2016;374:363-371. Available at: https://doi.org/10.1056/nejmra1511480.

25. Tsui JI, Lira MC, Cheng DM, et al. Chronic pain, craving, and illicit opioid use among patients receiving opioid agonist therapy. *Drug Alcohol Depend.* 2016;166:26-31 . Available at: https://doi.org/10.1016/j.drugalcdep.2016.06.024.

26. Stromer W, Michaeli K, Sandner-Kiesling A. Perioperative pain therapy in opioid abuse. *Eur J Anaesthesiol.* 2013;30:55-64. Available at: https://doi.org/10.1097/eja.0b013e32835b822b.

26 General Surgical Procedures and Considerations

Sylvia J. Baker, MSN, RN, CPAN (retired), FASPAN

LEARNING OBJECTIVES

A review of the content of this chapter will help the reader to:

1. Describe common general surgery procedures performed in the ambulatory setting.
2. Describe care requirements of the patient for various procedures.
3. Identify education that supports patient safety, as related to various procedures.
4. Describe relevant psychological factors affecting the decision to have general surgery.

OVERVIEW

The ambulatory and outpatient surgical settings provide a cost-effective and efficient means for patients to experience a myriad of procedures with the plan of returning to their homes shortly after the procedures. Recovering in the comfort of one's own home environment has been touted to improve patient outcomes and satisfaction. This chapter reviews various procedures performed in the ambulatory center and the recommended methods of nursing care. This chapter also highlights pertinent educational topics for patients and methods of providing them.

There are many reasons for individuals to pursue ambulatory general surgical procedures; the most common reasons are the relief of pain and the restoration of function or immobility in a setting that can mitigate the unease patients often feel when facing surgery.

FACTS AND FIGURES

According to the Centers for Disease Control and Prevention, approximately 48.3 million surgical and nonsurgical procedures were performed during 28.6 million ambulatory surgery visits to hospitals and ambulatory surgery centers in the mid 2010s.[1] These numbers have steadily increased since the advent of ambulatory centers in the early 1980s. Two factors that have impacted this increase are technologic advances (e.g., laparoscopic instrumentation) and improvements in anesthetic and analgesic techniques.

Patients of all ages undergo ambulatory procedures, with the majority being performed on those age 45–64 years, or approximately 39% of the population. Approximately 19% of procedures were performed on patients 65–74 years of age, and about 14% were performed on patients 75 years and older.[1]

PATIENT EDUCATION FOR GENERAL AMBULATORY SURGICAL PROCEDURES

Patient education begins with the first discussion of the surgical procedure and its plan, which often occurs in the provider's office. General patient education is presented here, and education about specific procedures follows for each type of procedure.

Not only is it vital that nurses provide education, but they also need to assess the retention and assimilation of information by patients. The teach-back method has been demonstrated to be the most effective means of ensuring the patient has understood information that will augment their recovery.[2] In addition to a verbal discussion, instructions need to be provided in a written format that the patient can read, understand, and refer to upon discharge. Highlighting the most important information is encouraged so that patients can refer to it if questions arise.

Patients should be given explanations of the procedure and its risks and benefits preoperatively. This is considered one aspect of informed consent, and the responsibility for it falls to the practitioner. The nurse's responsibility in informed consent is to verify that all questions have been answered to the patient's satisfaction. In addition, the nurse verifies that the signature on the consent is, in fact, that of the patient or legal representative.

For most ambulatory surgical procedures, preoperative patient education includes explaining how the skin will be prepared with an agent such as chlorhexidine and/or how nasal swabbing will be done. Information should also be given on physical therapy with assistive devices and exercises; dietary changes, including the expected NPO time before the procedure; activities such as isolation to prevent cross-contamination; and laboratory tests.

Postoperative care may also be explained during this phase of patient preparation. Patients need to be instructed on important aspects of their postoperative course, such as the appropriate clothing to wear at discharge (e.g., sweatpants, front-opening shirts or blouses, and foot coverings). Mobility expectations, weight limitations, and the use of assistive devices such as crutches or walkers are best introduced in preoperative plans rather than immediately prior to discharge from the center. Pain control modalities, both pharmacologic and nonpharmacologic, and instructions for taking opioids and properly disposing of unused dosages are equally important for the patient and significant others to understand. When opioids are part of the postoperative plan, it is prudent to encourage a diet that includes fiber to counteract the constipation that is often a side effect of opioids.

Preparation of the home is vital as the patient begins making preparations for a safe procedure and recovery. Patients should be instructed on how often to change bed linens and the care of pets during their convalescence. Safety of the environment should be assessed to ensure that hazards such as throw rugs and electrical cords are removed or replaced. Patients need to have an escort to take them home because after a procedure, the lingering effects of sedatives and anesthesia impact the ability to make decisions, as well as muscular coordination.

Postoperative instructions address activity levels (e.g., ambulation), bathing, wound care, pain control measures, proper disposal of unused medications, dietary changes, deep breathing exercises and the continued use of an incentive spirometer, antiembolic prophylaxis whether mechanical or pharmacologic, follow-up appointments, and when and who to call if unexpected conditions develop (Box 26.1).

GENERAL SURGICAL PROCEDURES AND ASSOCIATED NURSING CARE

Laparoscopic Procedures

Laparoscopic Appendectomy

Laparoscopic appendectomies (planned) to prevent perforation of friable tissue are frequently performed in an ambulatory setting. Removing an appendix via a laparoscope allows for a fast recovery, decreases the risk of infection, has a more aesthetically appealing outcome, and is reportedly associated with less pain (Figure 26.1).[3] Generally, this procedure is accomplished via three small incisions through the abdomen, one periumbilical, one suprapubic, and one in the left lower quadrant. The skin incisions are closed with steri-strips or skin glue. Local anesthetic infiltrated into the incisions generally provides adequate pain control, and a mild oral anti-inflammatory drug may be added. Some anesthesia providers augment the intraoperative medication with a calculated analgesic dosage of ketamine.

During the initial postoperative phase of care, the perianesthesia nurse needs to monitor dressings, assess the pain level, monitor the intake and output, administer antibiotics as necessary (and ordered), and assess the comfort level, including the presence of nausea. In addition to pharmacologic treatment for pain, nonpharmacologic therapies such as ice bags and ice packs, guided imagery, and repositioning can all be employed to promote patient comfort.

In preparation for discharge, the patient should receive instructions to ambulate regularly, rest frequently, and gradually increase activity as tolerated. Patients should avoid heavy lifting. Along with pulmonary toilet exercises, splinting of the abdominal region should be taught to promote an adequate cough and the prevention of atelectasis. Enemas need to be avoided unless approved by the surgeon.

Laparoscopic Cholecystectomy

A laparoscopic cholecystectomy is performed to relieve inflammation of the gallbladder, which may be caused by the formation of stones in the gallbladder that inhibit the emptying of bile into the small intestine. Scar tissue may also impede the exodus of bile from the gallbladder.

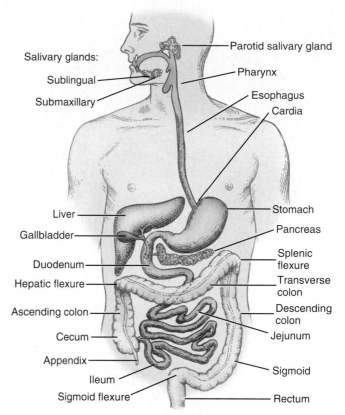

Fig. 26.1 Alimentary canal and its appendages. Devolder BE. Gastrointestinal surgery. Figure 11.1 in: Rothrock J. *Alexander's Care of the Patient in Surgery.* 16th ed. Elsevier; 2019.

Patients suffering with cholecystitis may present with episodic cramping pain in the right upper abdominal quadrant or epigastrium. This discomfort may radiate around to the back or shoulder. Attacks are often accompanied by nausea and vomiting. Patients may also present with jaundice, heartburn, flatulence, and/or fat intolerance. A differential diagnosis is accomplished via a physical examination, laboratory studies, and radiologic studies, which may include a flat plate of the abdomen, ultrasonograms, an IV cholangiogram, or an upper gastrointestinal series. Endoscopic retrograde cholangiopancreatography (ERCP) or computed tomography (CT) may also be employed to positively diagnose a problem.

Once general anesthesia has been provided, the cholecystectomy is accomplished with the use of a laparoscope, and the gallbladder is accessed via four small incisions through the abdomen (Figure 26.2). The abdomen is insufflated with carbon dioxide to move tissue aside for good visualization and access. Using trocar instrumentation with a camera, the surgeon can move vital structures to view the gallbladder clearly. During dissection the surgeon can provide hemostasis with a harmonic scalpel and remove the gallbladder through the abdomen using a specimen pouch.

Nurses should monitor dressings, assess pain levels, monitor intake and outtake, administer antibiotics if ordered, and make sure the patient is comfortable and is not nauseous. Pharmacologic treatments for pain and nonpharmacologic therapies such as ice bags and ice packs, guided imagery, and repositioning can be used to make patients comfortable.

One common complaint after this procedure is shoulder pain. This is due to a pneumoperitoneum that has developed during insufflation, when carbon dioxide is retained under

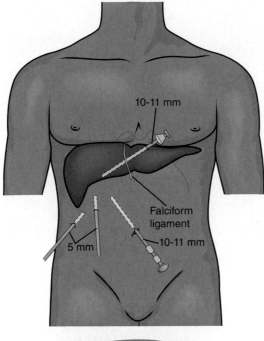

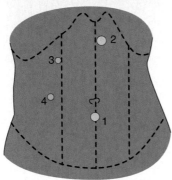

Fig. 26.2 Laparoscopic cholecystectomy incisions. Modified from: O'Brien D. Care of the gastrointestinal, abdominal, and anorectal surgical patient. Figure 40.6 in: Odom-Forren J, ed. *Drain's PeriAnesthesia Nursing: A Critical Care Approach.* Elsevier; 2018.

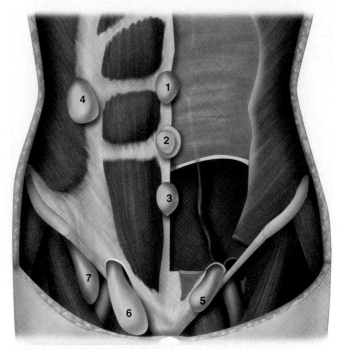

Fig. 26.3 Common sites of hernias. Smith JD. Hernia repair. Figure 13.1 in: Rothrock J. *Alexander's Care of the Patient in Surgery.* 16th ed. Elsevier; 2019.

the diaphragm. Patients should be reassured about the cause so they do not become alarmed. Repositioning may alleviate the symptoms, which may last for several days.

Postoperative instructions for a laparoscopic cholecystectomy should include regular ambulation, frequent rest periods, and a gradual increase in activity as tolerated. The patient should avoid heavy lifting. Pulmonary toilet exercises and splinting of the abdominal region should be taught to promote an adequate cough reflex and prevent atelectasis. Occasionally, short-term dietary changes may be necessary because the body is adjusting to the flow of bile directly into the small intestine.

Herniorrhaphy

A hernia is a sac lined by peritoneum that protrudes through a defect in the layers of a muscle wall. There are two types of hernias, acquired and congenital. Hernias are most commonly noted at inguinal canals, femoral rings, and the umbilicus (Figure 26.3). Contributing factors associated with hernia formation include older age, male sex, previous surgery, obesity, poor nutritional status, pulmonary and cardiac disease, and loss of skin turgor.[3]

Herniorrhaphies may be performed under general or regional anesthesia. Preoperative care and teaching include instructions for cleansing of the surgical site, maintaining preoperative NPO status, and reviewing anticipated changes in activity following surgery and during recovery. The perianesthesia nurse should focus on patient comfort and positioning following surgery. Attention to the pulmonary status is important in preventing atelectasis. In many cases, transversus abdominis plane blocks augment the comfort level for the patient and promote a timelier recovery.

Procedure-specific discharge teaching should include appropriate pain control measures, the expected progression of activity, and when to seek follow-up care. Deep-breathing exercises and/or the use of incentive spirometry should be taught. Splinting of the surgical site with the use of pillows decreases pain and improves compliance with pulmonary hygiene.

Anal-Rectal Procedures

There are several portions of the colon that may require surgical interventions in the ambulatory arena. Hemorrhoids, pilonidal cysts, and anal fistulas are three of the most common disorders requiring surgical repair that may be encountered in the outpatient setting. Procedures performed on a portion of the bowel require special preparation for the patient to experience the best outcomes. Enemas and oral bowel preparations may be part of the preparation for these surgical procedures.

For this group of surgeries, immediate postoperative care should be concentrated on monitoring dressings or the surgical site (should no dressings be employed) and controlling pain. Urinary retention is a potential complication, so intake and output should be monitored. Discharge instructions should focus on taking warm sitz baths as ordered, monitoring drainage, changing dressings, and bowel management. These patients should avoid constipation using a stool softener, adequate hydration, fiber intake, exercise, and a mild laxative if ordered.[3]

Hemorrhoidectomy

Hemorrhoids (also called piles) are swollen and inflamed veins around the anus or in the lower rectum.[4] There are two types of hemorrhoids, internal and external (Figure 26.4). Internal hemorrhoids are found above the internal sphincter, whereas external hemorrhoids are found outside the external sphincter of the rectum. Regardless of the type of hemorrhoid, these venous lesions may become engorged, inflamed, or thrombosed or may bleed. The patient may complain of pain, itching, and/or bleeding.

A hemorrhoidectomy is performed to remove the varicosities of veins or prolapsed mucosa to relieve pain or control bleeding. After excision of the hemorrhoid, the area may be packed with petroleum gauze. An alternate procedure to surgical excision may include a rubber-band ligation of the base of the hemorrhoid. If this process is utilized, the sloughing of the tissue is experienced in 7–10 days. Postoperative teaching specific to this procedure includes comfort measures, cleansing of the surgical area, and any dietary changes.

Pilonidal Cystectomy

Pilonidal cysts are pockets of skin that usually contain hair and skin debris. They are found at the base of the tailbone or top of the cleft of the buttocks. Patients who suffer with a pilonidal cyst note pain and may experience abscess formation.

Under local or general anesthesia, the surgeon resects the cyst/abscess and packs the wound with gauze. Occasionally, a drain may be placed to evacuate blood or exudate from the wound bed.[5]

Patients should be instructed on the proper care of the surgical site when gauze is placed and when to remove the packing. If a drain is placed, teaching needs to include care and emptying of the drain and monitoring of the drainage for amount, color, odor, and consistency. These assessments should be reported to the surgeon as recommended.

Anal Fistulectomy

Anal fistulas are the result of perianal abscesses inside the anal canal that had been drained by a physician or drained spontaneously through the perianal skin.[6] Unfortunately, a chronic sinus tract can develop, which causes pain and increased drainage. Fistulous tracts can be quite complex, arising from a myriad of preexisting conditions such as Crohn's disease, ulcerative colitis, fecal incontinence, trauma, radiation therapy, malignancy, and others.

The fistulous tract is excised under general or monitored anesthesia care with the patient in the prone or lithotomy position. Once the tract is excised, the surgeon may instill a local anesthetic, and a perineal dressing is applied.[7]

Patients should be taught that some leakage of stool and/or bleeding may occur. Cleaning instructions should be reinforced and signs and symptoms of infection should be noted, though infection is an uncommon complication.[7] These patients should also avoid postoperative constipation.

Endoscopic Procedures

Endoscopic procedures allow for visualization of the lumen of the gastrointestinal tract. These procedures are usually performed with the use of a flexible lighted fiberoptic scope or videoscope. The scope allows for the passage of instruments that give the practitioner the ability to take pictures, perform biopsies, remove polyps or foreign objects, and cauterize bleeding vessels.

Pre-procedural care includes appropriate bowel prep, maintaining NPO status, validation of the history and physical examination, and required laboratory tests.

Post-procedural care involves the monitoring of vital signs, control of discomfort, and a brisk return to the home environment. Patients should be instructed on dietary changes and follow-up requirements with the care provider, and their transportation for going home should be verified.

Esophagogastroduodenoscopy

An esophagogastroduodenoscopy (EGD) allows direct visualization of the esophagus, stomach, and proximal duodenum. A flexible scope is passed through the mouth and allows for direct visualization with still photos and videography (Figure 26.5).

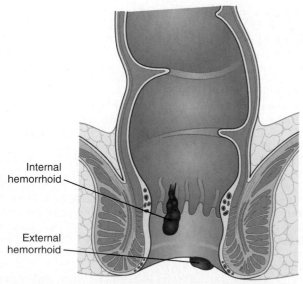

Fig. 26.4 Hemorrhoids. Kliegman RM, St Geme JW, Blum NJ, Shah SS, Tasker RC, Wilson KM. Surgical conditions of the anus and rectum. Figure 371.6 in: Kliegman RM, St Geme JW, Blum NJ, Shah SS, Tasker RC, Wilson KM, eds. *Nelson Textbook of Pediatrics.* Elsevier; 2020.

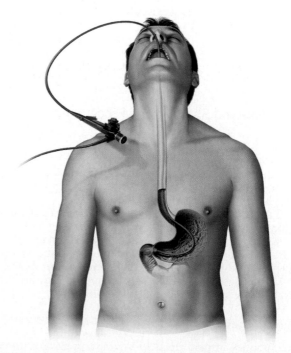

Fig. 26.5 Upper endoscopy. Clinical Key. Patient Education. Upper Endoscopy, Adult. Elsevier; 2022. https://www.clinicalkey.com/#!/content/patient_handout/5-s2.0-pe_1c408c54-4f2a-4b25-bbb8-4dffe96ef557?scrollTo=%235-s2.0-pe_1c408c54-4f2a-4b25-bbb8-4dffe96ef557-ID0EEIAE0

Conditions for which an EGD may be used include esophageal and stomach lesions, hiatal hernias, esophageal varices, ulcer disease, polyps, strictures, bleeding, and motility disorders, and it also can be a screening tool for specific preoperative evaluations such as bariatric procedures.[8]

Specific postprocedural nursing includes the assessment of the return of the gag reflex prior to providing liquids and nourishment. Patients may experience a sore throat following the procedure, but it will be self-limiting.

Colonoscopy

Using a flexible endoscope, a colonoscopy allows for direct visualization of the lower gastrointestinal tract from the rectum to the ileocecal valve.[8]

Patient conditions that may require a colonoscopy include screening, malignancy, polyps, inflammatory bowel diseases, diverticulitis, strictures, or bleeding.[8]

Specific preprocedure instructions include bowel preparation instructions.

Fecal Microbiota Transplantation

Human fecal suspension has been a practice since the fourth century in China to treat food poisoning and severe diarrhea. In 1983, the first documented *Clostridium difficile* infection was successfully treated.[9] Today, the introduction of healthy bacterial colonic flora into the gastrointestinal tract of an infected individual is becoming a more familiar treatment for refractory *C. difficile* infections. Specific preprocedure treatment includes vancomycin orally for three days. A factory-prepared fecal slurry is instilled via nasogastric tube or colonic instillation.

Specific post procedure care for esophageal instillation includes NPO for 5 hours, keeping the head of the bed elevated, and giving proton-pump inhibitors (e.g., pantoprazole) intravenously for 6–12 hours. If utilizing the colonic instillation, the patient should remain on bedrest for the remainder of the day and begin oral intake slowly while consuming a bland diet. For both routes, an antidiarrheal such as loperamide is administered at the end of the procedure and repeated six hours later to delay stool transit.[8]

Specific post procedure instructions include dietary changes and activity directions as noted.

Interventional Radiography Procedures

Endoscopic Retrograde Cholangiopancreatography

Endoscopic retrograde cholangiopancreatography (ERCP) is a procedure performed to evaluate the functioning of the pancreatic, hepatic, and common bile ducts. This procedure uses a flexible endoscope and a contrast medium.

The procedure is done to remove stones, perform a sphincterotomy, or dilate the ducts to facilitate the flow of bile.[8]

Preprocedural instructions should include NPO.

Postprocedural care includes monitoring of the vital signs, especially the temperature, as one complication of ERCP is cholangitis, which can lead to septicemia. Monitoring should also be done for patient comfort and bleeding.

Liver Biopsy

Liver biopsies are performed for a number of reasons, primarily to determine causal factors for hepatic dysfunction or lesions. When performed in the ambulatory setting, liver biopsies usually involve CT- or ultrasound-guided imaging. Using either of these adjuncts greatly decreases the chance of hemorrhage or damage to other organs such as the kidney, colon, or lung.

Liver biopsies are generally performed with a local anesthetic and, sometimes, moderate or conscious sedation. Specific laboratory work to be completed prior to this procedure includes obtaining the international normalized ratio and platelet count, though there is little evidence to support the validity of gathering these values.[10]

Patients should be instructed to withhold any anticoagulants prior to the procedure.

Positioning may play role in the delivery of postprocedural care. According to Costa et al., the traditional right-side position "appears to be less acceptable without any protective role in terms of adverse events."[11] Vital signs should be monitored and pain controlled. Patients should be instructed in how to self-monitor for hematoma formation and how to control pain.

Venous Surgical Procedures

Chronic venous insufficiency (CVI) is a long-term condition caused by malfunctioning of the venous valves, which allows blood to back-flow and thus create pooling or stasis within the vascular space or a deep vein thrombosis (DVT). Many patients who suffer with CVI also develop venous stasis ulcers. This condition tends to worsen over time.

Risk factors for CVI include age, family history of CVI, history of DVT in the legs, obesity, pregnancy, sitting or standing for long periods of time, and tall height. Patients who have CVI may complain of dull, aching discomfort in their legs, itching and tingling, pain that gets worse with longer periods of standing, and pain that lessens with leg elevation.

Treatment procedures include sclerotherapy (injection of saline or a chemical solution into the vein, which causes the vein to sclerose and disappear), phlebectomy (the damaged vein is removed through small incisions near the affected vessel), laser or radiofrequency treatments, or vein ligation and stripping (removing or tying off of the saphenous vein).[12,13]

Preprocedural and postprocedural treatments usually involve the use of compression stockings. The patient needs to have a clear understanding of the length of time this supplemental treatment should be continued. Dressings should be monitored and changed per physician order.

Thyroidectomy

Although thyroidectomy has traditionally been performed as an inpatient procedure, if the correct criteria are present, a safe total thyroidectomy may be performed at an ambulatory center. According to Compton et al., ambulatory centers may provide a safe, more accessible location for this procedure when strict adherence to guidelines and procedures are followed.[14]

The thyroid gland regulates the body's metabolism, energy, and growth and development and impacts virtually every organ. Reasons for thyroid surgery include Graves' disease, toxic multinodular goiter, thyroid cysts, and toxic adenomas (Figure 26.6).

To place the patient in the safest physiologic state, a euthyroid state should be achieved preoperatively. The goal of therapy is to inhibit the synthesis of thyroid hormone with antithyroid thionamides such as methimazole (which blocks the uptake of iodine) or propylthiouracil for pregnant women. The use of beta-blockers such as propranolol or esmolol or of calcium channel blockers may be incorporated into the treatment plan of symptomatic patients (i.e., patients with tachycardia and/or hypertension).

Postoperative care includes assessing for vocal cord impairment (due to laryngeal nerve damage) by asking the patient to enunciate the letters *a* and *e*, as well as for the ability to swallow. Assessment of the surgical site for hemorrhage is vitally important. Monitoring of the postoperative cardiac status aids

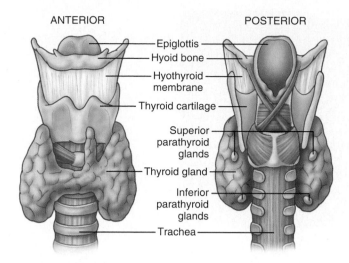

ANTERIOR   POSTERIOR

Epiglottis
Hyoid bone
Hyothyroid membrane
Thyroid cartilage
Superior parathyroid glands
Thyroid gland
Inferior parathyroid glands
Trachea

Fig. 26.6 Thyroid gland. Duffy C. Thyroid and parathyroid surgery. Figure 16.1 in: Rothrock J. *Alexander's Care of the Patient in Surgery.* 16th ed. Elsevier; 2019.

early treatment should any hypermetabolic or hyperdynamic issues develop, particularly in relation to the activation of the sympathetic system in response to the stress of surgery.

Specific postoperative instructions include the monitoring, measuring, care, and reporting of drainage from any drains placed. Patients should also be taught to have proper neck support by avoiding extreme head flexion or extension.

Skin Grafting or Excision of Lesions of the Skin or Subcutaneous Tissue

The skin is the largest organ of the body. It is comprised of the epidermis, dermis, and hypodermis. The skin serves as a protective barrier against physical, chemical, and bacterial agents. It is also instrumental in maintaining normothermia, and it functions as a sensory organ for pressure, touch, temperature, and pain. Skin prevents the loss of body fluids and excretes waste from sweat glands. Skin is instrumental in contributing to a person's self-concept and body image.[3] Excisions of skin lesions may be performed for the resection of basal cell, squamous cell, and malignant melanoma carcinomas and of a nonmalignant nevus or for cosmetic reasons. If large sections of skin must be resected during a procedure, skin grafting may need to be part of the surgery to promote wound closure and healing.

Preoperatively, patients should plan for a minimal level of sedation or anesthesia, depending on the location and extension of the lesion to be excised. NPO status should be determined by the anesthesia care provider should sedation be included in the surgical plan.

In addition to the general considerations of the immediate postoperative course, the perianesthesia nurse assesses the condition of the skin (e.g., blanching, expected amount of bleeding). Positioning of the operative site is also a prime consideration as pressure on the site needs to be avoided. It is generally a good rule of thumb to avoid placing ice packs on the site as the cold temperature may greatly impede circulation and thereby alter prompt and proper healing. Attention to the donor site, if one has been needed, should not be forgotten and should include the monitoring of the amount and color of drainage and the reporting of the findings to the provider.

Specific discharge instructions should include information regarding the drains that may be inserted to allow for appropriate approximation of the wound edges. It is vital to instruct

the patient in the technique for emptying and monitoring the drainage collected. The patient should demonstrate these techniques, as well as verbalize a method for documenting the output.

Breast Biopsy

According to the American Cancer Society, the overwhelming majority of breast biopsies do not result in a final diagnosis of cancer.[16] Patients who hear that breast cancer may be a possibility usually feel anxious and insecure, however. Patients (female and male) need to be presented with a caring, holistic treatment plan and ultimately require an interprofessional team approach.

The type of biopsy one has depends on several factors, including how suspicious the lesion appears, the size and location of the lesion, the number of lesions, and the family history and co-morbidities. A patient's personal preference for a procedure may also be a factor.

There are four basic types of breast biopsy to be considered. The first is a fine-needle aspiration (FNA), which entails the use of a hollow needle (of a smaller bore than one used for venipuncture) that is inserted into the suspicious area and through which tissue is aspirated with an attached syringe (Figure 26.7). A second type of biopsy is the core needle, for which a needle with a larger bore is used than for an FNA. This is the preferred type of biopsy when cancer is suspected and has been suggested by a mammogram, ultrasound image, or magnetic resonance image. A surgical biopsy is performed to excise all or part of a lump for testing. Usually, the entire suspicious lump is removed, as well as the surrounding margins of normal breast tissue.[16] On occasion, an axillary lymph node biopsy may be necessary; it can be performed as a needle biopsy, a sentinel lymph node biopsy, or an axillary lymph node dissection.

Evidence-Based Practice: Lump Localization

For many years the gold standard for localizing a non-palpable breast lump has been using a wire-guided method. Typically performed under local anesthetic and in the setting of radiology support, a wire is inserted into the center of the lump to ease the removing of the lump during surgery. The wireless technology, for example the use of radioactive seeds, allows for the localization process to occur at any time prior to the date of the surgery which improves patient satisfaction. In addition. The wireless technology is continuing to expand and includes radar reflector localization, magnetic seed localization, and radiofrequency tag identifier localization. Each wireless approach offers high success rates for surgical extraction of the breast lesion.

Source: Yeh ED, Portnow LH. Transitioning from the traditional wire localization to the wireless technology for surgical guidance at lumpectomies: Part A. Radioseed localization. Semin Ultrasound CT MRI. 2022;44(1):8-11. https://doi.org/10.1053/j.sult.2022.10.003

Potential complications of these procedures include hematoma, hemorrhage, and infection.

Patients should be instructed preoperatively on the length of time it will take after the biopsy to get the findings as this time frame can cause anxiety. Patients should be encouraged to ask questions.

Postoperatively, the perianesthesia nurse should continue to monitor drainage, whether it be directly into a dressing or via a drain. Postoperative comfort requires that both physical and emotional needs be taken into consideration. Patients should be positioned for comfort. An ice bag provides added

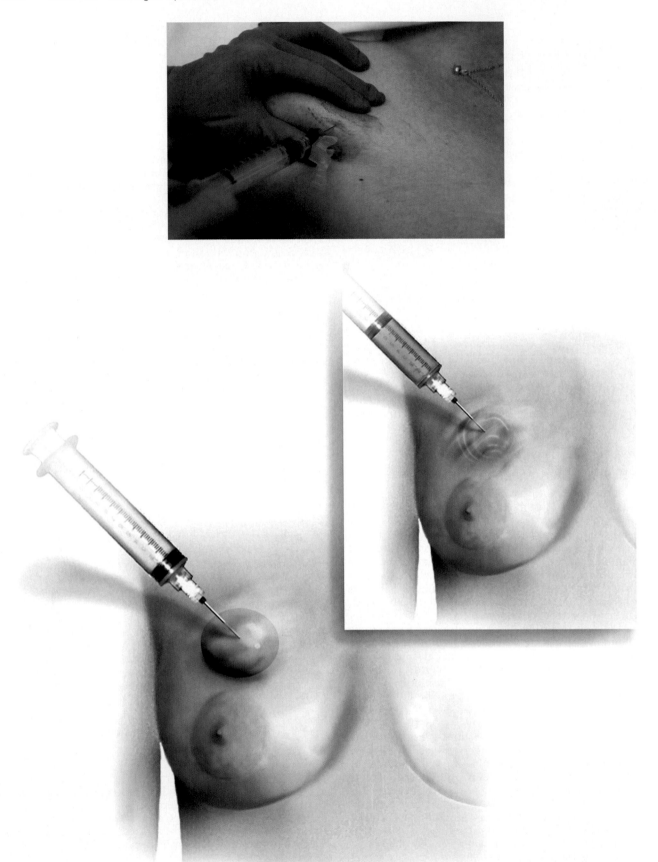

Fig. 26.7   Fine-needle aspiration. Stahl DL, Columbus KS, Baggish MS. The breast. Figure 103.21 in: Baggish MS, Karram MM, eds. *Atlas of Pelvic Anatomy and Gynecologic Surgery*. 5th ed. Elsevier; 2021.

comfort, as well as decreases the amount of ecchymosis. Supportive garments (e.g., a bra without underwires or an ace wrap bandage) may be ordered by the surgeon, and patients should be instructed to maintain these supportive garments as directed by the provider. Range-of-motion instructions should be verified, especially following a surgical biopsy or lymph node biopsy; these directions should be given by the provider.

GENERAL CONSIDERATIONS

Just the thought of surgery can be stressful for a patient, even if the outcome is expected to be positive. Incorporating the patient's emotional needs into the plan of care is important for the perianesthesia nurse.

Procedures performed by a general surgeon in an ambulatory setting are increasing in number and complexity. In addition to the variety of procedures being performed, patient acuity, or the intensity of patient care needed for a certain condition or procedure, is also increasing. It is vitally important that the ambulatory surgical staff be aware of special requirements for the preparation and discharge of ambulatory surgical patients.

CHAPTER HIGHLIGHTS

- Each surgical procedure requires planning and specific steps of care to have a final outcome that keeps patients safe.
- The teach-back method can ensure that patients understand the instructions that have been provided them by the perianesthesia nurse.

CASE STUDY

Mary Jane is a perianesthesia nurse working in the ABC Surgery Center's perianesthesia department. As Mary Jane surveys the schedule for the day, she finds that she will care for a variety of patients during her shift. Mary Jane anticipates that she will care for three patients who underwent, respectively, a laparoscopic cholecystectomy, inguinal herniorrhaphy, and hemorrhoidectomy, and also two breast biopsy patients.

What commonalities should Mary Jane expect in preparing her patients for their procedures? *(There will be a psychological impact of the procedure and a potential alteration in body image; each patient should have an NPO status; and skin asepsis will be necessary.)*

During the postoperative phase, Mary Jane will prepare her patients for discharge. What common discharge instructions will Mary Jane plan to deliver to her patients? *(She will discuss with them dietary changes, activity progression, pain control, appointments for follow-up visits to the practitioner, and the care of the surgical site.)*

What specific discharge instructions should Mary Jane provide her patients? *(Laparoscopic cholecystectomy: there is the potential for referred pain to the shoulder; inguinal herniorrhaphy: dietary changes will be needed and there will be restrictions on lifting; hemorrhoidectomy: sitz baths and stool softeners will be helpful; breast biopsy: wearing a supportive bra can be beneficial).*

Mary Jane will need to ascertain that her patients understand their instructions and that they have the tools to follow through on the instructions. What is the best way to verify her patients' understanding of their postoperative care? *(The teach-back method is a good way to verify understanding.)*

REFERENCES

1. Hall MJ, Schwarzman A, Zhang J, Liu X. Ambulatory surgery data from Hospitals and Ambulatory Surgery Centers: United States, 2010. *Natl Health Stat Report.* 2017;(102):1-15. Available at: https://www.cdc.gov/nchs/data/nhsr/nhsr102.pdf.
2. Yen PH, Leasure AR. Use and effectiveness of the teach-back method in patient education and health outcomes. *Fed Pract.* 2019;36(6):284-289. Available at: https://www.ncbi.nlm.nih.gov/pmc/articles/PMC6590951/.
3. Anicoche ML, Mamaril ME. General surgery. In: Schick L, Windle PE, Eds. *PeriAnesthesia Nursing Core Curriculum: Preprocedure, Phase I and Phase II PACU Nursing.* 4th ed. Elsevier; 2021.
4. National Institutes of Health. *Definition & Facts of Hemorrhoids.* NIH: US Department of Health and Human Services; 2016. Available at: https://www.niddk.nih.gov/health-information/digestive-diseases/hemorrhoids/definition-facts.
5. National Institutes of Health, National Library of Medicine. *Surgery for Pilonidal Cyst.* 2021. Available at: https://medlineplus.gov/ency/article/007591.htm.
6. Jayarajah U, Samarasekera DN. Predictive accuracy of Goodsall's rule for fistula-in-ano. *Ceylon Med J.* 2017;62(2):97-99. Available at: http://doi.org/10.4038/cmj.v62i2.8474.
7. Nottingham JM, Rentea RM. *Anal Fistulotomy.* StatPearls; 2022. Available at: https://www.ncbi.nlm.nih.gov/books/NBK555998/.
8. Dooley A, Aarne Grossman V. Ch 35: Interventional radiology and special procedures. In: Schick L, Windle PE, eds. *PeriAnesthesia Nursing Core Curriculum: Preprocedure, Phase I and Phase II PACU Nursing.* 4th ed. Elsevier; 2021.

9. Kelly CR, Kahn S, Kashyap P, et al. Update on fecal microbiota transplantation 2015: Indications, methodologies, mechanisms and outlook. *Gastroenterology.* 2015;149:223-237. Available at: https://doi.org/10.1053/j.gastro.2015.05.008.
10. Shaw C, Shamimi-Noori S. Ultrasound and CT directed liver biopsy. *Clin Liver Dis.* 2014;4(5):124-127. Available at: https://doi.org/10/1002/cld.437.
11. Costa RS, Cardoso AF, Ferreira A, et al. What recovery position should patients adopt after percutaneous liver biopsy? *Eur J Gastroenterol Hepatol.* 2019;31(2):253-259. Available at: https://doi.org/10.1097/meg.0000000000001290.
12. Heffline M. Care of the vascular surgical patient. In: Odom-Forren J, ed. *Drain's Perianesthesia Nursing A Critical Care Approach.* 7th ed. Elsevier; 2018.
13. National Institutes of Health, National Library of Medicine. *Venous Insufficiency.* 2022. Available at: https://medlineplus.gov/ency/article/000203.htm.
14. Compton RA, Simmonds JC, Dhingra JK. Total thyroidectomy as an ambulatory procedure in community practice. *OTO Open.* 2020;4(3):2473974X20957324. Available at: https://doi.org/10.1177/2473974x20957324.
15. Byrne M. Ch 21: Endocrine. In: Schick L, Windle PE, eds. *PeriAnesthesia Nursing Core Curriculum: Preprocedure, Phase I and Phase II PACU Nursing.* 4th ed. Elsevier; 2021.
16. American Cancer Society. *Breast Biopsy.* 2022. Available at: https://www.cancer.org/content/dam/CRC/PDF/Public/8579.00.pdf.

27 Genitourinary Surgery

Carre Smith, MSN, RN

LEARNING OBJECTIVES

A review of the content of this chapter will help the reader to:

1. Identify the role of the perianesthesia nurse in the preoperative, intraoperative, and postoperative phases of care of the patient having genitourinary (GU) surgery.
2. Describe the most commonly performed GU surgeries in the ambulatory outpatient setting.
3. Describe the most common risk factors of GU surgeries.
4. Identify the role of the nurse in discharge teaching for the GU patient.

OVERVIEW

Genitourinary (GU) surgery focuses on the kidneys, adrenal glands, bladder, prostate, urethra, and accessory structures of these organs. Since both the male and female urinary systems align closely with the genitalia, the genital system often needs to be accessed in order to treat the primary urologic problem.

GU surgeries are increasingly performed safely on an outpatient basis. Procedures such as prostate or bladder tumor resection, which less than a decade ago necessitated an inpatient stay of 1–three nights, are now routinely done in the ambulatory setting. In this setting, patients can be prepped for surgery, undergo the surgical procedures, recover, and be discharged to go home in a single morning. Regardless of the location of the procedure, the perianesthesia nurse is responsible for keeping patients safe, comfortable, and informed.

There are three main approaches to GU surgery: transurethral, laparoscopic, and open (or transabdominal). Robotic surgeries, although increasingly popular for general and gynecologic procedures, are not commonly done as same-day procedures for urologic disorders.[1] This chapter discusses the nurse's role in caring for the GU patient population in each phase of care and explores the most common GU surgeries carried out in the ambulatory surgery setting.

GENERAL CARE FOR GENITOURINARY SURGERY PATIENTS

Preoperative Care

Any planned surgery experience begins before the patient arrives at the hospital. Prior to the date of service, nurses who do preadmission testing should contact the patient and obtain a thorough health history to ensure that the patient has the best possible status for surgery. This includes following through with any co-morbidities that ought to be addressed, such as an elevated HgA1C level or recent episodes of chest pain. Preoperative instructions about the NPO status, any ordered bowel preps, and what medications are to be taken or held should be clarified in advance. On the date of service, the preoperative nurse should interview the patient again to ensure that all instructions have been followed. This includes ascertaining what the patient's current symptoms are and what the expectation is for relief of symptoms after surgery. This can be a good time to initiate discharge teaching because the patient is not under the influence of anesthesia or pain medication. Of course, all teaching should be repeated and reinforced after surgery, as well. It is normal for patients to feel embarrassment at discussing surgery involving these parts of their bodies. Therefore, the perianesthesia nurse in all phases of care should be cognizant of protecting the patient's dignity and modesty as much as possible while still speaking frankly and coherently about necessary issues. Providing skin preparation, including hair clipping, for patients prior to GU surgery is not routinely done in the preoperative area. If it is necessary, hair clipping can be carried out in the operating room.

Intraoperative Care

For most outpatient GU surgeries, antimicrobial prophylaxis is not indicated beyond a single dose or, at least, should be discontinued within 24 hours of the end of the procedure. To be optimally effective, the infusion of the first dose should begin within 60 minutes of the surgical incision (120 minutes for IV fluoroquinolones and vancomycin). This ensures that serum and tissue concentrations of the antimicrobial agent surpass the minimum inhibitory concentration of any target organisms. A longer duration of antimicrobials may be considered when prosthetic material or indwelling tubes are placed, or when there is already an existing infection.[2] Repeated dosing of antibiotics intraoperatively is indicated if the operative time exceeds two half-lives of the antibiotic chosen.

Patients undergoing urinary surgery are typically placed in lithotomy position. This poses a higher risk for damage to the lower extremity nerves (e.g., peroneal, saphenous, lateral femoral cutaneous, and sciatic nerves) and for compartment syndrome. The risk is higher if the procedure time is longer than 240 minutes and if the mean arterial pressure is maintained at less than 20% of baseline. Studies suggest that for every hour a patient is in lithotomy position, the risk for developing nerve injury increases by nearly 100-fold. Therefore, the operating room nurse should ensure that the patient is wearing sequential compression devices, carefully pad the lower extremities, note when the patient is nearing the 4-hour mark in lithotomy position, and collaborate with the surgical team to evaluate whether the patient's position can be changed. If the patient needs, additionally, to be in Trendelenburg position, early studies suggest that a supine Trendelenburg position may pose less risk of lower extremity nerve damage than a lithotomy Trendelenburg position.[3]

An uncommon but real risk of any GU surgery involving continuous irrigation is the risk that the bladder or surrounding organs may be perforated and that irrigation fluid may leak into the peritoneal cavity. The operating room nurse should collaborate with the surgeon to ensure that the intake and output of irrigation fluid are appropriately related. If there is a wide disparity (e.g., more fluid in than out), then perforation should be suspected and investigated. In this case, the patient may need to be held in the postoperative ambulatory care area several hours longer than usual to assess for hemodynamic changes or for further diagnostic testing.

Postoperative Care

Regardless of the type of GU surgery, every patient has certain postoperative needs in common. In the Phase I and Phase II PACU, the nurse should monitor vital signs carefully for tachycardia and hypotension, which, in combination, may be a sign of occult hemorrhage (Box 27.1).

The patient without an indwelling urinary catheter must be able to urinate with a normal stream before discharge, to ensure that edema of the urethra and urinary retention do not compromise voiding. If the patient is being discharged to go home with an indwelling urinary catheter, the perianesthesia nurse teaches the patient and caregiver to recognize when the catheter is draining properly and what the signs and symptoms of obstruction are. For patients who will remove their own urinary catheter at home, thorough teaching should be done, using written instructions, pictorials, demonstrations, and return demonstration methods. Home caregivers should be involved in the teaching when appropriate.

The nurse should explain to the patient the rationale for observing the color of urine. Bloody urine with small clots and burning when urinating may be experienced for a few voiding occurrences following the procedure. This usually resolves within two days to four weeks, depending on the type of surgery.

Encourage the patient to increase fluid intake. Fluids help flush the bladder to decrease the amount of bleeding and reduce the risk of infection. If the patient is not in a condition to drink well, the nurse may need to temporarily increase the rate of IV fluids.

Both the nurse and, later, the patient at home should assess for signs of serious complications (e.g., sepsis, bladder perforation, hematuria). Persistent, severe flank pain, a temperature over 38.5°C, and chills may signal the onset of infection. Copious bright-red blood, large and persistent clots in the urine, or urinary retention must be reported immediately to the surgeon.[4]

The kidneys and the prostatic bed are highly vascular; therefore, dressings applied after GU surgery may become soaked with blood and urine. These should be reinforced as necessary and the surrounding skin kept clean and dry to prevent breakdown. The postoperative nurse should monitor vital signs and the patient's presentation closely and assess the output of all tubes and drains frequently, collaborating with the surgical team in order to know how much drainage is safe to expect.

All patients undergoing procedures that involve abdominal or flank incisions should be assessed for abdominal distention after surgery. In addition, the patient should be assessed for bladder distention caused by an inability to void or the obstruction of catheters.

A healthy bladder holds 300–400 mL of urine,[5] but the urge to void is generally felt at 150–200 mL. Bladder volumes over 500 mL pose the risk of over distending the muscle fibers in the bladder wall. This can result in an inability to void or to empty the bladder completely, and this puts the patient at risk for permanent motility problems and urinary tract infections.[6] A bedside ultrasound bladder scanner can be used to assess whether a postoperative patient's bladder is full or if there is any postvoiding residual urine. Policies about when to intermittently catheterize a patient vary by institution, but the common guideline for this procedure is when volumes are between 400 and 600 mL (Figure 27.1).[7] Some algorithms put the threshold as low as 300 mL. The nurse should know the institution's policy regarding when a patient is at risk for urinary retention and when the patient should be scanned. In addition, guidelines should address the parameters for intermittent bladder catheterization. Depending on the volume and whether the patient is capable of voiding, straight catheterization should be performed to relieve urinary retention. Orders should be clear about when to contact the physician regarding residual urine volumes and recatheterization. If the patient needs to be discharged with a catheter in place, whether it will be self-removed at home or removed in the physician's office, the postoperative nurse should include teaching on how to care for the catheter in the discharge instructions.

NURSING CARE FOLLOWING SPECIFIC GENITOURINARY PROCEDURES
Cystoscopy

Cystoscopy is an invasive diagnostic procedure that allows direct visualization of the urethra, urinary bladder, and ureteral orifices through the insertion of a scope into the bladder.

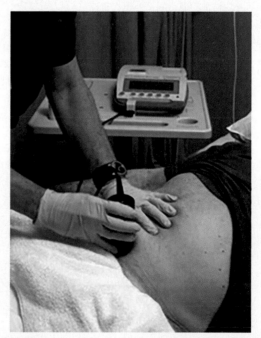

Fig. 27.1 Bladder scanner. Odom-Forren J. *Drain's PeriAnesthesia Nursing: A Critical Care Approach.* 7th ed. Elsevier; Kindle Edition. Figure 41.2.

BOX 27.1 Signs and Symptoms of Hemorrhage
Hypotension, especially when coupled with tachycardia
Dizziness and light-headedness
Nausea
Pallor
Headache, often severe
Frank bleeding
Abdominal distention or swelling around surgical site
Muscle and joint pain
Hypoxia
Decreased level of consciousness

There are two types of cystoscopes used, a rigid cystoscope and a flexible cystoscope. A rigid cystoscope is generally used for treatment. A thin tube with a lens and light system is inserted into the urethral meatus and advanced into the bladder. Biopsies can then be performed, as well as other types of surgeries. This is done under general anesthesia in an ambulatory care setting. A flexible cystoscope is more apt to be used for diagnostic purposes. With a flexible fiberoptic telescope the urologist can diagnose urinary abnormalities and evaluate the effectiveness of previous treatments. This is often performed under local anesthesia in an office setting.

Patients who have had operative cystoscopies normally experience urinary urgency in the PACU, either because of irritation of the urethra or because of incomplete emptying of the bladder intraoperatively. Providing these patients the opportunity to void as soon as possible reduces postoperative restlessness, agitation, and perceived pain or discomfort.

Ureteroscopy

Both flexible and rigid ureteroscopes are used for the diagnosis and removal of calculi (stones), fulguration of tumors, analysis of hematuria, and management of ureteral strictures (Figure 27.2). Complications are rare but may include perforation of the ureter. Close monitoring of the color and amount of urine output should be maintained.

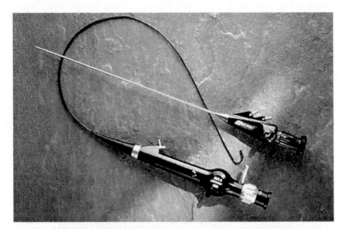

Fig. 27.2 Flexible and rigid ureteroscopes. Korey Marley HP. Genitourinary Surgery. Figure 15.12 in: Rothrock JC. *Alexander's Care of the Patient in Surgery*. 16th ed. Elsevier. 2019.

If the GU surgery being performed has the potential to produce significant swelling and inflammation around the ureter, a ureteral stent is used to facilitate the flow of urine and prevent obstruction or ureteral colic caused by edema. The stent may remain in place for several days or weeks postoperatively and is usually removed in the urologist's office. Patients with ureteral stents usually have marked colicky discomfort in the groin and/or flank areas. This is exacerbated with movement and urination and may not resolve until the stents are removed. These patients generally require more pain medication, including alpha-blockers such as tamsulosin, to decrease spasms and cramping in the ureters.

Certain ureteral stents have externalized sutures or strings that protrude from the urethra and are usually taped firmly to the patient's thigh. This is often done so that the patient may self-remove the stent at home after a certain interval. In this case, patients should be educated to avoid activities that pull on the suture, including care with dressing and undressing, wiping after urination, and sliding across furniture when sitting down. Bathing, swimming, and sexual activity should be avoided until the stent is removed. If the suture is left internally, the stent is removed later in the provider's office. The patient has the same restrictions as with an externalized stent.

Extracorporeal Shock Wave Lithotripsy

During extracorporeal shock wave lithotripsy (ESWL), high-energy sound waves from outside the body are directed at the precise location of a kidney stone (Figure 27.3). The waves break up the stone into smaller pieces without damaging the structures around it. These smaller pieces can pass more readily through the urinary system and out of the body. After ESWL, fluids should be increased and intake and output monitored carefully. Initially, the color of the urine may be cherry red to pink because of trauma from surgery; this condition may take several hours to clear. The surface skin over the area where the shock waves were delivered may show petechiae, redness, and bruising, and the patient may have mild pain from the force of the shock waves. This pain is usually localized to the skin and may be relieved with ice packs and nonsteroidal anti-inflammatory drugs (NSAIDs). Later, the patient may experience a different type of pain as the fragments of pulverized stones pass through the lower urinary tract.[8] Providers may or may not ask that patients strain their urine and save the stone fragments after surgery. If this is ordered, the patient should be provided with disposable filters to use when voiding at home.

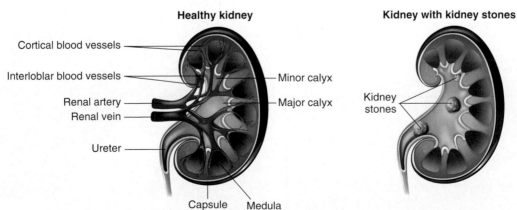

Human kidney stones

Healthy kidney   **Kidney with kidney stones**

Cortical blood vessels

Interloblar blood vessels

Renal artery

Renal vein

Minor calyx

Major calyx

Kidney stones

Ureter

Capsule   Medula

Fig. 27.3 Kidney stones. Espinosa G, Esposito R. Kidney stones. Figure 191.1 in: Pizzorno JE, Murray MT, eds. *Textbook of Natural Medicine.* Churchill Livingstone; 2021

Source: Elsevier Point of Care. Clinical overview: Nephrolithiasis. Updated August 12, 2022. https://www.clinicalkey.com

Prostate Surgeries and GreenLight Photoselective Vaporization of the Prostate

Benign prostatic hypertrophy is the most common prostate problem in men over age 50. About half of men in their 50s and as many as 90% of men in their 70s and 80s have enlarged prostates. This is problematic in that, as the prostate enlarges, it encroaches on the urethra and can be the cause of incomplete bladder emptying, as well as of urinary frequency, urgency, and lack of control.[9]

Photoselective vaporization of the prostate (PVP) is a treatment that uses a laser to vaporize prostate tissue, creating a channel in the urethra for free urination. Studies show that outcomes from GreenLight PVP are comparable to outcomes from traditional transurethral resection of the prostate (TURP) in smaller prostates. Patients with prostates larger than 70 mL in size have better results with TURP than PVP. Patients selected for the GreenLight procedure can be outpatients, but patients who require TURP, which has higher risks, still need an inpatient stay of 1 or 2 nights.[10]

As with other GU surgeries, the postoperative nurse caring for a patient after a GreenLight PVP should monitor the quantity and characteristics of the first urine voided, the quality of the patient's stream, and any signs or symptoms that point to possible hemorrhage.

Percutaneous Nephrolithotomy

Stones too large to remove via ureteroscopy can often be retrieved percutaneously. Using ultrasound, an incision is made in the flank and a nephrostomy tract is established. Stones smaller than 1 cm can be removed manually with a grasp forceps, using a nephroscope for guidance. For larger stones, lithotripsy is commonly used.

The perianesthesia nurse should be aware that blood loss from damage to an intrarenal artery is the most significant complication of percutaneous nephrolithotomy. The patient may be discharged with a nephrostomy tube that will stay in place for several days. Pain should be managed using a multimodal approach of rest, repositioning, warm packs, and NSAIDs as appropriate; this regimen can be supplemented by opioids. Adequate fluid intake helps to keep the kidneys flushed and promotes patient comfort.

Patients with refractory or recurring stones are candidates for a metabolic workup to determine whether dietary changes can make a difference. There are five types of renal stones: calcium oxalate (the most common), calcium phosphate, uric acid, struvite, and cysteine. Each stone has different dietary and fluid intake recommendations and restrictions. Knowledge of the chemical makeup of the stone allows the urologist to offer specific dietary recommendations. The discharge nurse should educate the patient about the importance of following through with the surgeon to ascertain the plan for preventing further stones.[11]

Transurethral Resection of the Bladder

Transurethral resection of the bladder is usually performed under general anesthesia in an outpatient setting. A scope, introduced into the bladder by way of a urethral catheter, is used to excise and fulgurate small, localized polyps and tumors, ulcers, or other areas of bleeding. Biopsy specimens can be obtained, calculi retrieved or crushed, and ureteral and urethral strictures dilated.

After surgery, some hematuria is normal. The urine may be fruit punch–colored with small clots, but both the color and clarity should resolve to normal over a period of up to 4 weeks. The patient should not be passing frank blood or large clots. The perianesthesia nurse should teach the patient to avoid heavy lifting (no more than eight pounds) and to monitor for excessive bleeding at home. Signs and symptoms of hypovolemia suggestive of hemorrhage should be reviewed. These include orthostatic dizziness, a new onset of activity intolerance, and abdominal or pelvic pain and distention.[12]

Hydrocele

A common and benign clinical finding in male patients is a testicular hydrocele.[13] The swelling caused by an accumulation of fluid surrounding the testicle can be painful. A hydrocelectomy is the typical surgical treatment for this condition. The incision is usually made in the scrotum; this allows the surgeon to remove the excess fluid and part of the sac or membrane, also known as the tunica vaginalis, that contained the fluid. Following surgery, the perianesthesia nurse monitors dressings, provides scrotal support, and applies ice to the area to reduce pain, swelling, and bleeding. Swift recognition of a hematoma can prevent interruption of the blood supply to the testes and subsequent testicular damage.[13]

Orchiectomy

The surgical removal of a testis or both testes is considered treatment for a number of conditions. These may include testes damaged by injury, infection, or malignant disease. Some individuals seek orchiectomy as part of a transitioning process for transgender women. Removal of the testes results in testosterone deficiency and sterility. Complications to monitor include hemorrhage, bruising, and pain. The perianesthesia nurse caring for this patient in the PACU may also need to provide emotional support as an orchiectomy permanently changes the appearance of the patient unless the option for testicular prostheses is included in the treatment plan. Postoperative discomfort and swelling are managed with the use of a scrotal support, multimodal analgesia, and ice to the surgical area.

Adult Male Circumcision

Circumcision is the surgical cutting away of the prepuce (foreskin) of the penis. This may be done under local anesthesia in the provider's office or in an ambulatory setting if the patient prefers to have the procedure under deeper anesthesia. There are many indications for circumcising an adult, including a patient history of painful sex, a short frenulum, and preference of appearance (Box 27.2). Recurring inflammations such as balanitis (inflammation of the glans), posthitis (inflammation of the foreskin), and balanoposthitis (inflammation of both the glans and the foreskin) are not only painful but are also associated with infections, including those that are sexually transmitted.

The patient should be taught to expect some swelling and bruising of the penis for 2–3 days after circumcision. This should be manageable with over-the-counter pain relievers such as ibuprofen or acetaminophen.

The patient will likely have a petroleum-based dressing over the glans to prevent the tissue from becoming too dry, covered by a dry sterile dressing that can be removed in a day or two. The penis should remain upright inside the underwear to mitigate swelling. Depending on patient comfort and provider preference, underwear can be loose-fitting or snug or may be replaced by an athletic supporter. The patient may resume activity as tolerated at home and expect any swelling to be resolved within 2–3 weeks.

Penile Implant

A penile implant, or penile prosthesis, is a treatment for erectile dysfunction usually reserved for patients who have failed more conservative treatments (Figure 27.4). The surgery involves placing either semi-rigid rods in the penis or inflatable rods in the penis with a saline pump in the scrotum. Inserting the semi-rigid rod allows the penis to remain firm, but it can be positioned away from the body for sexual activity and against the body at other times. The inflatable implant works when the patient presses the scrotal pump, sending saline solution to the device in the penis, inflating it and causing an erection. After intercourse, the device is deflated again.

After surgery, the patient can expect a course of antibiotics and pain medication for several days. The penis should be positioned upright inside clothing to reduce swelling, and the patient should be cautioned not to lift anything greater than eight pounds for four to six weeks following surgery. At that point, sexual activity can also be resumed as tolerated. The patient will have sutures that may be removed later in the provider's office.

Sacral Neuromodulation

The treatment of overactive bladder with an implanted sacral stimulator is a minimally invasive procedure performed under monitored anesthesia care or under procedural sedation (Figure 27.5). The surgical approach is staged. In stage 1, a wire is implanted along the sacral nerve and brought out through the skin of the buttock or flank, where it is connected to an electronic stimulator. This stimulator is worn on a belt and monitored for 2 weeks while adjusting stimulation up or down and keeping a voiding diary.

Following stage 1, the patient should be cautioned against heavy lifting or vigorous exercise. Bending at the waist, excessive twisting, and sexual activity should also be avoided, and care should be taken not to slide across furniture when sitting down so as not to dislodge the wire.

If there is significant improvement in the symptoms of overactive bladder (defined as ≥ 50% reduction in dysfunctional voiding symptoms from baseline), the patient returns to the operating room for stage 2. This is also done under monitored anesthesia care and involves the pacemaker and wire being placed completely under the skin. The patient then controls the electronic stimulator via a handheld programmer and can control the amount of stimulation required to manage symptoms.

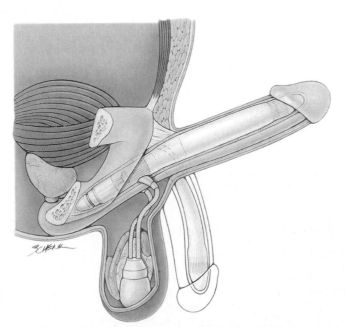

Fig. 27.4 Penile implant. Korey Marley HP. Genitourinary Surgery. Figure 15.20 in: Rothrock JC. *Alexander's Care of the Patient in Surgery.* 16th ed. Elsevier. 2019.

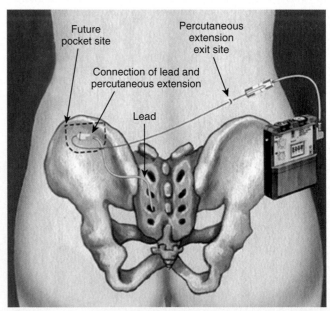

Fig. 27.5 Sacral nerve stimulation. Noblett KL, Cadish LA. Sacral nerve stimulation for the treatment of refractory voiding and bowel dysfunction. *Am J Obstet Gynecol.* 2014;201(2):99–106. Figure 2.

A 4- to 5-cm incision is made on either the right or left flank and a 1-cm incision is made over the sacrum. Any dressings can be removed after 48 hours, and the patient may shower. Activity should be restricted for 5–6 weeks. Too much activity before healing is complete can result in dislodging the wire, rendering the implant ineffective.

The potential complications of sacral nerve stimulators include pain at the insertion site, new pain, jolting or shocking sensations, worsening bladder problems, and infection.[14]

Botox Injection

Botulinum toxin is used to treat bladder dysfunction when treatment with anticholinergic medication has failed or cannot be tolerated. Under conscious sedation, botulinum toxin is injected directly into the detrusor muscle to block the efferent nerve impulses that stimulate the bladder to contract and empty. Potential complications include serious, immediate allergic reactions (e.g., itching, rash, wheezing, swelling). The patient may experience side effects such as dry mouth, discomfort at the injection site, fatigue, headache, neck pain, double or blurred vision, ptosis, and dry eyes. Adults being treated for urinary incontinence may experience other side effects, including urinary tract infection and painful urination. On a rare occasion the bladder may take several days to return to normal function. In this situation the patient may have to self-catheterize to achieve complete bladder emptying until normal function returns. Botox injection is not a permanent cure and must be repeated on average every 6 months.[15]

CHAPTER HIGHLIGHTS

- A wide variety of GU surgeries are performed in the outpatient setting.
- The highly vascular nature of the involved anatomy and postsurgical edema of small structures demand vigilance on the part of the perianesthesia nurse to ensure the patient is ready to be safely discharged to go home.
- Hemorrhage, infection, urinary retention, and pain are all important pitfalls for which assessment is needed.
- The highly private nature of the body parts involved require that the perianesthesia nurse be discreet and sensitive to the patient during the process, while also speaking frankly and clearly about the concerns and risks.
- When possible, teaching should be started preoperatively and repeated and reinforced postoperatively. The education of patients discharged with catheters or drains should include demonstration and return demonstration methods of teaching.

CASE STUDY

Andy S. is a 52-year-old male with a several-year history of urinary frequency, urgency, and retention unrelieved by treatment with alpha-blockers. Andy reports getting up "every 90 minutes" most nights to urinate and never feels he really empties his bladder. His family history includes a father with benign prostatic hypertrophy and diagnosed prostate cancer in his 60s. For 2 years, Andy's urologist has recommended a flexible cystoscopy to diagnose whether Andy would be a candidate for GreenLight PVP or TURP. Andy has resisted because he fears possible disfigurement and loss of sexual function. Finally, a friend who is a nurse convinces Andy that the benefits of the procedure outweigh the risks, and Andy reports to his urologist's office for the procedure.

On examination, the urologist concludes that the prostate is less than 70 mL in size and recommends a GreenLight PVP rather than a TURP. Preoperative teaching begins in the office with the understanding that Andy will go home with an indwelling urinary catheter, which he will need to remove at home on postoperative day one.

Several days before surgery, a preadmission nurse calls Andy at home to obtain his health history and give him preoperative instructions. On the day of surgery, Andy presents at the hospital, nervous but "ready to get this over with." The preoperative nurse prepares him for surgery and begins urinary catheter teaching.

After surgery, Andy emerges from anesthesia uneventfully in the PACU with initial vital signs of temperature 36.3°C, heart rate 82 bpm, respiratory rate 14 breaths per minute, and blood pressure 144/65 mm Hg. He has an indwelling 18 Fr. urinary catheter, which has put out 150 mL of cherry-red urine with small clots. Although Andy complains of an intense urge to void, he denies other pain. The PACU nurse medicates him with phenazopyridine 200 mg and acetaminophen 1000 mg. Forty minutes later, Andy's vital signs have trended upward to a heart rate of 102 bpm and a blood pressure of 175/80 mm Hg. He is restless and continues to report no relief. The nurse reassesses the urinary catheter and sees that the tubing is empty and no further urine has drained since Andy's arrival in the PACU. The nurse calls the surgeon and obtains an order to irrigate. She gently irrigates the bladder with 30 mL of normal saline and receives back 200 mL of bright-red urine with large clots in it. She reattaches the tubing, raises the head of the bed, and continues to monitor the drainage. Within 10 minutes, the urinary catheter bag contains 600 mL of urine. The urine in the tubing is lightening to pink, and Andy reports relief of urgency. He is transferred to the Phase II unit for discharge with a heart rate of 68 bpm and a blood pressure of 138/62 mm Hg.

In the Phase II unit, the discharge nurse reassesses Andy and determines that his pain level is 4/10, which he states is low enough to allow him to sleep at home. The nurse begins urinary catheter teaching again, demonstrating with a sample catheter and syringe how to remove the catheter at home. Andy demonstrates on the equipment that he can do this. The nurse gives him thorough written instructions, including a pictorial sheet in his discharge packet. She then explains to Andy how to empty his catheter at home and takes him to the bathroom so that he can practice emptying the bag. He demonstrates that he is able to do this by emptying 725 mL of pink urine. He is offered a leg bag but opts not to use it as the urinary catheter will be in place less than 24 hours and he has no plans to leave his house. Final vital signs show a heart rate of 65 bpm and a blood pressure of 140/67 mm Hg. Andy is discharged to go home with family care, denying further questions, needs, or complaints.

- Which clinical findings suggest that Andy is free of hemorrhage?
- What are signs that the urinary catheter is unobstructed and functioning properly?
- Can the nurse be confident that Andy is safe to manage his own urinary catheter at home? Why or why not?

REFERENCES

1. Sheetz KH, Claflin J, Dimick JB. Trends in the adoption of robotic surgery for common surgical procedures. *JAMA Netw Open.* 2020;3(1):e1918911. Available at: https://doi.org/10.1001/jamanetworkopen.2019.18911.

2. Lightner DJ, Wymer K, Sanchez J, Kavoussi L. Best practice statement on urologic procedures and antimicrobial prophylaxis. *J Urol.* 2020;203(2):351-356. Available at: https://doi.org/10.1097/ju.0000000000000509.

3. Vladinov GM, Glick B, Aguirre HO, Fiala RS, Maga JM. Lower extremity injury while undergoing urology procedures in the Trendelenburg with lithotomy position: three case reports. *J Perianesth Nurs.* 2021;36(3):214-218. Available at: https://doi.org/10.1016/j.jopan.2020.08.010.

4. Chrouser K, Foley F, Goldenberg M, et al. Optimizing outcomes in urologic surgery: intraoperative patient safety and physiological considerations. *Urol Pract.* 2020;7(4):309-318. Available at: http://dx.doi.org/10.1097/UPJ.0000000000000137.

5. Lukacz ES, Sampselle C, Gray M, et al. A healthy bladder: a consensus statement. *Int J Clin Pract.* 2011;65(10):1026-1036. Available at: https://doi.org/10.1111/j.1742-1241.2011.02763.x.

6. Brouwer TA, Rosier PFWM, Moons KGM, Zuithoff NPA, van Roon EN, Kalkman CJ. Postoperative bladder catheterization based on individual bladder capacity: a randomized trial. *Anesthesiology.* 2015;122:46-54. Available at: https://doi.org/10.1097/ALN.0000000000000507.

7. Stoffel JT, Chrouser K, Montgomery JS, et al. Optimizing outcomes in urological surgery: pre-operative care. *Urol Pract.* 2020;7(3):205-211. Available at: https://doi.org/10.1097/UPJ.0000000000000139.

8. Healthwise Staff. *Extracorporeal Shock Wave Lithotripsy (ESWL) for Kidney Stones. University of Michigan Health, Michigan Medicine Page.* Available at: https://www.uofmhealth.org/health-library/hw204232#:,:text=Extracorporeal%20shock%20wave%20lithotripsy%20(ESWL)%20uses%20shock%20waves%20to%20break,to%20precisely%20locate%20the%20stone.

9. National Institutes of Health. *National Institute of Diabetes and Digestive and Kidney Diseases Page. Prostate Enlargement (benign prostatic hyperplasia).* Available at: https://www.niddk.nih.gov/health-information/urologic-diseases/prostate-problems/prostate-enlargement-benign-prostatic-hyperplasia.

10. Elhilali MM, Elkoushy MA. Greenlight laser vaporization versus transurethral resection of the prostate for the treatment of benign prostatic obstruction: evidence from randomized controlled studies. *Transl Androl Urol.* 2016;5(3):388-392. Available at: https://doi.org/10.21037/tau.2016.03.09.

11. Anesthesia Key Page. *Care of the Genitourinary Surgical Patient.* Available at: https://aneskey.com/care-of-the-genitourinary-surgical-patient/.

12. Auvert B, Taljaard D, Lagarde E, Sobngwi-Tambekou J, Sitta R, Puren A. Randomized, controlled intervention trial of male circumcision for reduction of HIV infection risk: the ANRS 1265 trial. *PLoS Med.* 2005;2(11):e298. Available at: https://doi.org/10.1371/journal.pmed.0020298.

13. Lin L, Hong HS, Gao YL, et al. Individualized minimally invasive treatment for adult testicular hydrocele: a pilot study. *World J Clin Cases.* 2019;7(6):727-733. Available at: https://doi.org/10.12998%2Fwjcc.v7.i6.727.

14. SSSMHealth. *InterStim Therapy.* 2022. Available at: https://www.ssmhealth.com/urology/interstim-therapy-for-bladder-control-problems. Accessed August 18, 2022.

15. AbbVie. *Botox: What to Expect from Treatment.* 2022. Available at: https://www.botoxforoab.com/what-to-expect/. Accessed August 18, 2022.

28 Gynecologic Surgery

Brandy Rae Boissoneault, MSN, RN

LEARNING OBJECTIVES

A review of the content of this chapter will help the reader to:

1. Describe common obstetric and gynecologic surgeries.
2. Identify common complications associated with obstetric and gynecologic surgeries.
3. Identify nursing care throughout the perioperative continuum for specific obstetric and gynecologic procedures.
4. Identify ethical considerations unique to the obstetric and gynecologic population.

OVERVIEW

Advances in technology, anesthetics, and patient education have led to significant improvements in obstetric and gynecologic procedures and expanded the settings in which they are performed. Although most of these procedures still require an overnight stay, admission rates for these stays have been on a steady decline and the lengths of stays have become shorter. Procedures that were once performed in a hospital are now routinely performed in an office, and the more complex procedures, such as hysterectomies, are being performed in an outpatient setting. Deciding where a procedure should take place depends on the procedure's complexity, its anticipated complications, and the specific characteristics of patients. These topics are reviewed in this chapter.

The female reproductive system is a complex system with internal and external structures. The external structures, which are those that are visible externally, are the vulva, labia minora and labia majora, Bartholin's and skene's glands, clitoris, and vaginal opening (Figure 28.1). The internal structures are the vagina, uterus, ovaries, and fallopian tubes (Figure 28.2). The primary function of the female reproductive system is to produce and transport eggs needed for reproduction. The external structures aid in this process by enabling sperm to enter the body, as well as protecting the internal structures from organisms that can cause infection. Surrounding organs include the rectum, bladder, and intestines; they are often affected by obstetric and gynecologic conditions and the procedures performed to treat them (Figures 28.3 and 28.4). The complexity of the female reproductive system makes it susceptible to a variety of common conditions requiring surgical intervention (Table 28.1).[1,2]

Surgical procedures for the female reproductive system can be divided into three categories: obstetric, lower genital and vaginal, and abdominal gynecologic surgeries.[2] Obstetric surgeries are surgeries performed on pregnant women and include, but are not limited to, cervical cerclage, cesarean deliveries, treatment of ectopic pregnancies, and suction curettage.[2] Lower genital and vaginal surgeries include those related to organ prolapse (e.g., cystocele, enterocele, rectocele), dilatation and curettage (D&C), and hysteroscopies. Hysterectomies, laparotomies, oophorectomies, and salpingectomies fall into the category of abdominal gynecologic surgeries. This chapter explores common procedures performed in an outpatient surgery center with a greater focus on gynecologic procedures, followed by complications of the procedures and nursing care for them. Although the settings in which these procedures are performed may vary, the nursing care and complications related to gynecologic surgeries are similar and are therefore reviewed collectively.

COMMON OBSTETRIC AND GYNECOLOGIC SURGICAL PROCEDURES

Placement of Intrauterine Devices

An intrauterine device (IUD) is a type of long-acting, reversible contraceptive. The two types of IUDs are the copper-releasing device and the hormone-releasing device. The copper wire in the copper-releasing IUD prevents pregnancy by causing an inflammatory reaction that repels sperm. The hormone-releasing options are thought to prevent pregnancy by thinning the endometrium and thereby inhibiting ovulation and the activity of sperm. Due to its impact on the endometrial lining, which often minimizes or results in the complete absence of menstruation, the hormone-releasing IUD is often used to treat abnormal uterine bleeding.

Although easily placed in a doctor's office, IUDs may also be placed under anesthesia for a variety of reasons. This may be the best option if an IUD is being inserted at the same time as other procedures are being done or if patients have specific factors that recommend it (e.g., pain, failed attempts in an office setting, anxiety, trauma history). IUD-related complications are rare and may include infection, expulsion, or perforation. Expulsion is the most common complication, occurring in 2% to 10% of cases.[3] Perforation of the uterus is the next most common complication, occurring in 0.1% of cases, and is explored further in the section on Injury to Surrounding Organs and elsewhere in this chapter.[3] Patients should monitor for the displacement of an IUD by feeling for the attached strings regularly and should notify the provider if they are unable to locate the strings or if the device has fallen out.

Hysteroscopy

A hysteroscopy is performed to evaluate and diagnose common intrauterine conditions. The insertion of a small telescope through the cervix allows for the visualization of structures inside the uterus. The procedure can rule out common conditions, such as polyps or hyperplasia. A hysteroscopy can be performed in multiple clinical settings and is associated with the same complications as IUD insertion (e.g., infection, bleeding, perforation). To aid in a diagnosis, hysteroscopies are often combined with other procedures such as a D&C or endometrial sampling, or both.

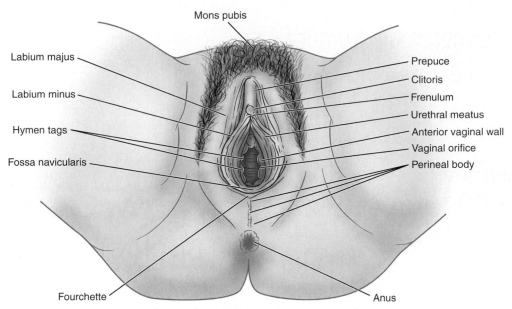

Fig. 28.1 Female external genital organs. (Carzo SA. Gynecologic and obstetric surgery. Figure 14.3 in: Rothrock J. *Alexander's Care of the Patient in Surgery.* 16th ed. Elsevier; 2019.)

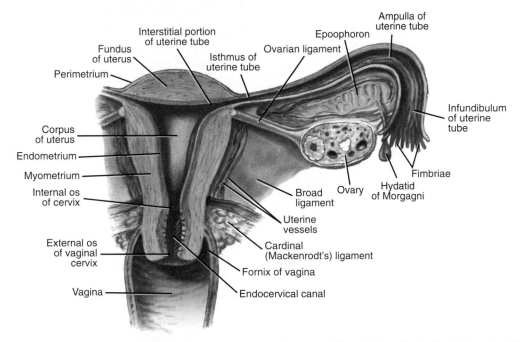

Fig. 28.2 Female reproductive organs. (Carzo SA. Gynecologic and obstetric surgery. Figure 14.1 in: Rothrock J. *Alexander's Care of the Patient in Surgery.* 16th ed. Elsevier; 2019.)

Evidence-Based Practice: Hysteroscopy and air embolism

Although the exact incidence of paradoxical air embolisms (PAE) resulting from the mechanical process involved with transvaginal hysteroscopies is not known, Han et al report that micro air emboli occur in nearly 98% of patients during this procedure. These micro emboli rarely arterialize. The formation of PAE is more likely to occur in the following situations: hysteroscopic myomectomies, prolonged length of surgery, excessive distention of the uterus, and extreme positioning in Trendelenburg. The perianesthesia nurse should be aware of the symptoms of PAE which include a sudden drop in end-tidal CO2, a drop in SpO2, and other signs of organ ischemia due to hypoxia. Postoperative treatment involves transfer to a higher level of care, intermediate critical care observation, echocardiograms and laboratory testing for evidence of myocardial damage. Chest x-rays or perfusion scans can serve to identify pulmonary emboli and magnetic-resonance imaging of the brain may be necessary to rule out neurological injury.

Source: Han K, Huang M-Q, Deng X, Shang Y-C. Remaining vigilant to paradoxical air embolism in patients undergoing hysteroscopic surgery: A case report and review of the literature. *J Perianesth Nurs.* 2021;36(6):606-611. https://doi.org/10.1016/j.jopan.2021.03.011

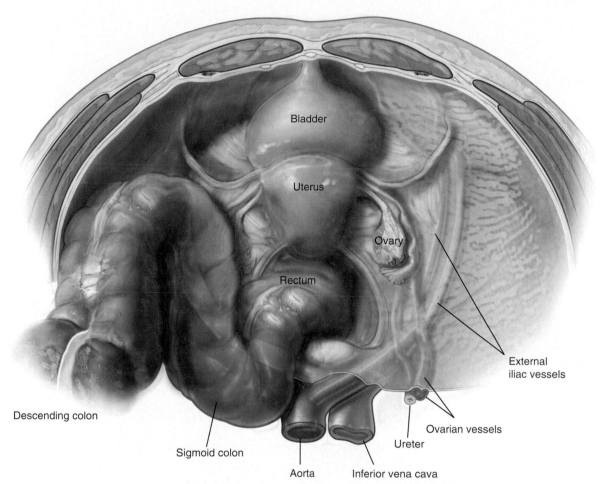

Fig. 28.3 Proximity of bladder and colon to reproductive organs. (Baggish MS. Advanced pelvic anatomy. Figure 2.6 in: Baggish MS, Karram MM, eds. *Atlas of Pelvic Anatomy and Gynecologic Surgery*. 5th ed. Elsevier; 2021.)

Dilatation and Curettage

A dilatation and curettage (D&C) procedure removes tissue from inside the uterus by dilation of the cervix and suctioning along the lining of the uterus. D&Cs may be done for therapeutic treatments (e.g., retained product, pregnancy terminations) or diagnostic reasons to evaluate abnormal uterine bleeding, postmenopausal bleeding, or abnormal cells.

Loop Electrosurgical Excision Procedure

A loop electrosurgical excision procedure (LEEP) is used to remove precancerous cells from the cervix. During a LEEP, a heated wire loop is used to shave off the cells on the cervix to prevent them from developing into cancerous cells. Although LEEPs are mostly performed in an office, they may be performed under anesthesia in an outpatient setting. Complications following a LEEP may include bleeding, infection, cervical stenosis, or persistent abnormal cells.

Endometrial Ablation

Endometrial ablation is a surgical procedure that cauterizes the endometrial lining. This is done to treat heavy or frequent menstrual bleeding and can be done via multiple methods, including radiofrequency, freezing, heated balloon, microwave energy, or electrocautery ablation.[4] Although the procedure can be performed in an office setting, it is routinely performed under anesthesia. Endometrial ablation is contraindicated in

women who have endometrial disorders, hyperplasia, uterine cancer, recent pregnancy, desire for future pregnancies, or uterine infections.[5,6] Most women have concurrent endometrial biopsies, hysteroscopies, or other diagnostic testing to rule out disorders prior to having an endometrial ablation.

Diagnostic Laparoscopy

Diagnostic laparoscopy is a minimally invasive surgical procedure performed to visualize and evaluate the reproductive and surrounding organs. This is often performed to confirm a diagnosis or evaluate a condition when other testing has been inconclusive. Common conditions leading to a diagnostic laparoscopy include exploration for causes of pelvic pain, confirmation of endometriosis, and diagnostic reasons for infertility. This procedure is performed through either a single incision or multiple small abdominal incisions. A small incision at the sub umbilical area serves as the site for the primary trocar, with additional sites added as needed in the right and left lower quadrants for additional instrumentation. The trocar insertions allow for instrumentation that can aid in tissue sampling or allow for other minor procedures to be performed.

Hysterectomy

A hysterectomy is the most common gynecologic procedure performed. It is estimated that 100,000 to 200,000 hysterectomies are performed yearly in an outpatient ambulatory setting.[7] This procedure is performed for a variety of benign

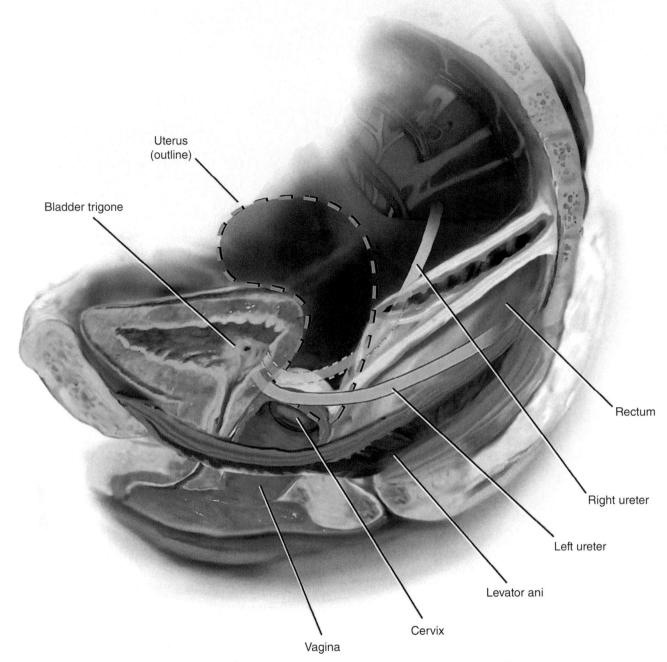

Fig. 28.4 Proximity of urinary structures to reproductive organs. (Baggish MS. Basic pelvic anatomy. Figure 1.37 in: Baggish MS, Karram MM, eds. *Atlas of Pelvic Anatomy and Gynecologic Surgery*. 5th ed. Elsevier; 2021.)

reasons (e.g., fibroids, endometriosis, pelvic support problems, abnormal uterine bleeding, chronic pelvic pain) and malignant reasons (e.g., cancers of the reproductive organs).[8] The types of hysterectomy include total, supracervical, and radical. A total hysterectomy removes the cervix and uterus, a supracervical hysterectomy removes the upper part of the uterus leaving the cervix in place, and a radical hysterectomy removes the uterus, cervix, and surrounding structures such as the ovaries and fallopian tubes.[8]

There are multiple ways a hysterectomy can be performed. The three broad methods include vaginal, abdominal, and laparoscopic. The approach performed has a direct impact on potential complications and patient morbidity.[9] The vaginal hysterectomy is the preferred method. Removal of the uterus through the vagina eliminates the need for an abdominal incision and allows patients to recover faster with fewer complications.[8] However, several contraindications exist (e.g., large uterine size, adhesions) with this approach, and they limit

TABLE 28.1 Common Obstetric and Gynecologic Conditions and Their Associated Symptoms

Condition	Description	Associated Symptoms
Abnormal uterine bleeding	Changes in frequency, duration, or amount of uterine bleeding from baseline (can be acute or chronic)	Bleeding between periods, more than 7 days, amenorrhea, postmenopausal bleeding
Dysmenorrhea	Pain with menstruation	Mild to severe pain before, during, or after menstruation
Amenorrhea	Absence of menstruation	Missing one or more menstrual cycles
Endometriosis	Abnormal growth of the endometrium outside of the uterus (e.g., ovaries or fallopian tubes)	Cyclic pain in the pelvis and uterus, dyspareunia, infertility, pain with urination or bowel movement
Adenomyosis	Abnormal growth of the endometrium into the muscles surrounding the uterus	Dysmenorrhea, pelvic pain abnormal uterine bleeding
Leiomyomas (fibroids or myomas)	Noncancerous tumors that develop in smooth muscle	Increased urination, pain, low back pain, dysfunctional uterine bleeding, dysmenorrhea, dyspareunia, miscarriages, infertility
Miscarriage	Spontaneous loss of pregnancy before 20 weeks' gestation	Mild to moderate pelvic and back pain, bleeding, passing of tissue
Retained product	Persistence of placental and/or fetal tissue in the uterus following pregnancy, miscarriage, or termination of pregnancy	Bleeding, pain, fever, infection
Ectopic pregnancy	Attachment of fertilized egg outside of the uterus (fallopian tube most commonplace)	Pain and bleeding; type and severity of pain can vary based on where attachment occurs
Ovarian cyst	Formation of cyst on the ovaries	Generally asymptomatic and can resolve on its own but can lead to torsion or rupture
Pelvic organ prolapse (cystocele, rectocele, uterine prolapse)	Loss of support to the uterus, bladder, and bowel, leading to their descent from the normal anatomic position toward or through the vaginal opening	Dyspareunia, pelvic pressure, or heaviness; cystocele is associated with urinary incontinence and retention
Infertility	Inability to conceive despite attempts for one year	Varies depending on the cause
Endometrial hyperplasia	Thickening of the endometrium	Abnormal uterine bleeding, postmenopausal bleeding
Gynecologic cancers	Cancer that starts in any of the female reproductive organs (ovarian, uterine, endometrial, vaginal, vulvar)	Pelvic pain and pressure, abnormal uterine bleeding, bloating, urinary frequency, constipation

Adapted from: Baggish MS, Karram MM. *Atlas of Pelvic Anatomy and Gynecologic Surgery*. 5th ed. Elsevier; 2021; and Winer WK. Care of the obstetric and gynecological surgical patient. In: Odom-Forren J (ed.). *Drain's PeriAnesthesia Nursing: A Critical Care Approach*. 7th ed. Elsevier; 2018.

this option for a variety of patients. An abdominal hysterectomy removes the uterus through an incision in the lower abdomen. This approach involves the greatest risk of complications, such as wound infection, bleeding, venous thromboembolism, and tissue damage.[8]

Minimally invasive hysterectomies (laparoscopic and robotic) have become the standard surgical approach. A laparoscopic hysterectomy incorporates the laparoscope along with small abdominal incisions to view and remove the uterus. This approach can be further divided into three categories: laparoscopic-assisted vaginal hysterectomy, laparoscopic hysterectomy, and total laparoscopic hysterectomy. Although laparoscopic surgery results in faster recovery, less pain, and shorter hospital stays, the procedure can take longer to perform and the potential for injury to surrounding organs is higher.[8]

Robotic Procedures

Robot-assisted hysterectomies allow the surgeon to remove the uterus with the use of a computer to control the surgical instruments. As robotic surgery techniques evolve, minimally invasive surgery is quickly becoming a choice for more patients. Robotic surgery is considered to be as successful as laparoscopic surgery for uncomplicated benign conditions, but it has been found to have its advantages in more complex cases, such as the removal of pelvic adhesions or fibroids, fulguration of endometriosis, surgical care of an obese patient or a patient with a large uterus, or treatment of gynecologic cancers.[10]

Surgeries for Gynecologic Cancer

Gynecologic cancer is defined as a malignancy involving a woman's reproductive organs as the primary site. Primary types of gynecologic cancer may include the cervix, ovaries, uterus, vagina, and vulva. Treatment is dependent on the type and stage of cancer and may include surgery, irradiation, or chemotherapy or a combination of these options. Most types of malignancies involving the female reproductive organs require a combination of treatments incorporating a variety of specialties in an interprofessional team approach.

Elective Female Genital Cosmetic Surgery

Elective female genital cosmetic procedures, such as labiaplasty and transgender surgeries, are performed by both obstetric and gynecologic surgeons and plastic surgeons. These types of surgeries can be reviewed further in the chapter on cosmetic surgeries.

Nonobstetric Surgery During Pregnancy

Nonobstetric surgery during pregnancy is rare and poses multiple risks to both the patient and the fetus. It is estimated that nonobstetric surgery is done in 0.2% to 2% of pregnancies.[11] The most common procedures, in order of occurrence, are appendectomy, cholecystectomy, adnexal surgery, trauma repair, surgery for small bowel obstructions, and breast surgery.[11] Although elective surgery should be postponed until after delivery, urgent or emergent surgery should not be denied. Ideally any antepartum (occurring before birth) surgery needing urgent attention should be postponed until the second trimester. In the event surgery is required during pregnancy, the patient's obstetrician should be consulted. If the provider does not have privileges at the facility, a provider who does should be consulted as part of the perinatal care plan. Preterm delivery is a risk associated with antepartum surgery, and, therefore, situations requiring anesthesia and surgery prior to delivery should be performed in an institution equipped for preterm deliveries, not in the outpatient setting. A nursing staff knowledgeable about and trained in fetal monitoring should always be available.

COMMON COMPLICATIONS OF OBSTETRIC AND GYNECOLOGIC SURGERIES

Cervical Injury

Cervical damage occurs when the cervix is torn. This often occurs with surgical instrumentation and is more common in the older population, in whom the aging cervical tissue is more pliable and fragile. In the presence of minimal bleeding, topical hemostatic agents can be used alone or as an adjunct to sutures (Table 28.2). If hemostatic agents are used, the patient should be informed of the impact these agents can have on the appearance and consistency of postoperative vaginal discharge.

Hemorrhage

Hemorrhage is a common complication that can occur regardless of the method or approach of the procedure being performed. Intraoperative hemorrhage is defined as blood loss exceeding 1000 mL or for which a blood transfusion is required.[12] A massive hemorrhage is one for which emergency lifesaving interventions are required or the acute blood loss is more than 25% of the patient's blood volume.[12]

To prevent the risk of hemorrhage, the preoperative evaluation should include the identification and treatment of preexisting anemia. An estimated 25% of patients presenting for a hysterectomy or myomectomy are anemic, and this is a risk factor that is a strong predictor of perioperative blood transfusions, infection, and a longer length of stay.[13] Elective outpatient surgery provides an opportunity for anemia to be identified and treated with iron or hormonal medications in preparation for the day of surgery. According to the American Association

of Gynecologic Laparoscopists, the goal of preoperative anemia management is to achieve a hemoglobin level greater than 12 g/dL prior to surgery.[13] The prophylactic administration of tranexamic acid (an antifibrinolytic administered orally or intravenously prior to incision) has also been associated with a reduction of intraoperative bleeding in obstetric and gynecologic surgeries.[12]

In the event bleeding occurs, direct pressure should be applied until the source is identified and controlled. This means that controlling the bleeding depends on determining the cause of the bleeding. Sutures, surgical clips, or coagulation can obtain hemostasis in smaller vessels; however, bleeding that involves the larger vessels (e.g., aorta, vena cava, iliac vessels) should be managed by a vascular surgeon.[12] In the presence of minimal bleeding, topical hemostatic agents may be used independently, as an adjunct, or when electrocautery or sutures cannot be used. These include physical agents such as oxidized regenerated cellulose (Surgicel) or microfibrillar collagen (Avitene), biologic agents such as topical tranexamic acid, and caustic agents such as silver nitrate or ferric subsulfate (Monsel solution) (Table 28.2).[14] Staff should be informed of the agents used within the facility, the mechanisms of action, and the potential side effects or complications. If homeostasis is not obtained and bleeding continues despite these interventions, a hysterectomy may be necessary, and the patient will require transfer to a higher level of care.

Infection

Infection is the most common complication following obstetric and gynecologic procedures. Not only are there a variety of operative and patient risk factors for infection, such as smoking and diabetes, but the types of gynecologic surgical site infections pose unique challenges because they are often polymicrobial. Micro-organisms that reside in the vagina, skin, or endocervix can contaminate the uterus and surrounding organs (e.g., urinary tract, vaginal cuff, intra-abdominal structures, bloodstream). This can occur at the time of surgery or in the postoperative period. The aim is prevention, which is achieved through a bundled approach involving skin preparation (e.g., clipping, not shaving, of hair; use of antiseptic preparations; use of surgical aseptic techniques) and the maintenance of normothermia, as well as selecting an appropriate antibiotic for the situation, to name a few.[13] This is a process that should start in the office with patient education and extend to the time well after discharge (Box 28.1).

TABLE 28.2 Topically Applied Hemostatic Agents and Nursing Implications for Their Use

Medication/Category	Purpose/Action	Nursing Implications
Thrombin/hemostatic agent	Applied directly to source of bleeding; causes conversion of fibrinogen to fibrin	Observe for fever or allergic reactions External use only
Gelatin matrix	May be mixed as granules or applied directly to source of bleeding to form a composite clot to seal bleeding vessel	Observe for anemia, atrial fibrillation, infection Not for intravascular use
Absorbable gelatin sponge	A film, powder, or sponge that can be cut to desired size and applied to site to absorb and hold blood and fluids to stop bleeding	Observe for infection at site Should not be used to close wounds as the application can interfere with skin healing at the edge of incisions
Collagen hemostat	A powder, sheet, or sponge applied directly to site of bleeding to attract platelets that will aggregate to form a physiologic clot	Observe for adhesion formation, allergic reaction, inflammation Should remove any excess with light irrigation and suction
Oxidized regenerated cellulose	Fibrous or weave-like fabric applied directly to site of bleeding to allow platelet aggregation to form a physiologic clot	Observe for encapsulation of fluid and foreign-body reactions Stored at room temperature

Adapted from: Murphy MP, Whitmore DM. Neurosurgery. Page 789 in: Rothrock J. *Alexander's Care of the Patient in Surgery*. 16th ed. Elsevier; 2019.

BOX 28.1 Steps for the Prevention of Surgical Site Infection

Preoperative Steps

Consider bacterial vaginosis and screening/treatment of urinary tract infection

Use of chlorhexidine 4% wipes/wash the night before and the morning of surgery

Cessation of smoking for ≥ 4 weeks

Glycemic control

Intraoperative Steps

Appropriate timing, selection, and dose of prophylactic antibiotics

Hair clipping

Skin/vaginal prep with chlorhexidine 4%

Sterile technique and meticulous hemostasis

If bowel resection or contaminated procedure performed, re-drape, re-gown/glove, and use only clean instruments for closing

Maintain normothermia and euvolemia

Limit duration of surgery

Discontinue urinary catheter at case end, unless otherwise indicated

Postoperative Steps

Remove dressings within 24 hours

Maintain euvolemia

Serum glucose < 180 mg/dL in patients with diabetes

Discontinue urinary catheter in the operating room or by midnight, unless contraindicated

---

Stone R, Carey E, Fader AN, et al. Enhanced recovery and surgical optimization protocol for minimally invasive gynecological surgery: An AAGL white paper. *J Minim Invasive Gynecol*. 2021;28(2):179–203. Table 5. https://doi.org/10.1016/j.jmig.2020.08.006

Injury to Surrounding Organs

Although rare, uterine perforation is a potential complication that can occur with any intrauterine procedure. Perforation occurs when surgical instruments perforate the organ wall. The clinical presentation may include pain and signs and symptoms of intra-abdominal bleeding such as vaginal bleeding, hypotension, tachycardia, and abdominal distention, rigidity, or pain. Often, however, perforations go undetected and resolve on their own. Treatment of perforations depends on the extent of the injury and associated clinical presentation.

Given the proximity of the genitourinary system to the female reproductive organs, urologic injuries, such as those involving the bladder or ureters, can occur (Figure 28.4). While bladder injuries are usually recognized immediately and repaired, ureteral injuries are often not discovered until the postoperative period (either immediately or after discharge). To mitigate rates of morbidity and mortality, early identification and intervention are vital. Nurses caring for this population of patients must have knowledge of risk factors, as well as the potential clinical presentations of patients with urologic injuries. Risk factors include obesity, previous laparotomy, abnormal anatomy, adhesions, adnexal masses, a large uterus, and intraoperative bleeding.[15] Assessment of the integrity of such organs intraoperatively via visualization, palpation, or cystoscopy prior to surgical closure is key to prevention and early recognition. If an injury is discovered, repair occurs during the same surgery via urologic consultation. In the postoperative course, patients should be observed for and instructed to report persistent, prolonged pain (of the back, abdomen, or flank), nausea (with or without vomiting), fever,

bladder dysfunction (e.g., distention, dysuria, hematuria, retention, low urine output), or signs and symptoms of an ileus.[15] If a surgical injury is present, additional signs may include rising or elevated laboratory results, including white blood cell counts and creatinine and blood urea nitrogen levels. However, such findings are not immediately evident.

Venous Thromboembolism

Venous thromboembolisms are deep vein thromboses and pulmonary embolisms. Preventing such complications through risk stratification and patient education is the goal. Recommendations for prevention in the outpatient setting for patients without a prior history of venous thromboembolisms include the standard application of mechanical compression devices, as well as early postoperative mobilization and ambulation.[13]

Local Anesthetic Systemic Toxicity

Paracervical blocks are often used for pain management. The aim of the paracervical block is to anesthetize the nerve bundles lateral to the cervix by injecting local anesthetics at 3 and 9 o'clock. Although the volume of lidocaine used for a paracervical block is low, systemic toxicity can still occur. Common LAST symptoms include tinnitus, numbness of the mouth, visual disturbances, confusion, seizures, or cardiorespiratory arrest. Perianesthesia nurses caring for patients who have had peripheral blocks should monitor for untoward symptoms and initiate LAST management and treatment with lipids per facility protocols.

NURSING CARE FOR OBSTETRIC AND GYNECOLOGIC SURGERY PATIENTS

Preoperative care, postoperative assessments, and patient education are vital for positive outcomes, particularly in the outpatient setting. Regardless of the type of procedure being performed, the nursing considerations for the obstetric and gynecologic population are similar. However, care should be customized to meet the specific needs of the patient.

Preoperative Care

Preoperative education and optimization should be initiated at the time of surgical booking. Patients should be engaged in interventions to reduce modifiable risk factors, set appropriate postoperative expectations, and participate in discharge planning. Optimization may include treatment of anemia, improving glucose control, smoking cessation, reduction in alcohol consumption, and participating in surgical clearance with providers when indicated. Discharge planning includes assessment of eligibility for same-day discharge, anticipated postoperative needs or concerns, pain management plans, infection prevention, and ongoing venous thromboembolism prophylaxis if indicated. The complexity and anticipated postoperative needs of the patient determine the setting in which the procedure is performed and the anticipated length of stay. Expectations must be clear, and the patient should be an active participant in decision making.

Laboratory work is common prior to obstetric and gynecologic procedures. Testing may be ordered at the preoperative visit or on the date of service. Nursing staff should be familiar with laboratory tests potentially impacting patient care, as well as specific provider preferences. Common pre-surgery blood tests may include pregnancy tests (serum or urine), coagulation studies, glucose levels, blood typing, and complete blood counts. Blood typing is often ordered to rule out the need for Rhogam or for more complex vascular procedures, such as hysterectomy, to not delay the administration of blood components in the event complications occur.

Depending on the facility guidelines, preoperative nurses may be responsible for phlebotomy. To mitigate risks (to staff and the patient), nurses must be knowledgeable about the best practices as well as the institutional policies on patient identification procedures, phlebotomy, blood collection, and specimen labeling. Unsafe phlebotomy can lead to patient injury or erroneous blood samples, which can result in inaccurate diagnoses and unwarranted interventions.

Patients undergoing obstetric and gynecologic procedures are at higher risk for postoperative nausea and vomiting (PONV). Gender, in this case female, is one of the strongest patient-specific predictors for PONV. As a result, all patients undergoing gynecologic surgeries are at risk. The potential for PONV increases with the presence of additional risk factors, such as a history of motion sickness, nonsmoker, age greater than 50 years, obesity, and delayed gastric emptying. Patients must be assessed for PONV and any risk factors reviewed with the anesthesia team to initiate the appropriate prophylactic interventions. Interventions may include application of a scopolamine patch, administration of dexamethasone and/or ondansetron intraoperatively, and limited use of opiates. If PONV persists postoperatively, the perianesthesia nurse can advocate for a prescription, such as for ondansetron, at discharge. A reactive rather than prophylactic approach to PONV management can prolong recovery, adversely impact the patient experience, and lead to an unplanned admission. Oral doxycycline is often ordered with uterine evacuations (e.g., D&C, ERS) and is known to cause nausea, vomiting, and upset stomach, particularly when patients have been fasting. The timing of administration of oral medications should be considered and antiemetics administered as needed preoperatively.

Preoperative optimization is the first step in preventing surgical site infection.[13] Patient-specific risk factors, which are often modifiable, include obesity, glycemic control, depressed immune system, history of drug-resistant organisms, malnutrition, and smoking. Operative risk factors include length of surgery, intraoperative blood transfusions, and wound classification. Mitigation of infection risk factors include educating patients to comply with preoperative showering (using antibacterial soap or chlorhexidine), avoid shaving prior to surgery, attempt smoking cessation, and actively work to optimize blood glucose levels.[13]

On the day of surgery, the perianesthesia nurse preparing the patient for surgery should reassess for risk factors and intervene when necessary. A consensus on the ideal target blood glucose levels is difficult to achieve; however, glucose levels should be checked and managed according to specific facility policies. Antimicrobial prophylaxis should be administered and timed according to evidence-based guidelines. Staff caring for this population of patients should be familiar with the recommended antibiotics based on the procedure being performed.

Pain management is a key factor in surgical recovery. The first steps in pain management are preoperative education and the establishment of postoperative expectations. Discussions should occur with the patient and support person with a focus on multimodal, opioid-sparing approaches. Both pharmacologic and nonpharmacologic interventions may include active or passive warming, positioning, application of cold or warm therapy, emotional support, or the administration of regional blocks (e.g., a paracervical or transverse abdominus plane block). Such discussions can further help to identify the psychosocial factors that can influence the patient's experience and perceptions of pain postoperatively.

In addition to physical symptoms with which the patient has presented, the perianesthesia nurse can also explore the concurrent psychological symptoms that this population of patients may be experiencing. This may include biases, belief symptoms, or values of the nurse regarding the type of patient situation. Patients may be triggered emotionally by the nature of obstetric and gynecologic surgery and experience varying emotions that can be expected with the potential loss of a fetus, hormonal therapy, sexual trauma, or cancer-related diagnoses. These emotions can range from sadness, anger, and resentment to fear, anxiety, and panic attacks. These emotions can be further heightened with anesthesia, the stress associated with surgery, or the experience of being in a vulnerable state. It is important to remember that surgery is a unique experience for each patient. Nurses must be aware of the varying emotions with which patients may present, the impact the emotions may have on the surgical experience, and the interventions that can be performed to provide support. The interventions include room placement, the reducing of external stimuli (when possible), active listening, therapeutic touch, and the involvement of partners or support persons when appropriate.

Postoperative Care

In the immediate postoperative period, most patients having obstetric and gynecologic surgery require phase I level care. This may or may not be in a separate postanesthesia care unit (PACU). In some outpatient settings, the recovery area is a hybrid unit where phase I and phase II are combined. Regardless of the physical location, the level of care required and the areas of focus remain the same as in traditional phase I and phase II units. In addition to immediate phase I assessments (e.g., respiration and ventilation, cardiac status, level of consciousness), patients should be assessed for bleeding, pain, the presence of PONV, and signs and symptoms consistent with common complications.

To mitigate the rates of morbidity and mortality associated with postoperative hemorrhage or uterine perforation, early identification is key. Throughout the recovery, visual inspection of the vagina and abdominal assessment must occur. The amount and consistency of bleeding should be assessed and documented. Inspect, palpate, and auscultate the abdomen to observe for the presence of hematomas and/or abdominal firmness. If vaginal packing is present, observe for active bleeding and follow the surgeon's orders for removal. Observe for signs and symptoms consistent with intra-abdominal bleeding, such as tachycardia, hypotension, oliguria (urine output < 20 mL/hour), confusion, or a firm abdomen.[12] The clinical presentation for uterine perforation is similar and includes abdominal distention, firmness of the abdomen, hypotension, or covert bleeding.[16] If hemorrhage or perforation is suspected and the patient is hemodynamically unstable, fluid resuscitation should be initiated and the patient prepped for a return to the operating room. In this case, the patient will require transfer to a higher level of care for prolonged monitoring.

Multimodal pain management is continued through the postoperative period. Although most gynecologic procedures can be managed with acetaminophen or a nonsteroidal anti-inflammatory drug, such as ibuprofen or ketorolac, opiates are sometimes prescribed and should only be administered as needed. Careful assessment can help rule out the presence of potential complications as the expected pain following obstetric and gynecologic procedures can often overlap with early signs of complications such as perforation or hemorrhage.

Follow-up phone calls are a key component of postoperative care. Postoperative phone calls impact patient satisfaction and patient outcomes and aid in early recognition of complications. These calls provide patients with an opportunity to ask clarifying questions regarding postoperative instructions and provide nurses with an opportunity to reinforce any additional teaching. Postoperative phone calls should be made within the first 24 hours after surgery, especially for hysterectomy patients who were discharged on the same day as surgery.

Patient Education

Patient education is paramount in outpatient surgery. Patients and their support person should be provided with both written and verbal instructions. These should include what to expect during recovery, signs and symptoms to report, and when to seek emergency care. Information on any new medications should be provided. Education should also include the importance of glucose control (especially within the first 48 hours), smoking cessation, venous thromboembolism prevention, and wound care. This is a process that should start in the surgeon's office and be reinforced preoperatively, postoperatively, during the follow-up phone call, and at the follow-up appointment as needed. Whenever possible, employ teach-back methods with demonstrations to ensure the patient and support person are understanding the instructions. This method also allows opportunities for questions and engages the patient and support person in preparation for the procedure and the postprocedural care.

Instructions should also incorporate multimodal pain management directions, including the use of over-the-counter analgesics, rest, nutrition, and comfort measures such as cold or heat therapy. Patients who are prescribed opiates should be instructed on their appropriate use, common side effects, how to minimize side effects, and how to destroy unused prescriptions. Patients should be instructed that applying heat, side lying, and walking can help alleviate chest, shoulder, and back discomfort associated with laparoscopic surgeries.

Minimal bleeding can be expected for 1 to 2 weeks following most obstetric and gynecologic procedures. Bleeding should not exceed that of a normal menstrual period, and patients should be instructed to report if they are soaking through an average-sized pad hourly or passing large clots. Providers may also recommend restrictions on heavy lifting and excessive activity. Additionally, to prevent infection, patients should refrain from sexual intercourse or inserting anything vaginally (e.g., tampons). Patients should be advised to report any concerns and not to self-diagnose or treat without contacting their surgeon first (e.g., yeast infections, dryness). If a LEEP or endometrial ablation was performed, patients should be informed that a watery discharge is normal but that a foul odor and/or vaginal irritation should be reported. Patients should also be reminded that amenorrhea, if that is the expectation following a LEEP or ablation procedure, may not be immediate.

The need for contraception should be discussed when applicable. Copper IUDs provide immediate contraceptive effects; however, patients should be instructed to avoid sexual intercourse for 24 hours and use an alternative contraceptive for at least 7 days following the placement of a hormone-releasing IUD. Although endometrial ablations may render the uterus unable to sustain a pregnancy, pregnancy is possible. For this reason, the use of contraceptive methods is recommended following an endometrial ablation given the high rates of complications with these pregnancies, such as miscarriage or prematurity.

Postoperative follow-up occurs for all patients and all procedures, but the timing and necessity are based on provider preference and the individualized needs of the patient. Patients who have undergone more complex procedures are typically seen by the surgeon 1–2 weeks following the surgery. Following IUD placement, it is recommended that patients have an appointment in 4 weeks to assess placement and to rule out the common complications of expulsion and perforation.[3]

ENHANCED RECOVERY AFTER SURGERY PROTOCOLS

To optimize patient outcomes following minimally invasive surgery, enhanced recovery after surgery (ERAS) protocols may be implemented. ERAS pathways are evidence-based interventions applied in a bundled approach across the surgical continuum. Potential interventions include preoperative patient education and engagement, fasting guidelines, analgesia, PONV prophylaxis, fluid optimization, thromboprophylaxis, antimicrobial therapy, normothermia maintenance, mobility, and diet. However, there is not currently a standardized approach. The concept supporting ERAS protocols is that the physiologic stress associated with surgery can be mitigated. Minimizing the stress response has been shown to reduce recovery times, shorten the lengths of stay, and decrease the overall costs of care.[13,17] When implemented, patients should be provided with both written and verbal education detailing the ERAS protocol. Patient guidebooks, one-on-one patient education sessions, group classes, access to nurse navigation and care coordination, and frequent multidisciplinary meetings can enhance success.

SAME-DAY DISCHARGE

The occurrence of same-day discharge, defined as discharge before midnight on the day of surgery, is on the rise for more complex procedures such as hysterectomies. Implementation of ERAS protocols, adoption of minimally invasive surgeries, advances in anesthetic options, and proper patient selection have contributed to the movement toward successful same-day discharge programs. Although consensus is currently lacking regarding patient inclusion criteria for the same-day discharge pathway, there is a clear consensus on the contraindications to same-day discharge, including the need for postoperative anticoagulation, poorly controlled chronic health conditions (e.g., noncompliant sleep apnea, unmanaged high blood pressure, mental health conditions), and poor home support or discharge plans.[13] Implementing a successful same-day discharge program requires an interprofessional approach, ongoing data collection, and concurrent modification of interventions based on the data. Although the success of same-day-discharge hysterectomies is variable in reports in the literature, studies have concluded that success is greater when patients are selected appropriately and ERAS protocols are followed.

ETHICAL CONSIDERATIONS IN OBSTETRIC AND GYNECOLOGIC SURGERY

Ethical decision making in the obstetric and gynecologic population is complicated by a variety of factors unique to the specialty. The greatest factor is the consideration that needs to occur of both the mother and the fetus, as there is a moral obligation to care for and protect both. Additional topics of ethical consideration include those surrounding reproductive health and technology. Decisions around reproductive health may include those related to sex (e.g., sexual violence, female genital mutilation), contraceptives, and abortion (e.g., therapeutic abortion, selective reduction). Reproductive technology includes "all reproductive treatments or procedures that manage human oocytes or embryos."[18] Recognizing and understanding these ethical considerations and how they can impact clinical decision making is key.

CHAPTER HIGHLIGHTS

- Advances in technology, anesthetics, and patient education have led to significant improvements in obstetric and gynecologic procedures and the settings in which they are performed.

- Procedures that were once performed in a hospital are now routinely performed in an office.
- More complex procedures, such as hysterectomies, are being performed in an outpatient setting.
- Perianesthesia nurses caring for these patients must have knowledge of the presenting conditions, actual procedures, and potential complications to effectively prepare and educate patients and their support persons for the experience.

CASE STUDY

Heather is a 45-year-old woman who has been experiencing irregular but heavy menses over the past two years. She has postponed her healthcare due to her active family lifestyle, but her symptoms of fatigue and pelvic discomfort have finally brought her to seek care. She reports that her mother went through menopause at an early age and has assumed this is what is happening to her now. Her gynecologist orders a standard panel of laboratory tests, including a pregnancy test (which is negative) and a hematocrit, which indicates mild anemia with a result of 29%. What therapy might the surgeon provide Heather prior to surgery to address her state of anemia? Heather reports she is not planning a future pregnancy and is now presenting to the ambulatory surgery center for an elective endometrial ablation.

The perianesthesia nurse preparing Heather overhears her tell her partner "I can't wait to never have to buy tampons again." Understanding that the ablation may not eliminate monthly uterine bleeding completely, how should the perianesthesia nurse respond to this comment?

As a female patient undergoing a gynecologic procedure, what PONV prophylaxis can be anticipated, if any? What are Heather's known risk factors for PONV?

Postoperatively, Heather discloses that she forgot about a deep vein thrombosis she experienced following orthopedic surgery while in her 30s. What recommendations should be made to mitigate Heather's risk for developing another blood clot?

REFERENCES

1. Baggish MS, Karram MM. *Atlas of Pelvic Anatomy and Gynecologic Surgery*. Elsevier; 2021.
2. Winer WK. Care of the obstetric and gynecological surgical patient. In: Odom-Forren J, ed. *Drain's PeriAnesthesia Nursing: A Critical Care Approach*. 7th ed. Elsevier; 2018.
3. Milton SH, Karjan NW, Isaacs C. Intrauterine device insertion. *Medscape*. 2021. Available at: https://emedicine.medscape.com/article/1998022-overview#a1.
4. American College of Obstetricians and Gynecologists. *Endometrial Ablation*. 2022. Available at: https://www.acog.org/womens-health/faqs/endometrial-ablation.
5. Famuyiide A. Endometrial ablation. *J Minim Invasive Gynecol.* 2017;25(2):299-307. Available at: https://doi.org/10.1016/j.jmig.2017.08.656.
6. Munro MG. Endometrial ablation. *Best Pract Res Clin Obstet Gynaecol.* 2018;46:120-139. Available at: https://doi.org/10.1016/j.bpobgyn.2017.10.003.
7. Kalogera E, Glaser GE, Kumar A, Dowdy SC, Langstraat CL. Enhanced recovery after minimally invasive gynecological procedures with bowel surgery: a systemic review. *J Minim Invasive Gynecol.* 2019;26(2):288-298. Available at: https://doi.org/10.1016/j.jmig.2018.10.016.
8. American College of Obstetricians and Gynecologists. *Hysterectomy*. 2021. Available at: https://www.acog.org/womens-health/faqs/hysterectomy.
9. Alshowaikh K, Karpinska-Leydier K, Amirthalingam J, et al. Surgical and patient outcomes of robotic versus conventional laparoscopic hysterectomy: a systematic review. *Cureus.* 2021;13(8):e16828. Available at: https://doi.org/10.7759/cureus.16828.
10. Smorgick N. Robotic-assisted hysterectomy: patient selection and perspectives. *Int J Womens Health.* 2017;9:157-161. Available at: https://doi.org/10.2147/IJWH.S99993.
11. Moises A, Castillo MYD, Garcia OFD. Perioperative management of pregnant women undergoing nonobstetric surgery. *Cleve Clin J Med.* 2021;88(1):27-34. Available at: https://doi.org/10.3949/ccjm.88a.18111.
12. Parker WH, Wagner WH. Management of hemorrhage in gynecologic surgery. *UpToDate.* 2022. Available at: https://www.uptodate.com/contents/management-of-hemorrhage-in-gynecologic-surgery#!
13. Stone R, Carey E, Fader AN, et al. Enhanced recovery and surgical optimization protocol for minimally invasive gynecological surgery: an AAGL white paper. *J Minim Invasive Gynecol.* 2021;28(2):179-203. Available at: https://doi.org/10.1016/j.jmig.2020.08.006.
14. American College of Obstetricians and Gynecologists Committee on Gynecologic Practice. Topical hemostatic agents at time of obstetric and gynecologic surgery. *Obstet Gynecol.* 2020;136(4):e81-e89. Available at: https://www.acog.org/clinical/clinical-guidance/committee-opinion/articles/2020/10/topical-hemostatic-agents-at-time-of-obstetric-and-gynecologic-surgery.
15. Jacob GP, Vilos GA, Al Turki F, et al. Ureteric injury during gynaecological surgery: lessons from 20 cases in Canada. *Facts Views Vis Obgyn.* 2020;12(1):31-42.
16. O'Brien D. Postanesthesia care complications. In: Odom-Forren J, ed. *Drain's PeriAnesthesia Nursing: A Critical Care Approach*. 7th ed. Elsevier; 2018:398-416.
17. American College of Obstetrics and Gynecologists Committee on Gynecologic Practice. Perioperative pathways: enhanced recovery after surgery. *Obstet Gynecol.* 2018;132(3):e120-e130. Available at: https://www.acog.org/clinical/clinical-guidance/committee-opinion/articles/2018/09/perioperative-pathways-enhanced-recovery-after-surgery.
18. Schweikart S. AMA code of medical ethics' opinions related to global reproductive health. *AMA J Ethics.* 2018;20(3):247-252. Available at: https://journalofethics.ama-assn.org/article/ama-code-medical-ethics-opinions-related-global-reproductive-health/2018-03.

29

Minimally Invasive Surgery, Laser Surgery, and Other Technologies

Katrina L. Bickerstaff, BSN, RN, CPAN, CAPA

LEARNING OBJECTIVES

A review of the content of this chapter will help the reader to:

1. Understand the history and general foundation of knowledge of ambulatory minimally invasive surgical procedures.
2. Describe common robotic and nonrobotic procedures, laparoscopic techniques, and endoscopic techniques performed in ambulatory settings.
3. Describe current laser techniques used for outpatient procedures.
4. Describe other nonsurgical minimally invasive modalities used in the ambulatory setting.
5. Describe the general nursing care for minimally invasive procedures.

OVERVIEW

Minimally invasive surgery is generally defined as an invasive procedure using natural orifice endoscopy and/or minimal surgical incisions to reduce damage and pain to the body. Minimally invasive surgery is quite different from open surgical techniques. Standard surgical procedures involve an incision through large areas of tissue to expose organs on which to operate. With minimally invasive surgery, the surgeon makes small incisions, called keyhole incisions, to gain access to the body and its internal structures so that operations can proceed rapidly with little injury and damage to the patient. Minimally invasive surgery has been made possible by small tubes called endoscopes and laparoscopes and tiny cameras and surgical instruments. Minimally invasive surgery reduces stress on the body because it proceeds much more rapidly and is less invasive than traditional surgical procedures. Hospital stays are reduced, and there are fewer complications. Most minimally invasive procedures are considered outpatient surgeries after which patients do not need to stay overnight in a medical facility.

There are many forms of minimally invasive surgery. Laparoscopy and endoscopy involve the passing of small instruments through one or more small incisions in the body or through natural openings into the digestive tract. Surgical robots provide magnified high-resolution, three-dimensional (3D) views of a surgical site and perform procedures that are guided by a surgeon.

Laser surgery incorporates the cutting power of a laser beam to make bloodless cuts in tissue or eliminate superficial lesions. There are many types of lasers in use today with variations in emitted wavelengths of light and power. Today's lasers have the ability to clot, cut, and vaporize tissue.

Evidence-Based Practice: Minimally invasive surgery
According to Mattingly, et al., the largest percent of minimally invasive surgeries (MIS), almost one in five outpatient surgeries, occurred in the ambulatory setting as recently as 2018. In order of frequency, laparoscopic cholecystectomies and appendectomies are the most common outpatient MIS procedures. These are followed by laparoscopic total hysterectomies, inguinal hernia repairs, and oophorectomies with or without salpingectomies. In comparison, it is estimated that only one in ten cases in the inpatient setting are considered MIS. The most common MIS surgeries in the inpatient setting also include laparoscopic cholecystectomies and appendectomies as well as vertical sleeve gastrectomies, gastric bypass procedures, and prostatectomies.

Source: Mattingly AS, Chen MM, Divi V, Holsinger FC, Saraswathula A. Minimally invasive surgery in the United States: Understanding its value using new datasets. *J Surg Res.* 2023;281:33-36. https://doi.org/10.1016/j.jss.2022.08.006

HISTORY OF MINIMALLY INVASIVE SURGERY

Minimally invasive procedures have been performed for a long time. Hippocrates, the father of medicine, detailed the use of a primitive anoscope for examining hemorrhoids in 400 BC. An Arabian named Abulkasim improved on Hippocrates's method around 1000 AD by reflecting light to examine the cervix. The main issue with these early attempts at endoscopy was finding an adequate light source. Fifteen hundred years passed without any major advancements in the field, until 1585, when Tulio Caesare Aranzi began focusing sunlight through a flask of water to project light into the nasal cavity.[1] It was not until the 19th century that Philipp Bozzini produced an endoscope with a light source. The device, the *Lichtleiter*, was a sharkskin-covered instrument housing a candle within a metal chimney.[2] A mirror on the inside reflected light from the candle through attachments into the urethra, vagina, or pharynx (Figure 29.1). One looked through a viewing window past the mirror down the funnel of the attachment. When the instrument was first tested in Vienna, examiners could see stones in a cadaver and were able to identify them as gallbladder stones. The light source used was from a series of mirrors and a candle. This was the basis of modern endoscopy.[2]

In 1901, the first experimental laparoscopy was performed on an animal model by Georg Kelling, a German surgeon. A visualizing scope was introduced into the peritoneum of a dog. Dr. Kelling made a small incision in the abdomen of a dog, insufflated the peritoneal cavity with sterile air, and was able to view the abdominal organs with a cystoscope. He had many goals for his new procedure, although his work found little support. Through his research, he established the importance of a sterile pneumoperitoneum to allow visualization, a basic principle for laparoscopic procedures.[1] The first laparoscopic procedure for humans was performed in 1910 by a physician named Hans Christian Jacobaeus. The technique was simple and relied on a syringe to instill air into the abdomen for insufflation. Air

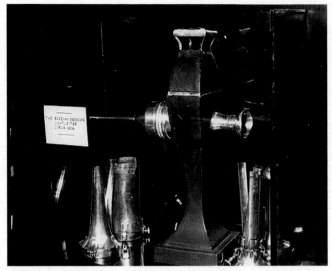

Fig. 29.1 Early endoscope. Philipp Bozzini called his device a "Lichtleiter," or light conductor. (Hanlon CR. Bozzini endoscope returns home. *Bull Am Coll Surg* 2002;87(7):39–40. https://www.facs.org/about-acs/archives/pasthighlights/bozzinihighlight)

emboli were a concern, and by 1938, a specific type of spring-loaded blunt-tip needle was developed by János Veres for drainage of ascites and evacuation of fluid and air from the chest. The application of the Veres needle was deemed safe for the instillation of gases into the abdomen, and thus it became an indispensable tool for many laparoscopic procedures. The Veres needle is still in use today.

The initial years of laparoscopic and endoscopic procedures were plagued by the limited lighting necessary for visualization. In 1954, two physicists named Harold Hopkins and Narinder Kapany developed the first functional fiberoptic prototype. With an adequate light source, visualization within the body cavity was limited to one physician hunched over and peering into the eyepiece of the scope. In 1982, practices changed with the evolution of a real-time high-resolution video camera that could be attached to the end of any endoscope. Once the image was projected onto the monitor, the surgeon could stand upright and work with both hands without handling the camera. The monitor was a game changer. At that point, the only constraints to minimally invasive surgery were suddenly shifted to the creativity, inspiration, and willingness of surgeons far and near.

Approximately five years after this key innovation, the revolution of minimally invasive surgery began. The first laparoscopic cholecystectomy was reported in 1987 by Philippe Mouret in Lyon, France. The evolution toward laparoscopy and thoracoscopy was a monumental shift in surgical capacity akin to the advent of general anesthesia and antiseptic agents. In the five years that followed, surgeons from every subspecialty began applying the surgical principles found in those original cholecystectomies.[1]

The first robotic surgical procedure was described in 1985. A modified industrial robot was used to guide a needle for a brain biopsy. This industrial robot, with an accuracy of 0.05 mm, served as a prototype for the neuromate, a modern stereotactic robot, which received approval from the Food and Drug Administration (FDA) in 1999 for nonlaparoscopic, image-guided, stereotactic, surgeon-controlled brain surgery.[3] This system allowed for the first successful robotic surgery. Robots now allow for great precision when used in minimally invasive surgeries, such as laparoscopies that use flexible fiberoptic cameras.

Robotic brain surgery in 1985 was the first laparoscopic procedure involving a robotic system; a cholecystectomy was performed in 1987; and in the following year a robot performed a transurethral resection. In 2000, the da Vinci system, a robotic surgical system using minimally invasive techniques, broke new ground by becoming the first robotic surgery system approved by the FDA for general laparoscopic surgery in both adults and children. The extent to which robotic surgery has been embraced by the surgical community has been unmatched. It has been driven in part by rapid advances in technology and by the ease with which adjustments have been made to existing laparoscopic procedures and techniques.

The term *laser* is an acronym for light amplification by stimulated emission of radiation. The laser would not have been possible without an understanding that light is a form of electromagnetic radiation. Medical lasers are medical devices employing precisely focused light sources to treat or remove tissues. Ordinary light, such as that from a lightbulb, has many wavelengths and spreads in all directions. Laser light, on the other hand, has a specific wavelength. It is focused on a narrow beam and creates an extremely high intensity light. In 1917, Einstein proposed the process that makes lasers possible, called stimulated emission. He theorized that, besides absorbing and emitting light spontaneously, under the proper circumstances atoms could release excess energy as light either spontaneously or when stimulated by light. It would take nearly 40 years before scientists would be able to amplify those emissions and put lasers on the path to becoming the powerful tools they are today.

In 1961, the first medical treatment using a laser on a human patient was performed at Columbia-Presbyterian Hospital in Manhattan by Dr. Charles J. Campbell of the Institute of Ophthalmology at Columbia-Presbyterian Medical Center and Charles J. Koester of the American Optical Company. An American Optical Company ruby laser was used to destroy a retinal tumor. Multiple gas lasers were developed by 1962, and the laser had already been applied in dermatologic and vocal cord surgery via the use of the surgical microscope.[4]

MINIMALLY INVASIVE SURGICAL PROCEDURES
Laparoscopic Procedures

There are several different techniques that surgeons can use to perform minimally invasive surgery. The goal of all these techniques is to decrease pain and speed recovery by eliminating the need for a large incision. Almost all minimally invasive surgeries are performed with the patient asleep under a general anesthetic apart from orthopedic minimally invasive procedures, for which a patient may opt for regional anesthesia.

Laparoscopic surgery is a technique in which the surgeon makes several small incisions about one-half inch in size instead of a single large incision. For most colon and rectal operations, three to five incisions are needed. Small tubes called trocars are placed through these incisions and into the abdomen. Carbon dioxide gas is used to inflate the abdomen to give the surgeon room to work and better visualize structures. This allows the surgeon to use a camera attached to a thin metal telescope (called a laparoscope) to watch a magnified view of the inside of the abdomen on operating room monitors. Special instruments have been developed for the surgeon to pass through the trocars to take the place of the surgeon's hands and traditional surgical instruments. Surgical stapling devices for dividing and reconnecting the intestine, as well as energy devices for cutting and cauterizing tissues and blood vessels, have also been adapted for laparoscopic use. For most operations, one slightly larger incision (2–four inches in length) must be made so that tissue can be removed from the abdomen.

Laparoscopic-assisted surgery is the term used to describe a procedure that is mainly performed laparoscopically and then completed through a small abdominal incision. Strictly speaking, many "laparoscopic" procedures are actually laparoscopic-assisted ones because some part of the operation is performed through the incision for specimen removal. For example, *hand-assisted laparoscopic surgery* is one variation of laparoscopic surgery in which a device is placed through a small, 2- to 3-inch incision that allows the surgeon to pass a hand into the abdomen to assist in performing the operation. The surgeon still uses the laparoscope to view the operation on monitors and uses the same instruments, staplers, and energy devices as in traditional laparoscopic surgery. The specimen is removed through the device used by the surgeon to place a hand in the abdomen. The main advantage of this procedure is that the ability to use the surgeon's hand may be necessary to complete the operation. The disadvantage is that the incision required might be slightly larger than would otherwise be necessary.

Single-incision surgery, also known as *single-site surgery*, is another minimally invasive option. With this technique, both the laparoscopic camera and the operating instruments are passed through a single small incision of approximately two inches in length that can also be used for removing the specimen. The primary advantage of this technique is that it results in less visible scarring since no additional small trocar incisions are necessary. The disadvantage is that most surgeons find this technique more difficult than traditional laparoscopic surgery because the instruments are placed so closely together.[5]

Over the past two decades, laparoscopic surgery has become extremely popular and offers advantages for patients over open surgery. Laparoscopy can also be used for diagnostic purposes, to examine organs, to check for abnormalities, or to obtain tissue samples. The main advantages are less pain, shorter recoveries, fewer hospital stays, and earlier returns to routine activities.[6]

Many surgeons of all specialties have embraced laparoscopic minimally invasive surgery. Today there are a multitude of minimally invasive ambulatory laparoscopic surgical procedures performed.

Video-Assisted Laparoscopic Thoracoscopic Procedures

Video-assisted thoracoscopic surgery involves the insertion of a tiny camera and surgical instruments through small incisions in the chest or neck to diagnose and treat problems affecting the lung, esophagus, and other areas in the chest.

Laparoscopic Surgery of the Biliary Tract

In most general surgeons' laparoscopic practices, laparoscopic cholecystectomy is the main procedure performed. Patients who undergo this procedure usually have symptomatic gallstones and a positive preoperative assessment for symptoms and signs of biliary tract disease.

Laparoscopic Appendectomy

An appendectomy is the surgical removal of the appendix, a finger-shaped sac attached to the beginning part of the colon (cecum). The appendix is in the lower right abdomen. Laparoscopy for suspected appendicitis is a straightforward procedure and is a common emergency surgery performed when the appendix is inflamed with infection. A laparoscopic appendectomy may also be done electively when the condition is chronic rather than acute.

Laparoscopic Herniorrhaphy

A hernia may be umbilical or inguinal, and it occurs when the inside layers of the abdominal wall have weakened and tissue (such as the intestine) becomes trapped in the wall and causes a bulge or tear. The minimally invasive laparoscopic approach involves multiple small incisions on the abdomen. The surgeon uses images from the laparoscope as a guide for repairing the hernia either by sewing the abdominal wall together or, often, using a prosthetic mesh placed over and covering the hernia defect.

Laparoscopic Gynecologic and Pelvic Procedures

During the last half century, laparoscopy has evolved from a limited gynecologic surgical procedure used only for diagnosis and tubal ligations to a major surgical tool used for a multitude of gynecologic indications. Like upper abdominal laparoscopic procedures, gynecologic laparoscopic pelvic surgery requires several small incisions, insufflation, and insertion of the laparoscope. Pelvic organs such as the uterus, ovaries, and fallopian tubes can be visualized. As a diagnostic tool, the procedure may determine the cause of pelvic pain; examine an abnormality such as a tissue mass, ovarian cyst, or tumor; confirm the presence of endometriosis; identify a pelvic inflammatory disease; examine the fallopian tubes for obstructions or an ectopic pregnancy; investigate conditions that might cause infertility; and observe the extent of ovarian, endometrial, or cervical cancer. Laparoscopy is not only used as a diagnostic tool but it can be used for many pelvic surgical procedures.

Examples of laparoscopic surgery include:

- Myomectomy (removal of uterine fibroids)
- Hysterectomy (removal of uterus)
- Endometrial ablation (destruction of uterine lining)
- Oophorectomy (removal of ovaries)
- Cystectomy (removal of ovarian cyst)
- Repair of pelvic organ prolapse
- Tubal ligation or reversal of tubal ligation

Arthroscopic Procedures

Although surgeons often use a gas to expand the surgical cavity for many minimally invasive laparoscopic procedures, they also use fluid as a medium for distention and irrigation. Orthopedic surgery is one procedure for which an irrigating fluid is infused. An orthopedic surgeon inserts a thin, flexible fiberoptic video camera called an arthroscope through an incision the size of a buttonhole near a joint (such as the knee or shoulder) to examine, diagnose, and sometimes repair joint damage. Arthroscopy is used to identify and treat tears, lesions, inflamed tissue, bone spurs, and other damage inside joints. The procedure is commonly performed on the shoulder, elbow, wrist, hip, knee, ankle, and foot. Minimally invasive spine surgery also uses a form of an endoscope to treat certain spinal conditions. Several endoscopic surgical techniques may be used to stabilize the spine and remove damaged tissue, bone spurs, or spinal discs that are compressing the spinal cord and causing pain.

Natural Orifice Transluminal Endoscopic Surgery

Natural orifice transluminal endoscopic surgery (NOTES) has emerged as one of the most exciting areas in the field of minimally invasive surgery during the last decade. This is a surgery that allows access to the body cavity through natural orifices, such as the oral, rectal, urethral, or vaginal openings, with little to no scarring. Since polypectomy was first performed in 1955, major advances in technology and refinements of endoscopic technique have allowed endoscopic surgeons to perform complex endoscopic interventions.[7] NOTES comprises a wide spectrum of procedures. They use various natural accesses such as transgastric or transvaginal routes. They also can focus on different direct-target or distant-target organs. For instance, a transvaginal approach can be used for gallbladder removal in patients who have suffered traumatic intentional puncture of an organ (e.g., stomach, rectum, vagina, or urinary bladder); an endoscope is used to gain access to the abdominal cavity and perform an intra-abdominal operation.

NOTES has been theorized to offer benefits such as decreased postoperative pain with less need for postoperative analgesia, shorter hospital stays, faster recoveries, and less scarring. Additionally, NOTES may provide easy alternative access to the body cavity in morbidly obese patients, in whom traditional open or laparoscopic access can be difficult because of the thickness of the abdominal wall. Lastly, NOTES may reduce the lifetime risk of incision-related complications in children.

Bronchoscopy

Bronchoscopy is the use of a flexible tube with a light and a camera called a bronchoscope. This scope is inserted through the nose or mouth to look inside the lungs and airways. Bronchoscopy helps to evaluate and diagnose lung problems, assess blockages, obtain samples of tissue or fluid, and help remove a foreign body.

Hysteroscopy

Hysteroscopy uses a small, narrow, thin, lighted tube (hysteroscope) inserted through the vagina to allow visualization of the inside of the uterine cavity, cervix, and vagina without the need for any incisions. This is often done to evaluate uterine bleeding. Specialized hysteroscopes are also used for treatment in some cases, such as the removal of fibroids, polyps, or scar tissue.

Endoscopy

Endoscopy is used to examine the inside of the digestive tract by means of a small, flexible tube (endoscope) with a light and a camera lens at the end. Tissue samples from inside the digestive tract may also be taken for examination and testing. The endoscope may be passed orally to view and diagnose conditions of the upper gastrointestinal system. A sigmoidoscopy is a procedure that examines the rectum and lower part of the large intestine, and a colonoscopy examines the entire colon.

Laryngoscopy

An indirect laryngoscopy uses a light source and a small mirror to observe the inside of a patient's throat. The mirror usually has long handles, which help to place the mirror safely against the roof of a patient's mouth. A direct flexible laryngoscopy involves a small telescope located at the end of a cable. The cable and telescope are inserted through the nose and then down the patient's throat. Both procedures allow the surgeon to view the larynx, including the vocal cords, as well as nearby structures such as the back of the throat. Like other scopes, these instruments can be used to take biopsy samples of the vocal cords or nearby parts of the throat.

Cystourethroscopy

The cystourethroscopy is a procedure used to examine the entire bladder lining and take biopsies of any areas that look questionable, view the lower urinary tract, collect urine samples, and examine the prostate gland. The cystoscope is a thin tube with a light and a lens or small video camera on the end. The tube is passed through the urethra.

The Future of Natural Orifice Transluminal Endoscopic Surgery

NOTES is considered a new type of hybrid endoscopic surgery. There are many procedures currently being studied at hospitals and research facilities around the world. NOTES represents the next frontier of surgical principles and endoscopic techniques. Currently, the standard approach to reaching the peritoneal cavity is via a surgical incision through the skin, which allows the introduction of a small camera deep into the abdomen. The NOTES surgical technique offers a new modality with which organs such as the gallbladder can be removed without external incisions or scars. As research results in advances in techniques, NOTES is evolving and becoming more commonplace in surgical centers around the world.

Minimally Invasive Robotic Procedures

Robotic surgery, or *robotic-assisted surgery*, is a newer variation on minimally invasive surgery that has revolutionized the way many surgical procedures are being performed. Robotic procedures represent a new standard of care that has resulted from rapid developments in technology and, also, modifications made to existing laparoscopic procedures and surgical techniques. The ease with which these modifications have been made has contributed to the rapid pace of advancement. Robotic surgery is a form of laparoscopy. Small incisions about a half inch each are made through which a surgeon can place a laparoscope and instruments for surgical procedures. In traditional laparoscopy, a surgeon holds the instruments and directly places them through the incisions. The instruments can move forward and backward and can be opened and closed manually. In robotic surgery, the same incisions are made and the same instruments placed but the instruments are usually held in place by robotic arms. The surgeon controls the robotic arms and instruments from a control center or console while tracking his or her progress using a 3D image on a monitor and operating controls to maneuver robotic arms that perform the surgery. The console is usually several feet away from the patient but in the same operating room. The console can also be controlled from a remote location.

While robotic surgery is relatively new, it has proven useful for treating areas of the body that are difficult to navigate, such as the head and neck and deep abdominal or genital areas. Use of the robotic arms allows surgeons to work with precision and dexterity. There are differences between the techniques of open surgical procedures, minimally invasive laparoscopic procedures, and robotic surgical procedures[8] (Table 29.1).

There are many different procedures, from oral surgery to rectal procedures, being performed by surgical robots. The minimally invasive nature of robotic surgery is being used for many ambulatory procedures that would have required long hospital stays if performed traditionally. Some of the more common robotic procedures are listed in Box 29.1.

Robotic Gynecologic Procedures

Surgeons have been using robots to assist with female reproductive surgeries since 2005. Hysterectomies and procedures for treating pelvic organ prolapse, fibroids, and problems with ovaries or fallopian tubes are commonplace.

TABLE 29.1 Differences Between Robotic, Laparoscopic, and Traditional Open Surgical Procedures

Aspect	Laparoscopic Surgery	Robotic Surgery	Open Surgery
Incision	Small multiple	Small multiple	One larger
Instrumentation	Cameras Laparoscopes Small instruments	Cameras Robot console Small natural dexterity instruments	General surgical hand instruments
Visualization	Direct visualization 2D imaging	3D visualization Good geometric accuracy Motion scaling	Direct visualization Hand-eye coordination
Level of dexterity	Limited due to incisional constraints Loss of depth perception Poor ergonomics	Stable No fatigue	Touch enhanced
Access to body cavity	Able to reach areas not reached by human hands Limited range of motion	Able to reach inaccessible areas of the body	Full access via incision
Recovery time	Shorter recovery	Shorter recovery	Longer recovery
Advantages	Less inpatient stays Less recovery time Increased patient satisfaction Enhanced cosmetic outcome Less infection Less blood loss Lower cost	Surgeon directly in the field Less inpatient stays Less infection Less blood loss Shorter recovery time Increased patient satisfaction Enhanced cosmetic outcome Able to use qualitative information	Surgeon directs the robots via a console in real time Generally short total surgical time
Disadvantages	Touch decreased Surgeon prone to fatigue/tremor	Touch absence Learning curve Unable to use qualitative information Procedure time No judgment Surgeon away from bedside, directs robot from console	Surgeon prone to fatigue/tremor Less sterile, high infection rate More traumatic More painful Increased blood loss Large scar, disfigurement

Lanfranco AR, Castellanos AE, Desai JP, Meyers WC. Robotic surgery: A current perspective. *Ann Surg.* 2004;239(1):14–21. https://doi.org/10.1097/01.sla.0000103020.19595.7

BOX 29.1 Ambulatory Minimally Invasive Robotic Surgical Procedures

Bariatric surgery

Gastric bypass
Gastric sleeve
Gastric banding

General surgery

Cholecystectomy
Herniorrhaphy

Gynecologic surgery

Hysterectomy
Sacrocolpopexy
Myomectomy
Endometriosis resection

Urologic surgery

Partial nephrectomy
Prostatectomy

Orthopedic surgery

Joint (hip, knee) replacement

Lanfranco AR, Castellanos AE, Desai JP, Meyers WC. Robotic surgery: A current perspective. *Ann Surg.* 2004;239(1):14–21. https://doi.org/10.1097/01.sla.0000103020.19595.7d

Robotic Genitourinary Procedures

Male patients with prostate cancer may have the prostate removed using the robotic surgery system. This means less pain, minimal blood loss, and a faster recovery than with open surgery. Traditional laparoscopic prostate surgery and robotic prostate surgery seem similar in these regards. Other operations on the urinary tract can also be done robotically.

- Pyeloplasty: repairs an abnormality of the kidney and nearby ureter.
- Cystectomy: removes all or part of the bladder to treat bladder cancer.
- Nephrectomy: treats kidney cancer, kidney stones, or kidney disease by removing all or part of the kidney.
- Ureteral reimplantation: disconnects the ureter from the bladder and reconnects it to keep urine from flowing backward from the bladder into the kidneys

Robotic Head and Neck Surgeries

Surgeons often have difficulty reaching some areas of the mouth and throat with typical minimally invasive techniques. The robot's smaller, more flexible instruments assist the surgeon using techniques such as transoral robotic surgery, which is performed through the mouth using three robotic arms, to treat cancer and other conditions.

Robotic Colorectal Surgeries

Surgery can help patients with many conditions in the colon and rectum, including colorectal cancer, inflammatory bowel disease, and hemorrhoids. Robotically assisted surgery proves particularly valuable for rectal operations, performed within the tight confines of the pelvis. Other surgeries include colon resection, rectal resection, and rectopexy.

Robotic Gastrointestinal Surgeries

Gallbladder surgery was one of the first procedures to be performed with a laparoscope, and it is now commonly done with robotic assistance. Robotic surgery is also used to help surgeons treat people with gastrointestinal cancers, remove lymph nodes, remove and reconstruct organs and tissues, and conduct bariatric weight loss procedures.

Robotic Joint Replacement Surgeries

Two slightly different robotic surgical systems have been developed to perform hip and knee replacements. In some cases, they perform specific tasks that a surgeon would otherwise do by hand, including making a space in the bone to insert part of an artificial joint. In others, they help the surgeon do this work more precisely. Robotic joint replacements use computer software to convert anatomic information into a virtual patient-specific 3D reconstruction of the joint.[9]

Laser Surgical Procedures

There are several types of laser surgeries, and most have resulted in better wound healing than the same surgeries done with conventional surgical instruments; the type of laser, wavelength used, and delivery system chosen are part of this improvement.[10] Surgeons use lasers to cut, coagulate, and remove tissue. Laser therapy is an attractive alternative to common excision due to its minimally invasive effect. Today, lasers are widely used in the diagnosis and treatment of many diseases. Lasers produce bloodless cuts in tissue and can eliminate superficial lesions such as skin tumors.

Lasers emit different wavelengths of light and have various levels of power and ability to clot, cut, or vaporize tissue. Lasers can relieve the bleeding or obstruction resulting from some diseases. For example, lasers can shrink or destroy colon polyps and tumors that have created intestinal or gastric obstructions. Laser therapy is sometimes used alone, but it is also often used with traditional surgical methods, chemotherapy, or radiation therapy. Lasers can close nerve endings to relieve postoperative pain and seal lymph vessels to decrease swelling and slow the growth of tumor cells.

Most lasers have an energy source, an active medium, and a resonant cavity. The energy source can be electrical current, a high-powered lamp, or a chemical reaction. As the light beam passes through the active medium, photons stimulate each other and energy is continually built up. The active medium may be a solid, a liquid, or a gas.

The beam can be pulsed or continuous. A laser delivery system can use fibers, an articulated arm, or fixed optics. It can be connected to an operating microscope or used through an endoscope.[11]

The three types of lasers most often used in medical treatment are the carbon dioxide laser, neodymium:yttrium-aluminum-garnet (Nd:YAG) laser, and argon laser. The carbon dioxide laser is primarily a surgical tool. It converts light energy to heat that is strong enough to minimize bleeding while it cuts through or vaporizes tissue. The neodymium:yttrium-aluminum-garnet laser is capable of penetrating tissue more deeply than other lasers.

It causes blood to clot quickly and can enable surgeons to see and work on parts of the body that could otherwise be reached only through open surgery.

The argon laser provides the limited penetration needed for eye surgery and superficial skin disorders. In a special procedure known as photodynamic therapy, this laser uses light-sensitive dyes to shrink or dissolve tumors.

Because minimally invasive techniques are continually being sought for the treatment of different pathologic processes, the use of lasers has become increasingly popular in modern medicine. Often referred to as *bloodless surgery*, laser procedures usually involve less bleeding than conventional surgery. The heat generated by the laser keeps the surgical site free of germs and reduces the risk of infection. Because only a small incision is required, laser procedures often take less time (and cost less money) than traditional surgery. Sealing off blood vessels and nerves reduces bleeding, swelling, scarring, pain, and the length of the recovery period.[12] In addition to their practical usefulness in the operating room, lasers have a wide range of applications in almost every part of the body (Figure 29.2).

Endovenous Laser Ablation

Endovenous laser ablation is a new method of treating varicose veins. Instead of tying and removing the abnormal veins, as was done with traditional methods, the veins are heated by a laser. The heat kills the walls of the veins, and the body then naturally absorbs the dead tissue. Endovenous treatment is currently one of the most frequently used methods for varicose veins.

Laser Surgeries for Laryngeal Disorders

Laser surgery through the mouth is a treatment for early stage and locally advanced laryngeal cancers. Laser vocal cord surgery is an endoscopic procedure used to remove and treat several conditions that affect the vocal cords, including vocal cord dysplasia, benign nodules, polyps, laryngeal papillomas, and some laryngeal malignancies. This style of minimally invasive surgery is becoming increasingly popular in the United States and abroad.

Laser Photo Vaporization of the Prostate

Laser photo vaporization of the prostate (PVP) is a minimally invasive treatment for an enlarged prostate. During laser PVP surgery, a tube with an imaging system (cystoscope) is inserted into the penis. A surgeon places a laser through the cystoscope to burn away excess tissue blocking urine flow through the prostate.[13]

Femtosecond Laser-Assisted Cataract Surgery

Cataract surgery is one of the most common operations in healthcare. Femtosecond laser-assisted cataract surgery enables more precise ocular incisions and lens fragmentation than does phacoemulsification cataract surgery. The femtosecond laser creates a round opening in the anterior capsule by dissecting it with a circular laser pattern crossing the anterior capsule. This has several advantages over the manual creation of openings, which is the most technically challenging aspect of cataract surgery.[14]

Laser Surgery for Cutaneous Lesions

Laser/light therapy is a nontoxic and noninvasive therapy that uses light energy to repair and regenerate skin cells. The procedure reduces the need for medication, improves the outcomes for skin conditions treated, and increases the recovery rates of

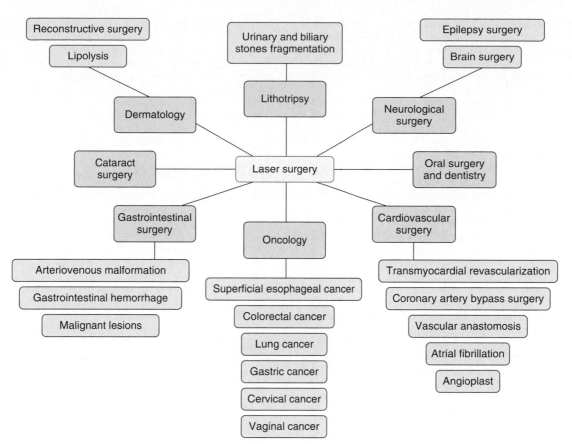

Fig. 29.2 Laser applications in surgery. Khalkhal E, Rezaei-Tavirani M, Zali MR, Akbari Z. The evaluation of laser application in surgery: A review article. *J Lasers Med Sci*. 2019;10(Suppl 1):104–111. Figure 1. https://doi.org/10.15171/jlms.2019.s18

affected tissues. Therapeutic indications include, but are not limited to, actinic and seborrheic keratoses, warts, moles, skin tags, epidermal and dermal nevi, scar treatment, keloids, skin cancers, and neurofibromas.

Hemorrhoidectomy with the Carbon Dioxide Laser

Laser hemorrhoidectomy is a new laser procedure for the outpatient treatment of hemorrhoids. The hemorrhoidal arterial flow feeding the hemorrhoidal plexus is stopped by means of Doppler-guided laser coagulation. The narrow laser beam is precise and accurate and the procedure results in rapid, unimpaired healing.[15] It seals small blood vessels and thereby allows a bloodless field. The laser approach also seals superficial nerve endings, giving the patient no or minimal postoperative discomfort.

OTHER MINIMALLY INVASIVE TECHNOLOGIES
Radiofrequency Ablation Procedures

Radiofrequency ablation is a minimally invasive procedure and is considered a modified electrocautery technique that has emerged as the frontrunner among the many choices for local, minimally invasive tissue ablation. It is effective, adaptable, and relatively inexpensive. Radiofrequency ablation has been used for years in the treatment of cardiac dysrhythmias from aberrant conduction pathways, osteoid osteoma, prostate hypertrophy, and chronic pain. More recent clinical applications include tumor ablation in the liver, kidney, adrenal gland, bone, lung, and breast, as well as soft tissue debulking and pain palliation.[16] Radiofrequency ablation works by passing electrical current in the range of radio waves between a needle electrode positioned in the tumor and grounding pads placed on the patient's skin. The radiofrequency current produces a prominent level of heat within the tumor tissue surrounding the electrode.

Cryotherapy

Cryotherapy is a minimally invasive therapy that removes damaged or diseased tissue in a variety of medical conditions. Cryotherapy uses imaging guidance, a needle-like applicator called a cryoprobe, and liquid nitrogen or argon gas to create intense cold to freeze and destroy diseased tissue, including cancer cells. Physicians use image-guidance techniques such as ultrasound, computed tomography scanning, or magnetic resonance imaging to help guide the cryoprobes to treatment sites inside the body. The technique is used to treat a variety of skin conditions, as well as tumors in the liver, kidneys, bones, lungs, and breasts.

GENERAL CONSIDERATIONS IN MINIMALLY INVASIVE PROCEDURES

Minimally invasive surgery is becoming increasingly popular. The term *minimally invasive surgery* is not a description of surgery that is trivial or easy. The method does offer the benefits of less postoperative pain, early ambulation, and shorter hospital stays, as well as better cosmetic results. The anesthetic management is aimed at getting the patient safely through the procedure and minimizing the specific risks arising from the laparoscopy and the patient's coexisting medical problems. Appropriate anesthetic techniques help to ensure a quick recovery and a relatively pain-free postoperative course with early return to normal function.

There are many challenges for the anesthesia provider during minimally invasive surgeries. There is often restricted access to the surgical site, and the insufflation of gas into the peritoneum or extraperitoneal space may pose unique challenges associated with the creation of a pneumoperitoneum or the absorption of the carbon dioxide. These challenges may result in severe complications such as pulmonary embolism, pneumothorax, pneumomediastinum, and hemodynamic instability. Specific positioning and monitoring of a patient to whom the anesthesia provider often has restricted access, often in a poorly lit environment, can contribute to anesthetic complications.

As laparoscopic and robotic surgical procedures become more refined and commonplace, anesthesia providers are being presented with patients from higher-risk groups, including obese patients, elderly patients, and patients with advanced cardiac and respiratory disease. Many of these patients were once deemed unsuitable for laparoscopic techniques.

The overall anesthetic management is aimed at getting the patient safely through the procedure and minimizing the specific risks arising from the laparoscopy and the patient's coexisting medical problems.

All patients presenting for minimally invasive robotic or nonrobotic surgeries must be thoroughly assessed with respect to issues inherent to the planned surgical approach and the patient's medical status. Since a quick recovery and minimal disruption to the patient's everyday routine are desirable goals for minimally invasive surgeries, the anesthetic technique focuses on these goals, as well. Controllable IV and volatile anesthetics with a favorable pharmacokinetic and pharmacodynamic profile are usually used for both the induction and maintenance of anesthesia. The ideal anesthetic for minimally invasive surgery should have a quick onset and short duration of action and should be free of adverse effects.[17]

Preoperative Considerations

When a patient is deemed a candidate for a robotic or a laparoscopic operation, the specific history relevant to this approach includes the acuity and complexity of the patient's disease process and a history of chronic obstructive pulmonary disease, cardiac disease, or prior abdominal surgeries. Pulmonary function testing and assessment of the hypoxia baseline and hypercarbia may be necessary and may make laparoscopy more precarious than laparotomy in borderline cases. Cardiac risk factors are relevant to the patient's anesthetic risk, as well as the suspected insult of the planned procedure, but the reduction of cardiac output caused by pneumoperitoneum may also need to be a factor. No amount of prior abdominal surgery contraindicates laparoscopy, but the location of scars and any history of adhesions encountered in prior surgeries are considered. Patient-specific variations in adhesion formation, inflammatory and infectious processes, foreign bodies such as mesh, and immunosuppression may all impact the degree of intra-abdominal scar formation.[18]

Postoperative Considerations

The complications unique to robotic and laparoscopic surgeries include those related to the creation of a pneumoperitoneum, patient positioning, and surgical instrumentation. Intraperitoneal carbon dioxide insufflation and changes in patient positioning during laparoscopic surgery have several hemodynamic, pulmonary, and endocrine consequences. In addition, several surgical complications, including subcutaneous emphysema, pneumothorax, pneumomediastinum, gas embolization, acute hemorrhage, and bowel or bladder perforation, can occur during either the robotic or laparoscopic approach. Postoperative complications include pain, nausea, vomiting, pulmonary impairment, wound infection, peritonitis, delayed hemorrhage, incisional hernia, and metastases at the trocar insertion sites.[19]

CHAPTER HIGHLIGHTS

- Minimally invasive surgery reduces stress on the body by taking less time and being less invasive than traditional surgical procedures.
- Forms of minimally invasive surgery include laparoscopy, arthroscopy, natural orifice transluminal endoscopic surgery, robotic procedures, laser procedures, radiofrequency ablation, and cryotherapy.
- The ideal anesthetic for minimally invasive surgery should have a quick onset and short duration of action and should be free of adverse effects.

CASE STUDY

Arthur is a 74-year-old patient of a newly hired urologist. He presents with a history of chronic pain, arthritis, failed spinal fusions, and mild hypertension. On a recent annual checkup his prostate-specific antigen test was normal, but he continues to have complaints of urinary frequency and "dribbling." He never feels as though he is able to empty his bladder. The surgeon informs Arthur that his condition is benign prostatic hypertrophy and he should have no fear of cancer. The surgeon is recommending that Arthur be scheduled for a laser photo vaporization of the prostate.

Arthur has many questions. The preoperative perianesthesia nurse is prepared to answer the following questions from this patient:

Will I be asleep for this procedure?
How is this procedure performed?
What should I expect for pain postoperatively?
Will I have to stay overnight for this procedure?

REFERENCES

1. St. Peter SD, Holcomb GW. History of minimally invasive surgery. *Atlas of Pediatric Laparoscopy and Thoracoscopy.* Elsevier; 2016.
2. Engel R. Development of the modern cystoscope: an illustrated history. *Medscape.* 2007. Available at: https://www.medscape.com/viewarticle/561774.
3. Hockstein NG, Gourin CG, Faust RA, Terris DJ. A history of robots: from science fiction to surgical robotics. *J Robot Surg.* 2007;1(2): 113-118. Available at: https://doi.org/10.1007/s11701-007-0021-2.
4. Rose M, Hogan H. A history of the laser: 1960 – 2019. *Photonics Media.* 2019. Available at: https://www.photonics.com/Articles/AHistory_of_the_Laser_1960_-_2019/a42279.
5. American College of Colon and Rectal Surgeons. *Minimally invasive surgery expanded version.* 2020. Available at: https://fascrs.org/patients/diseases-and-conditions/a-z/minimally-invasive-surgery-expanded-version.
6. Lee-Kong S, Feingold DL. The history of minimally invasive surgery. *Semin Colon Rectal Surg.* 2013;24(1):3-6. Available at: https://doi.org/10.1053/j.scrs.2012.10.003.
7. Hon-chi Y, Wai-yan Chiu P. Recent advances in natural orifice transluminal endoscopic surgery. *Eur J Cardiothorac Surg.* 2016;49(1): 25-30. Available at: https://doi.org/10.1093/ejcts/ezv364.

8. Lanfranco AR, Castellanos AE, Desai JP, Meyers WC. Robotic surgery: a current perspective. *Ann Surg.* 2004;239(1):14-21. Available at: https://doi.org/10.1097/01.sla.0000103020.19595.7d.

9. Kayani B, Haddad FS. Robotic total knee arthroplasty. *Bone Joint Res.* 2019;8(10):438-442. Available at: https://doi.org/10.1302%2F2046-3758.810.BJR-2019-0175.

10. Khalkhal E, Rezaei-Tavirani M, Zali MR, Akbari Z. The evaluation of laser application in surgery: a review article. *J Lasers Med Sci.* 2019;10(suppl 1):104-111. Available at: https://doi.org/10.15171/jlms.2019.s18.

11. Miller G. Minimally invasive surgery, laser, and other technologies. In: Burden N, Quinn DMD, O'Brien D, Dawes BSG, eds. *Ambulatory Surgical Nursing.* 2nd ed. Elsevier; 2000.

12. Encyclopedia of Surgery. *Laser Surgery.* 2022. Available at: https://www.surgeryencyclopedia.com/La-Pa/Laser-Surgery.html.

13. Berquet G, Corbel L, Della Negra E, et al. Prospective evaluation of ambulatory laser vaporization of the prostate for benign prostatic hyperplasia. *Lasers Surg Med.* 2015;47(5):396-402. Available at: https://doi.org/10.1002/lsm.22363.

14. Lawless M, Bala C. Femtosecond laser-assisted cataract surgery. *US Ophthalmic Review.* 2014;7(2):82-88. Available at: https://doi.org/10.17925/USOR.2014.07.02.82.

15. Agbo SP. Surgical management of hemorrhoids. *J Surg Tech Case Report.* 2011;3(2):68-75. Available at: https://doi.org/10.4103/2006-8808.92797.

16. Friedman M, Mikityansky I, Kam A, et al. Radiofrequency ablation of cancer. *Cardiovasc Intervent Radiol.* 2004;27(5):427-434. Available at: http://dx.doi.org/10.1007/s00270-004-0062-0.

17. Dec M, Andruszkiewicz P. Anesthesia for minimally invasive surgery. *Video Surgery and Other Miniinvasive Techniques.* 2015;10(4):509-514. Available at: http://dx.doi.org/10.1007/s00270-004-0062-0.

18. Tsuda S. *Preoperative Considerations for Minimally Invasive Surgery.* Society of American Gastrointestinal and Endoscopic Surgeons. n.d. Available at: https://www.sages.org/wiki/preoperative-considerations-minimally-invasive-surgery/.

19. Joshi GP. Complications of laparoscopy. *Anesthesiol Clin North Am.* 2001;19(1):89-105. Available at: https://doi.org/10.1016/s0889-8537(05)70213-3.

Ophthalmic Surgery

Angelique Weathersby, MSN, MBA, RN

LEARNING OBJECTIVES

A review of the content of this chapter will help the reader to:

1. Describe common ophthalmic surgery procedures performed.
2. Identify medications frequently used in ophthalmic surgery.
3. Discuss implications of ophthalmic surgery for pediatric and geriatric patients.
4. Identify nursing care for specific surgical procedures.

OVERVIEW

Ophthalmology is a medical specialty concerned with the diagnosis and treatment of disorders of the eye. Though more common in the elderly, ophthalmic surgery is performed on people of all ages to treat injuries and diseases of the eye. Caring for the ophthalmic surgical patient presents unique challenges to the perianesthesia registered nurse. Not only does the nurse need to possess a thorough knowledge of postoperative care but she or he must also be familiar with all aspects of ophthalmic surgery to provide quality care. In addition, the perianesthesia nurse needs to understand the normal anatomy of the eye. The basic anatomy of the eye is illustrated in Figure 30.1.

Due to technologic advances and increasing pressures to contain costs, many ophthalmic surgery procedures are being performed in free-standing ambulatory surgery centers rather than hospitals. Patients can return home within 24 hours of surgery. The perianesthesia nurse must have strong assessment and communication skills to provide care for the patient's needs preoperatively. The nurse must be vigilant and able to recognize and treat postoperative complications, provide patient education and emotional support, and maintain patient safety in a fast-paced environment.[1-4]

FACTS AND FIGURES

Cataracts are the leading cause of vision loss in the United States and of blindness worldwide. The risk of cataracts increases with age. In 2010, White Americans 40 years of age and older had the highest prevalence rate of cataracts (18%), followed by Black Americans (13%) and Hispanic Americans (12%). By 2050, it is expected that the number of people in the United States with cataracts will double. Most cases will be seen in White people, though Hispanic Americans are expected to have the most rapid increase in prevalence.

Glaucoma is the second leading cause of blindness. In 2010, glaucoma affected about 1.9% of people in the United

States age 40 and older. Black Americans had the highest prevalence rate (3.4%), followed by Americans of other races (2.1%), White Americans (1.7%), and Hispanic Americans (1.5%). By 2050, the number of people in the United States with glaucoma is expected to increase by more than double.

Refractive errors are the most frequent eye problems in the United States. More than 23.9% of Americans aged 40 and older have nearsightedness (myopia), and 8.4% have farsightedness (hyperopia). More than 150 million Americans use corrective eyewear to compensate for refractive errors, at a cost of more than $15 billion each year. Approximately 800,000 surgeries to correct refractory errors were done in 2010.[5,6]

ANESTHESIA CONSIDERATIONS

The plan for the type of anesthesia to be used for a patient's surgery is determined by the anesthesiologist together with the surgeon and the patient. The decision is based on the type of surgical procedure, the length of the surgery, the patient's preference, and the patient's age and health status. Risk factors for co-morbidities such as hypertension, diabetes mellitus, renal insufficiency, chronic heart failure, advanced age, and chronic obstructive lung disease place the patient at higher risk for anesthetic complications.[7]

Illicit drug use is increasingly frequent in the general population and in those requiring anesthesia for surgery.[8-10] The anesthesia plan must include consideration of potential drug interactions and a strategy to alleviate the effects of drug withdrawal.

There are four types of local anesthetics used for ophthalmic surgery: retrobulbar, peribulbar, sub-Tenon's, and topical.[11,12] For patients with the ability to lie still during the procedure, a local anesthetic may be a good choice. The retrobulbar and peribulbar approaches are needle-based techniques. The differences between these two blocks are in the insertion site and the depth and angles of the needle placement. The retrobulbar block (Figure 30.2) involves blocking the ciliary nerves, ciliary ganglion, and cranial nerves III, IV, and VI. Cranial nerve VII is not blocked, allowing the patient to close the eye (see Figure 30.2). The peribulbar block involves blocking the ciliary nerves and cranial nerves III and IV. Cranial nerve II (optic nerve) is not blocked, so vision is unaffected. Most complications related to these blocks are due to needle misplacement and include hemorrhage, subconjunctival edema, perforation of the globe, optic nerve atrophy, central spread of the local anesthetic, brainstem injury, and allergic reaction. The risk of hemorrhage and atrophy of the optic nerve is lower with the peribulbar technique. The technique for the sub-Tenon's block involves instillation of a local anesthetic in the space under the Tenon's capsule (dense connective tissue surrounding the globe) and blocks the ciliary nerves. It is considered a safe alternative to the two needle blocks. Complications related to the sub-Tenon's technique are mainly subconjunctival swelling and subconjunctival hemorrhage.[13]

Topical anesthesia involves instilling local anesthetic eye drops on the cornea. In addition to being quick and easy to perform, this technique avoids the potential complications

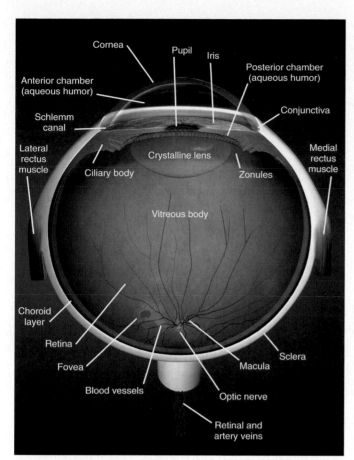

Fig. 30.1 Anatomy of the eye. Horizontal section through left globe. Mielcarek ED. Ophthalmic Surgery. Figure 18.1 in: Rothrock JC. *Alexander's Care of the Patient in Surgery*. 16th ed. Elsevier. 2019.

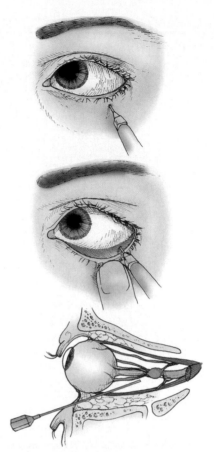

Fig. 30.2 Retrobulbar block. Mielcarek ED. Ophthalmic Surgery. Figure 18.9 in: Rothrock JC. *Alexander's Care of the Patient in Surgery*. 16th ed. Elsevier. 2019.

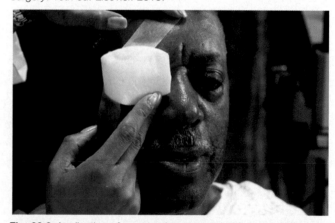

Fig. 30.3 Application of a protective eye patch. Mielcarek ED. Ophthalmic Surgery. Figure 18.13 in: Rothrock JC. *Alexander's Care of the Patient in Surgery*. 16th ed. Elsevier. 2019.

related to needle blocks. Limitations of topical anesthesia include the possibility of incomplete anesthesia, shorter duration, and mobility of the eyeball and the lids.

General anesthesia is used for patients without the ability to lie still (e.g., uncooperative patients or children), patients with a frequent cough, and unstable critical care or trauma patients.

GENERAL NURSING CARE
Preoperative Care

"The scope of perianesthesia nursing practice involves the cultural [and] social complexities [and the] developmental and age-specific assessment, diagnosis, intervention, and evaluation of individuals across the perianesthesia continuum and phases of care."[14] Assessment of the patient's physical and emotional status prior to surgery is an important part of preoperative care.[15-17] The nurse providing preoperative care is focused on preparing the patient for surgery. Clear, complete communication between the patient, family or caregiver, and perianesthesia nurse is essential to promote patient safety and enhance patient satisfaction. A medically approved interpreter should be used if there is a language barrier. Definitions of ophthalmic terms are shown in Table 30.1. Quality patient care requires respect for and acceptance of the patient's cultural values, beliefs, and behaviors toward their health care and treatment. Focusing on the patient's needs prevents misunderstandings.

Preparation for surgery also involves reviewing and validating existing information, such as the presence of allergies, medical and anesthesia history, length of fasting, laboratory test results, and current medications. It is important to know whether anticoagulants and nonsteroidal and other anti-inflammatory medications are being used because they have the potential for causing intraoperative bleeding. The patient's name, operative eye, and surgical procedure to be performed are confirmed. Surgery consents and medical clearances are verified. Co-morbidities or concerns that may impact the surgery outcome are communicated to

TABLE 30.1 Ophthalmic Definitions

Ophthalmic Term	Definition
Amblyopia	Decreased vision in one or both eyes due to abnormal vision development in infancy or childhood. In the first few years of life, the brain must learn to see or interpret the images provided by the eyes. In amblyopia, the brain receives a poor image from the eye and thus does not learn as well. Vision loss occurs in this case because nerve pathways between the brain and the eye are not properly stimulated.
Blepharoplasty	Removal of excess tissue, fatty deposits, or tightening of the skeletal muscles of the eyelids. Performed to improve the appearance of the eyelids or to increase the field of vision.
Cataract	A medical condition in which the lens of the eye becomes progressively opaque, resulting in cloudy or blurred vision.
Chalazion	A small, usually painless lump on the edge of the eyelid caused by blockage of the meibomian gland at the base of an eyelash.
Cicloplegia	Paralysis of the ciliary muscle of the eye, causing an inability of the curvature of the lens to be adjusted to focus on nearby objects.
Dacryocystorhinostomy	A surgical procedure to create a new passage from the lacrimal sac through the lacrimal bone, to the inside of the nose to restore tear drainage when the nasolacrimal duct is blocked.
Depth perception	The ability to see things in three dimensions (length, width, and depth) and to judge the distance of an object.
Entropion	A medical condition in which the eyelid turns inward so that the eyelashes and skin rub against the eye surface, causing irritation and discomfort. More common in the lower eyelid.
Enucleation	A surgical procedure that involves removal of the entire globe. The muscles that control eye movement are left intact.
Evisceration	A surgical procedure that involves removal of the cornea and inner contents of the eye; however, the sclera and the attached extraocular muscles remain intact.
Exenteration	An extensive surgical procedure that involves removal of the eye, including the adjacent structures of the eye, the orbit, the surrounding soft tissues, and the eyelids.
Glaucoma	A group of diseases that damage the eye's optic nerve and can result in vision loss and even blindness. Open-angle glaucoma, the most common form, results in increased eye pressure.
Goniotomy	A surgical procedure, performed for congenital glaucoma, in which the first layer of the natural drain system (trabecular meshwork) is cut, allowing the fluid to leave the eye more easily and lowering the intraocular pressure.
Hydroxyapatite implant	An implant composed of calcium phosphate derived from the exoskeleton of marine coral. It is used to replace the volume of the orbit when the eye has been surgically removed. Because its structure and chemical makeup is almost identical to the hydroxyapatite of human bone, it is less likely to be rejected.
Intraocular lens (IOL)	A tiny artificial lens for the eye. It replaces the eye's natural lens when the natural lens is removed during cataract surgery.
Intraocular pressure (IOP)	The fluid pressure inside the eye. The normal range for eye pressure is between 10- and 20-mm Hg. Eye pressure that is too low or too high can damage vision.
Keratoplasty	Partial or total excision of cloudy corneal tissue and its replacement by clear corneal tissue from a human donor. • In deep lamellar endothelial keratoplasty (DLEK) the outer corneal layers of the recipient are left intact. • In Descemet membrane endothelial keratoplasty (DMEK) no additional stromal tissue is transplanted from the donor. • In Descemet stripping endothelial keratoplasty (DSEK) a small amount of posterior stromal thickness from the donor is transplanted.
LASIK	Laser in situ keratomileusis (LASIK) is a surgical procedure that combines keratomileusis with the accuracy of the excimer laser to correct of a broad range of refractive abnormalities.
Miosis	Constriction of the pupil of the eye resulting from a normal increase in light, or by certain drugs or pathologic conditions.
Mydriasis	Dilation of the pupil of the eye resulting from a normal decrease in light or caused by certain drugs, pathologic conditions, or trauma.
Pars plana vitrectomy	A technique in vitreoretinal surgery in which vitreous is removed using instruments introduced into the eye through the pars plana.
Penetrating keratoplasty	A surgical procedure in which a full-thickness resection of the patient's cornea, followed by placement of a full-thickness donor corneal graft, is placed to minimize postoperative astigmatism.
Phacoemulsification	A surgical technique in which the cataract is emulsified with an ultrasonic handpiece and aspirated from the eye.
Plaque therapy	The most common form of radiation therapy used to treat eye melanomas. Small seeds of radioactive material are placed directly into or very close to the cancer. The radiation from the seeds is focused only on the tumor.
Pneumatic retinoplexy	A surgical procedure done to repair a detached retina and restore vision by injecting a gas bubble into the eye. The gas bubble presses against the area of torn retina, forcing it back into place.
Pterygium	A raised, wedge-shaped, benign growth of the clear mucous membrane lining of the inner eyelids and the sclera that extends onto the cornea; may cause decreased or distorted vision.
Ptosis	A drooping of one or both eyelids.
Scleral buckling	A surgical procedure used to repair retinal detachments. It involves placing a silicone band around the outside of the eye that pushes the wall of the eye slightly inward. This creates a counterforce inside the eye that pushes the detached retina back against the inner wall, allowing it to re-attach. The encircling band remains on the eye but is not visible after the surgery.

TABLE 30.1 Ophthalmic Definitions—cont'd

Ophthalmic Term	Definition
Strabismus	A medical condition in which the eyes are not aligned properly and point in different directions.
Tarsorrhaphy	A surgical procedure in which the upper and lower eyelids are sewn together, either partially or completely, to protect the cornea.
Trabeculectomy	A surgical procedure in which a small portion of the trabecular tissue lying between the anterior chamber of the eye and the canal of Schlemm is excised to facilitate drainage of aqueous humor and relieve intraocular pressure caused by glaucoma.
Vitrectomy	A surgical procedure in which some or all the vitreous gel from the middle of the eye is removed and replaced with either a salt water (saline) solution or a bubble made of gas or oil.

Adapted from: Baddely CG. Care of the ophthalmic surgical patient. Pages 473–474 in: Odom-Forren J. *Drain's Perianesthesia Nursing: A Critical Care Approach.* 7th ed. Elsevier; 2018.

the appropriate clinical team members and documented. A designated driver is identified.

Patients with a fever, cough, runny nose, or vomiting are at risk for respiratory complications such as laryngospasm or aspiration. Strategies to manage postoperative pain in patients with chronic pain are predetermined by the surgeon together with the anesthesiologist. The nurse documents the patient's vital signs, oxygen saturation, height, weight, pain level, and spiritual, psychosocial, and cultural status. An allergy wristband is applied per institutional protocol. Intravenous access is established.

The ophthalmic surgery patient is often experiencing heightened anxiety. Promote trust and help the patient to cope with fears with empathy, open communication, active listening, reassurance, and a positive attitude. Providing the patient with the opportunity to ask questions helps to allay fears.[18,19] Always alert patients with reduced vision when approaching the bedside, prior to doing a procedure, or when stepping away.

Review perioperative education and postoperative instructions related to pain control, activities, diet, wound care, and topical medications with the patient and family. Discuss the patient's feelings and beliefs about the surgical outcomes as it is important for the patient to have realistic expectations. Offer patients the chance to use the bathroom just before surgery.

Patient care for pediatric patients is a team effort as the parents know and understand their child's specific needs. Parents must be involved in decision-making and their questions must be answered to allay fears. Detailed preoperative education is essential. Provide information about the anticipated length of surgery, the time parents will be brought to the bedside after surgery, the type of dressings that will be in place, and the home care requirements. Parents should remain at the bedside to soothe a child until the child is taken to surgery.[20]

Evidence-Based Practice: Patient education to reduce preoperative anxiety

Overview:

Anxiety related to an upcoming ophthalmic surgery is common and experienced by many patients and their families. The patient may share fears about being awake or experiencing pain during the procedure. The patient may not understand the surgery fully. The patient may be terrified by the thought of possible vision loss. Addressing anxiety prior to surgery is extremely important for both the surgery outcome and the patient's safety and satisfaction.

Establishing trust and providing information based on the patient/family needs enhances understanding, encourages active involvement in self-care, reduces pain, and aids in compliance.

Implications for Nursing Practice:

Patient-focused education is effective in decreasing anxiety, reducing pain, increasing satisfaction, and improving outcomes.

Data from:

Rajala M, Kaakinen P, Fordell M, Kaariainen M. The quality of patient education in day surgery by adult patients. *J Perianesth Nurs.* 2018;33(2):177–187;

Socea SD, Abualhasan H, Magen OR, et al. Preoperative anxiety levels and pain during cataract surgery. *Curr Eye Res.* 2020;45(4):471–476;

Yahya Al-Sagarat A, Al-Oran HM, Obeidat H, Hamlan AM, Moxham L. Preparing the family and children for surgery. *Crit Care Nurs Q.* 2017;40(2):99–107; and

Wongkietkachorn A, Wongkietkachorn N, Rhunsiri P. Preoperative needs-based education to reduce anxiety, increase satisfaction, and decrease time spent in day surgery: A randomized controlled trial. *World J Surg* 2018;42(3):666–674.

It is essential that nurses understand the actions of ophthalmic medications frequently used in the perianesthesia setting, the potential alterations to the patient's reaction to anesthetic drugs, and the systemic effects of all drugs taken, and anesthetics used (Table 30.2). Closely monitor geriatric patients because they are at a higher risk for severe systemic effects. Elderly patients tend to take a higher number of medications and undergo more surgeries than other age groups (see Chapter 23). Anti-infective, anti-inflammatory, constricting, or dilating ophthalmic drops are frequently ordered to be given prior to ophthalmic surgery. Reassure the patient by discussing the reason for the drops in a calm manner. Providing the patient with explanations reduces fear of the unknown. Verify that the correct medication is instilled in the correct eye to prevent a delay or cancellation of surgery. To help both clinicians and patients distinguish between the various topical ophthalmic medications, a universal color-coding system was established by a partnership of the U.S. Food and Drug Administration, the American Academy of Ophthalmology, and the pharmaceutical industry. The patient is able to use the color-coded caps and labels on the bottles to verify that the correct eye drops are being taken when at home (Table 30.3).

Postoperative Care

Patients who have had general anesthesia are transported to the Phase I postanesthesia care unit (PACU). Postanesthesia care begins with a physical and emotional assessment on arrival, with emphasis on the patient's respiratory status. A thorough handoff report is given to the PACU nurse by staff from the operating room and anesthesia care teams.[21,22] The patient's history, surgical procedure, type of anesthesia given, allergies, vital signs, and oxygen saturation are reported. It is important to know the patient's preoperative anxiety level and coping mechanisms, any problems during surgery, the type of dressings used, the postoperative positioning requirements, and whether the patient can see in the unoperative eye.

TABLE 30.2 Selected Ophthalmic Medications

Category/Name	Indication	Systemic Effects
ADRENERGIC AGONISTS		
Alphagan P Combigan	Decreases intraocular pressure via decrease in aqueous humor	Oral dryness Visual disturbance, dizziness Bradycardia, hypotension, nausea
α-ADRENERGIC AGONIST		
Epinephrine	Mydriasis	Bradycardia Tachycardia Hypertension
β-ADRENERGIC AGONIST		
Phenylephrine	Potent vasoconstrictor Decreases intraocular pressure	Dysrhythmias Headache Sedation
ANTICHOLINERGIC		
Cyclopentolate	Cycloplegia	Central anticholinergic syndrome
ANTI-INFECTIVES		
Gentamicin Neomycin Ciprofloxacin Ofloxacin	Bactericidal	Itching, hives
MUSCARINIC AGONISTS		
Tropicamide Atropine Scopolamine	Prolonged mydriasis	Tachycardia Flushing, dry skin, thirst Elderly may display agitation, confusion, or central nervous system excitation May precipitate attack of narrow-angle glaucoma
ANTICHOLINESTERASES		
Echothiophate Phospholine iodine	Induces miosis Increases aqueous drainage	Bradycardia, bronchospasm Reduction in plasma cholinesterase for up to 3–7 weeks after discontinued Prolongation of duration of action of procaine, chloroprocaine, and succinylcholine
ANTI-INFLAMMATORY, NONSTEROIDAL		
Diclofenac Nevanac Ketorolac	Decreases postoperative inflammation and pain	Burning sensation Headache Rhinitis, facial edema Abdominal pain, nausea Delayed wound healing
ANTI-INFLAMMATORY, STEROIDAL		
Alrex Maxidex Pred Forte Zylet	Decreases inflammation	Increased intraocular pressure Delayed wound healing Rare hypercorticoidism
β-ADRENERGIC ANTAGONISTS		
Betimol Combigan Cosopt Timolol	Mydriasis	Light-headedness, fatigue, disorientation General central nervous system depression Bradycardia, palpitations, syncope, increase in heart block, and congestive heart failure Bronchospasm
CARBONIC ANHYDRASE INHIBITORS		
Azopt Acetazolamide Diamox	Decreases intraocular pressure via decreased production of aqueous humor	Confusion, tinnitus Flushing, headache, polyuria Electrolyte imbalance Dyspepsia with long-term use IV administration can cause acute hypotension Tingling of extremities
CHOLINERGIC AGONISTS		
Acetylcholine Pilocarpine Miochol-E	Induces miosis	Headache, bradycardia, hypotension, flushing, and bronchospasm May inhibit focusing

TABLE 30.2 Selected Ophthalmic Medications—cont'd

Category/Name	Indication	Systemic Effects
PROSTAGLANDINS		
Lumigan Travatan Z Xalatan	Decreases intraocular pressure via increasing outflow of aqueous humor	Ocular dryness, visual disturbances Headache, increased risk of infections May change the color of the iris
MISCELLANEOUS		
Fluorescein	IV dye for evaluation of retinal vasculature	Urticaria, rhinorrhea, dizziness, pharyngoedema Nausea and vomiting

Adapted from Prescriber's Digital Reference. https://www.pdr.net; Mielcarek ED. Ophthalmic surgery. Pages 1396–1401 in: *Alexander's Care of the Patient in Surgery.* 16th ed. Elsevier; 2019; and Baddeley, CG. Care of the ophthalmic surgical patient. Page 475 in: Odom-Forren J. *Drain's Perianesthesia Nursing: A Critical Care Approach.* 7th ed. Elsevier; 2018.

TABLE 30.3 Color-Coding System for the Caps and Labels of Topical Ophthalmic Medications*

Color	Class
Light green	Adrenergic agonist combinations
Purple	Adrenergic agonists
Tan	Anti-infectives
Gray	Anti-inflammatory, nonsteroidal
Pink	Anti-inflammatory, steroids
Olive green	Anti-inflammatory, immunomodulators
Dark blue	Beta-blocker combinations
Yellow	Beta-blockers
Orange	Carbonic anhydrase inhibitors
Black	Cytotoxic
Dark green	Miotics
Red	Mydriatics and cycloplegics
Turquoise	Prostaglandin analogues

*The objective of the color-coding system for topical ophthalmic medications is to help patients distinguish among the various medications to minimize the risk of patients selecting the incorrect medication.
Adapted from: American Academy of Ophthalmology: Color Codes for Topical Ocular Medications. https://www.aao.org/about/policies/color-codes-topical-ocular-medications

The perianesthesia nurse provides care for the patient's immediate postoperative needs and treats any complications. The nurse also documents the patient's vital signs, oxygen saturation, level of consciousness, pain level, and condition of the surgical site. The adult patient is usually awake with the head of the bed elevated on admission. A patch, shield, dressing, or eye mask may be in place over the operative eye (Figure 30.3). Caution the patient not to disturb the dressing or try to rub the eye. The patient would likely need to return to the operating room if the sutures were broken or the site began to bleed. Patients sometimes report mild to moderate pain after eye surgery. A multimodal approach to pain control is useful. Severe pain is unusual and should be reported to the surgeon.

Postoperative nausea and vomiting (PONV) occur more frequently. Treat pain, nausea, or vomiting promptly as these conditions could increase the intraocular pressure in the operative eye and trigger bleeding.

Children are at high risk for postoperative complications (see Chapter 22). Perianesthesia nurses should be certified in pediatric advanced life support. Airway support and emergency equipment must be readily accessible. Pediatric patients are often positioned in the lateral position to allow drainage of oral secretions. Closely monitor the patient for airway obstruction, hypoxia, laryngospasm, bradycardia, emergence delirium, pain, and nausea.

The *oculocardiac reflex*, a sudden decrease in heart rate and blood pressure, is a risk with any ophthalmic surgery.[8,23] It can occur in response to manipulation of the extraocular muscles or surrounding ocular tissues, as in vitreoretinal and eye muscle surgeries. Pediatric patients are at significant risk during surgery to correct strabismus. Atropine, retrobulbar blocks, anticholinergic drugs, or a ketamine infusion may be used by the anesthesiologist to suppress the oculocardiac reflex. Continuous monitoring for bradycardia, respiratory depression, hypotension, and dysrhythmias is essential. Immediate removal of pressure from the globe and surrounding structures usually restores the sinus rhythm and allows the surgery to continue. If symptoms persist, IV atropine and cardiovascular support are indicated.

The nurse's role in Phase I is one of constant vigilance, supporting basic life-sustaining needs, and transitioning the patient to the intensive care unit, to an inpatient ward, or to Phase II. The Ophthalmic Surgery Competency Tool is shown in Table 30.4.

Evidence-Based Practice: Postoperative nausea and vomiting

Overview:

PONV remains a major concern following ophthalmic surgery and can delay discharge from the hospital or ambulatory surgery center, increase patient discomfort, decrease patient satisfaction, and increase costs. Giving aromatherapy consisting of isopropyl alcohol, peppermint, ginger, lavender, peppermint, and spearmint, used singly or in various combinations, has been reported to have a positive effect on PONV.

Implications for Nursing Practice:

A multimodal approach of aromatherapies used in conjunction with pharmacologic antiemetics may help to relieve PONV and deserves further study.

Data from: Asay K, Olson C, Donnelly J, Perlman E. The use of aromatherapy in postoperative nausea and vomiting: A systematic review. *J Perianesth Nurs.* 2019;34(3):502–516;
Brown L, Danda L, Fahey TJ. A quality improvement project to determine the effect of aromatherapy on postoperative nausea and vomiting in a short-stay surgical population. *AORN J.* 2018;108(4):361–369;
Hunt R, Dienemann J, Norton HJ, Hartley W, Hudgens A, Stern T, Divine G. Aromatherapy as treatment for postoperative nausea: A randomized trial. *Anesth Analg.* 2013;117(3):597–604; and
Karsten M, Prince D, Robinson R, Stout-Aguilar J. Effects of peppermint aromatherapy on postoperative nausea and vomiting. *J Perianesth Nurs.* 2020;35:615–618.

TABLE 30.4 Ophthalmic Surgery Competency Tool

The nurse can demonstrate the knowledge, skills, abilities, and behavior necessary to provide safe, competent, and efficient nursing care to the post-ophthalmic surgery patient.

Competency	Evidence (Code)	Action Plan/Follow-up Comments
Performs an assessment on the patient who undergoes ophthalmic surgery on admission, discharge, and as condition warrants	V/O/R	
Discusses potential adverse effects of anesthesia and verbalizes nursing considerations: • Topical • Local block • Moderate sedation • General	V/O/R	
Demonstrates appropriate interventions to prevent complications; ensures patient safety: • Identifies risk factors/co-morbidities • Monitors airway status • Assesses presence of dizziness, nausea, bleeding, pain, and other conditions	V/O/R	
States understanding of oculocardiac reflex pathophysiology and nursing care: • Identifies risk factors • Monitors heart rate, respiratory status, blood pressure, and cardiac rhythm • Nursing considerations	V/O/R	
States understanding of route, onset, duration of action, dose ranges, peaks, interactions of medications used in ophthalmic surgeries: • Antibiotics • Corticosteroids • Miotics • Mydriatics	V/O/R	
Discusses nursing care for common ophthalmic-specific procedures and interventions: • Blepharoplasty • Cataract extraction • Evisceration and enucleation • Excision of pterygium • Keratoplasty • Trabeculectomy • Vitrectomy	V/O/R	
Discusses nursing care for special/vulnerable populations who have had ophthalmic-specific procedures, including: • Geriatrics • Pediatrics	V/O/R	
Provides patient/family teaching related to self-care and prevention of complications, at time of discharge or transfer	V/O/R	
Conducts follow-up telephone calls; reinforces patient/family education and provides information as needed	V/O/R	
Effectively communicates with clinical team members as needed	V/O/R	
Effectively documents all pertinent information	V/O/R	
Competency Evidence Codes: **V = Able to verbalize understanding** **O = Competency confirmed by direct observation** **R = Reviewed references and resources**	Date: _____ Staff Nurse Signature: _____ Nurse Manager Signature: _____	

Adapted from: Appendix 3: Competency assessment tools. In: Shaw ME, Lee A. *Ophthalmic Nursing*. CRC Press; 2016.

In Phase II, the perianesthesia nurse's focus is on preparing the patient for discharge and self-care. Each ophthalmic surgical procedure has specific instructions for home care. Reinforce the instructions with the patient and family. Emphasize the importance of protecting the operative eye after surgery. The patient is not to rub the eye or to get water in it. The covering over the eye must remain clean and in place. Dressings over the operative eye are frequently taped in place. The tape should not extend past the jaw because the action of chewing may loosen the tape and cause the covering to move or come off. Remind the patient to always wear the dressing over the eye and for the duration specified by the surgeon. Any restrictions to activity, such as swimming, bathing, shampooing, driving, sleeping position, operating heavy machinery, or lifting heavy objects, should be explained. Activities that could stress the operative site or increase eye pressure should be avoided.

Depth perception is lost when one eye has a dressing, patch, or shield over it. Vision is sometimes blurred postoperatively due to the type of procedure done, topical medication given, and increased tear production. In addition, the unoperated eye may also have poor vision. Remind the family that the patient will need assistance negotiating steps and getting to the bathroom. Assistance in reaching for hot items, such as a cup of coffee, will be needed to avoid a burn. Evaluate the patient's balance and equilibrium. Advise the patient to wear sunglasses when outside during the day to minimize light sensitivity. Tell the patient that reading may be uncomfortable because the muscles of the operative eye move in tandem with the unoperative eye, but that the patient will be able to watch television comfortably.

Therapeutic eye drops or ointments are frequently prescribed for the patient to administer at home. Teach the patient the proper instillation of eye drops and ointments and provide the schedule on and order in which they are to be administered. Most eye drops and ointments are placed in the lower fornix. However, other locations include the cornea, lids, periocular wounds, and socket. The patient should understand the action and side effects of the medications. Advise the patient that eye drops may sting and may leave an unpleasant taste in the mouth. Review the proper way to store the medications. Caution the patient not to use over-the-counter pain medications containing aspirin or nonsteroidal anti-inflammatory drugs as these can increase the risk of bleeding in the eye.

Instruct the patient to call the clinic for questions and go to the emergency department if there is redness, swelling, bleeding or drainage from the eye; changes to vision; severe pain not relieved by prescribed medication; fever; or prolonged nausea and vomiting while recuperating at home. Discuss strategies with the patient and family about possible alterations to the home environment that can be done to promote the patient's safety, self-confidence, and independent living.

To confirm understanding, ask the patient to restate the instructions and demonstrate self-administration of medications. Place a printed copy of all instructions in the patient's preferred language, the date and time of the follow-up appointment, and the prescription for discharge medications in the discharge packet. Verify the name of the designated driver who will accompany the patient home.

Postanesthesia care continues until discharge criteria have been met. Discharge criteria are facility-specific and developed by the medical and anesthesia departments. However, the perianesthesia nurse's physical assessment of the patient is equally as important for safe discharge as a standardized score. Prior to discharge, the patient's vital signs should have returned to baseline. Pain, nausea, and vomiting should be relieved or at a level acceptable to the patient. It is not always necessary for the patient to take fluids or void prior to discharge. If there is any doubt related to the patient's physical status or safety, delay the discharge and report concerns to the surgeon.[24]

SURGICAL PROCEDURES

Ophthalmic surgical procedures and the nursing implications for them are described as follows.[1,2,25]

Surgery of the Lens

A cataract is an opacity in the lens that causes vision loss. Though mainly seen in the elderly, cataracts can occur in any age group.[26] Cataracts are considered among the main causes of blindness around the world. Children may be born with congenital cataracts or develop them later. Traumatic cataracts are formed following an eye injury or an electric shock. Secondary cataracts develop after eye surgery or are associated with other health issues such as diabetes, steroid use, smoking, and prolonged exposure to sunlight. The only treatment for cataracts is surgery.

Preoperative preparation involves telling the patient what to expect during the perioperative process. Discuss how the cataract will be treated and whether an intraocular lens will be implanted. Tell the patient how long the surgery will take and how long the patient will be in the postanesthesia area. Review plans for the management of the patient's postoperative pain and nausea. Patients may express the expectation that they will see well without glasses right after surgery. Discuss healing times related to the surgical procedure to manage expectations.

Cataract extraction is one of the most frequently performed surgeries in the ambulatory setting. The procedure is usually performed under local anesthesia with a needle block or by instilling local anesthetic eye drops on the cornea. The lens is removed and often replaced with an intraocular crystalline lens. Having an intraocular lens in place obviates the need for contact lenses or cataract eyeglasses.

There are several techniques for removing the lens. *Intracapsular cataract extraction* is rarely used. It involves removing the entire lens and capsule. This leaves no structure to support the intraocular lens, so it is placed in front of the iris. *Extracapsular cataract extraction* involves removing the lens but leaving the posterior portion of the capsule intact. The intraocular lens is placed behind the iris and the pupil constricted.

The technique most commonly used is *phacoemulsification cataract extraction*. In this technique, the lens is broken up into tiny pieces by ultrasonic vibrations and removed by irrigation and aspiration through a small incision. The posterior capsule is used to support the intraocular lens.

As with any surgery, there is a risk of complications. Postoperative edema causes a rise in intraocular pressure; however, it normally resolves without treatment within 24 to 72 hours. Secondary glaucoma (optic nerve damage and vision loss) could develop from prolonged increased intraocular pressure. Leaking damaged retinal blood vessels contribute to macular edema. Other potential complications are retinal detachment, corneal opacification, intraocular hemorrhage, infection, and sterile endophthalmitis.[27-30]

Pain should be minimal and manageable with acetaminophen or a similar analgesic. Patients are usually seen the first morning after surgery in the outpatient clinic for follow-up. Remind the patient not to bend at the waist or to lift heavy objects. Encourage the patient to relax for the first 24 hours after surgery. Remind the patient that watching television is fine; it will not harm the eye.

The patient should be advised to sleep on the back or on the unoperated side with the head slightly elevated. Antibiotic and steroidal anti-inflammatory eye drops may be prescribed. Review the drops' actions, proper methods of instillation, and administration schedule with the patient.

Surgery of the Retina

Retinal detachment is the separation of part of the retina from the vascular layer of the eye. Causes of this condition include previous eye surgery, vascular disease, and intraocular neoplasm. Detachment may also be congenital or related to severe myopia or the normal aging process. An injury to the retina is often considered emergent as it poses a serious threat to vision. As the retina separates, the affected part causes vision loss in the corresponding visual field. Surgical procedures of the retina, usually done under general anesthesia, are intended to return the retina to its correct position. Mydriatic drops are administered preoperatively to enable the surgeon to examine the retina and locate the exact number, size, and types of detached areas, holes, and tears. Each eye is examined as retinopathies can affect both eyes. The patient and family need to understand that this surgery may be lengthy.

Vitrectomy is the removal of vitreous humor by aspiration and is done to repair extremely large retinal tears, retinal detachment with scarring, a macular hole, or a penetrating injury or to remove vitreous opacities, fibrous tissue, retained foreign bodies, or membranes. The vitreous humor is replaced with therapeutic gas, air, or silicone oil. Aqueous humor will gradually fill the eye's chamber and replace the air or therapeutic gas as it is absorbed. Silicone oil must be removed later. The patient will experience farsightedness while the silicone oil is in place. Complications of vitrectomy include infection, corneal edema, and hemorrhage. Strong analgesics are required postoperatively.[31,32]

In *scleral buckling* surgery, segments of silicone sponge (scleral buckle) are sutured onto the sclera over the site of the hole, causing an indentation and bringing the separated layers of the retina together to close the areas where the retina is detached and to reduce the chances of further detachment. Rarely, solid silicone is shaped into bands to encircle the eye underneath the extraocular muscles and to support the width and height of the buckle in targeted areas. Monitor the cornea for clarity, as cloudiness is an indicator of ischemia. The accumulation of subretinal fluid, displacement of the buckle, distorted vision, and infection are complications of scleral buckling surgery.

Pneumatic retinopexy involves introducing an air or therapeutic gas bubble into the eye. The bubble, weighing less than the vitreous humor, floats over the detached area and acts as a splint to push it against the detached part of the eye. The air or gas bubble is absorbed within a few weeks of the surgery. Emphasize the importance of the prescribed dependent face-down position (Figure 30.3). The dependent face-down position maintains the gas bubble in the correct location, maximizes the tamponade effect of the bubble, and promotes healing. Advise the patient that the position may need to be maintained for two weeks to ensure retinal reattachment. Remind the patient that travel in airplanes or to high elevations or scuba diving is prohibited. The gas bubble will expand due to cabin pressurization or changes in atmospheric pressure, causing increased intraocular pressure and pain (Figure 30.4).

The lids and conjunctiva are usually swollen after surgery due to the amount of movement of the eye required during the operation. Stress on the area of detachment is to be avoided. Review activity limitations with the patient. The patient will experience moderate to severe ocular pain; give analgesics promptly. The physician may check the eye pressure in the PACU to rule out anterior segment ischemia. Provide ice compresses to enhance comfort and control swelling.[33] Antibiotic, mydriatic, steroidal, and nonsteroidal anti-inflammatory eye drops may be prescribed. Review the actions, proper method of instillation, and administration schedule with the patient. Encourage the patient to wear an eye shield at night to prevent accidental rubbing of the operated eye while asleep.

Surgery for Glaucoma

Glaucoma is a group of eye diseases that can cause vision loss and blindness. Almost three million Americans have glaucoma, and it is the second leading cause of blindness worldwide. From 2010 to 2050, the number of people in the United States with glaucoma is expected to increase by more than double, from 2.7 million to 6.3 million.

The eye constantly makes aqueous humor. The aqueous humor flows between the posterior and the anterior chambers of the eye through a space between the cornea and the iris called the angle. When in equilibrium, the intraocular pressure is stable.

The two main types of glaucoma are open-angle glaucoma and closed angle glaucoma. Open-angle glaucoma is the most common type in the United States. In open-angle glaucoma, increased resistance to aqueous outflow through the angle causes pressure to build up in the eye, damage the optic nerve, and result in vision loss. In the less common closed angle glaucoma, access to the drainage pathways is obstructed by the iris, causing increased eye pressure, damage to the optic nerve, and vision loss. The only treatment for glaucoma is to reduce intraocular pressure. When pressure-reducing medications are not effective, surgery is indicated. The patient should understand that surgery for glaucoma is done to prevent the disease from progressing but that it cannot restore vision already lost.

Trabeculectomy involves making a scleral flap and removing a strip of trabecular meshwork from below the flap. The scleral flap is sutured back into place to create a fistula through which the aqueous fluid can drain from the inside of the eye into the scleral vessels. The tissue that forms a fluid reservoir over this surgically created area is called a bleb. Examine the area surrounding the bleb. The anterior chamber should be shallow but not flat. Notify the surgeon if the anterior chamber is flat as it could be an indication that the bleb is draining too much aqueous fluid. Trabeculectomy can also be performed using a laser. This method results in scarring of the tissue, which then stretches the trabecular meshwork and facilitates aqueous drainage. Complications of trabeculectomy surgery include the overdrainage or underdrainage of aqueous fluid, misdirection of aqueous fluid into the posterior segment of the eye, cataract formation, infection, or hyphema (a collection of blood in the anterior chamber of the eye).

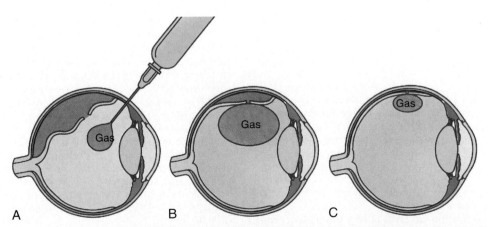

A   B   C

Fig. 30.4 Pneumatic retinopexy. Mielcarek ED. Ophthalmic Surgery. Figure 18.23 in: Rothrock JC. *Alexander's Care of the Patient in Surgery*. 16th ed. Elsevier. 2019.

30

In closed angle glaucoma, an *iridectomy* can be performed to remove a section of tissue from the outer edge of the iris, creating an opening of the angle and improving aqueous fluid outflow.

When filtering surgical procedures are not successful, placement of a *drainage device* into the posterior subconjunctival space may be done. The device is usually implanted under local anesthesia using a retrobulbar or peribulbar block. Canaloplasty is a method in which a small microcatheter is inserted into the eye around the trabecular meshwork. The catheter is dilated using an injection of a viscoelastic to enlarge the Schlemm canal, a vessel supporting the flow of fluids within the eye. The catheter is then removed, and a suture is placed within the channel and tightened to keep the channel open and facilitate aqueous fluid flow out of the eye.

Discuss medications to be used at home. A mydriatic drop is usually used for the operated eye, while a miotic drop is used to treat the patient's chronic glaucoma in the unoperated eye. Remind the patient of the importance of continuing to use the eye drops for the unoperated eye, as well as the eye drops for the operative eye. Emphasize the importance of making certain that the correct eye drops are placed in the correct eye. A mix-up would cause severe harm. The patient will experience surgical pain; verify that the patient has received a prescription for an analgesic.

Pediatric patients with unilateral glaucoma are at risk for amblyopia (also known as lazy eye). The patient should wear a patch over the unaffected eye following surgery. Though it is sometimes difficult for children to tolerate wearing a covering over the eye, emphasize its importance to the parents. Patching the unaffected eye forces the brain to pay attention to the image coming from the operative eye, prompting the brain to learn to see better from the weaker eye.[33-36]

Excision of Pterygium

The conjunctiva is a transparent and elastic membrane that lines the inner surface of the eyelids and covers the sclera. A pterygium is a degenerative condition characterized by a thick fibrovascular growth of epithelial tissue over the cornea. The cause is unclear but is thought to be related to increased exposure to wind, dust, or ultraviolet light. A pterygium may grow over the pupillary opening and compromise vision. Surgical treatment is usually done under topical or peribulbar anesthesia and involves excision of the growth off the conjunctiva and cornea down to the sclera. Pterygia tends to reoccur. The goal of surgery is to not only remove the growth but also to prevent recurrences. Low-dose radiation may be used on the surgical wound as an adjunct therapy. Instruct patients to wear polarized sunglasses when outside during the day. Complications of surgery include graft detachment, corneal thinning, or granulomas.

Surgery of the Cornea

The cornea is a transparent, avascular outer layer that covers the front of the eye and with the anterior chamber and lens, refracts light. Corneal transparency may be compromised by scars, infections, burns, corneal dystrophies, or edema after intraocular surgery. *Corneal transplantation*, in which corneal tissue from one human eye is grafted to another, is done to improve or restore vision when the retina and optic nerve are functioning properly. The transplant can also reduce pain and improve the appearance of a diseased cornea. "Since 1961, more than 1,000,000 men, women, and children have had their sight restored through a corneal transplant."[6] The Eye Bank Association of America (EBAA) member eye banks in the United States provided 85,601 corneas for transplant in 2019.[6,37]

Prior to surgery, the pupil may be constricted to prevent damage to the lens during the operation unless a cataract is to be removed at the same time. Mannitol may be given to lower intraocular pressure.

There are several techniques for corneal transplantation. *Penetrating keratoplasty* surgery is performed to treat a full-thickness pathologic condition. The central two thirds of the damaged cornea are removed and replaced with clear, healthy donor tissue. The transplant may be done under local or general anesthesia. For local anesthesia, a retrobulbar or peribulbar block is used together with a facial block to prevent procedural pain. Adequate akinesia (absence of movement) and anesthesia are required to prevent the patient from squeezing the eyelids after removal of the host cornea. The anesthesia provider must keep the patient comfortable during the transplantation. Any posterior pressure during this time can lead to suprachoroidal hemorrhage or expulsion of the intraocular contents. With this method, postoperative recovery is very long. It is sometimes years before the best-corrected visual acuity is achieved. Complications include graft rejection, astigmatism of the graft, and infection. A rigid gas-permeable contact lens may be required to correct the astigmatism. Patients with a full-thickness graft have a lifetime risk of wound dehiscence owing to the loss in tectonic strength of the repair.[38] Teach the patient the symptoms of graft rejection and the necessity of seeking immediate treatment for it.

Lamellar keratoplasty, a more technically difficult surgery, is used to treat a partial-thickness pathologic condition. With this method, the corneal stroma and epithelium are replaced but the host endothelium is kept; this decreases the risk of transplant rejection and improves the graft's stability.

Descemet stripping endothelial keratoplasty (DSEK) surgery is done for patients who have Fuchs endothelial dystrophy, corneal edema caused by intraocular surgery, or failed corneal transplants. It involves replacing only the endothelium without transplanting the entire cornea; this results in improved corneal clarity, less astigmatism, shorter healing times, and less chance of wound dehiscence and tissue rejection.

Deep lamellar endothelial keratoplasty (DLEK) surgery consists of replacing the endothelium without transplanting the full cornea to restore vision, preventing astigmatism of the graft. The transplanted endothelium is inserted into the host through a small incision, reducing the risk of infection.

Injury to the eye results when an object such as glass, metal, sand, plastic, or wood enters the eye under force. The foreign body could lodge itself in any of the structures of the eye. A thorough patient history is necessary because the object may not be seen on physical examination. *Foreign body removal* should be done as soon as possible to prevent inflammation, scarring, infection, or vision loss. A corneal foreign body is usually removed in an office or emergency room setting using a topical anesthetic. However, deeply imbedded objects are removed in the operating room. The patient must know how to protect the eye from further injury following surgery. Advise the patient to wear protective glasses any time there is potential for damage. Eye drops are prescribed to prevent infection and to ease pain and discomfort.

Refractive corneal procedures are done to correct myopia, hyperopia, and astigmatism by reshaping the cornea to change the refractive power of the eye.[39-41] For myopia, the cornea is flattened by removing more tissue from the center of the cornea than from the periphery. Hyperopia is corrected by removing more tissue from the sides of the cornea than from the center. Astigmatism requires that corneal tissue be removed from the wider sides to make the surface of the eye spherical. The need for eyeglasses and contact lenses is reduced or eliminated after refractory surgery. Most of these surgeries take only minutes and are done in the outpatient setting.

Preoperative preparation for refractive surgery includes reviewing the postoperative instructions with the patient and explaining what to expect during the surgical procedure. A mild sedative is given to help the patient relax, and eye drops are administered to numb the eyes.

Complications of refractive surgery include scarring or cloudiness of the cornea, thinning of the cornea, dry eyes, and corneal infection. Following surgery, patients should be reminded not to rub their eyes. Preservative-free artificial tears are used for several weeks to reduce dry eye symptoms. Sunglasses should be worn when outside during the day. The patient may experience glare and halos around lights, especially at night. Patients return for a follow-up appointment the following day.

Laser-assisted in-situ keratomileusis (LASIK) is the most common outpatient ophthalmic refractory surgery. In LASIK surgery, a microkeratome is used to create a flap. An excimer laser is used to reshape the cornea. The flap is then smoothed back into place. The healing process is fast; the patient may be able to resume normal activities after 24 hours. Visual acuity is established within a few hours. There is little pain; over-the-counter medications may be used for pain control. Patients should be encouraged to keep their eyes closed and rest or take a nap after surgery. Steroid and antibiotic eye drops are used for 4–10 days.

The *photorefractive keratectomy (PRK)* method is done for patients with thin corneas, previous corneal scarring, or other corneal diseases. The outer layer of cells on the cornea is manually removed using a special brush, blade, laser, or alcohol solution. The cornea is then reshaped using a laser. A contact lens is placed in the eye to act as a bandage. The patient may experience pain from the regrowth of corneal epithelium and should avoid strenuous activity for one week.

Laser epithelial keratomileusis (LASEK) surgery is done on the epithelial surface of the cornea. After the eye is numbed with topical anesthetic drops, the epithelium is loosened with a diluted alcohol solution and mechanically pushed aside. The cornea is then reshaped using a laser. The loosened epithelium is returned to its original position, and a contact lens is placed to act as a bandage. This technique avoids problems creating or reattaching the flap, and the patient experiences less dry eye discomfort. It may take 1–2 weeks to achieve full visual acuity. Patients experience more pain than with LASIK surgery but less pain than with PRK surgery. Steroid eye drops are used several weeks longer than with LASIK surgery.

Strabismus

There are six extraocular muscles that control eye movement. These muscles work in pairs to move the eye up, down, right, left, or at an angle. When the eyes look at an object, an image from each eye is sent to the brain. The brain combines the two images into one single, three-dimensional image when the muscles are working together, and the distance of an object can be determined. Strabismus is a condition in which the eyes do not point in the same direction because the extraocular muscles lack coordination. One eye may look straight ahead while the other eye looks in a different direction.

Children with strabismus may have a family history of it. Less often, a child may have a disorder that affects the brain, such as Down syndrome, hydrocephalus, brain tumor, or cerebral palsy. When one eye is out of alignment, two different images are sent to the brain. The brain does not combine the two images into one single, three-dimensional image. Instead, the brain learns to ignore the image from the eye looking in a different direction. Instead, it sees only the image from the eye looking straight ahead. If the condition is left untreated, the child does not develop normal vision and loses depth perception.

Adults with strabismus may have had it since childhood, or they may have an injury or disorder that affects eye muscles such as muscular dystrophy, head trauma, Bell palsy, or stroke. An adult who develops strabismus after childhood often has double vision because the brain has already learned to receive images from both eyes. The brain is unable to ignore the image from the eye looking in a different direction, so two images are seen.

Eye muscle exercises and prism eyeglasses are used to focus the eyes inward; eye drops to make the eye blurry and wearing a patch are other treatments for strabismus. If treatments are ineffective, surgery is indicated. *Surgery for strabismus* is usually done under general anesthesia on children six years of age or less to allow normal vision and depth perception to develop. Surgery on adults eliminates double vision and is usually done with topical anesthesia. The patient and family should be informed that PONV may be a complication of this surgery, and there should be a plan in place to manage it. They should also understand that more than one surgery may be needed to treat strabismus.

The surgical procedure involves the separation and relocation of the extraocular rectus muscles to adjust their tension on the eye (creating more or less pull) as necessary to straighten the eye position. This may need to be done in both eyes. When the muscles are repositioned, they are reattached with dissolvable sutures.[42-44]

Adjustable sutures are often used in surgery. The surgeon may, in the PACU, adjust the extraocular muscles until the eye is perfectly positioned by gently pulling on the sutures. The oculocardiac reflex can occur in response to manipulation of the extraocular muscles, particularly in children. Monitor the patient for bradycardia, respiratory depression, hypotension, and dysrhythmias.[45]

PONV and pain must be treated promptly. The patient should not experience severe pain. The patient may have double or blurred vision. An eye patch may be in place over the operative eye. Children are more comfortable without an eye patch. Home care instructions should be reviewed.

Surgery of the Lacrimal Gland

Lacrimal glands are located at the upper outer aspect of each orbit and produce tears. Tears spread across the eyeball by blinking. They keep the eyes from drying out, clean the eyes, and protect the eyes against infection. The tears cover the cornea and then drain out the punctum in the medial eyelids and flow down the canaliculi into the lacrimal sac. They then drain down the nasolacrimal duct into the nose. Lacrimal surgery is performed for treatment of obstruction to tear flow due to trauma, tumors, or infection.

Dacryocystorhinostomy is a surgical procedure performed to treat infections of the lacrimal sac. The goal of the surgery is to restore the normal flow of tears through the tear ducts to the nose and alleviate excessive tearing. It involves the creation of a new tear passageway for drainage directly into the nasal cavity. A small tube may be inserted into the passageway to keep it open until healing is complete (3–6 months).

Following surgery, an antibiotic ointment and drops for pain control are given. The patient is to avoid blowing the nose or sneezing for one week. Cold compresses may be applied four to six times each day for no longer than fifteen minutes at a time until swelling subsides. Sleeping with the head elevated with two or three pillows helps decrease swelling. The patient is to avoid heavy lifting for 7–10 days following surgery. This eases any extra pressure and blood flow to the sutures. If the inside of the nose feels dry, patients may use a pure saline nasal spray to restore some moisture. Advise the patient to avoid air travel during this period as the pressure differences can add extra strain to the operative area as well. Tell the patient to notify the surgeon if the tube becomes dislodged. *Conjunctivodacryocystorhinostomy* is a surgical procedure done to treat canalicular obstruction. Lacrimal drainage is done under endoscopic visualization to place a plastic or glass tube to stent a passageway created from the conjunctival sac through the lacrimal sac to the nasal cavity. A mustache dressing to catch drainage may be used as the surgery site is near the medial canthal area or inside the nose.[46-49]

Remind the patient to avoid blowing the nose for one week. After 1 week, the patient can place a finger over the opening of the tube to prevent dislodgement when sneezing, blowing the nose, or coughing. Advise the patient that it will take 3–6 months for the medial canthal tissue to contract around the tube. A pressure dressing will remain in place until the morning after surgery. Monitor the patient carefully for any bleeding on the dressing or epistaxis as blood loss from this procedure can be catastrophic. The hemorrhage may be readily apparent or could be via the back of the throat. For this reason, pulse, blood pressure, and respiratory rate should be closely monitored. Watch for excessive swallowing.

Surgery of the Eyelids

An eyelid is a fold of skin that closes over the eye to keep the eye moist. Eyelids serve to protect the eye from injury, excessive light, and foreign objects. There are both upper and lower eyelids.

Oculoplastic procedures performed on the eyelids include treatment of droopy upper eyelids, extra eyelid skin, or eyelids that turn inward or outward.

Obstruction of the meibomian gland caused by secretions may lead to a chalazion, manifesting as a firm bump in the eyelid. *Removal of chalazion surgery* is usually done with a local anesthetic. A small incision is made on the eyelid. The incision is made on the outer eyelid for a larger chalazion and made on the inner eyelid for a smaller one. The contents of the chalazion are scraped out. The incision is closed with dissolvable stitches. After the chalazion is removed, the wound is left open for drainage. A pressure eye patch may be applied to keep the eye closed.

An entropion occurs when the eyelid margin inverts. It may be congenital or caused by scarring or aging and weakness of muscles. It is more common in women and those over the age of 60. It may cause significant corneal irritation due to the rubbing of in-turned lashes against the surface of the eye. The only way to permanently treat entropion is with surgery. *Everting suture correction* is a surgical procedure that turns the eyelid outward. It involves removing part of the outer lid or shortening tendons and muscles with stitches to tighten them and decrease laxity of the eyelid. The skin is closed with dissolvable sutures. Scar tissue holds the eyelid in place after the stitches are removed.

An ectropion is a condition where the eyelid sags or turns outward, causing irritation in the inner eyelid. It is more common in men and those over the age of 60. The only way to permanently correct ectropion is with surgery. A *lateral tarsal strip procedure* involves tightening the lower eyelid and rotating the eyelid margin back into normal position. A small incision is made in the outside corner (lateral canthus) of the eyelid. The eyelid is tightened by reattaching the tarsus (the thick, middle layer of the eyelid) to the bone of the lateral orbital

rim. A full-thickness skin graft or local skin–muscle (myocutaneous) flap may be required. Skin may be taken from in front of or behind the ear or just above the clavicle.

Surgical treatment of chalazions, entropions, and ectropions is usually done in an office setting with local anesthesia and IV sedation; however, general anesthesia in the hospital may be required for children and very anxious patients. A topical antibiotic is typically applied to the operated areas during the first postoperative week. Ice packs are recommended for swelling and comfort for 2–3 days. The patient should understand the importance of protecting the tightened eyelid from injury during the first 3 weeks of healing. A protective eye shield should be worn while sleeping.

With age, eyelids stretch and the muscles supporting them weaken. As a result, excess fat may gather above and below the eyelids, causing sagging eyebrows, drooping upper lids, and the formation of bags under the eyes. Excess fat and skin around the eyes can sometimes impair vision. *Blepharoplasty* is a surgical procedure performed to repair drooping eyelids by removing excess skin, muscle, and fat. The surgery may be done on the upper eyelids only, the lower eyelids only, or on all four eyelids. The procedure is often performed in the outpatient setting with local anesthesia.

After surgery, the patient should be monitored for increasing periorbital inflammation because this may be an indication of infection or an allergy to topical medication. Severe pain, increased swelling, a feeling of pressure behind the eye, or vision loss should be reported to the surgeon as they may indicate retrobulbar hemorrhage.[50,51]

Discharge instructions are reviewed with the patient and family. Patients should avoid heavy lifting, bending at the waist, or operating heavy machinery to prevent stress on the surgical site. Iced compresses for control of swelling and comfort are encouraged. Antibiotic/steroid ointments are usually applied twice a day. Patients are advised to sleep with their head elevated. The patient may experience mild to moderate pain that can be managed with acetaminophen or a similar over-the-counter analgesic. Artificial tears or eye lubricants are recommended to relieve dry eyes. Patients should be told that the bruising and swelling normally lasts for 10–14 days after surgery. Cosmetics and contact lenses should not be worn until the surgeon clears their use.

Ptosis is when the upper eyelid droops over the eye. The upper eyelid may droop a small amount or so much that the pupil is covered, and vision is affected. It may be congenital or result from aging, be a side effect of eye surgery, or result from injury. The goal of surgery is to create a natural-appearing upper lid fold with elevation of the lid. Outpatient surgery for adults is done under a general or local anesthetic with sedation. Surgery for children is done under general anesthesia to prevent amblyopia. There are three types of surgery to treat ptosis.[52] The surgical procedure performed is based on the amount of ptosis and strength of the muscles in the eyelid that raise the lid.

The *levator resection* uses an external approach and is done for patients with minimal to moderate droopy eyelids and good to excellent strength in the muscles. An incision is made in the skin of the eyelid. Then the attachment of the levator muscle is repositioned by suturing it to the connective tissue in the eyelid. The surgical scar is hidden in the fold of the eyelid.

Surgery may be performed using an *internal approach*. This procedure is done for patients with minimal to moderate droopy eyelids and excellent strength in the levator muscles. The eyelid is turned inside out, and the eyelid muscle is shortened from the inside of the eyelid. The levator muscle is shortened when more of the eyelid needs to be lifted. The Mueller muscle is shortened when less of the eyelid needs to be lifted.

The *frontalis sling fixation* is performed for patients with severe ptosis and poor muscle strength. In this procedure, the upper eyelid is attached to the frontalis muscle, the muscle just above the eyebrows, using a small silicone rod that is passed through the eyelid, underneath the skin. By connecting the upper eyelid to the frontalis muscle with the rod, the forehead muscles can be used to elevate the eyelid. This surgery is usually done under general anesthesia. Patients should be advised that they will be unable to completely close the eye for 2–3 months. Lubricant eye drops and ointments are used to keep the eye moist and to prevent irritation and infection.

Surgery of the Globe and Orbit

Surgery of the globe and orbit involves removal of the eye. It is a life-changing procedure performed as a last resort. Removal of an eye is done for patients with malignant tumors so large they cannot be treated effectively with radiation or other therapy. After surgery, a small sample of the tumor is removed to analyze the appearance and genetic characteristics of the tumor cells. This information can help determine the tumor's risk of spreading. Surgery is also done to remove a degenerated blind, painful eye that is irreversibly damaged, cancerous, or affected by nonresponsive glaucoma.

Surgery is done more frequently for patients after trauma. Rupture of the globe occurs when the integrity of the outer membrane of the eye is damaged by a blunt or penetrating injury. When the eye is damaged beyond repair, surgery is indicated. There are three types of surgery for removal of the eye: evisceration, enucleation, and exenteration. Surgery is performed on an outpatient basis and may be done under general anesthesia or monitored anesthesia care. Patients should be informed about what to expect immediately after surgery, including management of pain, nausea, and vomiting. The patient should understand that a conformer will be placed and that a large pressure dressing will cover the surgical site. Instructions for home care should be discussed. The patient should be encouraged to schedule an ocularist appointment soon after surgery for a fitting to start the insurance verification process and get the desired prosthetic made in a timely manner.

Evisceration is removal of the contents of the eye but leaving the sclera and attached muscles intact. Evisceration will allow normal eye movement. *Enucleation* is removal of the entire eyeball, severing its muscular attachments and optic nerve. It is preferred over evisceration for malignancies, traumatic injury, and infection of the eye.

In both evisceration and enucleation, a spherical implant is placed into the orbit to maintain orbital volume. In an evisceration, the implant is wrapped by the sclera with the extraocular muscles still attached. In an enucleation, the extraocular muscles are detached from the sclera and then attached to the implant. The tissues surrounding the eye are then closed over the implant. At the end of surgery, a plastic conformer is placed to maintain the shape of the eye. The eyelids are sometimes sewn shut to keep the conformer in place. A pressure dressing with eye pads is taped over the eye socket to protect the wound and prevent bleeding.

For extensive malignancies of the globe or orbit, an *exenteration* will be done to try and clear all residual tumor cells. This surgery consists of removing the entire orbital contents, including the periosteum, the muscles, the lacrimal gland system, and the optic nerve. The procedure may also include removal of the external structures of the eyelids. The socket is usually reconstructed with the use of a split-thickness skin graft taken from the thigh. Extensive plastic reconstruction surgery will be required.

Complications of these surgeries include bleeding, scarring, infection, and eyelid droopiness. The implant could fall out after evisceration or enucleation surgery.

Instructions for home care are reviewed with the patient and family prior to discharge. The pressure dressing is to be kept clean and dry and in place until it is removed by the doctor at the follow-up clinic appointment. The patient is to avoid dirty environments and to do no heavy lifting, using heavy equipment, bending at the waist, or strenuous activities for at least two weeks. The surgical site is to be kept dry; the patient cannot shower, swim, or use a hot tub for at least three weeks. The patient should be instructed to use the antibiotics, steroids, or analgesics as prescribed. Emphasize the importance of shielding the unoperated eye with protective glasses any time there is potential for damage, such as participating in sports, yard work, or housework.[53-57]

REPAIR OF TRAUMATIC AND BURN INJURIES TO THE EYE

Injuries that penetrate or perforate the eye, blunt traumas, and ocular burns are considered ophthalmic emergencies and can result in vision loss. Most individuals sustaining these injuries are males with an average age in the 30s. These injuries occur most frequently in the home and workplace. Common sharp objects such as sticks, knives, scissors, screwdrivers, and nails can cause penetrating and perforating injuries.

Blunt trauma can result in serious damage to the structures of the eye, such as the cornea, iris, lens, and retina. The patient may sustain an orbital fracture. Common blunt objects that cause injury are rocks, fists, and baseballs. Paintball and BB gun injuries are increasingly noted in teenage patients. Blunt trauma may accompany a penetrating injury.

Ocular burns can be classified as chemical or thermal. Chemical burns may result from exposure to common household items such as oven cleaners, laundry detergents, bleach, and ammonia. Industrial exposure to fertilizers, industrial acids, lye, lime, and cement may also cause chemical burns. Thermal ocular injuries may result from accidents with cooking oil, an electric arc, and an explosion from an e-cigarette. Accidents with fireworks can cause both thermal and chemical burns.

The patients are likely to be terrified about the threat of vision loss. Postoperatively, they require reassurance, information on the extent of the injuries, and information on treatments. Prompt administration of analgesics is important.[58]

Children admitted with ocular trauma, and whose history is not appropriate for the injury sustained, must be carefully assessed for signs of child abuse. Appropriate action must be taken, if found, to protect the child.[59]

CHAPTER HIGHLIGHTS

- Ophthalmic surgery may be done on patients of any age, from pediatric to geriatric.
- Cataract is the leading cause of blindness worldwide and the leading cause of vision loss in the United States.
- Glaucoma is the second leading cause of blindness worldwide.
- Refractive errors are the most frequent eye problems in the United States.
- Increasingly, ophthalmic surgeries are performed in an ambulatory setting.
- Attention to psychosocial support helps to minimize fear and anxiety in this patient population.

CASE 30.1

Daniel Rodriguez, age 5, is admitted to the preoperative care unit to prepare for surgery. He is scheduled to have strabismus surgery. He has never had surgery before. Daniel has no allergies. The surgery will be done with general anesthesia. Baseline vital signs are within normal limits. Daniel lives with his parents and two sisters in an upstairs apartment. His mother does not work outside the home. The nurse is assessing the patient and interviewing the parents. Daniel speaks English but his parents do not. Daniel is tearful and admits to being scared. Mrs. Rodriguez appears nervous.

- What are some of the challenges in caring for this patient?
- Identify two methods that the nurse can use to communicate with Daniel's parents.
- What nonpharmacologic interventions can the nurse use to help Daniel and his mother cope with his anxiety?
- What educational information would be useful for the nurse to provide to his mother at this time?

Daniel has an uneventful surgery and is taken to the Phase I recovery area. He is sleeping with an oral airway in place. He is breathing oxygen at 6l/m via mask. His vital signs are within normal limits. His cardiac rhythm is a normal sinus rhythm, at a rate of 84 bpm.

- Describe the postoperative goals of nursing care for Daniel.

Daniel is waking up. The oral airway is removed. His parents are brought to the bedside. The nurse checks the cardiac monitor and notes the sinus rhythm, which now has a rate of 59 bpm.

- What are the priorities for Daniel's care?

After 2 hours, Daniel meets the facility's discharge criteria. The perianesthesia nurse is preparing him for discharge.

- Discuss instructions and information that the PACU nurse must be sure to include in the discharge teaching for Mr. and Mrs. Rodriguez to meet Daniel's individual needs.

CASE 30.2

Mr. Smith, age 76, has been admitted to the preoperative care unit to prepare for surgery. He is scheduled to have excision of a cataract from the left eye with an intraocular lens implant. He will return in two months to have surgery to remove a cataract from his right eye. Mr. Smith is hard of hearing and wears hearing aids in both ears. He has a history of diabetes and has been receiving insulin for the past five years. He had hip surgery 30 years ago and uses a cane. He smokes one pack of cigarettes daily. Mr. Smith has no allergies. The surgery will be done with a peribulbar block with sedation. Baseline vital signs are within normal limits, and his blood sugar is 136 mg/dL. He lives with his elderly wife in an upstairs apartment. During his interview, Mr. Smith expresses feelings of anxiety about being awake during the surgery.

- What are some of the challenges in caring for this patient?
- What nonpharmacologic interventions can the nurse use to help Mr. Smith cope with his anxiety?
- Identify potential concerns about the patient's ability to recuperate safely at home.

Mr. Smith has an uneventful surgery and is taken to the Phase II recovery area. He has a patch taped over the left eye. He is awake and alert. His vital signs are within normal limits. His blood sugar level is 98 mg/dL. He denies surgical pain but does report mild nausea.

- Describe the postoperative goals of nursing care for Mr. Smith.

Mr. Smith meets the facility's discharge criteria. The perianesthesia nurse is preparing Mr. Smith for discharge. His wife is brought to the bedside.

- Discuss instructions and information that the PACU nurse must be sure to include in the discharge teaching for Mr. Smith to meet his individual needs.

REFERENCES

1. Mielcarek ED. Ophthalmic surgery. In: Rothrock JC, McEwen DR, eds. *Alexander's Care of the Patient in Surgery*. 16th ed. Elsevier; 2019.
2. Shaw, ME, Lee A. *Ophthalmic Nursing*. CRC Press. Kindle Edition. 2016.
3. Badderley CG. Care of the ophthalmic surgical patient. In: Odom-Forren J, ed. *Drain's Perianesthesia Nursing: A Critical Care Approach*. Elsevier; 2018.
4. Russell KM, Warner ME, Erie JC, Kruthiventi SC, Sprung J, Weingarten TN. Anesthesia recovery after ophthalmologic surgery at an ambulatory surgical center. *J Cataract Refract Surg*. 2019;45(6): 823-829. Available at: https://doi.org/10.1016/j.jcrs.2019.01.017.
5. National Eye Institute. *Cataract Data and Statistics*. Available at: https://www.nei.nih.gov/learn-about-eye-health/eye-health-data-and-statistics. Accessed July 31, 2021.
6. American Academy of Ophthalmology. *Eye Health Statistics*. Available at: https://www.aao.org/newsroom/eye-health-statistics. Accessed July 31, 2021.
7. American Academy of Ophthalmology, Fang ZT. *Anesthesia Management of Ophthalmic Surgery in Geriatric Patients*. Available at: https://www.aao.org/Assets/0985ab39-20ce-4779-9322-e718972edd86/635711977904770000/anesthesia-management-of-ophthalmic-surgery-in-geriatric-patients-pdf. Accessed July 31, 2021.
8. Arnold RW. The oculocardiac reflex: a review. *Clin Ophthalmol*. 2021;15:2693-2725. Available at: https://doi.org/10.2147/opth.s317447.
9. Ead H. Caring for the patient who uses cannabinoids. *J Perianesth Nurs*. 2018;33(3):360-362. Available at: https://doi.org/10.1016/j.jopan.2018.03.006.
10. Horvath C, Bowman Dalley C, Grass N, Tola DH. Marijuana use in the anesthetized patient: history, pharmacology, and anesthetic considerations. *AANA J*. 2019;87(6):451-458.
11. Gayer S, Kumar CM. Ophthalmic regional anesthesia techniques. *Minerva Anestesiol*. 2008;74(1):23-33.
12. Nouvellon E, Cuvillon P, Ripart J, Riou B. Regional anesthesia and eye surgery. *Anesthesiology*. 2010;113(5):1236-1242. Available at: https://doi.org/10.1097/ALN.0b013e3181f7a78e.
13. Kumar CM, Eid H, Dodds C. Sub-tenon's anaesthesia: Complications and their prevention. *Eye*. 2011;25(6):694-703. Available at: https://doi.org/10.1038/eye.2011.69.
14. American Society of PeriAnesthesia Nurses. Part One: The Scope of Perianesthesia Nursing Practice. In: 2021-2022 Perianesthesia Nursing Standards, Practice Recommendations, and Interpretive Statements. ASPAN; 2020.
15. Clifford T. Preoperative optimization. *J Perianesth Nurs*. 2018; 33(6):1006-1007. Available at: https://doi.org/10.1016/j.jopan.2018.09.006.
16. Tuohy D. Effective intercultural communication in nursing. *Nurs Stand*. 2019;34(2):45-50. Available at: https://doi.org/10.7748/ns.2019.e11244.
17. Wright PR. Care of culturally diverse patients undergoing ophthalmic surgery. *Insight*. 2011;36(1):7-10.
18. Clair C, Engstrom A, Stromback U. Strategies to relieve patients' preoperative anxiety before anesthesia: Experiences of nurse anesthetists. *J Perianesth Nurs*. 2020;35(3):314-320. Available at: https://doi.org/10.1016/j.jopan.2019.10.008.
19. Ross J. Effective communication improves patient safety. *J Perianesth Nurs*. 2018;33(2):223-225. Available at: https://doi.org/10.1016/j.jopan.2018.01.003.
20. American Society of PeriAnesthesia Nurses. Practice Recommendation 9: Family Presence in the Perianesthesia Setting. In: 2021-2022 Perianesthesia Nursing Standards, Practice Recommendations, and Interpretive Statements. ASPAN; 2020.
21. American Society of PeriAnesthesia Nurses. Practice recommendation 6: Safe transport of care: Handoff and transportation. In 2021-2022 Perianesthesia Nursing Standards, Practice Recommendations, and Interpretive Statements. ASPAN; 2020.
22. American Society of PeriAnesthesia Nurses. Practice Recommendation 2: Components of assessment and management for the perianesthesia patient. In: 2021-2022 Perianesthesia Nursing Standards, Practice Recommendations, and Interpretive Statements. ASPAN; 2020.
23. Yoo JJ, Gishen KE, Thaller SR. The oculocardiac reflex: Its evolution and management. *J Craniofac Surg*. 2021;32(1):e80-e83. Available at: https://doi.org/10.1097/scs.0000000000006995

24. Zhu Y, Yang S, Zhang R, et al. Using clinical-based discharge criteria to discharge patients after ophthalmic ambulatory surgery under general anesthesia: An observational study. *J Perianesth Nurs.* 2020;35(6):586-691. Available at: https://doi.org/10.1016/j.jopan.2020.04.012.

25. Hussain SS. Ophthalmology. In: Schick L and Windle PE, eds. *Perianesthesia Nursing Core Curriculum: Preprocedure, Phase I and Phase II PACU Nursing.* ASPAN; 2021.

26. American Academy of Ophthalmology, Boyd K. *Cataract Surgery.* 2021. Available at: https://www.aao.org/eye-health/diseases/what-is-cataract-surgery. Accessed July 31, 2021.

27. Glaucoma Research Foundation. *What Is Secondary Glaucoma?* Available at: https://www.glaucoma.org/glaucoma/secondary-glaucoma.php. Accessed July 31, 2021.

28. Abdelmassih Y, Beaujeux P, Dureau P, Edelson C, Caputo G. Incidence and risk factors of glaucoma following pediatric cataract surgery with primary implantation. *Am J Ophthalmol.* 2021;224:1-6. Available at: https://doi.org/10.1016/j.ajo.2020.09.025.

29. Petousis V, Sallam AA, Haynes RJ, et al. Risk factors for retinal detachment following cataract surgery: The impact of posterior capsular rupture. *Br J Ophthalmol.* 2016;100(11):1461-1465. Available at: https://doi.org/10.1136/bjophthalmol-2015-307729.

30. Wielders LHP, Schouten JSAG, Nuijts RMMA. Prevention of macular edema after cataract surgery. *Curr Opin Ophthalmol.* 2018;29(1):48-53. Available at: https://doi.org/10.1097/icu.0000000000000436.

31. McCloud C, Harrington A, King L. A pre-emptive pain management protocol to support self-care following vitreo-retinal day surgery. *J Clin Nurs.* 2014;23(21-22):3230-3239. Available at: https://doi.org/10.1111/jocn.12572.

32. Li Z, Wang Q. Ice compresses aid the reduction of swelling and pain after scleral buckling surgery. *J Clin Nurs.* 2016;25(21-22):3261-3265. Available at: https://doi.org/10.1111/jocn.13362.

33. National Eye Institute. *Glaucoma.* Available at: https://www.nei.nih.gov/learn-about-eye-health/eye-conditions-and-diseases/glaucoma. Accessed July 31, 2021.

34. National Eye Institute. *Glaucoma Surgery.* Available at: https://www.nei.nih.gov/learn-about-eye-health/eye-conditions-and-diseases/glaucoma/glaucoma-surgery. Accessed July 31, 2021.

35. Hua L, Yingjuan L, Jingshu Z, Wei C. The effect of health education video on ocular massage after trabeculectomy. *Comput Inform Nurs.* 2014;32(6):294-298. Available at: https://doi.org/10.1097/cin.0000000000000062.

36. Weinreb RN, Aung T, Medeiros FA. The pathophysiology and treatment of glaucoma: a review. *JAMA.* 2014;311(18):1901-1911. Available at: https://doi.org/10.1001/jama.2014.3192.

37. Eye Bank Association of America. *Facts & Statistics.* Available at: https://restoresight.org. Accessed July 31, 2021.

38. Ang M, Mehta JS, Htoon HM, Tan DTH. Indications, outcomes, and risk factors for failure in tectonic keratoplasty. *Ophthalmology.* 2012;119(7):1311-1319. Available at: https://doi.org/10.1016/j.ophtha.2012.01.021

39. American Academy of Ophthalmology. *EyeWiki. Refractive Surgery.* Available at: https://www.aao.org/eye-health/treatments/photorefractive-keratectomy-prk. Accessed July 31, 2021.

40. Benatti CA, Vinciguerra R. *LASEK. American Academy of Ophthalmology. Eyesmart.* Available at: https://eyewiki.aao/LASEK. Accessed July 31, 2021.

41. National Eye Institute. *Surgery for Refractive Errors.* Available at: https://www.nei.nih.gov/learn-about-eye-health/eye-conditions-and-diseases/refractive-errors/surgery-refractive-errors. Accessed July 31, 2021.

42. *American Association for Pediatric Ophthalmology and Strabismus. Strabismus Surgery.* Available at: https://www.aao.org/eyenet/article/performing-endoscopic-conjunctivodacryocystorhinos. Accessed July 31, 2021.

43. American Academy of Ophthalmology. *Adult Strabismus Surgery - 2017.* Available at: https://www.aao.org/clinical-statement/adult-strabismus-surgery. Accessed July 31, 2021.

44. Boyd K. *Strabismus in Children.* Available at: https://www.aao.org/eye-health/diseases/strabismus-in-children. Accessed July 31, 2021.

45. Waldschmidt B, Gordon N. Anesthesia for pediatric ophthalmologic surgery. *J AAPOS.* 2019;23(3):127-131. Available at: https://doi.org/10.1016/j.jaapos.2018.10.017.

46. American Academy of Ophthalmology. *EyeWiki. Conjunctivodacryocystorhinostomy with Glass Tube (Endoscopic).* Available at: https://eyewiki.org/Conjunctivodacryocystorhinostomy_with_Glass_Tube_(Endoscopic). Accessed July 31, 2021.

47. American Academy of Ophthalmology. Servat JJ, Levin F, Nesi-Eloff FD, Nesi FA. Performing an endoscopic conjunctivodacryocystorhinostomy. *Eyenet Magazine.* 2013;43-44. Available at: https://www.aao.org/eyenet/article/performing-endoscopic-conjunctivodacryocystorhinos. Accessed July 31, 2021.

48. Eshraghi B, Ghadimi H. Lacrimal gland prolapse in upper blepharoplasty. *Orbit.* 2020;39(3):165-170. Available at: https://doi.org/10.1080/01676830.2019.1649434.

49. American Academy of Ophthalmology. *EyeWIKI. Dacryocystorhinostomy.* Available at: https://eyewiki.aao.org/Dacryocystorhinostomy. Accessed July 31, 2021.

50. Neves JC, Medel Jiménez R, Arancibia Tagle D, Vásquez LM. Postoperative care of the facial plastic surgery patient—forehead and blepharoplasty. *Facial Plast Surg.* 2018;34(6):570-578. Available at: https://doi.org/10.1055/s-0038-1676354.

51. Gomez J, Laquis SJ. Blepharoptosis: Clinical presentation, diagnosis, and treatment. *Insight.* 2015;40(2):5-9.

52. American Academy of Ophthalmology. EyeSmart. *What Is the Surgical Procedure for Eyelid Ptosis?* Available at: https://www.aao.org/eye-health/ask-ophthalmologist-q/droopy-eyelid-surgery. Accessed July 31, 2021.

53. Dodge-Palomba S. Providing compassionate care to the pediatric patient undergoing enucleation of the eye. *Insight.* 2008;33(1):10-12.

54. American Academy of Ophthalmology, EyeWIKI. *Enucleation.* Available at: https://eyewiki.aao.org/Enucleation. Accessed July 31, 2021.

55. American Academy of Ophthalmology, EyeWIKI. *Exenteration.* Available at: https://eyewiki.aao.org/Exenteration. Accessed July 31, 2021.

56. American Academy of Ophthalmology, EyeWIKI. *Evisceration.* Available at: https://eyewiki.aao.org/Evisceration. Accessed July 31, 2021.

57. Leclerc R, Olin J. An overview of retinoblastoma and enucleation in pediatric patients. *AORN J.* 2020;111(1):69-79. Available at: https://doi.org/10.1002/aorn.12896.

58. Patel SJ, Feldman BH, Shah VA, Murchison A, et al. *Ocular Penetrating and Perforating Injuries.* American Academy of Ophthalmology. EyeWIKI. Available at: https://eyewiki.aao.org/ocular_penetrating_and_perforating_injuries. Accessed July 31, 2021.

59. Christian CW, Levin AV. The eye examination in the evaluation of child abuse. *Pediatrics.* 2018;142(2):1-8. Available at: https://doi.org/10.1542/peds.2018-1411.

ADDITIONAL RESOURCES

American Academy of Ophthalmology
www.aao.org
American Association for Pediatric Ophthalmology and Strabismus
https://aapos.org/home
American Society of Ophthalmic Registered Nurses
www.asorn.org
American Society of Ophthalmic Registered Nurses. *Scope and Standards of Ophthalmic Clinical Nursing Practice.* San Francisco, California. 2019, ASORN.
American Society of PeriAnesthesia Nurses
www.aspan.org
Eye Bank Association of America
https://restoresight.org
Patterson K, Grenny J, McMillan R, Switzler A. *Crucial conversations: Tools for talking when the stakes are high.* 2nd ed. McGraw-Hill Education. 2011.

31 | Oral and Maxillofacial Surgery

*Denise O'Brien, DNP, RN, ACNS-BC, CPAN (retired), CAPA (retired), FAAN, FCNS, FASPAN;
Kristen Lemorie, MSN, RN, AGCNS-BC, CPAN, CAPA*

LEARNING OBJECTIVES

A review of the content of this chapter will help the reader to:

1. Describe the physiology associated with oral and maxillofacial surgery.
2. Describe common oral and maxillofacial procedures.
3. Identify nursing care for specific surgical procedures.

OVERVIEW

Surgeries on oral and maxillofacial structures are performed by surgeons who specialize in oral and maxillofacial, otorhinolaryngologic, or plastic and reconstructive surgery. Specialists in oral and maxillofacial surgery are specifically trained to manage the various patient diagnoses and conditions that result in the need for surgery. The conditions for which procedures are performed in the outpatient setting and the procedures themselves are discussed in this chapter. It is important for the nurse to understand the surgeon's plan of care to anticipate the patient's needs.

FACTS AND FIGURES

The structures involved in oral/maxillofacial procedures are the oral cavity and skeletal components of the face, including the mandible, maxilla, zygoma, naso-orbital ethmoid complex, and supraorbital structures (Figures 31.1 to 31.3). The oral cavity includes the lips, teeth, gums, buccal mucosa, tongue, hard and soft palate, tonsils, pharynx, and temporomandibular joint (TMJ). Jaw bones (mandible, maxilla), muscle, and mucosa surround the oral cavity. The cavity forms the beginning of the digestive system and is a major organ of speech and emotional expression.

The trigeminal nerve (cranial nerve V) splits into the maxillary division, which supplies sensation to the upper teeth, and the mandibular division, which supplies sensation to the lower teeth (Figures 31.4 to 31.6). There are three branches that supply sensation to other areas of the mouth and face. The lingual nerve provides sensation to the anterior two thirds of the tongue and the floor of the mouth and gums. The inferior alveolar nerve provides sensation to the premolar and molar teeth of the mandible, and the mental nerve provides sensation to the lower lip and chin.

The mandible and maxilla constitute the bony structure of the jaw. The mandible is a horseshoe-shaped bone that forms the lower jaw and is the largest and strongest bone in the face. This bone articulates with the TMJ. The maxilla is an irregularly shaped bone that forms the upper jaw. This bone touches every other facial bone except the mandible. It forms the orbit, the nasal cavity, and the palate and supports the upper teeth.

Although the TMJ can be compared with other joints in the body, there are distinct differences. The TMJ is a bicondylar joint, also called a condylar joint, formed by the glenoid fossa of the temporal bone and the mandibular condyle. The meniscus (disk) of connective tissue lies between the bone structures. A capsule of the joint is reinforced laterally by the temporomandibular ligament, which limits the anterior and posterior condylar movements.

Oral and maxillofacial procedures can be restorative, therapeutic, elective, or urgent. Examples include dental extractions (odondectomy) or implants, fracture reduction, incision and drainage of abscesses or cysts, and excision of tumors or lesions (Table 31.1). Lasers are used for oral and maxillofacial surgical procedures. Uses include coagulation of angiomatous lesions or TMJ arthroscopy.[1,2] The nursing care needs of patients undergoing oral and maxillofacial procedures include maintaining the airway, managing nausea and vomiting related to swallowed blood, halitosis (bad breath), and an unpleasant taste in the mouth. Patients may also experience

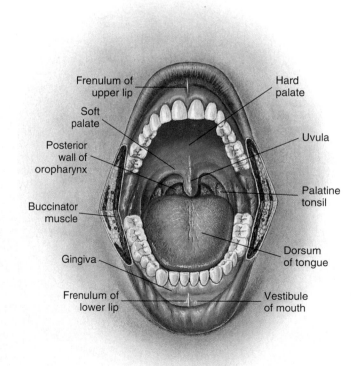

Fig. 31.1 Anatomic structures of the oral cavity. (Flanagan AL. Otorhinolaryngologic surgery. Figure 19.7 in: In Rothrock J. *Alexander's Care of the Patient in Surgery*. Elsevier; 2019.)

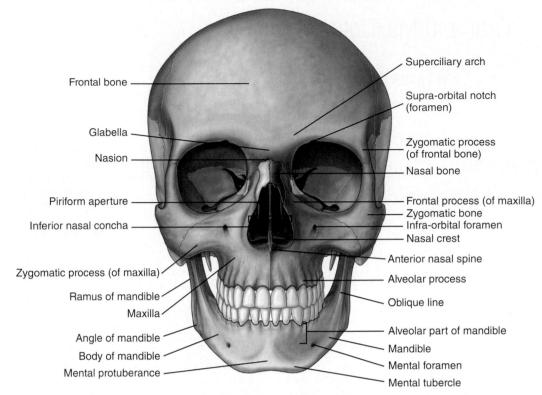

Fig. 31.2 Anterior view of the skull. (Drake RL, Vogl AW, Mitchell AWM. Head and neck. Figure 8.3 in: *Gray's Basic Anatomy*. 3rd ed. Elsevier; 2023.)

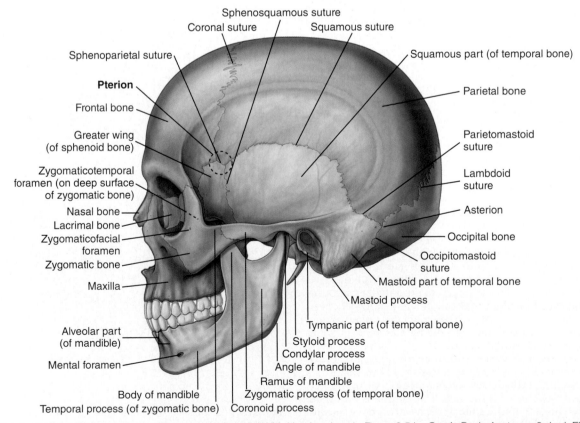

Fig. 31.3 Lateral view of the skull. (Drake RL, Vogl AW, Mitchell AWM. Head and neck. Figure 8.5 in: *Gray's Basic Anatomy*. 3rd ed. Elsevier; 2023.)

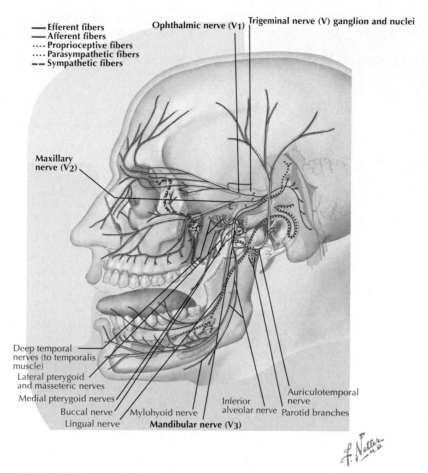

Efferent fibers
Afferent fibers
···· Proprioceptive fibers
···· Parasympathetic fibers
−− Sympathetic fibers

Ophthalmic nerve (V₁)

Trigeminal nerve (V) ganglion and nuclei

Maxillary nerve (V₂)

Deep temporal nerves (to temporalis muscle)

Lateral pterygoid and masseteric nerves

Medial pterygoid nerves

Buccal nerve

Lingual nerve

Mylohyoid nerve

Inferior alveolar nerve

Auriculotemporal nerve

Parotid branches

Mandibular nerve (V₃)

Fig. 31.4 Trigeminal (V) nerve. (Norton NS. Temporal and infratemporal fossae. Figure 7.12 in: *Netter's Head and Neck Anatomy for Dentistry.* 3rd ed. Elsevier; 2017.)

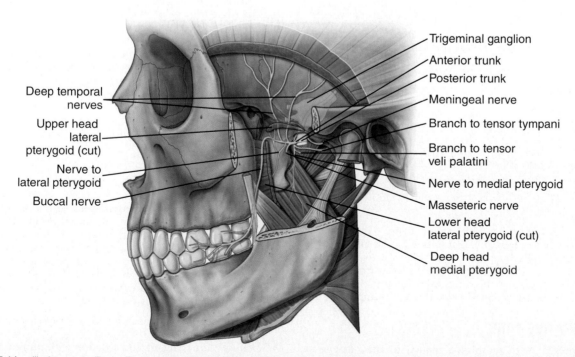

Deep temporal nerves

Upper head lateral pterygoid (cut)

Nerve to lateral pterygoid

Buccal nerve

Trigeminal ganglion

Anterior trunk

Posterior trunk

Meningeal nerve

Branch to tensor tympani

Branch to tensor veli palatini

Nerve to medial pterygoid

Masseteric nerve

Lower head lateral pterygoid (cut)

Deep head medial pterygoid

Fig. 31.5 Mandibular nerve. (Drake RL, Vogl AW, Mitchell AWM. Head and neck. Figure 8.130 in: *Gray's Basic Anatomy.* 3rd ed. Elsevier; 2023.)

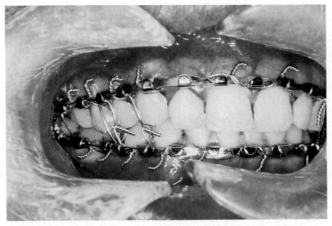

Fig. 31.6 Teeth in occlusion with arch bars in place. (McEwen DR. Reconstructive and aesthetic plastic surgery. Figure 22.25 in: Rothrock J. *Alexander's Care of the Patient in Surgery*. Elsevier; 2019.)

TABLE 31.1 Terminology of Oral/Maxillofacial Surgery

Term	Definition
Alveolectomy	Radical surgical reduction or removal of the alveolar process
Alveoplasty	Bone conserving, surgical contouring, or remodeling of the residual ridge to achieve a denture-bearing surface
Arch bars	Rigid metal bars used to splint and fix the teeth, maxilla, or mandible
Dental implant	A prosthetic implant with an anchoring subperiosteally or endosteally
Genioplasty	Correction of chin deformities
Gingivectomy	Removal of all loose, infected, and diseased gingival tissue
Intraoral biopsy	Excisional or incisional removal of abnormal tissue for histopathologic examination
Marsupialization	Creating an accessory cavity to encourage repair and regeneration; used to eliminate the closed condition of a cyst
Odontectomy	Tooth extraction; can be single or multiple; may be needed because of trauma, recurrent infections, or nonresorbable teeth or to prepare for implants
Vestibuloplasty	Alveolar ridge augmentation for the purpose of marking a residual ridge available to use as a denture-bearing surface

Adapted from: Fonseca RJ. *Oral and maxillofacial surgery*. 3rd ed. Elsevier; 2018; and O'Brien D. Oral/maxillofacial/dental. Pages 675-685 in: Schick L, Windle PE, eds. *PeriAnesthesia Nursing Core Curriculum: Preprocedure, Phase I and Phase II PACU Nursing*. 4th ed. Elsevier; 2021.

difficulty chewing and talking after surgery. Uncooperative patients, small children, and patients who are physically or mentally frail or disabled may be unable to withstand procedures that, under normal circumstances, are performed in an office. These people may be candidates for ambulatory surgical procedures, such as dental extractions or fillings.

PREOPERATIVE CARE

Patients present with symptoms related to their diagnoses. After a review of systems, the perianesthesia nurse assesses the facial and oral structures to determine a baseline status. During the preoperative assessment, the perianesthesia nurse additionally observes how far the patient can open his or her mouth and assess for trismus (limited opening), lumps, facial swelling, and skin color and texture. This includes examining the intraoral cavity and the tongue for size, mobility, color, and texture, as well as the oral mucosa, alveolar ridges, gingivae, and general condition of the teeth. Nutritional status, including that during the preoperative fasting period, is also assessed since pain or injury to the oral and maxillofacial structures might result in decreased desire or inability to eat. Patients should be adequately hydrated before the procedure.

Relevant laboratory values for coagulation or other studies and radiographs or computed tomography scan results must be available. Patients are asked about previous problems with bleeding and a history of oral surgery procedures to determine reactions to local anesthesia, delayed healing, or alveolalgia (dry socket). The perianesthesia nurse then reviews the consent form with the patient to obtain verbal recognition that the procedure and risks are understood. One risk surgeons often explain involves the potential for transient or permanent numbness due to nerve damage.

The use of prophylactic antimicrobial therapy may be considered for patients with certain cardiac conditions, including rheumatic heart disease, mitral valve prolapse, valve replacement histories, and other congenital heart diseases that render patients at highest risk for infective endocarditis.[3] Prescribed antibiotics should be initiated prior to the start of the surgical procedure in accordance with facility surgical antimicrobial prophylaxis guidelines.[3] Maintaining good oral health and regular dental care should be emphasized due to the critical role in postoperative infection risk reduction.[4]

Patient education includes preparing the patient for the possibility of bloody oral drainage and the need to secure appropriate supplies for home, including cool and soft foods and beverages, medications prescribed by the physician, and cold therapy (e.g., an ice pack), although this may be provided to the patient at the surgery center. Discharge planning should also include general postoperative instructions related to pain management, symptoms to report, activities, and follow-up care.

Patients might be concerned, anxious, or fearful about their resultant body image or might show concern about undergoing a surgical procedure. Many procedures can be done through an incision in the oral cavity; therefore, scarring is not an issue. Altered appearance due to soft tissue changes related to the surgical procedure may be distressing to patients even if only temporary.[5] Patient teaching is important to increase the patient's and family member's understanding of the expected outcomes and participation in postoperative care. The perianesthesia nurse should assess the patient's and family member's need for information and ability to understand instructions.

INTRAOPERATIVE CARE

Patients are anesthetized using monitored anesthesia care or general anesthesia. Nasal or nasotracheal intubation is commonly used to eliminate interference with the surgical procedure and to provide better access to the operative field. A moist packing is used to occlude the posterior pharynx to prevent inadvertent aspiration of fluids. If monitored anesthesia care is required, the following sedative-hypnotic, analgesic, and anesthesia agents may be utilized[6]:

- Benzodiazepines (midazolam) for anxiolysis, sedation, and amnesia
- Ketamine, for analgesia and sedation with minimal respiratory depression

- Opioids (fentanyl, morphine, hydromorphone) for analgesia
- Propofol for hypnosis/sedation with antiemetic properties
- Alpha-2 agonists (dexmedetomidine) for sedation, anxiolysis, analgesia, and prevention of emergence delirium

Local anesthesia can be used as an adjunct during general anesthesia to ease dissection, allow for less anesthetic agent, and minimize immediate postoperative pain. The addition of epinephrine to the local agent helps to minimize bleeding in the operative field and prolong the anesthetic effect of the injection. Nurses should be aware of the signs and symptoms of local anesthesia systemic toxicity and ensure that treatment (e.g., IV lipids) is immediately available.[7]

Although every effort is made to maintain aseptic technique, the mouth is an area that harbors pathogens. Prevention of infection is important because a postoperative infection can result in the loss of bone and teeth, endocarditis, loss of implants, or scarring. In some oral surgical practices, the patients are provided antimicrobial mouth rinses to complete prior to the induction of anesthesia.[8] Corticosteroid medications, such as dexamethasone, are often given intravenously to reduce pain, inflammation, edema, and trismus. A sterile field is created, and sterile instruments are used to prevent the introduction of pathogens and to prevent cross-contamination. Ointments or balms can be used to lubricate the patient's lips to prevent them from cracking. When retracting the mouth to gain operative access, attention must be given to avoid injury to the lips and tongue, because it is easy for them to be pinched given the small area of visualization. Hemostatic agents may be required to manage intraoral bleeding.

At the end of the procedure, the oral cavity is suctioned, and pressure packs are placed. The perioperative nurse should document the removal of the throat pack and the accuracy of the sponge count because the patient's airway could be fatally compromised if any foreign object is inadvertently left in place. Sponges may be placed between the patient's teeth or gums and the lip to provide pressure on incisions, but they must be monitored constantly until the patient is alert enough to be aware of their presence and to maintain an adequate airway. An oral or nasal airway may be inserted for transfer to the postanesthesia care unit (PACU).

POSTOPERATIVE CARE

The postoperative nurse receives handover reports from the anesthesia care provider and perioperative nurse. Information shared includes the type of procedure, the presence and type of splints, and the location of packing and sutures that were used. If the jaws are wired or secured with elastics, wire cutters or scissors should be immediately available if the patient vomits or respiratory distress occurs.

Postoperative monitoring of respiratory and cardiac status, vital signs, and bleeding and observation of internal and external facial and oral structures for changes are critical. Suction should be available if bleeding occurs or secretions collect in the oral cavity; gentle use of suctioning is imperative because vigorous suctioning can impair clot formation and prevent hemostasis. The patient is positioned to facilitate drainage of saliva or bloody secretions. Because of the procedure or local anesthesia that is used, the patient may experience difficulty swallowing. After some oral and maxillofacial procedures, pressure may be maintained on the surgical sites by having the patient bite gently on folded gauze pads of 4-by-4 inches or sponges of 2-by-2 inches. Gauze should not be cut for this use because frayed edges could allow threads to come off in the mouth. Swallowed blood can result in nausea and vomiting. The pressure resulting from vomiting or retching can increase the chance of bleeding and suture dehiscence.

Other potential problems after oral and maxillofacial procedures include infection;[9] nerve damage with temporary or permanent paresis of the lips, mouth, or face;[9] inadvertent puncture of the maxillary sinus; damage to other teeth;[10] edema, and, rarely, fracture of the jaw,[9,11] Analgesics should be given to minimize pain. Physicians should be consulted about the use of ice packs directly on the surgical site due to the possibility of a rebound effect (increased blood flow) that might occur after the ice pack is removed.

Postoperative edema is expected. External cryotherapy (e.g., ice packs) may be prescribed for intermittent use at home over the first 24-48 hours to reduce postoperative pain and edema. Periorbital ecchymosis, swelling of the jaw and cheeks, mouth discomfort, and inability to open the mouth wide are common occurrences. An oral analgesic is usually prescribed for pain, and the patient is warned to avoid taking aspirin in the early postoperative period due to a potential risk for bleeding. Antiemetics, antibiotics, and analgesics (nonsteroidal anti-inflammatory medications) are usually ordered; medication regimens should be reviewed with the patient and family member/caregiver.

Unintentional swallowing of blood may result in nausea and vomiting. In turn, patients may avoid eating, and their nutritional status and hydration can be compromised. Patients should understand the need to meet nutritional requirements for healing, and they should be encouraged to use antiemetics or other strategies to reduce nausea. Patients will resume a diet appropriate for their procedure. If the procedure is aggressive, the patient can have a clear-liquid to full-liquid high-calorie diet as tolerated. Some patients might begin with a soft (nonchewing) diet and progress to a regular diet as recommended by the surgeon. The patient should avoid temperature extremes in food and beverages. Soft foods may or may not be allowed depending on the type of surgery performed. Patients should be taught oral hygiene. For bad breath or taste and to reduce biofilm formation and gingival inflammation, the physician may allow the patient to gently rinse with salt water or a commercial or prescription mouthwash, but a specific physician's order should be obtained before this instruction. After a tooth extraction, the protective blood clot over the socket may be lost with vigorous gargling or rinsing, resulting in a dry socket; this implies that bone has become exposed at the extraction site and causes severe pain.

Evidence-Based Practice: Treating "Dry Socket"

Dry socket, also known as alveolar osteitis (AO), is a common postoperative complication following dental extractions. The incidence of AO is reportedly as high as 68%. Several factors have been identified as potentially contributing to the etiology of AO. These include the presence of bacteria often related to poor oral hygiene, local tissue trauma, smoking, oral contraception, and the actual location of the extraction (higher % in mandibular extractions). Chow et al., report a number of interventions to treat AO including topical and local anesthesia, systemic analgesics, medicated local dressings, and the use of low-level later therapy (LLLT).

Source: Chow O, Wang R, Ku D, Huang W. Alveolar osteitis: A review of current concepts. *J Oral Maxillofac Surg.* 2020;78(8):1288-1296. https://doi.org/10.1016/j.joms.2020.03.026

The patient may be wearing a prosthetic device in the mouth postoperatively. The nurse should check its proper position and ensure that it does not compromise the airway prior to the patient's discharge. The patient must understand the proper use and care of any device that has been fitted, including whether removal of the device is allowed, necessary cleaning, and the potential problems or restrictions while the prosthesis is in place. If the jaw is stabilized with wires or bands, the patient should be taught how to cut the wires or bands in the event of respiratory distress or vomiting. The patient may also be instructed on how to use dental wax to reduce mucosal irritation (Box 31.1).

COMMON ORAL AND MAXILLOFACIAL PROCEDURES

Dental Extraction, Incision and Drainage, and Excision of Nonmalignant Tumors or Lesions

The extraction of teeth involves bony and soft tissues of the oral cavity. Patients may require surgery in an ambulatory surgical center (ASC) because of their systemic conditions, the extent of the procedure, or anticipated difficulties in removing the teeth that can be managed more easily and more comfortably with sedation or anesthesia. Reasons for the extraction might include severe loss of bone structure supporting the teeth, teeth that interfere mechanically with placement of a restorative appliance (e.g., dentures), fractured roots, or nonvital pulps. An alveoplasty (procedure to smooth the jawbone) or vestibuloplasty (surgical reshaping of the patient's anatomy.

An abscess or infected cyst, tumor, or lesion can form in any area of the oral cavity. Abscesses that will not respond to antibiotics and must be drained or cysts that must be excised are examples of symptoms of patients who might require surgical intervention in the ASC for the benefit of having monitored anesthesia care or general anesthesia. Patients might present with symptoms of swelling or pain, depending on the size and location of the abscess or cyst. It is common to obtain a culture of drainage to identify the specific bacteria causing the problem. If an abscess is large and there is concern that healing might be difficult, a wound drain might be inserted.

A cyst is a pouch or sac without an opening that contains fluid. Cysts form in various sizes and locations. Types of cysts include developmental (lined with epithelium), neoplastic (abnormal growth of cells), and mucous retention cysts (most common). Most cysts are harmless, although some may become swollen, tender, and infected. Treatment can require complete extraction or the creation of a window in the bone to allow permanent drainage and regrowth of the area (marsupialization).

Nonmalignant tumors or abnormal growths can be found in numerous areas of the oral cavity. These lesions can form in the soft tissue (e.g., gingiva, buccal mucosa, tongue) or bone (e.g., maxilla, mandible, palate). Examples include hyperplasia, fibromas, chondromas, papillomas, or dermoid cysts.[1] An incisional (removing a representative area) or excisional (removing the total lesion) biopsy might require a histopathologic (frozen section) examination. Exostoses or tori (bone outgrowths) might also occur on the alveolar ridges, palate, or other bone areas requiring excision.

The parotid, submandibular, sublingual, and accessory glands supply saliva through ducts to the oral cavity. The lingual nerves are in close relationship to the submandibular ducts. Tumors, cysts, stones, or trauma may affect salivary glands. Surgery on the ducts is the method of choice to treat lesions of accessory salivary glands, to manage malignant lesions, or to correct traumatic injuries. Postoperative care of these patients varies based on the patients' needs for surgery. Airway management is a priority initially and on a long-term basis because edema could result and requires immediate attention.

Dental Restorations and Implants

The placement of dental implants is a restorative procedure for the permanent anchoring of prosthetic teeth. Implants are placed to improve function, provide comfort, and improve esthetics and emotional and psychological attitudes.[12] The procedure provides more natural-appearing and natural-feeling teeth than that provided by traditional dentures. Patients must understand the risks, limitations, cost, and time commitment of implant restorations.[13]

Implant fixtures can be used to anchor single or multiple replacement teeth. The implant fixtures are either buried beneath the mucosal layer or implanted in the periosteal layer (subperiosteally) or in the bone. The dental implant (replacement tooth) fixture is inserted approximately 4 weeks to several months after the insertion of implant fixtures, depending on the time appropriate for the type of implant being used. Implant fixtures are made of titanium, ceramic, or polymer.[14]

Patients undergo the procedure with monitored anesthesia care or a general anesthetic. A local anesthetic with epinephrine is often injected to aid hemostasis and postoperative analgesia. The bone canal is prepared using specialized drills. Screws, commonly called implant fixtures, are screwed into the bone of the mandible and maxilla very gently to avoid damage to the bone surrounding the implant.[14] Because the local anesthesia for dental work can spread to nearby structures, the nurse must ensure that the patient is able to swallow properly prior to discharge from the ASC.

The benefits of dental implants over traditional dentures include decreased pain from ill-fitting dentures, improved sense of taste, better dentition and digestion, improved psychological attitude, a more natural look and feel, and sometimes a reduction in problems involving the TMJ. Oral hygiene is imperative for the success of implants.

Temporomandibular Joint Arthroscopy

TMJ diseases and dysfunctions are several; congenital or developmental deformities of the condylar head, early ankylosis, neoplasia, septic arthritis, or degenerative disease might cause symptoms. The TMJ can also be injured by trauma. The TMJ is like other joints in that it requires satisfactory function between the disk and bone elements of the joint for maximum function and comfort.

Arthroscopic intervention for TMJ dysfunction has been used in the United States since 1983. Both diagnosis and treatment are possible arthroscopically. It has been reported as an effective technique for treating various stages of internal derangement.[15] Fibrous adhesions in the joint can be lysed, debridement performed, and the disk repositioned through the arthroscope. Often, simple lavage of the joints seems to have a therapeutic effect on decreasing joint symptoms.[16]

Patients who are treated arthroscopically have usually tried more conservative medical treatments without success. Jaw pain, persistent headaches, mechanical restrictions, and difficulties in chewing and opening the mouth are typical presenting symptoms. Counseling is important before surgery so that the patient is well informed of the expected outcomes of surgery and the potential risks (e.g., perforation of the external auditory canal and damage to cranial nerve VII with resultant facial paralysis.)[15] Insurance reimbursement for TMJ surgery may be restricted; this restriction may create financial hardship for the patient.

Before the patient's procedure, an occlusive splint is fitted and the patient, surgeon, or the splint production specialist usually brings the customized device to the ASC. This appliance is worn in the mouth postoperatively to relieve pressure on the jaw muscles and to maintain proper occlusion. Intraoperatively, the patient's position is supine. Procedure times vary, depending on the amount of work that is required.

Postoperative discomfort may require the use of analgesics. Elevation of the patient's head helps to relieve feelings of pressure, and ice is used to reduce or prevent swelling and reduce pain after the surgery. Physiotherapy to correct trismus may be required after the patient is discharged. Generally, diets are restricted to full liquids for the first 7-10 days and are then advanced to foods that require no chewing, often based on patient comfort. It is important for the patient to wear the occlusal splint as directed, to follow instructions regarding diet and activity restrictions, and to take all prescribed medications.[17]

Fracture Reduction and Facial Reconstruction

Closed and open reductions of the mandible can be done in the outpatient setting. A simple fracture can be repaired using general anesthesia and with the application of a stabilizing device, such as elastic bands or wires. Arch bars, which are small strips of metal secured to the teeth, may be applied to ensure proper alignment, and provide maxillomandibular fixation while the bones heal. Numerous interdental eyelet wires (e.g., Ivy loop technique) can be placed on the posterior teeth to serve as attachment sites for wires or elastic bands. The wires or splints secure the mandible and maxilla to bring the teeth into normal occlusion.

Open reduction of fractures with plates, screws, or wire might be used to repair a fractured mandible or maxilla or a zygomatic fracture. Frequently, the incision can take place through the oral cavity. The fracture site is exposed, and bone is approximated. The securing devices are applied. Although the patient's tissue is manipulated to implant the securing devices, unless there is concern about the patient's ability to care for himself or herself, airway management, or postoperative bleeding, these patients are candidates for the outpatient setting.

Airway assessment throughout the perioperative event as well as immediately postoperatively is important, because the jaws are potentially wired to reduce movement or elastic bands are applied to secure the jaw in a closed position (see Figure 31.6). Patients are taught about diet and nutrition because they are unable to eat a regular diet, perform oral hygiene, or take action in the event of airway difficulties. The use of adequate pain control and cold therapy (ice packs) should be reviewed.

Orthognathic Surgery

Orthognathic surgery serves a number of patients for a variety of purposes. Patients who have either acquired or congenital defects associated with the mechanics of oral and facial structures (e.g., malocclusion), as well as clinical deformities impacting the patient's psychosocial status, may require surgical treatment. The surgical approach to these deformities requires either a reduction or an enhancement of the maxilla or the mandible, depending on the actual deficit. Advances in surgical techniques have improved the options for patients so they can undergo orthognathic surgery on an outpatient basis. In addition, successful same-day discharges require that the patient and family are well prepared and motivated to provide home-based postoperative care.[18]

CHAPTER HIGHLIGHTS

- Oral and maxillofacial procedures can be restorative, therapeutic, elective, or urgent.
- Procedures may include, but are not limited to, dental extractions (odondectomy) or implants, fracture reduction, incision and drainage of abscesses or cysts, and excision of tumors or lesions.
- Thorough preoperative assessment and patient education are crucial for optimizing patient outcomes.
- Postoperative nursing care needs of patients undergoing oral and maxillofacial procedures include maintaining the airway and managing nausea and vomiting related to swallowed blood, halitosis (bad breath), and an unpleasant taste in the mouth.

CASE STUDY

A 63-year-old female is a self-described dental phobic. As a young child, she vividly recalls a terrible experience with a dentist. As a result of this impressionable episode, she has struggled with routine oral and dental care over the past two decades. A quick exam by a new dental hygienist revealed a suspicious lesion on the lateral surface of her tongue. Aware of the anxiety, her dentist determined that she would need extensive laser therapy to the affected surfaces of the tongue. Although the procedure would be quick, the anxiety of the patient was a huge factor in determining where and how the procedure should occur.

She was given a preoperative physical and otherwise was found to be in good health. Since she had no issues with obesity, sleep apnea, diabetes, asthma, limited mouth opening, restricted airway, or the use of psychiatric drugs she was determined to be a good candidate for the outpatient surgery center. In addition, her preanesthesia assessment revealed no clinical contraindications for general anesthesia.

As the perianesthesia nurse, what issues are anticipated to impact this patient's experience and recovery? Consider the following:

- How is the patient dealing with the diagnosis of a 'suspicious lesion'?
- What are the implications for patient education related to both pain management and nutrition following laser ablation of the tongue?
- What other needs should be discussed in terms of discharge and follow-up upon preparation for returning home?

REFERENCES

1. Fonseca RJ. *Oral and Maxillofacial Surgery*. 3rd ed. Elsevier; 2018.
2. Solderer A, Kaufmann M, Hofer D, Wiedemeier D, Attin T, Schmidlin PR. Efficacy of chlorhexidine rinses after periodontal or implant surgery: a systematic review. *Clin Oral Investig*. 2019;23(1):21-32. Available at: https://doi.org/10.1007/s00784-018-2761-y.
3. Anderson DJ. Antimicrobial prophylaxis for prevention of surgical site infection in adults. *UpToDate*. November 2022. Available at: https://www.uptodate.com/contents/antimicrobial-prophylaxis-for-prevention-of-surgical-site-infection-in-adults#H852308389.
4. Wilson WR, Gewitz M, Lockhart PB, et al. Prevention of viridams group streptococcal infective endocarditis: A scientific statement from the American Heart Association. *Circulation*. 2021;143(20):e963-e978. Available at: https://doi.org/10.1161/cir.0000000000000969.
5. Moorthi RK, Kumar MPS. Pre- and post-operative anxiety in patients undergoing dental extractions. *Drug Invention Today*. 2018;10:2445-2449. Available at: https://www.researchgate.net/publication/328869016_Pre-_and_post-operative_anxiety_in_patients_undergoing_dental_extractions.
6. Rosero EB. Monitored anesthesia care in adults. *UpToDate*. November 2022. Available at: https://www.uptodate.com/contents/monitored-anesthesia-care-in-adults#H2720012704.
7. El-Boghdadly K, Pawa A, Chin KJ. Local anesthetic systemic toxicity: Current perspectives. *Local Reg Anesth*. 2018;11:35-44. Available at: https://doi.org/10.2147/lra.s154512.
8. Hassan S, Dhadse P, Bajaj P, Sethiya K, Subhadarsanee C. Pre-procedural antimicrobial mouth rinse: A concise review. *Cureus*. 2022;14(10):e30629. Available at: https://doi.org/10.7759/cureus.30629.
9. Askar H, Di Gianfilippo R, Ravida A, Tattan M, Majzoub J, Wang HL. Incidence and severity of postoperative complications following oral, periodontal, and implant surgeries: a retrospective study. *J Periodontol*. 2019;90(11):1270-1278. Available at: https://doi.org/10.1002/JPER.18-0658.
10. Molina A, Sanz-Sanchez I, Sanz-Martin I, Ortiz-Vigon A, Sanz M. Complications in sinus lifting procedures: Classification and management. *Periodontol 2000*. 2022;88(1):103-115. Available at: https://doi.org/10.1111/prd.12414.
11. Dos Santos Silva W, Silveira RJ, de Araujo Andrade MGB, Franco A, Silva RF. Is the late mandibular fracture from third molar extraction a risk towards malpractice? Case report with the analysis of ethical and legal aspects. *J Oral Maxillofac Res*. 2017;8(2):e5. Available at: https://doi.org/10.5037/jomr.2017.8205.
12. Block MS. Dental implants: the last 100 years. *J Oral Maxillofac Surg*. 2018;76(1):11-26. Available at: https://doi.org/10.1016/j.joms.2017.08.045.
13. Nishimura RD, Beumer J, Perri GR, Davodi A. Implants in the partially edentulous patient: Restorative considerations. *Oral Health*. 1998;10:19-28.
14. American Association of Oral and Maxillofacial Surgeons. Introduction to implant dentistry: a student guide. *J Maxillofac Oral Surg*. 2017;75(2):28-41. Available at: https://doi.org/10.1016/j.joms.2016.09.034.
15. Chowdhury SKR, Saxena V, Rajkumar K, Shadamarshan RA. Complications of diagnostic TMJ arthroscopy: An institutional study. *J Maxillofac Oral Surg*. 2019;18(4):531-535. Available at: https://doi.org/10.1007/s12663-019-01202-3.
16. Bergstrand S, Ingstad HK, Moystad A, Bjornland T. Long-term effectiveness of arthrocentesis with and without hyaluronic acid injection for treatment of temporomandibular joint osteoarthritis. *J Oral Sci*. 2019;61(1):82-88. Available at: https://doi.org/10.2334/josnusd.17-0423.
17. Altaweel AA, Ismail HA, Fayad MI. Effect of simultaneous application of arthrocentesis and occlusal splint versus splint in management of non-reducing TMJ disc displacement. *J Dent Sci*. 2021;16(2):732-737. Available at: https://doi.org/10.1016/j.jds.2020.08.008.
18. Mcewen DR. Reconstructive and aesthetic plastic surgery. In: Rothrock J, ed. *Alexander's Care of the Patient in Surgery*. Elsevier; 2019:810-852.
19. Pekkari C, Weiner DK, Marcusson A, Davidson T, Naimi-Akbar A, Lund B. Patient safety with orthognathic surgery in an outpatient setting. *Int J Oral Maxillofac Surg*. 2023;52(7):806-812. Available at: https://doi.org/10.1016/j.ijom.2022.12.001.

32 Orthopedic and Podiatric Surgery

Theresa L. Clifford, DNP, RN, CPAN, CAPA, FASPAN, FAAN

LEARNING OBJECTIVES

A review of the content of this chapter will help the reader to:

1. Describe common outpatient orthopedic surgery procedures performed.
2. Identify nursing care for specific surgical procedures.
3. Identify potential complications related to outpatient orthopedic surgery.

OVERVIEW

Treatment of orthopedic and podiatric conditions in an ambulatory surgery setting is extremely common in contemporary times. Procedures are generally performed for congenital, traumatic, or acquired conditions that may have resulted in acute or chronic disorders. These conditions include musculoskeletal disorders caused by abnormality of development, structural disease, degenerative changes, or injury. The disorders might affect any of the bones or supporting structures of the skeletal system (Figure 32.1).

Caring for patients undergoing procedures on bones or associated structures requires thorough assessments, patient preparation, and planning to ensure that the procedure is completed in the safest and most efficient manner. The ability to decrease the length of stay is a benefit of less invasive procedures but does not preclude the need to spend time preparing for the procedure and teaching the patient. This is particularly true regarding procedures that have traditionally been performed in an inpatient setting such as total joint arthroplasty. Facilitating successful transition from operating room to home requires an understanding of the anatomy and associated physiology, specific patient conditions, co-morbidities and needs, the plan of care to be provided by other team members (e.g., surgeon, anesthesiologist, physical therapist), intraoperative interventions, and expected outcomes.

The anatomy of the musculoskeletal system includes bony structures, ligaments, tendons, and nerves. The specific patient condition and needs influence the plan of care. Understanding and relating the structures involved and the physiologic condition enables individualized patient and procedure preparation, teaching, and discharge planning. Patients undergoing orthopedic and podiatric procedures are various ages, with varying physical conditions. Their needs provide a challenge to the perioperative and perianesthesia nursing personnel.

Knowledge of the patient's needs and the plan of care being provided by others complements the preparation for the procedure. Surgeon preferences vary based on level of familiarity with instrumentation and choice of operative technique. This includes implant and repair types. An example includes positioning the patient for a surgical procedure. The position selected is expected to provide exposure without compromising the patients' respiratory, circulatory, or neurovascular status. The nursing intervention is aimed at preventing patient injury. Understanding the position and equipment specifically used by a physician increases the ability to assess, plan, implement, and evaluate the patient's perianesthesia plan of care.

FACTS AND FIGURES

A 2010 data report from the Centers for Disease Control and Prevention 15% of surgical procedures (7.1 million) that were performed in outpatient hospital centers were musculoskeletal surgeries.[1] There are many drivers for the expanding volume of orthopedic surgeries being done in outpatient or office-based settings. These include lower costs, advanced surgical techniques, progressive opioid-sparing pain control measures, improved patient and provider satisfaction, and fewer complications. Workflow efficiencies in the outpatient setting have also driven higher volumes and improved experiences. These include the ability to perform the same or similar procedures repeatedly, faster turnover times, more selective patient criteria, and optimized pain and comfort measures.[2] As insurers follow Medicare reimbursement rules which have removed primary total joint arthroplasties from the inpatient list, most patients presenting for orthopedic procedures should now be evaluated to consider receiving care in the ASC setting.[3]

GENERAL ORTHOPEDIC SURGICAL PROCEDURES

Perianesthesia care of the patient undergoing outpatient orthopedic surgery includes, but is not limited to, basic clinical interventions applying to all surgical candidates. These preparatory actions consist of a preoperative assessment involving a general review of the medical and surgical histories, medications, allergies, the family history, and social determinants, to name a few. Any relevant preoperative testing, including verification of preoperative diagnostic imaging and selective laboratory tests, must be documented. During the preoperative phase, providers as well as members of the anesthesia team determine the appropriateness of the patient for an outpatient setting based on previously established criteria. The criteria for surgery in an outpatient setting may include the complexity of surgery, management of co-morbidities, and other surgical risks. The preoperative period is the best time to initiate patient education related to the procedure, expected recovery, and ultimate outcomes, as well as postoperative care needs, such as the use of durable medical devices (e.g., crutches, walkers, slings) and pain management (Box 32.1). A critical component of successful outpatient surgery is the engagement and commitment of the patient to be an active member of the care team and assume personal responsibility for following instructions for pre- and postoperative care.[4]

Chapter 19 in this book provides a thorough overview of the principles of enhanced recovery after surgery (ERAS). These same pathways have been explored for their applicability to orthopedic patients. Overall, ERAS has been shown to improve patient outcomes following anesthesia and surgery,

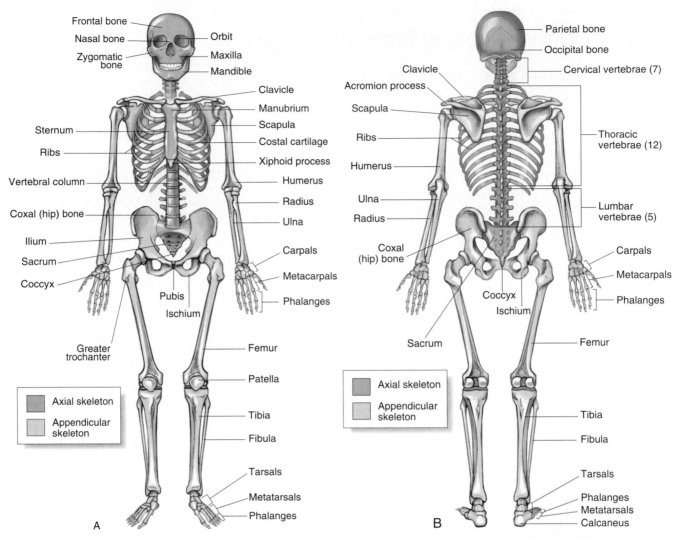

Fig. 32.1 Anterior view (A) and posterior view (B) of the skeleton. Bowen BA. Orthopedic surgery. Figure 20.1 in: Rothrock JC. *Alexander's Care of the Patient in Surgery.* 16th ed. Elsevier; 2019.

BOX 32.1 Demonstration of Education Outcomes by Orthopedic Surgery Patients

Demonstrate proper use of supportive devices (e.g., crutches, walkers, and/or walking shoes)

Describe proper dosage procedure for prescribed analgesic medications and report uncontrolled pain

Report excessive drainage on dressings

Describe signs and symptoms of infection and report findings to the physician immediately

Report any neurologic or circulatory impairment

Describe understanding of the need for limited mobility for 6–8 weeks

Cannon S. Orthopedics and podiatry. Box 29.3 in: Schick L, Windle PE, eds. *Perianesthesia Nursing Core Curriculum: Preprocedure, Phase I and Phase II PACU Nursing.* 4th ed. Elsevier; 2021.

---

as well as to reduce the length of stay.[5] The goals for each phase of ERAS, including the preoperative, intraoperative, and postoperative phases, apply to the orthopedic patient. These goals include preoperative interventions aimed at optimizing patients physically to better manage the stress associated with the surgical experience, to improve the patient's knowledge and expectations for the experience through comprehensive preoperative education, and to reduce the impact of prolonged fasting on insulin resistance and hyperglycemia.[5] Interoperative techniques aim for the least invasive approach and application of contemporary opioid-sparing pain management interventions (e.g., liposomal nerve blocks). Efforts to optimize fluid balance help to reduce postoperative nausea and vomiting, support the best oxygenation of tissues, and support enhanced wound healing.[5] Early mobilization and multimodal analgesia round off the postoperative phase of care to reduce pulmonary complications and barriers to comfort that are likely to impede recovery.[5]

Total Joint Arthroplasty: Hip and Knee

Total joint arthroplasty is fast becoming an outpatient option for many patients. A wide variety of surgical vendors supply an improved assortment of implant components for joint replacement surgery. Management of patient expectations for the surgical experience and the ultimate outcome related to total joint replacement surgery is important in terms of discharge planning for same-day procedures. The advent of nerve blocks for pain management and the option of care management to assess and plan for early rehabilitation and home support can better prepare the patient for the optimal experience.[6]

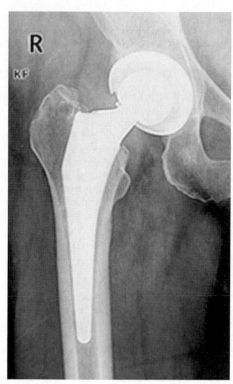

Fig, 32.2 Example of hip replacement implant. Bowen BA. Orthopedic surgery. Figure 20.51 in: Rothrock JC. *Alexander's Care of the Patient in Surgery.* 16th ed. Elsevier; 2019.

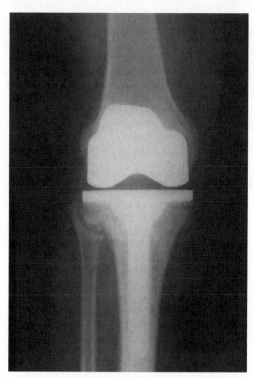

Fig, 32.3 Total knee arthroplasty. Adapted from: Scott RD. Total knee arthroplasty after osteotomy. Figure 8.6C in: Scott RD, ed. *Total Knee Arthroplasty: A Technique Manual.* 3rd ed. Elsevier; 2020.

There are a number of surgical methods for replacing arthritic, worn, or injured hip and knee joints. Minimally invasive surgery designed to minimize the size of incisions and avoid major surgical trauma to supporting muscles and tissues around the joint has resulted in shorter recovery times.[7] Additionally, applying the science of peripheral nerve blocks and the improved action of local analgesics and anesthetics, as well as improved physical therapies, has enabled the development of same-day clinical pathways for certain patients. Some clinical settings have benefitted from the introduction of robot- or computer-assisted procedures.

The traditional posterior hip replacement requires a slightly longer incision on the back and side of the hip; to accomplish this, some muscles must be cut to gain access to the joint. A more contemporary approach is the anterior or anterior-lateral method, which separates rather than incises the muscles for joint access, thereby allowing faster surgical recoveries in the appropriate patient population (Figure 32.2).

Patients requiring knee replacements also benefit from minimally invasive techniques. The knee is composed of three compartments, and the pathologic conditions of these compartments may mend themselves by several different procedures. Total knee replacements can now be completed with incisions that are half the length of the traditional procedures; Figure 32.3 shows a total knee arthroplasty.[7] Some patients may be candidates for partial or unicompartmental replacements, depending on the location of the bony defects or area of arthritis. Certain criteria must be met for selecting patients for successful same-day pathways for any joint replacement (Table 32.1).

Shoulder Procedures

There are several common surgeries performed for shoulder conditions. An arthroscopy is often done when conservative

TABLE 32.1 Inclusion and Exclusion Criteria for an ASC Surgical Procedure

Inclusion Criteria	Exclusion Criteria
Age < 70 years	Chronic obstructive pulmonary disease
Primary total knee arthroplasty	Coronary artery disease
Body mass index < 40	Preoperative hemoglobin < 10 g/dL
Independent ambulation preoperatively	Preoperative pain syndrome or opioid dependence
ASA score I or II	Congestive heart failure
Appropriate assistance at home	Chronic renal disease

Eason T, Toy P, Mihalko WM. Setting up an outpatient or same-day discharge total knee arthroplasty (TKA) program. In: Mihalko WM, Mont MA, Krackow KA, eds. *Technique of Total Knee Arthroplasty.* 2nd ed. Elsevier; 2023.

measures for a frozen shoulder have been unsuccessful (e.g., adhesive capsulitis manifesting as stiffness and pain). This procedure allows the surgeon to incise the tightened sections of the shoulder capsule and to manipulate the joint while the patient is under anesthesia to help loosen the joint and scar tissue. Another common shoulder procedure is the open or arthroscopic repair of torn rotator cuff muscles (i.e., the supraspinatus, infraspinatus, teres minor, and suscapularis muscles).[8] Impingement syndrome, also called rotator cuff tendonitis, can be treated by a subacromial decompression to increase space between the acromion (the bony process on the scapula) and the rotator cuff.

Cimino et al. report dramatic increases in the number of shoulder arthroplasty cases being performed annually.[9]

Their data were for traditional total shoulder arthroplasties and also reverse total shoulder arthroplasties and hemiarthroplasties. The systematic review revealed no statistical differences in patient outcomes for outpatient and inpatient shoulder arthroplasties when patients were selected appropriately.[9] Several key advances in surgical care have made it possible for shoulder procedures to be performed in the outpatient setting. As previously mentioned, carefully determined clinical criteria for selecting outpatient candidates must be established and followed by the healthcare team. Adherence to these criteria is crucial for mitigating the risks of surgical complications.

Hand Procedures

Trigger finger and Dupuytren contractures (which are a tightening of the muscles, tendons, skin, and tissues causing joint stiffening) are common finger and hand disorders. Chronic irritation of the tendon sheath leads to a narrowing of the space between the sheath, causing finger stiffness and temporary locking of the finger joints. Patients generally present for surgical intervention when conservative measures such as corticosteroid injections or splinting fail.[10] The surgical treatment consists of open or percutaneous divisions of the A1 pulley (one of five flexor tendons). The patient is usually able to use the digit following the surgery but should not do heavy lifting or gripping for 2 weeks. Scar massage is encouraged once the incision is healed to avoid painful scarring.[10]

Carpal tunnel release is another common outpatient hand procedure for patients who have failed nonsurgical therapies such as wrist splinting or physical therapy. During carpal tunnel release, extra space is provided for the median nerve by dividing the transverse carpal ligament, which has trapped the nerve due to thickening tissues or injury (Figure 32.4).[8] Incisional massage is encouraged after this surgery, as it was for trigger finger repair, to avoid painful scarring and tissue contracture.

Carpometacarpal joint arthroplasty is another common surgical option for arthritis located at the base of the thumb (Figure 32.5). The condition is more common in females and with advancing age. Many patients begin treatment using analgesics, activity modification, splints, and steroid injections. Surgeons have options for several approaches to address the pain and dysfunction of this joint, including removal of the

trapezium, adding implants to fill the gap, replacing the joint, or interposition of the tendon to fill the bone space.[11] Postoperative care varies according to the surgeon. However, most patients are splinted or casted until the wound is healed enough to begin physical therapy, usually at 4–6 weeks following surgery.

There are several additional hand procedures appropriate for the outpatient setting. These include hand and wrist arthroscopies, fracture and trauma repairs, excisions of bone and soft tissue tumors, and procedures for the management of vascular injuries. Guidelines for surgical selection should be established and followed, and, when possible, protocols for enhanced recovery processes should be maintained. In a survey reported by Thompson and Calandruccio, 37% of patients sought hand surgery to manage moderate to severe pain affecting both their ability to function as well as their associated quality of life.[2]

Sports Injuries

Most orthopedic surgeons are trained to provide surgical care for both sports and trauma-related injuries, although some prefer to specialize. Minimally invasive arthroscopic procedures have reduced surgical trauma and expedited the healing of certain joint-related conditions often associated with the "weekend athlete," as well as with the superiorly trained and conditioned athlete. These conditions can include tears of the meniscus of the knee or anterior cruciate ligament, tears of the labrum of the shoulder or rotator cuff injuries, injuries to the ankle ligament or cartilage, soft tissue injuries to the elbow from repetitive ball pitching, and tears of the labrum of the hip (Figure 32.6).

Trauma and fracture care are also common outpatient procedures. Reportedly 20% of patients who visit a sports medicine clinic present with common stress and sports-related fractures.[12] The location of, extent of, and mechanical stress placed on the fracture determine the course of treatment. This may include simple splinting or immobilization with rest and analgesics. In more complex situations, fracture care requires surgical repair. The goal of any chosen therapy is to support healing and rehabilitation of the fractured bone. Athletes are prone to certain fractures depending on their preferred activities; Box 32.2 lists some of the most common stress and sports injuries.

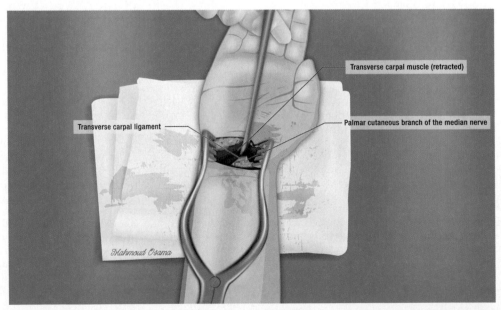

Fig. 32.4 Carpal tunnel release. Borekci A, Selahi O, Tanriverdi N, et al. Accessory hand muscles over the transverse carpal ligament: An obstacle in carpal tunnel surgery. *World Neurosurg.* 2023;170:e402-e415. https://doi.org/10.1016/j.wneu.2022.11.045.

changes in both bowel and bladder function. Common signs of cervical degenerative disc disease include neck pain, stiff neck, sharp shock-like nerve pain radiating down the shoulder and arm, numbness and weakness of the affected extremity, and worsening pain upon movement. Box 32.3 lists a glossary of terms for the spinal anatomy and diseases.

Naessig et al. report that the number of lumbar surgeries has more than doubled over the past few decades and that there has been a similar increase in the volume of corrective cervical surgeries.[14] Contemporary trends in spinal surgery have leaned toward outpatient settings as a more cost effective and safe clinical environment. For a list of spine procedures currently being done in the ASC setting, see Box 32.4. Pressure on the spinal cord causes sensory and motor complaints; this is often the result of degeneration from repetitive activities, aging, trauma, or injury. Herniation of the disc, also known as herniated nucleus pulposus, is the most common diagnostic finding (Figure 32.8).[15]

Choosing the outpatient setting for orthopedic neurologic procedures requires appropriate patient selection based on solid criteria that will have the best outcomes. The success of outpatient spine programs in part can be attributed to improved technologic advances for orthoneurologic procedures, as well as the advantages of multimodal and progressive pain and comfort management measures. While each facility may have developed a specific protocol for deeming specific surgeries and specific patients appropriate for outpatient procedures, these protocols are usually quite similar. The exclusion criteria for keeping patients out of outpatient centers and admitting them as inpatients to a hospital-based practice may include, but not be restricted to, age over 65 years, body mass index over 30 kg/m[2], American Society of Anesthesiologists patient classification higher than 2, current dialysis dependency, anticipated prolonged anesthesia times, and recent sepsis.[16]

The general postoperative care of the spinal patient includes early ambulation and frequent neurologic assessments. The perianesthesia nurse does a neurologic assessment for sensation and motion of the extremities, including the presence of numbness, sensations of "pins and needles," and motor function, including the ability to move and the strength of movements. Patients are told to avoid bending, twisting, lifting, pushing, or pulling until advised to do so by the surgeon. Comfort measures include the avoidance of prolonged sitting or standing, propping oneself up with pillows, and taking analgesics as prescribed. Intermittent cold therapy to the incisional site is also helpful for promoting comfort and reducing swelling.

Podiatric Procedures

Podiatrists commonly perform procedures for the foot and ankle in the outpatient setting. These surgeries are often performed to

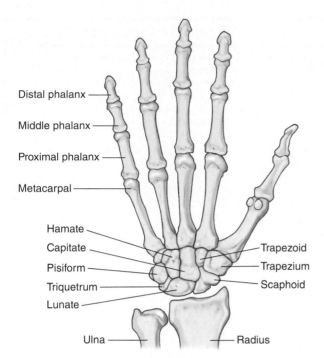

Distal phalanx
Middle phalanx
Proximal phalanx
Metacarpal
Hamate
Capitate
Pisiform
Triquetrum
Lunate
Ulna
Trapezoid
Trapezium
Scaphoid
Radius

Fig. 32.5 Carpometacarpal joint arthroplasty. Bowen BA. Orthopedic Ssurgery. Figure 20.5 In: Rothrock JC. *Alexander's Care Of the Patient in Surgery.* 16th ed. Elsevier; 2019.

Nonathletic individuals also risk fractures related to a variety of activities or accidents. Ankle fractures make up 10% of all adult injuries treated in trauma settings.[13] Surgical care is indicated when conservative, nonoperative treatment fails or when the viability of the limb is at risk due to the nature of the fracture. Fractures deemed stable respond to casting and immobilization for four or more weeks, but this approach can result in a poor union of the bone (nonunion) and skin breakdown. Operative repairs may include simple realignment while the patient is under anesthesia, internal fixation (e.g., plates and screws), external fixation (e.g., ring external fixators) or a combination of all these techniques (Figure 32.7).

Orthopedic Neurologic Procedures

The incidence of degenerative disc disease in the American population in general has risen.[14] Patients with lumbar disease typically present with intermittent or continuous back pain and spasms. This pain is often made worse when sitting or bending forward. Other signs include sciatica, muscle weakness, peripheral numbness, reduced reflexes, and potential

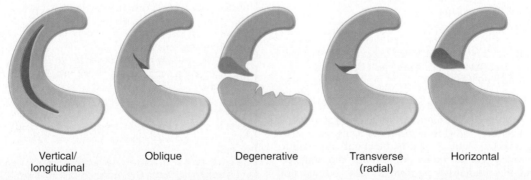

Vertical/   Oblique   Degenerative   Transverse   Horizontal
longitudinal   (radial)

Fig. 32.6 Meniscal tears. Ruzbarsky JJ, Maak TG, Rodeo SA. Meniscal injuries. Figure 94.6 in: Miller MD, Thompson SR, eds. *Delee, Drez, & Miller's Orthopaedic Sports Medicine.* 5th ed. Elsevier; 2020.

BOX 32.2 Sports Medicine Fractures

Femoral neck stress fracture	Runners
	Present with groin pain
	Requires imaging, including MRI, bone scans
	Risk developing avascular necrosis
Tibia stress fracture	Endurance athletes
	Running
	Focal tibial pain
Proximal fifth metatarsal stress fracture	Runners or marchers
	Pain along lateral border of foot
	Usually require surgical stabilization
Other metatarsal stress fractures	Involve 1st to 4th metatarsals
	Runners and dancers
	Distal fractures heal more readily
Navicular stress fractures	Present with dorsal foot pain
	More common in sprinting and jumping sports
	More common in males
	Weight bearing is prohibited for healing to occur
Pars stress fractures	Lumbar spine fracture from repetitive lumbar extension
	Common in gymnasts and football linemen
	Often have hamstring spasms
Rib fractures	Secondary to trauma or stress injury
	Localized pain worsens with direct pressure or deep breathing
	Rest, ice, analgesia
Clavicle fractures	Midshaft fractures most common
	Direct shoulder blows, collisions, falls
	Rowing, diving, baseball, weightlifting, gymnastics
	Recent trend to surgically fixate rather than provide conservative treatment

Adapted from: Kim C, Kaar SG. Commonly encountered fractures in sports medicine. In: Miller MD, Thompson SR, eds. *DeLee, Drez, & Miller's Orthopaedic Sports Medicine.* 5th ed. Elsevier; 2020.

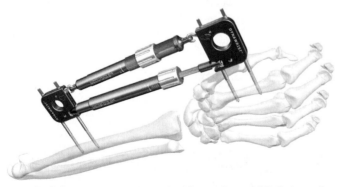

Fig. 32.7 Dynawrist dynamic external fixator. Bowen BA. Orthopedic surgery. Figure 20.27 in: Rothrock JC. *Alexander's Care of the Patient in Surgery.* 16th ed. Elsevier; 2019.

correct anatomic deformities resulting from genetic pathologies, injuries such as fractures, and chronic health or aging issues such as arthritis (Figure 32.9). Table 32.2 lists the common podiatric conditions for which procedures are done in an outpatient setting. Procedures that podiatrists perform include, but are not limited to, the treatment of inflamed or injured ligaments and tendons (e.g., plantar fasciitis), care of foot fractures, management

---

BOX 32.3 Glossary of Spinal Anatomy and Disease Terms

Annulus: the fibrous outer portion of an intervertebral disc
Arthritis: inflammation of a joint
Artificial disc surgery: surgical replacement of a diseased or herniated disc
Bone spur: a bony growth or the rough edge of a bone
Centrum: the body of a vertebra
Cervical myelopathy: compression of the spinal cord in the neck causing pain, numbness, or weakness in the neck or arms and coordination issues
Cervical radiculopathy: an irritated pinched nerve causing pain, numbness, or weakness radiating into the arm or chest
Cervical spine: the first seven vertebrae of the spine located in the neck
Coccyx: the bone below the sacrum (i.e., tailbone)
Disc degeneration: the deterioration or breakdown of a disc
Discectomy: the surgical removal or partial removal of an intervertebral disc
Foramen: the opening in the vertebrae of the spine through which the spinal nerve roots travel
Foraminotomy: the removal of a small portion of bone and joint that overlie the spinal nerve and soft tissue causing neural compression
Herniated disc: a condition in which the jelly-like material of a disc bulges or ruptures out of its normal position
Intervertebral disc: a tough elastic cushion located between the vertebrae in the spinal column that acts as a shock absorber for the vertebrae
Joint: the junction of two or more bones that allows varying degrees of motion between the bones
Ligament: fibrous connective tissue that connects bones together at joints or that passes between the bones of the spine
Lumbar spine: five vertebrae of the spine located in the lower back
Nerve: neural tissue that conducts electrical impulses from the brain and spinal cord to all other parts of the body and conveys sensory information from the body to the central nervous system
Nerve root: the initial portion of a spinal nerve where the nerve originates from the spinal cord
Nucleus pulposus: the gelatinous inner portion of an intervertebral disc
Sacrum: part of the pelvis located below the lumbar spine and above the coccyx
Spinal canal: a bone-composed channel located in the vertebral column protecting the spinal cord and nerve roots
Spinal cord: bundles of nerve fibers enclosed in the spinal canal; a pathway for nerve impulses to and from the brain and a center for operating and coordinating reflex actions independent of the brain
Spinal fusion: a surgical procedure in which bone is grafted onto the spine creating a solid union between two or more vertebrae
Spinal stenosis: narrowing of the vertebral column that may result in pressure on the spinal cord, spinal sac, or nerve roots
Spine: the flexible bone column extending from the base of the skull to the coccyx
Spondylitis: the inflammation of vertebrae
Spondylolisthesis: the forward displacement of one vertebra onto another
Thoracic spine: the 12 vertebrae located between the cervical and lumbar spine
Vertebrae: the 33 bones that make up the spine (divided into four sections: cervical, thoracic, lumbar, and sacral)

Karasin B, Grzelak M. Anterior cervical discectomy and fusion: A surgical intervention for treating cervical disc disease. *AORN J.* 2021;113(3): 237–251. Page 239. https://doi.org/10.1002/aorn.13329

BOX 32.4 Current Spine Procedures Performed in the ASC Setting

Microlumbar discectomy
Lumbar laminectomy
Vertebroplasty
Kyphoplasty
Anterior cervical discectomy and fusion (ACDF) at one or two levels
Posterior cervical foraminotomy
Cervical disc arthroplasty at one or two levels
Lumbar fusions at one or two levels (MIS-TLIF and LLIF)*
Posterior cervical fusion*
ACDF at three or more levels*
Lumbar fusions at three or more levels*

*More recent procedures done in the ASC setting rather than hospital setting.
LLIF, lateral lumbar interbody fusion; MIS-XLIF, minimally invasive surgery extreme lateral lumbar interbody fusion.
Gerling MC, Hale SD, White-Dzuro C, Pierce KE, Naessig SA, Ahmad W, Passias PG. Ambulatory spine surgery. *J Spine Surg*. 2019;5(Suppl 2):S1147-S153. Table 1. https://doi.org/10.21037/jss.2019.09.19

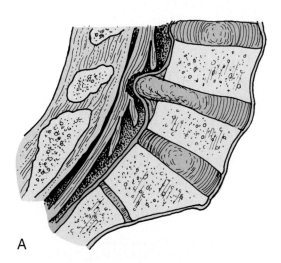

A

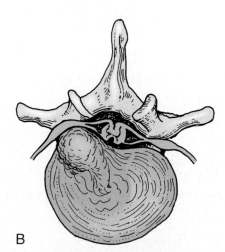

B

Fig. 32.8 Ruptured intervertebral disk. Modified from: Thomas ML. Care of the neurosurgical patient. Figure 38.9 in: Odom-Forren J, ed. *Drain's PeriAnesthesia Nursing: A Critical Care Approach.* Elsevier; 2018.

of diabetic foot conditions and general wound care, correction of bunions and hammertoes, removal of bone spurs, and biopsy and removal of tumors.

POSTOPERATIVE ISSUES

Quality outpatient orthopedic programs monitor the rates of patient returns to an emergency department, readmissions, reoperations, and overall notable complications. The postoperative complications often associated with orthopedic cases include the development of deep vein thrombosis, pulmonary embolism, fat embolism, compartment syndrome, shock, urinary retention, and infection, depending on the type of surgery being performed.[17] Other reported challenges include prolonged nausea and vomiting and uncontrolled pain.[18] Obviously, some complications can manifest immediately, while others may develop over a period of time following the procedure. Table 32.3 lists common orthopedic complications. Recent studies confirm that standardized postoperative follow-up can help to mediate a patient's postoperative concerns and fears.[19]

> **Evidence-Based Practice: Benefits of follow-up care for patients**
> The following recommendation is made based on a recent qualitative, nonexperimental, descriptive study aimed at revealing patients' perceptions of their postoperative recovery experiences after orthopedic surgery.[19] Healthcare systems providing outpatient orthopedic experiences can best address patient anxiety and fears by offering a standardized follow-up process. This may include a postoperative phone call from the perianesthesia registered nurse between two and five days after the procedure to help address any concerns and to reduce reported feelings of isolation and loneliness.[19]

Patient discharge to go home requires careful planning and patient teaching. The recovery process following orthopedic and podiatric procedures can be complex, depending on the degree to which patients require immobilization and rehabilitation. Patients and their caregivers and families should be prepared with knowledge of the following[8,17,20]:

- Pain management methods, including medications, rest, elevation, and cold or heat therapies
- Prevention of constipation
- Adequate hydration and nutrition
- Care of the operative site, including neurovascular status of limb. incision site, and drains, casts, and splints
- Signs of infection
- Mobility restrictions such as weight-bearing and driving
- Use of assistive devices and medical equipment
- Environmental safety
- Self-care
- When to call the surgeon

CHAPTER HIGHLIGHTS

- Patient preparation for outpatient orthopedic surgery includes proper clinical assessments, determination of conformity to established criteria, patient education, and relevant preoperative testing.
- Perianesthesia nurses providing perianesthesia care to orthopedic patients have knowledge of the anatomic and physiologic conditions being treated.
- Perianesthesia nurses providing perianesthesia care to orthopedic patients have knowledge of potential complications and subsequent nursing interventions.

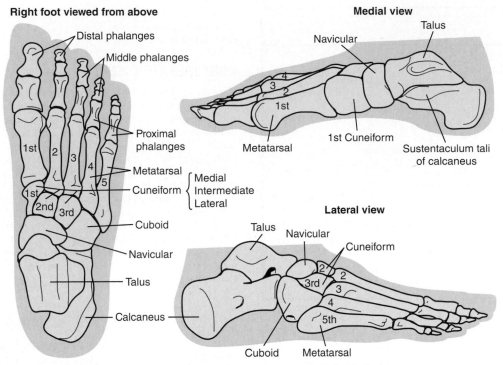

Fig. 32.9 Bones of the right foot. Cannon S. Orthopedics and podiatry. Figure 29.1 in: Schick L, Windle PE, eds. *Perianesthesia Nursing Core Curriculum: Preprocedure, Phase I and Phase II PACU Nursing.* 4th ed. Elsevier; 2021.

TABLE 32.2 Common Podiatric Procedures

Condition	Definition	Information
Arthrodesis	Surgical immobilization or fusion of a joint	Excision of bone wedges with fusion Indicated for severe compromise of muscle function, digital and metatarso-phalangeal joint stability inadequate Treatment for hallux valgus (method: divide tendon, resect cartilage, provide stability to joint with k-wire or other means) Triple arthrodesis: subtalar joint, talonavicular joint, and tarsometatarsal joint (treatment for equinus deformity, cavus deformity, flatfoot, or forefoot cavus)
Arthrolysis	Surgical procedure in which mobility is restored to an ankylosed (fused/immobile) joint	
Arthroplasty	Surgical repair or reformation of a joint	Resection or replacement of bony structure of joint Indicated for alleviation of pain and correction of digits with flexor to rigid deformity caused by: Inflammatory arthritis Degenerative arthritis Congenital deformity Flail toes Revision of previous surgery Keller resection arthroplasty for bunions: Tissues released around the joint Articular surface exposed Medial eminence resected Implant (k-wire) seated Capsulorrhaphy completed
Arthrotomy	Incision into a joint	
Bunion	Enlargement and inflammation of the joint bursa at the base of the great toe, usually causing the toe to displace laterally; usual etiology is long-term wearing of tight-fitting shoes	Revision of soft tissue structures and/or bone to correct deformity Soft tissue procedures correct muscle imbalance: McBride, DuVries, Mann, and Silver Soft tissue and bone procedure: Keller resection arthroplasty, Chevron osteotomy, and Akin procedure Purpose: simple treatment of hallux valgus causing impaired function and/or pain; cosmetic improvement
Capsulotomy	Incision into the joint capsule	Incision of capsule Treatment of equinovarus foot Performed in conjunction with other procedures Method: Incision through superficial fascia, expose joint, and incise capsule

TABLE 32.2 Common Podiatric Procedures—cont'd

Condition	Definition	Information
Corns	Conical thickening of skin in areas of constant irritation	

Exostosis	A bony growth on the surface of a bone, also called osteoma or hyperostosis	Exostectomy:
		   Resection of lateral prominences (callus) of toes
		   Commonly fifth toe

Hallux	The great toe	

Hallux valgus	Displacement of the great toe laterally toward the other toes; often coexists with a bunion, but often the two terms are inaccurately used synonymously	Foot deformity involving first metatarsal and great toe (hallux)
		Lateral angulation of great toe
		Progresses, resulting in medial deviation of first metatarsal
		Often accompanied by multiple disorders and symptoms; commonly affects lesser toes
		Occurs in females nine times more often than males; may be congenital or a result of rapid growth
		Symptoms:
		   Adults: pain or dull ache over metatarsal head
		   Adolescents: chief complaints are unrelenting pain, altered body image; may have family history
		Radiographs show exostosis with subluxation or dislocation of first metatarsal head

Hallux varus	First metatarsal deviates medially, and the great toe deviates laterally Flexion and varus rotation	Condition may start late in childhood or in early adult life More common in females Curly or overlapping toes Commonly affects third, fourth, and fifth toes May be agitated by improperly fitting footwear
Hallux rigidus (stiff big toe)	Painful stiffness of first metatarsophalangeal joint of the toes when walking; toe becomes rigid	Caused by arthritis

Hammer toe	A deformity in which there is dorsiflexion of the metatarsophalangeal joint (joint between the foot and toe) or plantar flexion of interphalangeal (IP) joints	Abnormal flexion posture of the proximal IP joint of one of the lesser four toes
		Second toe most frequently affected
		Metatarsophalangeal joint
		Stage of deformity depends on joint involvement and degree of contracture
		Treatment:
		   Soft tissue procedures: Girdlestone, Taylor, Parrish, Mann, and Coughlin
		   Soft tissue and bone procedures

Mallet toe	A deformity in which the most distal IP joint is involved
	Usually genetic
		Flexion posture of the distal IP join
		Second toe most frequently affected
		Etiology:
		   Pressure at tip of toes, possibly caused by shoes
		   Persons with peripheral neuropathy; no known reason
		Treatment:
		   Flexor tenotomy at distal IP flexion crease
		   Subtotal or total resection of middle phalanx

Morton neuroma	Interdigital nerve entrapment within a metatarsal interspace that causes pain between the distal to third and fourth metatarsal head, particularly with weight bearing	Symptoms and common findings:
		   Pain in plantar forefront area (sharp, dull, throbbing, burning sensation)
		   Swelling of plantar metatarsal
		   More common in women
		   Affects overweight person
		Following may play a role:
		   Abnormal positioning of toes
		   Flat feet
		   Forefoot problems, including bunions and hammertoes
		   High foot arch
		   Tight shoes with high heels

Osteotomy	Incision into a bone	Removal or addition of a bone wedge Extra-articular or intra-articular Extra-articular most commonly in the calcaneus for cavovarus heel Metatarsal osteotomy for plantar calluses, hallux valgus: many types including wedge resection, Chevron, "Z," Reverdin, and Mitchell Mitchell osteotomy: capsular incision, medial eminence removed, drill holes offset, and suture passed; double osteotomy completed with excision of bone between, capital fragment displaced, and suture tied; medial capsulorrhaphy completed
Pes planus	Flatfoot with loss of normal medial longitudinal arch	Initial treatment is conservative therapy with shoes with arch supports Surgical treatment with onset of disabling pain Correction procedures include Miller, Durham flatfoot plasty, triple arthrodesis, and calcaneal displacement osteotomy

Continued

TABLE 32.2 Common Podiatric Procedures—cont'd

Condition	Definition	Information
Pes cavus	Hollow foot, clawfoot occurs with neuromuscular conditions such as spina bifida, cerebral palsy, muscular dystrophy, or congenital clubfoot	Muscular weakness in foot Several procedures required for repair Soft tissue release, decrease contracture Tendon transfer to correct muscle imbalance Osteotomy: incision into a bone Arthrodesis: surgical immobilization or fusion of a joint
Plantar	Regarding the sole of the foot	Endoscopic plantar fasciotomy Operative tissue repair using a less invasive procedure Completed using fluoroscopy Procedure: stab incision, blunt dissection to create a channel, pass a trocar, and release the plantar fascia Open procedure more invasive; appropriate procedure for fascia release
Tenotomy	Incision of a tendon, eliminates tendon function, relieves contracture	Incision of tendon; eliminates tendon function and relieves contracture Completed in conjunction with other procedures

Adapted from: Cannon S. Orthopedics and podiatry. Table 29.1 in: Schick L, Windle PE, eds. *Perianesthesia Nursing Core Curriculum: Preprocedure, Phase I and Phase II PACU Nursing*. 4th ed. Elsevier; 2021.

TABLE 32.3 Common Orthopedic Complications

Complication	Cause	Nursing Assessment and Care
Deep vein thrombosis (DVT)	Obstruction of deep venous circulation by a blood clot Causes: venous stasis, trauma to vascular wall, hypercoagulable state (e.g., injury) Occurs in 40% to 60% of patients with lower-extremity surgery	Assessment: Edema, warmth, redness, tenderness/pain Care: Early ambulation Maximize mobility Adequate hydration Compression devices (e.g., sequential compression, antiembolic hose) Anticoagulants as ordered
Compartment syndrome	Neurovascular collapse due to increased pressure within the closed fascia space covering muscle, blood vessels, nerves	Assessment: Pain, pallor, paresthesia (e.g., burning, numbness), pulselessness of the limb, paralysis due to compression of nerves, rigid or "tight" limb due to tissue engorgement, rhabdomyolysis from muscle injury Care: Perform frequent neurovascular checks, maintain limb at neutral heart level position, remove ice, notify surgeon, loosen any dressings or constrictive devices Prepare for transfer to higher level of care and reoperation for fasciotomy
Fat embolism	Mobilization of fat and free fatty acids leading to acute pulmonary insufficiency	Assessment: Confusion, agitation, anxiety, change in level of consciousness, tachypnea, dyspnea, hypoxemia, pulmonary edema, petechial rash of head/neck/thorax/conjunctiva Care: Treat sepsis and shock Hydrate to prevent hypovolemia and circulatory compromise Prepare for transfer to higher level of care
Pulmonary embolism (PE)	Complete or partial obstruction of pulmonary artery thrombus or foreign body	Assessment: Rapid onset of chest pain, dyspnea, tachypnea, tachycardia, restlessness, cough with or without bloody sputum, syncope Care: Same as DVT Elevate head of bed Supplement with oxygen Prepare for intubation and transfer to higher level of care
Postoperative urinary retention (POUR)	Inability to empty urine from the bladder due to spinal anesthesia or anesthesia medications	Assessment: Pain and discomfort in lower part of abdomen, restlessness, hypertension, tachycardia, anxiety, tachypnea, diaphoresis Care: Palpation of bladder for distention or use of bedside ultrasound to assess volume Catheterize per protocol

Adapted from: Cannon S. Orthopedics and podiatry. In: Schick L, Windle PE, eds. *Perianesthesia Nursing Core Curriculum: Preprocedure, Phase I and Phase II PACU Nursing*. 4th ed. Elsevier; 2021; and Thomas ML. Care of the orthopedic surgical patient. In: Odom-Forren J: *Drain's PeriAnesthesia Nursing: A Critical Care Approach*. 7th ed. Elsevier; 2018.

CASE STUDY

Larry is a 62-year-old male who underwent a total shoulder arthroplasty 9 months ago. His original surgery and recovery were uneventful until he instinctively reached to help a disabled family member who was falling. As a result, the rotator cuff on his operative shoulder fully tore, causing excruciating pain and limited movement of his arm. His surgeon recommended revision surgery consisting of a reverse total shoulder arthroplasty. Although Larry resisted and opted for additional physical therapy, he eventually consented to outpatient surgery for the revision.

What analgesic techniques will benefit Larry?

What is the difference between a traditional total shoulder replacement and a reverse total shoulder arthroplasty?

How would Larry benefit from care management given that he provides care to a disabled family member at home?

REFERENCES

1. Hall MJ, Schwartzman A, Zhang J, et al. Ambulatory surgery data from hospitals and ambulatory surgery centers: United States, 2010. *Natl Health Stat Rep.* 2017;(102):1-15. Available at: https://www.cdc.gov/nchs/data/nhsr/nhsr102.pdf.
2. Thompson NB, Calandruccio JH. Hand surgery in the ambulatory surgery center. *Orthop Clin North Am.* 2018;49(1):69-72. Available at: https://doi.org/10.1016/j.ocl.2017.08.009.
3. Becker's ASC Review. Overcoming obstacles to surgery migration. *Becker's Healthcare.* November 8, 2022. Available at: https://www.beckersasc.com/leadership/overcoming-obstacles-to-surgery-migration.html.
4. Specht K, Agerskov H, Kjaersgaard-Andersen P, Jester R, Pedersen BD. Patients' experiences during the first 12 weeks after discharge in fast-track hip and knee arthroplasty—a qualitative study. *Int J Ortho Trauma Nurs.* 2018;31:13-19. Available at: https://doi.org/10.1016/j.ijotn.2018.08.002.
5. Kaye AD, Urman RD, Cornett EM, et al. Enhanced recovery pathways in orthopedic surgery. *J Anaesthesiol Clin Pharmacol.* 2019;35(suppl 1):S35-S39. Available at: https://doi.org/10.4103/joacp.joacp_35_18.
6. Sandler AB, Scanaaliato JP, Narimissaei D, McDaniel LE, Dunn JC, Parnes N. The transition to outpatient shoulder arthroplasty: a systematic review. *J Shoulder Elbow Surg.* 2022;31(7):e315-e331. Available at: https://doi.org/10.1016/j.jse.2022.01.154.
7. MacKenzie CR, Su EP. Surgical treatment of joint diseases. In: Goldman L, Schafer AI, eds. *Goldman-Cecil Medicine.* 26th ed. Elsevier; 2020:1783-1788.
8. Bowen BA. Orthopedic surgery. In: Rothrock JC, ed. *Alexander's Care of the Patient in Surgery.* 16th ed. Elsevier; 2018; 666-754.
9. Cimino AM, Hawkins JK, McGwin G, Brabston EW, Ponce BA, Momaya AM. Is outpatient shoulder arthroplasty safe? A systematic review and meta-analysis. *J Shoulder Elbow Surg.* 2021; 30(8):1968-1976. Available at: https://doi.org/10.1016/j.jse.2021.02.007.
10. Wolf JM. Tendinopathy. In: Wolfe SW, Pederson WC, Kozin SH, Cohen MS, eds. *Green's Operative Hand Surgery.* 8th ed. Elsevier; 2022:2105-2120.
11. Newton A, Talwalkar S. Arthroplasty in thumb trapeziometacarpal (CMC joint) osteoarthritis: An alternative to excision arthroplasty. *J Orthop.* 2023;35:134-139. Available at: https://doi.org/10.1016/j.jor.2022.11.011.
12. Kim C, Kaar SG. Commonly encountered fractures in sports medicine. In: Miller MD, Thompson SR, eds. *DeLee, Drez, & Miller's Orthopaedic Sports Medicine.* 5th ed. Elsevier; 2020:131-142.
13. Qin C, Dekker RG, Helfrich MM, Kadakia AR. Outpatient management of ankle fractures. *Orthop Clin North Am.* 2018;49(1):103-108. Available at: https://doi.org/10.1016/j.ocl.2017.08.012.
14. Naessig S, Kapadia BH, Ahmad W, et al. Outcomes of same-day orthopedic surgery: Are spine patients more likely to have optimal immediate recovery from outpatient procedures? *Int J Spine Surg.* 2021;15(2):334-340. Available at: https://doi.org/10.14444/8043.
15. Thomas ML. Care of the neurosurgical patient. In: Odom-Forren J, ed. *Drain's PeriAnesthesia Nursing: A Critical Care Approach.* 7th ed. Elsevier; 2018:565-588.
16. Gerling MC, Hale SD, White-Dzuro C, et al. Ambulatory spine surgery. *J Spine Surg.* 2019;5(suppl 2):S1147-S153. Available at: https://doi.org/10.21037/jss.2019.09.19.
17. Thomas ML. Care of the orthopedic surgical patient. In: Odom-Forren J, ed. *Drain's PeriAnesthesia Nursing: A Critical Care Approach.* 7th ed. Elsevier; 2018:549-564.
18. Darrith B, Frisch NB. Avoiding complications with outpatient total hip and knee arthroplasty. In: Courtney PM, Fillingham YA, Thompson SR, eds. *Complications in Orthopaedics: Adult Reconstruction.* Elsevier; 2023:34-43.
19. Larsson F, Stromback U, Gustafsson SR, Engstrom A. Postoperative recovery: experiences of patients who have undergone orthopedic day surgery. *J Perianesth Nurs.* 2022;37:515-520. Available at: https://doi.org/10.1016/j.jopan.2021.10.012.
20. Cannon S. Orthopedics and podiatry. In: Schick L, Windle PE, eds. *Perianesthesia Nursing Core Curriculum: Preprocedure, Phase I and Phase II PACU Nursing.* 4th ed. Elsevier; 2021.

LEARNING OBJECTIVES

A review of the content of this chapter will help the reader to:

1. Describe the common otorhinolaryngologic surgeries completed in an ambulatory surgical setting.
2. Cite common statistics related to otorhinolaryngologic procedures.
3. Identify postoperative nursing care for those surgeries.
4. Describe situations where a head/neck surgery might be contraindicated in an ambulatory surgical setting.

OVERVIEW

Otorhinolaryngologic surgeries, often colloquially referred to as ear, nose, and throat (ENT) procedures, are performed on the skin, soft tissues, and glands of the ears, nose, and throat, as well as the upper portion of the respiratory tract. Because they are comparatively noninvasive, many such surgeries are ideal for the outpatient surgical setting, and they make up 21% of all cases completed in ambulatory surgery centers (ASCs).[1] This chapter discusses these surgeries, which clinicians perform on both children and adults, as well as certain head and neck procedures that can frequently be performed in ASCs. Each section treats a specialty area and elaborates on its common procedures (performable in the ambulatory setting), the associated risks, and proper patient care.

FACTS AND FIGURES

Twenty-one percent of the procedures performed in ASCs are otorhinolaryngologic in nature.[2] The average net revenue per surgical case is $2492.[2] Twenty-seven percent of the patients are under the age of 24, and 21% are over the age of 64.[2] The percentage of surgical ear procedures performed in the outpatient setting is 91.8%, and the percentage of surgeries performed on the nose, mouth, and pharynx in the outpatient setting is 86.7%.[3]

OTORHINOLARYNGOLOGIC SURGICAL PROCEDURES
Procedures of the Ear

Most surgical procedures performed on the ear are safe enough to be completed in an outpatient surgery center. In fact, more than 90% of ear surgeries are performed in these centers because the risk for complications is comparatively low.[3] Postoperative concerns primarily depend upon the location of the surgical site, with surgeries located closer to the brain carrying more serious risks. Surgeries involving the inner ear—anatomically closer to the brain—should be observed for

the leakage of cerebrospinal fluid, a clear fluid, from the ear.[4] Additionally, there is a risk for facial nerve injury (Box 33.1). Once the patient is awakened from anesthesia, postoperative assessments of the cranial nerves should be conducted. All abnormal findings need to be reported to the surgical team. Common postoperative side effects of ear surgeries are nausea, nystagmus, and dizziness. Care should be taken to instruct the patient to move the head and change positions slowly to help alleviate these side effects (Figure 33.1).[5]

Cochlear Implants

Some deaf clients are candidates for cochlear implant surgery, which allows for the auditory processing of sound. While this cannot restore hearing in the classic sense, with sufficient training and therapy, deaf patients can be taught to recognize and process auditory stimuli received via a cochlear device. During the procedure, a receiver is implanted in the mastoid and the device is inserted into the cochlea, allowing stimulation of the auditory nerve (Figure 33.2).[4]

These patients do not have the ability to hear immediately after surgery, and it is important to ensure that they have an interpreter or another effective means of communication available as they awaken. Their preferred method of communication should be discussed preoperatively and given in handoff to the postanesthesia nurse and care team members. Although the postoperative care is straightforward, it is important to ensure that follow-up appointments have been scheduled with the surgeon and occupational therapist. The latter ensures that they are taught how to use the implant properly.

Evidence-Based Practice: Post-lingual deafness and cochlear implants

A study published by Saeedi et al., confirmed that patients who became deaf after having acquired both speech and language skills demonstrated that cochlear implants significantly enhance the function of hearing in these post-lingual patients. Factors that impact the success of cochlear implants include the original cause of hearing loss, the length of time an individual used hearing aid devices prior to surgery, and the presence of any postoperative complications following the implantation.

Source: Saeedi M, Amirsalari S, Dadgar S, Khosravi MH. Outcomes of cochlear implantation in post-lingually deaf patients. *Int Tinnitus J.* 2021;25(1):18-22. https://doi.org/10.5935/0946-5448.2020005

Myringotomy

A myringotomy is a procedure performed on the middle ear to correct eustachian tube dysfunction. It is the second most commonly performed surgery in the pediatric population.[3] In children, recurrent ear infections often precipitate this surgery. Frequent fluid collection caused by infections coupled with poor drainage can create long-term problems, including

BOX 33.1 Facial Nerve Assessment

Smile enough to show teeth
Wrinkle forehead
Pucker lips
Wrinkle nose
Squeeze eyelids shut
Stick out tongue

Marshall R. Otorhinolaryngology. In: Schick L, Windle PE, eds.
*Perianesthesia Nursing Core Curriculum: Preprocedure, Phase I
and Phase II PACU Nursing.* 4th ed. Elsevier; 2021.

hearing loss and delays in speech development.[5] In infants and children, the procedure is often completed bilaterally. While it is more commonly done in children, adults can also undergo this surgery, though it is typically unilateral.[4]

To perform a myringotomy, the surgeon creates an opening in the tympanic membrane and then places a tube to allow the continuation of fluid equalization.[4] In acute situations such as trauma or infection, this simple drainage of the fluid trapped behind the tympanic membrane can restore hearing. In situations that require tube insertion, the tubes can be placed for a few months or for multiple years based on the chronicity of the problem (Figure 33.3).[5]

Tympanoplasty

A tympanoplasty is the surgical correction of an injured tympanic membrane. A tympanoplasty repairs a perforated tympanic membrane that cannot heal on its own. Unrepaired membrane ruptures can cause hearing loss and can make it unsafe for a person to be submerged in water because water would then be able to enter the middle ear.[5] Informally referred to as "eardrum ruptures," perforations can result from infections, direct injury as from an object inserted too forcefully into the ear, or indirect injury from head trauma.

Mastoidectomy

When squamous cells accumulate around the mastoid process or space, this accumulation can form a cholesteatoma. A cholesteatoma is a cyst-like structure that can cause necrosis in the mastoid bone and in the structures of the middle ear. A mastoidectomy removes the diseased mastoid, as well as the surrounding affected tissues. Historically, before antibiotics were common, this was also done for control of infection, but infection is rarely an instigating factor in the modern surgical climate.[5]

Stapedotomy

Some conductive hearing loss is caused by otosclerosis, the condition in which abnormal bone growth forms around the foot of the stapes and does not allow for movement and prevents the transmission of sound waves. A stapedotomy is the partial removal of the stapes structure while preserving the foot of the stapes. The surgeon creates an opening in the stapes foot and places a prosthesis to allow sound wave transmission. In the past, a stapedectomy was the more common procedure.[5] During a stapedectomy, the complete stapes structure is surgically removed, and a prosthesis is placed for sound wave conduction.[4]

Procedures for the Nose and Sinuses

Nasal and sinus surgeries are ideal options for a surgery center. These surgeries are usually performed with the goal of resolving chronic problems, such as chronic sinusitis, or to correct structural variances that might affect breathing. While serious risks exist, severe side effects are rare, and most such surgeries are considered minimally invasive. Vision loss is one symptom of a serious complication, the unintended entrance into the orbital cavity and would necessitate surgical intervention.[4] Almost 95% of plastic or reconstructive procedures for the nose are completed in the ambulatory setting.[3]

Postoperative care of this patient population should focus on airway management, bleeding control, and symptom relief.

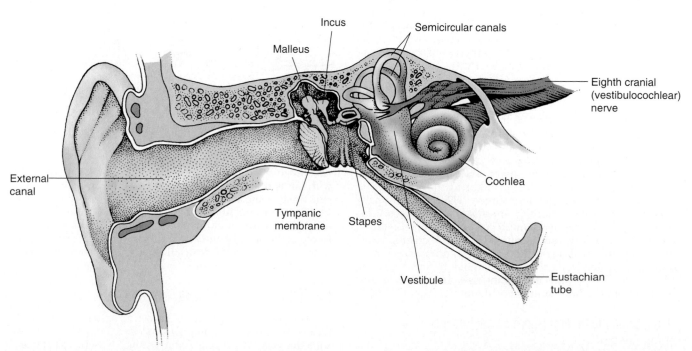

Fig. 33.1 Anatomic structures of the external ear, middle ear, and inner ear. Flanagan AL. Otorhinolaryngologic surgery. Figure 19.1 in: Rothrock JC. *Alexander's Care of the Patient in Surgery.* 16th ed. Elsevier; 2019.

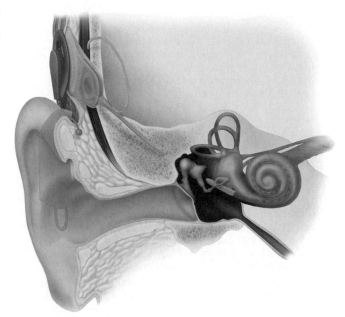

Fig. 33.2 Cochlear implant. Flanagan AL. Otorhinolaryngologic surgery. Figure 19.19 in: Rothrock JC. *Alexander's Care of the Patient in Surgery*. 16th ed. Elsevier; 2019.

Often nasal and sinus surgeries require some form of nasal packing or splints, and they can make it difficult to breathe through the nose. The perianesthesia nurse should observe airway patency closely, especially before the patient fully wakes. Special care should be taken with patients who have a history of obstructive sleep apnea (OSA). Anesthesia is known to potentiate the effects of OSA, and the side effects of these surgeries can exacerbate that potentiation.

The preferred position of patients after nasal surgery is the semi-Fowler position. Some drainage is expected, but the nurse should observe the patient for uncontrolled or significant bleeding. Patients often have a dressing below the nose, sometimes referred to as a mustache dressing, in addition to nasal packing. Since drainage of blood down the back of the throat can cause nausea, antiemetics should be available, and the patient should be instructed to expectorate secretions instead of swallowing them (Figure 33.4).[4]

Sinus Surgery and Sinus Endoscopy

Sinus surgery is indicated when traditional treatment of sinusitis, including appropriate antibiotic regimes, is ineffective. Surgical intervention to drain the sinuses can be minimally invasive with the use of endoscopy. Depending on the scope of the problem, open sinus surgery inclusive of ethmoidectomy and sphenoidotomy can be indicated.[5]

Functional endoscopic sinus surgery (FESS) is a minimally invasive surgical correction for sinusitis or nasal polyps.[4] This surgical approach results in improved healing times, reduced morbidity, and decreased surgical trauma to existing structures compared with previous methods. It does, however, require a high degree of surgical technique by the physician. This procedure presents significant risks as it is performed close to both the brain and the ocular orbits (Figure 33.5).[5]

Nasal Septoplasty and Submucosal Resection of the Septum

The septum can require surgical correction for multiple reasons, including trauma, fracture, or abnormal formation.

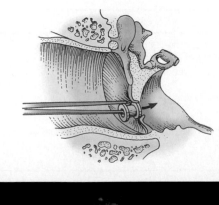

A

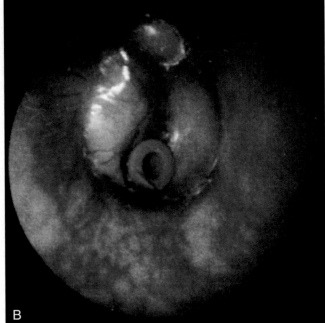

B

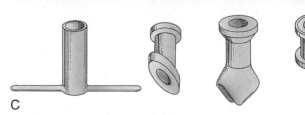

C

Fig. 33.3 Myringotomy and tube placement. Flanagan AL. Otorhinolaryngologic surgery. Figure 19.17 in: Rothrock JC. *Alexander's Care of the Patient in Surgery*. 16th ed. Elsevier; 2019.

Any irregular positioning of the septum may cause difficulty with sinus drainage or breathing mechanisms. Chronic obstructions of the sinus cavity caused by septal deviations can lead to the formation of sinus disease and nasal polyps. A nasal septoplasty or submucosal resection of the septum allows for the straightening of cartilage and osseous structures of the septum with the removal of extra or obstructing tissues as necessary.[5]

Nasal Cautery and Epistaxis

The control of nasal bleeding, known as epistaxis, commonly results in a surgical rhinology procedure, and 93% of these surgeries occur in an outpatient setting.[3] Nosebleeds are usually minor and can usually be controlled in the home setting with direct pressure. In cases where the bleeding is significant

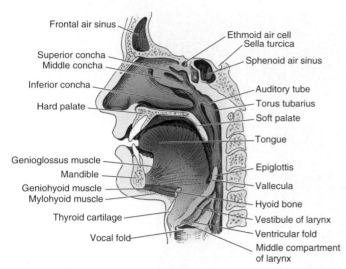

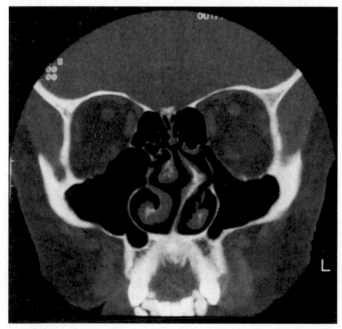

Fig. 33.4 Sagittal section of the face and neck. Flanagan AL. Otorhinolaryngologic surgery. Figure 19.4 in: Rothrock JC. *Alexander's Care of the Patient in Surgery.* 16th ed. Elsevier; 2019.

Fig. 33.5 CT scan of sinuses. Flanagan AL. Otorhinolaryngologic surgery. Figure 19.24 in: Rothrock JC. *Alexander's Care of the Patient in Surgery.* 16th ed. Elsevier; 2018.

and intractable, emergency room visits may be required. If those measures fail, surgery becomes necessary. Nasal packing and balloon nasal packing are two common surgical approaches. In some instances, endoscopy can be used with the application of cautery directly to the bleeding vessels.[5]

Procedures for the Head and Neck

Surgical Procedures for Cancers of the Head and Neck

While several otorhinolaryngologic surgeries are ideal for the outpatient setting, some must be evaluated quite carefully by

the surgeon to ensure safety. The procedure itself must be considered: How invasive is the surgery? How close does it get to major blood vessels? How will it affect the airway? What risks of complications exist? Consideration of the patient's medical history also plays a critical role: Is there a history of OSA? Is the patient taking anticoagulants, which can increase the risk of bleeding?

For cancers affecting the head and neck, as well as lymph nodes to varying degrees, many of the surgeries are far too invasive and have much too high a risk to be completed in an outpatient setting. Even thyroid or parathyroid surgeries should be considered carefully by the surgeon. If a complete thyroidectomy is not necessary, the case might be considered for an outpatient setting. A more complex case, such as invasive thyroid cancer, will most likely be completed in an inpatient setting. Airway concerns, including the inability to manage secretions, swelling, and hematoma formation, can be a major factor when assessing the safety of a surgery completed on the neck.

Thyroidectomy

As previously mentioned, these cases should be carefully evaluated by the surgical team for appropriateness in an ambulatory surgery setting. A skillful surgeon paired with a healthy patient presenting with few co-morbidities could certainly be considered for an outpatient setting.[1] Nearly 62% of partial or complete thyroidectomies are performed in the outpatient setting (Figure 33.6).[3]

The thyroid is the largest gland of the endocrine system and houses significant blood flow. Because the thyroid is positioned near many critical vascular, airway, and nervous system structures, the risk of complications in thyroid surgeries is concerning. Thyrotoxicosis and thyroid malignancy are the main indications for complete or partial thyroidectomies. Because dysfunctional secretion of thyroid hormones can be dangerous during the surgical period, preoperative assessments of the patient's thyroid hormone levels (to ensure that the patient is euthyroid) is of utmost concern.[6] Unlike most other surgeries discussed in this chapter, this surgery requires a general anesthetic. Surgical complications can be significant, including hypocalcemia, thyroid storm, injury to the laryngeal nerve, pneumothorax, and hematoma (Box 33.2). The risk associated with a surgical site hematoma is airway obstruction, and it constitutes a true surgical emergency.[6]

Recently, work has been done to create robotic approaches to thyroid and parathyroid surgeries. These include axillary, facelift, and transoral approaches. The primary goal of such robotic use appears to be cosmetic in nature, avoiding the neck scarring sometimes resulting from traditional surgical approaches. Originating in South Korea, adoption into the western medical cultures has been slow. The main barriers are cost, steep technical knowledge requirements, and an increased operative and anesthesia time, among others. Research does suggest that the oncologic outcomes and overall surgical safety are like those of traditional surgeries, with the added perk of an improved cosmologic outcome.[7]

Procedures for the Mouth and Throat

Salivary Gland Surgery

Salivary gland surgery is done to correct problems that are either obstructive, inflammatory, or neoplastic in nature. Most tumors of the salivary glands are benign and can be corrected with simple excision, but a rare malignancy may be found on biopsy. These procedures include excision of the submandibular gland

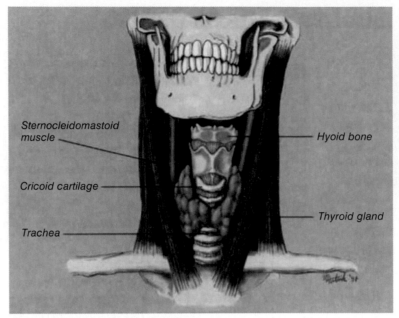

Fig. 33.6 Thyroid gland. Moore S, Haughey BH. Surgical treatment for thyroid cancer. *AORN J.* 1997;65(4):710–725. Figure 1.

or parotidectomies. Bacterial inflammatory disorders are most typically found in the parotid glands, and this is thought to be due to the glands' close proximity to the oral cavity. Prior to modern-day vaccination regimes, mumps was the primary cause of salivary disorders with viral origins. Postoperative complications should be monitored based on the knowledge that facial nerves can be damaged depending upon the mechanism of approach.[5]

Tonsillectomy and Adenoidectomy

This is one of the most common surgeries in the pediatric population (see Chapter 22), though its popularity has waned in the last few years.[3] It is also sometimes completed in adults. Typically, this surgery manages OSA or Pickwickian syndrome with a concurrent uvulopalatopharyngoplasty (UPPP) (Figure 33.7).[6] In adult patients, the perioperative team should consider co-morbidities and how they will affect the surgical course. The preferred postoperative positioning

for these patients, particularly pediatric patients, is side lying with the head tilted slightly downward, allowing secretions to flow out of the mouth rather than onto the vocal cords. Adults often prefer the high Fowler position on awakening, and if they can self-manage their secretions and airway, this is acceptable.[7]

Although the procedure is comparatively simple, some significant risks are associated with it. Airway compromise should be the postoperative nurse's number one concern. Swelling and exudate can both cause airway compromise. The risk of bleeding is significant and should be monitored carefully. Estimated blood loss for this procedure is 4 mL/kg, with that rate increasing if a UPPP is also performed.[7] The drainage onto the vocal cords, as well as the need for frequent suctioning, risks causing bronchospasms or laryngospasms. Suction should be kept to the minimum necessary amount to prevent spasm or rebleeding. Due to blood loss during surgery and the blood's subsequent collection in the gastrointestinal system, postoperative nausea and vomiting can also be a concern. The anesthesiologist should consider orogastric suctioning before the surgery's end, as well as prophylactic antiemetics, to manage this concern.[7]

Laryngoscopy

A laryngoscopy is the passage of a laryngoscope into the throat to allow direct examination of the larynx; it can also include biopsies or polypectomies. Often performed under procedural sedation, the duration is typically short. The main concern in the postoperative period is the considerable risk of laryngospasm. Airway monitoring should be maintained until the patient is fully awake and able to appropriately manage the airway and secretions. Positioning while the patient is sedated should be side lying to allow for secretion drainage. Once awake, the patient may assume a side-lying semi-Fowler position. Other common side effects are coughing, throat irritation, and bleeding. The nurse should attempt to promote vocal rest, manage discomfort, and monitor for increased bleeding.[4]

BOX 33.2 Emergency Care During Thyroid Storm

Maintain a patent airway and adequate ventilation
Administer supplemental oxygen
Establish vascular access for fluid resuscitation or medication administration
Monitor intake and output
Give antithyroid drugs as prescribed
Initiate continuous cardiac monitoring
Monitor vital signs every 30 minutes or more frequently
Control hyperthermia with application of ice packs and cooling blankets
Provide reassurance to patient and family
Prepare for transfer to a higher level of care

Adapted from: Duffy C. Thyroid and parathyroid surgery. Table 16.1 in: Rothrock JC. *Alexander's Care of the Patient in Surgery.* 16th ed. Elsevier; 2019.

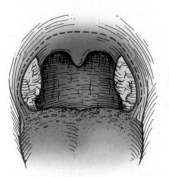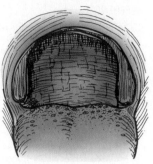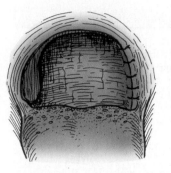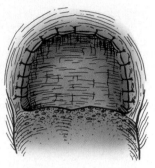

Fig. 33.7 Technique of palatopharyngoplasty. Flanagan AL. Otorhinolaryngologic surgery. Figure 19.36 in: Rothrock JC. *Alexander's Care of the Patient in Surgery.* 16th ed. Elsevier; 2019.

TABLE 33.1 Discharge Instructions for Otorhinolaryngologic and Head and Neck Procedures

Procedure	Instructions*
Adenoidectomy and tonsillectomy	Avoid throat clearing, coughing, and vigorous nose blowing No bending, straining, or lifting Consume bland, soft diet Expect bloody or tarry stools secondary to swallowed blood Observe voice rest Expect that throat discomfort may increase between postprocedural days four and eight secondary to separation of eschar from pharyngeal bed
Laryngoscopy/esophagoscopy	Review patient education Avoid throat clearing and coughing Bland, soft diet when gag reflex returns Voice rest Avoid lifting and straining
Oropharyngeal neck surgery	Avoid throat clearing, coughing, and vigorous nose blowing No bending, straining, or lifting Consume bland, soft diet Expect bloody or tarry stools because of swallowed blook Observe voice rest Expect that throat discomfort may increase between postprocedural days four and eight secondary to separation of eschar from pharyngeal bed
Septoplasty	Change moustache dressing when soiled; maintain count of change frequency if excessively soiled or saturated Use a humidifier as ordered/needed to moisten air Avoid nose blowing; sniff secretions to back of nose and swallow or expectorate Avoid bending, straining, or lifting Sneeze with mouth open Avoid use of straws for drinking liquids Smoking increases recovery time and risk of septal perforation Expect nausea and bloody or tarry stools secondary to swallowed blood
Tympanoplasty	Avoid getting ears wet Avoid sudden turning; encourage slow, smooth movements Sneeze with mouth open to avoid eustachian tube pressure Gentle nose blowing only Smoking increases risk of postprocedural tympanic perforation Noises such as popping and/or cracking may be heard in the ear by the patient and are considered normal

*Discharge instructions vary by surgeon

Adapted from: Marshall R. Otorhinolaryngology. In: Schick L, Windle PE, eds. *Perianesthesia Nursing Core Curriculum: Preprocedure, Phase I and Phase II PACU Nursing.* 4th ed. Elsevier; 2021.

DISCHARGE INSTRUCTIONS

Discharge instructions for patients who have undergone otorhinolaryngologic and head and neck surgeries are summarized in Table 33.1.

CHAPTER HIGHLIGHTS

- This chapter discussed how common it is for otorhinolaryngologic surgeries to be performed in the ambulatory care setting.

- It also noted that most of these cases are considered minimally invasive, with a few exceptions, making them ideal for the ASC.
- Even minimally invasive surgeries should be undertaken in the outpatient setting only after the patient history, surgeon's skill, and availability of specialty equipment are considered by the perioperative team.
- Otorhinolaryngologic surgeries are common in both adults and children.

CASE STUDY

A patient is presented to an ASC for a procedure to correct deafness. What procedure should the nurse expect to occur? What is a critical piece of information for this patient population that should be obtained on registration?

The nurse knows that the patient's communication preference is a critical piece of data for the recovery period. The patient affirms fluency in American Sign Language (ASL) and asks that an interpreter be present on awakening. The nurse then ensures that a medical interpreter fluent in ASL will be available.

While completing the preoperative evaluation, the patient's support person expresses how exciting it will be that the patient will be able to hear right after surgery. How should the nurse respond to this statement?

The patient is awakening in the postoperative area, and the nurse has ensured that an interpreter is at the bedside. How should the nurse direct the patient to move and be positioned?

REFERENCES

1. Neirengarton MB. Benefits of ambulatory surgical centers for otolaryngology. *ENT Today*. 2020. Available at: https://www.enttoday.org/article/benefits-of-ambulatory-surgical-centers-for-otolaryngology/.
2. Dyrda L. *73 Facts and Statistics in ENT and ASCs*. Becker's ASC Review; 2017. Available at: https://www.beckersasc.com/asc-news/73-facts-and-statistics-on-ent-and-ascs.html.
3. Weir LM, Steiner CA, Owens PL. *Surgeries in Hospital-Owned Outpatient Facilities 2012*. Agency for Healthcare Research and Quality. 2015; Statistical Brief #188
4. Flanagan A. Otorhinolaryngologic surgery. In: Rothrock JC, ed. *Alexander's Care of the Patient in Surgery*. Elsevier; 2019.
5. McEwen DR. Care of the ear, nose, throat, neck, and maxillofacial surgical patient. In: Odom-Forren J, ed. *Perianesthesia Nursing: A Critical Care Approach*. 7th ed. St. Louis, MO: Elsevier; 2018.
6. Gill CJ. Anesthesia for the ear, nose, throat, and maxillofacial surgery. In: Nagelhout JJ, Elisha S, eds. *Nurse Anesthesia*. 7th ed. St. Louis, MO: Elsevier; 2018.
7. Tamaki A, Rocco JW, Ozer E. The future of robotic surgery in otolaryngology head and neck surgery. *Oral Oncology*. 2020;101:104510. Available at: https://doi.org/10.1016/j.oraloncology.2019.104510.

34 Cosmetic and Reconstructive Surgery

Theresa L. Clifford, DNP, RN, CPAN, CAPA, FASPAN, FAAN

LEARNING OBJECTIVES

A review of the content of this chapter will help the reader to:

1. Describe common cosmetic and reconstructive procedures performed in the ambulatory surgery setting.
2. Describe the impact of common medical conditions on surgical outcomes.
3. Describe relevant psychological factors affecting the decision to have cosmetic or reconstructive surgery.
4. Identify nursing care for specific surgical procedures.

OVERVIEW

In the setting of an ambulatory surgery practice, plastic and reconstructive surgery is performed for a wide variety of reasons. There are two broad categories of plastic surgery. The first is the elective procedure, which is often aimed at changing the physical appearance. The cosmetic procedure is perceived by the individual as an opportunity to enhance self-esteem and increase the sense of emotional well-being. Studies have shown that scores for body image and satisfaction increased after aesthetic procedures.[1,2]

The second category of plastic surgery is reconstructive procedures. Some are performed to correct congenital abnormalities. Certain medical or physiologic conditions, such as cancers, can alter the body's shape or ability to function properly. Accidental or catastrophic events causing bodily injury can also result in unusual or grotesque changes in physical appearance or functionality. In some circumstances, reconstructive surgery can help to restore the functional aspect of the body impaired by the alteration. Examples include minor or pervasive birth defects, scars resulting from oncologic procedures for skin or breast cancers, and treatment for injuries sustained in accidents or from burns.

FACTS AND FIGURES

The American Society of Plastic Surgeons (ASPS) publishes annual statistics related to plastic surgery and other procedures.[3] Although a large number of minimally invasive cosmetic procedures are office-based, many cosmetic and reconstructive procedures are performed in the setting of a hospital-based or free-standing surgery center. Office-based procedures include the use of botulinum toxin type A (Botox), facial rejuvenation procedures such as chemical peels and soft tissue fillers, and laser hair removal, to name a few. In 2019, the ASPS reported 18.1 million cosmetic procedures of which 1.8 million were surgical procedures (Box 34.1). In the same year, 5.9 million reconstructive procedures were reported (Box 34.2). The demographics of patients seeking cosmetic procedures is also captured in the data: the vast majority are female (Figure 34.1), nearly half of patients are between the ages of 40 and 54 (Fig. 34.2); Caucasians make up nearly 72% of the total number of patients having procedures in this multibillion-dollar industry.

COSMETIC PROCEDURES
Augmentation Mammaplasty

The most common cosmetic surgery performed in the ambulatory setting is the augmentation mammaplasty. This procedure is primarily done to electively increase the size of the breasts, enhance the shape and contour of the breasts, or correct abnormalities in shape related to physical development or surgical defects. An added benefit of the augmentation mammaplasty is an enhanced self-image and subsequent self-confidence. The procedure involves the insertion of prosthetic implants or fat transfers either just above (submammary) or below the pectoral and serratus anterior muscles of the chest wall (submuscular) (Figure 34.3).[4] The types of implants vary according to the manufacturer, the preference of the plastic surgeon, and the choice of the patient. These include saline-filled, silicone-filled, round, smooth, and textured implants, to name a few. Several approaches have been developed to ensure proper placement of the implant. Surgeons can elect to insert the implant through an inframammary incision (along the bottom of the breast contour), a transaxillary approach, a periareolar incision, or an endoscopic approach.

The breast augmentation procedure is typically performed under general anesthesia. Occasionally the surgery can be done with a peripheral block or local anesthetic and total intravenous anesthesia. During phase I recovery and prior to discharge, the perianesthesia registered nurse should check frequently for the presence of a developing hematoma. Upon visual inspection, the breasts should remain equal in size, and upon palpitation, the surrounding tissue should remain soft to touch. Also, when assessing for a hematoma, gentle palpation of the superior aspect of the pectoralis muscle can detect a diffuse migration of blood into soft tissues. Additionally, lung auscultation can detect signs of a pneumothorax. A collapsed lung is a potential complication, particularly when the transaxillary approach has been used.

In the absence of a preoperative nerve block or the injection of local anesthetics to reduce pain, discomfort immediately following the augmentation procedure is typically described as moderate to severe. The multimodal approach to pain and discomfort management is best and can include nonpharmacologic means. Depending on the preference of the surgeon, breast compression garments or large ace wraps provide some relief. The application of cold therapy (e.g., ice packs) can also provide comfort but should be approved by the provider. Preventative measures for postoperative nausea to reduce the incidence of postoperative vomiting further promote patient comfort.

Postoperative patient education may vary according to surgeon preferences but can generally address common issues.

BOX 34.1 Five Most Commonly Performed Surgical Cosmetic Procedures in 2019 According to the American Society of Plastic Surgeons

Breast augmentation
Liposuction
Nose reshaping
Eyelid surgery
Facelift

Data from: American Society of Plastic Surgeons. *Plastic Surgery Statistics Report.* ASPS; 2019. https://www.plasticsurgery.org/documents/News/Statistics/2019/plastic-surgery-statistics-full-report-2019.pdf

BOX 34.2 Five Most Commonly Performed Reconstructive Procedures in 2019 According to the American Society of Plastic Surgeons

Tumor removal
Laceration repair
Maxillofacial surgery
Scar revision
Hand surgery

Data from: American Society of Plastic Surgeons. *Plastic Surgery Statistics Report.* ASPS; 2019. https://www.plasticsurgery.org/documents/News/Statistics/2019/plastic-surgery-statistics-full-report-2019.pdf

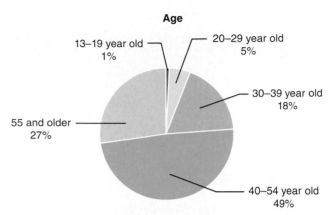

Age

13–19 year old 1%
20–29 year old 5%
30–39 year old 18%
40–54 year old 49%
55 and older 27%

Fig. 34.2 Age distribution. Data from: American Society of Plastic Surgeons (ASPS). Plastic Surgery Statistics Report. ASPS; 2019. https://www.plasticsurgery.org/documents/News/Statistics/2019/plastic-surgery-statistics-full-report-2019.pdf

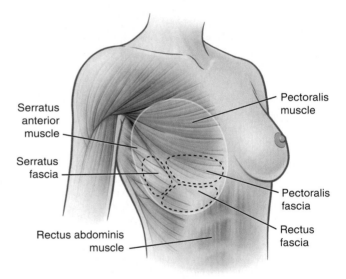

Fig. 34.3 Placement of breast implant below the pectoralis major muscle. © 2017, Memorial Sloan Kettering Cancer Center. Image source: Clinical Key, IMAGE. Nelson JA, Cordeiro PG, Immediate implant breast reconstruction with total muscle coverage-two-stage. Figure 11.4 in: Pu LLQ, Karp NS, eds. *Atlas of Reconstructive Breast Surgery.* Elsevier; 2019.

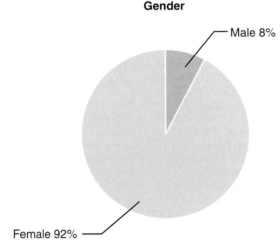

Gender

Male 8%
Female 92%

Fig. 34.1 Female to male ratio. Data from: American Society of Plastic Surgeons (ASPS). Plastic Surgery Statistics Report. ASPS; 2019. https://www.plasticsurgery.org/documents/News/Statistics/2019/plastic-surgery-statistics-full-report-2019.pdf

The patient should be taught how to detect signs of a developing hematoma and be instructed to notify the surgeon immediately. Breast compression garments in the form of either a soft support bra or ace wrap should be worn for the first week. As the site begins to heal, capsule formation, or the development of scar tissue surrounding the breast implant, is a potential complication that should be reported to the surgeon. Gentle breast massage may help to prevent capsular scarring or contracture by keeping the implant mobile under the tissue and the breast tissue pliable. Massage instructions may vary according to provider practice. Normal patient activities can be resumed at the direction and advice of the surgeon.

Liposuction and Fat Grafting

The second most common cosmetic procedure is known as liposuction and may include the harvesting of adipose tissue for reimplantation or fat transfers. Currently there are a number of noninvasive office-based procedures that are popular amongst select patients and may, at times, be used to augment the traditional and more invasive liposuction.[5] Patients seek liposuction as a solution for enhancing the physical appearance by removing unwanted adipose tissue. This procedure helps add contour to sculpt a body shape for desired lines and curves. In addition to adding more definition to a shape, fat can be transferred (in a procedure known as liposculpture or liposhifting), providing accentuation to certain areas of the body. In general, patients who undergo large-volume liposuction are candidates for ambulatory surgery settings as opposed to office-based settings for the support of intraprocedural and postoperative care.

The procedure itself involves the removal of adipose tissue from areas such as the face, neck, abdomen, thighs, buttocks, flanks, and extremities. There are several common techniques available depending on the preference of the cosmetic surgeon.[6] Tumescent liposuction involves the injection of a tumescent solution into the tissue. This solution includes local anesthetics that have been diluted to help reduce immediate discomfort and blood loss. Ultrasound and laser-assisted procedures use the technology to help break up the fatty tissues, allowing for easier removal. Suction-assisted liposuction involves the use of a vacuum-like device to remove the fat. To reduce any superficial scarring, small incisions are used to introduce the suction device. Tissue is removed and the volumes recorded. In some cases, the procedure can be done under general anesthesia; however, more often local anesthesia with or without procedural sedation has been associated with good patient compliance and satisfaction.

Liposuction, as a cosmetic procedure, tends to have a low incidence of complications. Major complications include hematoma development, surgical site infections, pulmonary issues such as dyspnea and atelectasis, and venous thromboembolism.[7] Secondary complications, which are non–life threatening in nature, include contour irregularities, skin discoloration, tissue and wound breakdown, and patient reports of dissatisfaction with results. Perianesthesia nursing care following the procedure includes interventions for managing patient-reported pain and discomfort. Monitor for signs of hypovolemia, and encourage active oral hydration as tolerated. Compression garments are applied immediately postoperatively to control microbleeding and to reduce the potential for hematoma and seroma formation.[7] The use of compression also supports the healing process, and this minimizes uneven surfaces. These garments are worn starting at 24 hours following surgery to several weeks following surgery.

Preparing the patient for home care includes instructions on keeping hydrated to reduce complications from third-spacing of fluids and avoiding any aspirin-containing products to prevent unwanted bleeding. Depending on the preference of the surgeon, most patients are advised to maintain minimal activities for the first week following the procedure and to avoid any strenuous activity for a month while healing continues. Patients can be taught that bruising, swelling, and copious leakage of serosanguineous drainage are normal postoperative findings. A patient should be instructed to report signs of a hematoma or seroma (e.g., large swelling near a surgical site, warmth, redness) to the surgeon.

Rhinoplasty

The third most common cosmetic procedure is the rhinoplasty, also known as a "nose job." Patients who seek this procedure have opted for surgical reshaping of the nose to improve the appearance from natural or injury-related causes. During a rhinoplasty, the nasal bones may be fractured and cartilage, fat, and/or skin can be removed to reshape the nose. Occasionally, the septum is reconstructed to improve the work of breathing. Like many other cosmetic procedures, this can be performed using local anesthesia, procedural sedation, or general anesthesia.

Postoperatively the perianesthesia nurse assesses the patient for pain and discomfort, as well as for ease of breathing and postoperative bleeding. Keeping the head of the bed elevated and applying a facial ice mask support the reduction of pain and swelling. If nasal packing is used, the patient may need reassurance to mouth breathe and stay calm. If a nasal drip pad is in place, change it as needed. The patient may need to be taught to raise or spit out any postnasal drainage to

avoid postoperative nausea. For patients at risk of postoperative nausea and vomiting, prophylactic antiemetics are warranted. Breathing through the mouth may cause dryness of the oral mucosa, and frequent mouth care or sips of fluids can be helpful.

Patient education for the post rhinoplasty procedure includes activity restrictions while the surgical site is healing. Advise the patient to avoid any strenuous activity for a month and to limit flexing from the waist to minimize pressure on the incisions. If nasal packing has been used, the surgeon usually removes it the following day or within three days. For comfort and swelling control, the patient should be encouraged to continue applying the ice mask at home. The patient should be informed that any postoperative swelling or bruising can appear worse over the first 24–72 hours before receding. Other patient tips include the use of a humidifier while at home to reduce the amount of tissue dryness of the mucous membranes. Extra oral fluids can promote mucosal comfort.

Blepharoplasty

The fourth most sought after cosmetic surgery is the removal of fat or excess tissue from the eyelids. Blepharoplasty is often performed to provide patients with a refreshed, younger appearance. Two common complaints lead the patient to a cosmetic surgeon. The first is the decision to correct either upper or lower eyelid puffiness or to remove sagging excess tissue. Secondly, excess skin and lax tissues surrounding the eyes can lead to impaired vision, and the surgery becomes essential for improving the field of vision. The actual procedure involves the surgical removal of unnecessary skin and adipose tissue. Occasionally, the procedure requires a shortening of the muscles of the upper and lower eyelids done through incisions placed in the crease of the upper lid and in the lower lid below the lash margin (Figure 34.4).[8]

The procedure itself can safely be performed in the office setting under local anesthesia. However, the patient's ability to cooperate, as well as the presence of co-morbidities, may necessitate a surgical setting. Postoperatively the perianesthesia nurse assesses the patient for risks associated with retrobulbar hematomas. Signs of medical emergencies include a complaint of pressure behind the eye and loss of vision. The nurse observes for complaints of pain or tightness around the eye, bruising, swelling from hematoma, obvious bulging of the eye, and ecchymosis. Maintaining normotension helps to reduce the potential for hematomas, as does the prevention of straining, lifting, or bending for approximately one week following surgery. The patient should be taught to use facial ice packs to reduce swelling and to avoid the use of aspirin-containing products while healing.

Self-care tips at home include keeping the head elevated for the first five days to minimize edema. Gentle skin cleansing with warm water or saline can help remove crusty debris from the incisions, and the generous use of eye lubrication drops can alleviate the discomfort of temporary dryness of the eye. Female patients should avoid the application of makeup for up to two weeks so that the fragile tissues can heal. Other options for reducing scar formation include the application of vitamin-enriched cream, light topical massage, and active sun protection using sunglasses or sunscreens.[8] The patient should always be advised to call the surgeon for any visual changes, including loss of vision or the development of posterior eye pressure.

Rhytidoplasty, Rhytidectomy, and Browlift

The traditional facelift, also known as the rhytidoplasty or rhytidectomy, is generally used to provide rejuvenation to the

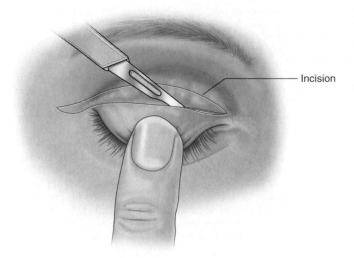

Fig. 34.4 Minimally invasive upper blepharoplasty. Adapted from: Spinelli HM, Lewis A, Elahi E. *Atlas of Aesthetic Eyelid and Periocular Surgery.* Saunders; 2003. Image source: Clinical Key, IMAGE. Few E, Ellis M. Blepharoplasty. Figure 9.25 in: Rubin JP, Neligan PC, eds. *Plastic Surgery: Volume 2: Aesthetic Surgery.* 4th ed. Elsevier; 2017

appearance of wrinkled, lax facial skin. The procedure alone requires the removal of redundant facial skin and management of underlying muscles and fat. A facelift is often done in concert with other procedures, such as the browlift or forehead surgery, blepharoplasty, and/or liposuction, in order to achieve the desired results. In addition, nonsurgical interventions can further support the final outcome, including the use of neurotoxins or laser resurfacing of the skin. Traditional facelifts involve small incisions behind the hairline along the temporal region.

Depending on the complexity of the planned procedure, the surgery can be performed under procedural sedation or general anesthesia. During the immediate phase of recovery, the perianesthesia nurse assesses for the development of a hematoma, readily identified by palpation of the soft surrounding tissues of the neck and forehead. The use of bulky head wrap dressings is fairly common. In complex cases, the surgeon may use either a closed-suction type drain or a wicking-type drain. In either case, the drain patency must be ensured to avoid the formation of hematomas and subsequent swelling. Cool or iced compresses can be helpful to provide comfort and to control swelling. Sedentary activities and positioning to elevate the head are also encouraged. In addition to assessing for a hematoma, the perianesthesia nurse should monitor cranial nerve VII, the facial nerve responsible for motor function. Patients often report a temporary numbness of the ears and cheeks secondary to the surgical manipulation of tissues. Local anesthetics in the wounds and operative sites may cause temporary alterations in the function of cranial nerve VII; however, any aberrant findings should be reported to the surgeon. These include facial asymmetry noted when instructing the patient to smile, frown, or wrinkle the forehead or nose.

In preparation for home care, the perianesthesia nurse provides education to the patient that includes activity restrictions and positioning recommendations. If drains are present, drain care should be taught with teach-back demonstrations. To minimize the use of facial muscles and tissues that must heal, the patient should be encouraged to choose soft foods. If postoperative pain should increase, numbness be progressive, or signs of infection such as fever and chills develop, the patient should report immediately to the surgeon. In addition, evidence of increased swelling and asymmetry or signs of a hematoma should be conveyed to the surgeon immediately.

Body Contouring

The procedures that for body contouring are primarily performed to shape areas of the body after surgical weight loss. Other factors that impact the decision to pursue body contouring procedures include effects of aging, pregnancy, and prior surgical scars. Excess skin and muscle laxity resulting from these conditions can impact the abdomen, back, upper arms, breasts, and inner and outer thighs. The tissue can cause discomfort and skin irritations such as chafing or infections due to moisture retention or the rubbing of redundant tissue against the body. In addition, excess skin can be the source of musculoskeletal and postural tension and strain. Ultimately, body contouring can improve the sense of well-being and confidence. Procedures generally performed to reduce excess and redundant tissue are often done in combination and follow 1 or 2 years of weight loss stability. These include, but are not limited to, abdominoplasty, panniculectomy, brachioplasty, thigh lift, buttock lift, mastopexy, mammaplasty, and liposuction. When done in combination, these procedures can take from 2–10 hours of operating and anesthesia time.

Abdominoplasty is the fifth most common cosmetic procedure. Removal of hanging excess abdominal skin and tissue, also known as the pannus, is called a panniculectomy. An abdominoplasty includes the repair of underlying abdominal muscles that have been weakened by time or conditions such as pregnancy. In most cases, the procedure ends following a repositioning of the umbilicus made necessary by the removal of loose abdominal skin and tissue. Also known as a "tummy tuck," the abdominoplasty can provide a flatter, firmer contour to the abdomen. Additional procedures designed to remove excess and sagging skin include the buttock lift (gluteoplasty), inner or outer thigh lift (thighplasty), and upper arm lift (brachioplasty).

A *mastopexy*, or breast lift, is the common term for the reshaping and lifting of the contour of a female breast that has excess, sagging skin. The reduction mammaplasty is performed to reduce breast tissue in the patient with macromastia, or mammary hyperplasia. A similar procedure for removing excess tissue and skin from the male breast is known as a *gynecomastectomy*. There are several techniques a surgeon can use to accomplish procedural goals. Most are nerve-sparing, nipple-preserving techniques including a peri-areolar incision, as well as the classic inverted-T incision involving the bottom edge of the areola, from the lower portion of the areola to the breast crease and along the fold of the breast. In some cases, the breast lift is combined with an augmentation.

The perianesthesia care and teaching of a patient is the same for any type of body contouring surgery. The perianesthesia nurse promotes comfort and best ventilation efforts by positioning the patient either supine or in a semi-Fowler position. To reduce tension on abdominal incisions, the patient may be encouraged to rest with pillows under the knees to relieve undue pressure and to walk in a stooped position. Other activity restrictions should be reinforced per surgeon preferences. This often includes no heavy lifting, straining, or exercising for at least 4–6 weeks. The patient is taught to maintain compression or support garments for several days to several weeks postoperatively. In addition to promoting comfort, the compression garments can also reduce hematoma formation and help maintain the position of dressings if needed. If drains have been used, either bulb suction drains or wicking drains, drain care is needed and includes the emptying and measuring of the output.

The patient requires education regarding pain and comfort management. Adequate pain and nausea control is necessary for optimal mobility, postoperative coughing, and deep breathing. If indicated, ice or cold compress routines can help with swelling and comfort, as well. Finally, patients must be taught to assess for the development of a hematoma, which is indicated by a large, uneven area of swelling and increased tenderness. Any signs or symptoms of an infection, including fever and chills, must also be reported to the surgeon.

Labiaplasty

An emerging option in the field of cosmetic surgery involves treatments for vaginal rejuvenation. The goals of vaginal rejuvenation include vaginal tightening and tissue restoration, decreased incidence of incontinence, and reduction of vaginal dryness (atrophic vaginitis). However, labiaplasties are performed to reduce excess tissue in the labia minora, often as result of childbirth, aging, sex, and genetic hyperplasia.[9] Postoperative patients are advised to limit showers and to avoid wearing form-fitting clothing until the surgeon ensures that the surgical wound has healed. Other activities, such as strenuous exercise, running, or riding a bicycle, should be avoided for several weeks. Patients should be advised to refrain from sexual intercourse for at least four weeks.

ADDITIONAL COSMETIC PROCEDURES
Genioplasty/Mentoplasty

The procedure for enhancing the shape of a chin by using the patient's own bone or silicone implants is a *genioplasty*, and the procedure for removing excess mandibular bone for the overprojected chin is a *mentoplasty*. Since facial symmetry is socially appealing, patients yearn for proportionate facial features. When a chin is too short, too long, or crooked in appearance, patients seek cosmetic solutions for a more natural look. For these procedures, incisions are placed inside the mouth or in the slight crease beneath the chin. A secondary gain for a well-designed approach is an aesthetically pleasing jawline alignment. Patients having the oral incisions need careful oral hygiene until the incisions are healed. A liquid or soft diet helps reduce tension on the operative site.

Otoplasty

An otoplasty is performed to reshape and/or reposition the ears. The procedure is typically used to correct ears that are either malformed (e.g., due to microtia) or very prominent. Microtia, the malformation of the external ear, occurs in 1 of 2,000 to 10,000 babies in America.[10] It has been determined that by age 5, a child's ear is 90% of the size it will be when the child is an adult.[11] In the case of a malformed ear, the surgeon may use cartilage harvested from the ribs to give shape and form to a reconstructed helix or outer rim of the ear. Surgeons performing an otoplasty reshape existing cartilage and skin of the outer ear and bring the outer portion of the ear closer to the head.

The perianesthesia nurse caring for the patient recovering from cosmetic ear surgery assesses for signs of developing hematomas. If drains are present, the drain must remain patent and drain care must be taught to the patient and family. Depending on the age of the patient, a bulky head dressing is often maintained for the first postoperative week and a headband is worn for the following 2–3 weeks. Advise the patient to sleep with extra pillows to keep the head elevated and to avoid any vigorous activities for 2–4 weeks following surgery.

RECONSTRUCTIVE PROCEDURES
Skin Lesions and Tumor Removal

Under the umbrella of reconstructive procedures, the removal of skin lesions and tumors ranks number one. The removal of skin lesions, either benign or malignant, may require an ambulatory surgery setting as opposed to an office-based setting because of the size and extent of the excision and ability of the patient to cooperate during the procedure. There are three primary malignant skin lesions requiring clinical attention. They are the basal cell carcinoma, which is the most common form of skin cancer; squamous cell carcinoma, which can be more invasive to underlying tissue; and malignant melanoma, which is the most serious form of skin cancer.[12] Most often a simple excision of the lesion addresses the concerns for any recurrent or residual cancer. In some situations, outpatient treatment with laser or radiation therapy or topical preparations can provide adequate treatment.

In cases where the spread or location of the cancer is more challenging, the surgical approach to treating skin lesions may involve wide excision procedures or the Mohs procedure.[13] For more invasive cases, the area of excision may require skin grafts or flaps to bring the wound to closure. Certain head and neck skin cancers, when invasive, may destroy the form and appearance of facial structures. Some situations may require reconstructive surgery to address defects left by wide excisions. To stage a lesion that is suspected to have metastasized, node dissection may be performed and can provide information for future treatment planning.

Evidence-Based Practice: What is Mohs surgery?
Mohs surgery is a procedure that relies on the ability to examine small samples of tissue under a microscope throughout the procedure. The goal is to stop removing tissue when the tissue margins are clear of signs of cancerous cells. Once the clear margins are found, the resulting wound can be closed or reconstructed.

Data from: Etzkorn JR, Alam M. What is Mohs surgery? *JAMA Dermatol.* 2020;156(6):716. doi:10.1001/jamadermatol.2020.0039

The perianesthesia nurse caring for the patient having surgery for skin cancer must be able to offer reassurance and the opportunity for the patient to verbalize anxiety related to the diagnosis, as well as any fears concerning potential scarring. In the postoperative phase, encourage the patient to keep the affected area elevated to reduce swelling and to maintain dressing or wound care as instructed. The patient with skin cancer benefits from the reinforcement of educational prevention measures. This includes a discussion regarding the careful application of sunscreens, the donning of protective clothing and headwear, and efforts to avoid prolonged direct sun exposure.[12] The patient should also be encouraged to comply with frequent skin checks for early detection of new lesions or recurrence.

Laceration Repair and Scar Revisions

The second most common reconstructive procedure is surgery to repair lacerations, and the fourth most common procedure is performed to revise scars. Canine bites are the most common laceration requiring surgical repair. Procedures regarding scar revisions are intended to remove unsightly scars, or at least, reduce scar tissue. Surgical consultation is implicated for the following conditions[14]:

- Extensive or complex lacerations or scars
- Lacerations requiring prolonged repair times

- Lacerations requiring grafting for full closure
- Profoundly contaminated wounds requiring extensive washouts
- Wounds with the potential for concurrent nerve or vascular damage
- Injury involving additional structures, such as fractures
- Injuries with obvious cosmetic implications involving facial or head and neck features

Common approaches to repairing skin defects help to restructure a scar to be better aligned with natural skin.[15] The technique chosen by the surgeon best matches the situation based on the characteristics of the injury or scar. Some sutures are absorbable, while others may require removal depending on the location and tension on skin edges. Topical ointments and wound dressings also vary. Patients should be taught wound care, activity restrictions, bathing directions, and other self-care instructions per surgeon preference. Signs of wound infections should be reported immediately to the surgeon.

Cleft Lip and Palate Repair

Maxillofacial surgery ranked third for all reconstructive surgeries in 2019. Cleft lip and palate repair is included in this category of reconstructive surgery. Cleft lip occurs when the facial tissues forming the lip in utero fail to join, leaving a gap that can extend through the lip into the nose.[16] The same phenomenon occurs in cleft palate when the tissue developing the roof of the mouth fails to join together, creating a gap in the roof of the mouth. Children born with these conditions can have one or the other or a combination of both. Feeding issues and speech development lead parents to seek repair of congenital lip defects within the first 12 months of life and congenital palate defects within the first 18 months of life.[16] In some cases, the repairs can be done simultaneously. In other cases, staged procedures are warranted; the staging depends on the extent of the repairs and the potential for skeletal reconstruction (Figure 34.5).

The perianesthesia nurse caring for the postoperative child must pay particular attention to the pediatric airway to assess for swelling, drainage, and the potential for aspiration. These patients should be positioned side to side with the head of the bed elevated, and pronation must be avoided. Comfort measures, including parental presence, are useful for minimizing crying and restlessness that might cause undue stress and tension on suture lines. Cool compresses, if tolerated, can help reduce swelling and promote comfort. Parental instructions for feeding routines per the surgeon's preference should be reinforced.

Gender Confirmation Surgery

The ASPS reports a 15% increase in gender confirmation surgery between 2018 and 2019.[3] The population of individuals who self-describe as transgender or gender nonbinary (TGNB) is growing as the social culture and norms have become more accepting.[17] Gender confirmation surgery, or sex reassignment surgery, often entails transmasculine changes (female to male) or transfeminine changes (male to female). These individuals seek surgery as a means of securing the physical appearance that best matches the gender they identify with internally.

Simplified surgical procedures involve either "top surgery" (e.g., mastectomy or breast augmentation) or "bottom surgery" (e.g., surgical alteration of birth genitals). Regardless of the nature of transgender patients, chest reconstruction procedures are more common.[17] In some cases, the surgical transition requires several stages, as well as complementary procedures such as blepharoplasty, rhytidectomy, liposuction, and thyroid chondroplasty (removal of the prominent laryngeal cartilage or Adam's apple). To feminize male genitalia, surgery may include labioplasty, orchiectomies, penectomy, clitoral reduction, and/or vaginoplasty. To masculinize female genitalia, in addition to removal of the vagina and labia, penile reconstruction and scrotoplasty may be performed. Additionally, these patients may elect to have a hysterectomy and salpingo-oopherectomy. In a staged approach, penile implants as well as testicular prostheses may be added.

Perianesthesia nurses providing care to the TGNB patient must begin by establishing the patient's preferred identity and pronoun. An effort to create and maintain an environment of acceptance begins with setting assumptions aside. Recommendations from the American Society of PeriAnesthesia Nurses position statement on gender diversity include ensuring that staff are provided training and education to promote awareness of the unique health needs of transgender individuals.[18] Routine postoperative care and associated patient education should be reinforced.

BREAST RECONSTRUCTIVE PROCEDURES
Reduction Mammaplasty

The purpose of a reduction mammaplasty is to remove excess breast tissue (macromastia), which is usually disproportionate to the body shape, or to correct asymmetric breasts (e.g., Poland syndrome). Many individuals with an excessive volume of breast fat and glandular tissue experience chronic issues related to back, neck, and shoulder discomfort caused by the weight of the chest. In addition, some report chronic skin irritations or rashes under the breast resulting from retained moisture and tissue friction. Often a patient reports a poor self-image, poor self-confidence, and shame issues due to large breasts.

The surgical approach to a reduction mammaplasty mirrors the approach used for body-contouring purposes. Excess tissue can be removed by way of nerve-sparing and nipple-preserving techniques. These include a variety of incisional techniques such as a peri-areolar incision, a keyhole incision that traces the areola down to the breast crease, as well as the classic inverted-T incision (shaped like an anchor) involving the bottom edge of the areola, from the lower portion of the areola to the breast crease and along the fold of the breast. Usually, the nipple and areola can be kept intact and sutured into an aesthetically appropriate location; however, with extremely large breasts and reductions, the nipple and areola are sometimes removed and transplanted as a free graft.[19]

The perianesthesia nurse caring for the patient following a breast reduction carefully assesses the patient for an early hematoma. This is best assessed by palpating the superior aspect of the pectoralis muscle near the third rib above the soft breast tissue toward the clavicle. In some cases, the surgeon may use wicking or bulb suction drains. The patient needs to be taught drain care and provided with ample supplemental dressings to reinforce areas of drainage. Applying surgical support or compression bras helps to provide comfort, maintain dressings, and minimize the collection of fluid and swelling in the soft surrounding tissues.

Postoperatively, patients should be encouraged to drink fluids liberally to replace any volume losses during surgery. While walking and moving around are important, routine strenuous exercising and heavy lifting should be avoided for at least the first month following breast reduction surgery to prevent undue tension on delicate sutures and to support healing. Patients are often advised to wear a compression bra or a regular sport bra to provide support and added comfort while recuperating. Tenderness and increased breast sensitivity are normal postoperative findings, as are bruising and some swelling.

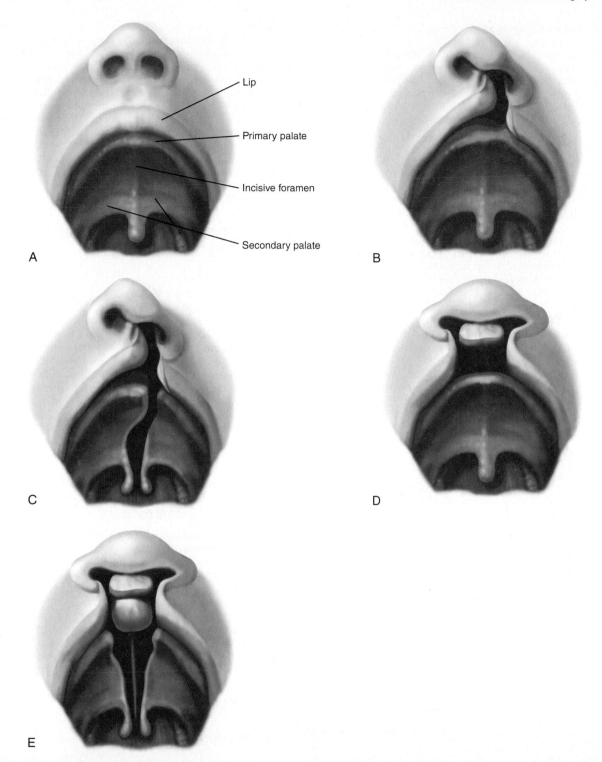

Fig. 34.5 Surgical repair of cleft lip and cleft palate. **A.** Normal lip and palate. **B.** Unilateral cleft lip. **C.** Unilateral cleft lip and palate. **D.** Bilateral cleft lip. **E.** Bilateral cleft lip and palate. Illustration by James A. Cooper, MD, San Diego, CA. Image source: Clinical Key, IMAGE. Pettit KE, Tran NV, Pretorius DH. Ultrasound evaluation of the fetal face and neck. Figure 10.10 in: Norton ME, ed. *Callen's Ultrasonography in Obstetrics and Gynecology.* 6th ed. Elsevier; 2016.

Breast Reconstruction

Breast reconstruction is typically performed when surgical excisions or oncologic treatments such as radiation for breast cancers have resulted in breast asymmetry. Nononcologic reconstructions can be required due to trauma, injuries, and congenital malformations or asymmetries. The simplest approach to breast reconstruction is the insertion of breast implants, much like the breast augmentation procedure previously described. In some cases, prior to the final implants, tissue expanders may be required to increase the pocket space under the remaining breast tissue so that a prosthetic implant can be placed.

An alternative to breast implants involves the creation of live tissue flaps. Using an autologous donor site, the surgeon transplants skin, muscle, and tissue from the patient's body to the area being reconstructed.[20] There are five common tissue flap procedures. The first, the transverse rectus abdominis muscle flap (TRAM), uses abdominal muscle and tissue to reconstruct the breast. Two primary TRAMs are possible. The first, called the pedicle TRAM flap, tunnels the resected tissue from the abdominal skin to the chest wall while maintaining the original blood supply. The free TRAM flap moves the same resected tissue without the original blood supply, necessitating microvascular revascularization of the tissue (Figure 34.6).

Other common tissue flap surgeries include the deep inferior epigastric perforator flap (DIEP). The DIEP differs from the TRAM in that abdominal muscle is not used for the restoration of breast form. The latissimus dorsi flap incorporates tissue from the upper back through a skin tunnel to the chest wall. The gluteal artery perforator flap uses buttock tissue, and the transverse upper gracilis flap uses tissue from the inner thigh. Surgeries involving the patient's own tissue for reconstruction often choose this approach because of the natural appearance it gives to the breast. In some situations, the surgeon may include an implant or fat transfer to provide better breast shape.

The nurse caring for the patient following a flap procedure prioritizes several assessments and interventions to support optimal perfusion of the transplanted tissues (Box 34.3). This includes maintaining normothermia to avoid vasoconstriction of the blood supply to the flap. Early recognition and treatment of hypotension and hypovolemia also serve to maintain a robust blood perfusion to the transplant. These assessments include monitoring of the temperature of the skin on the transplanted tissue, as well as the capillary refill. Prolonged refill may indicate compromised perfusion, while capillary refill that is too rapid may be an indication of venous engorgement.[21] The color of the flap is equally important. A pale flap is an indication of insufficient perfusion, while a bluish tone suggests venous congestion. Gentle palpation of surrounding tissue can detect an early hematoma. Thorough pain and comfort management, including the minimization of nausea, can help to reduce wound tension.

GENERAL CONSIDERATIONS IN COSMETIC AND RECONSTRUCTIVE SURGERY

Co-morbidities

The choice of anesthesia varies based on the complexity of the surgery, the ability of the patient to tolerate the procedure, and the need for the patient to actively participate in positioning, as well as the various underlying medical conditions of the patient. Successful cosmetic and reconstructive surgery requires preemptive optimization of medical co-morbidities that impact the ability to heal. In general, mature adults tend to heal slower because of the effects of aging on circulation and the presence of chronic conditions. Nutritional deficits may impair the healing process. Individuals who use products that are inhaled or who have substance use disorders, including alcohol, may recover poorly. Other factors that have an impact on healing include, but are not limited to, diabetes, peripheral vascular disease, cardiopulmonary disorders, obesity, and hematologic disorders impacting bleeding and clotting factors.[21]

Psychological Background

The psychology involved with body image and self-confidence cannot be understated. The principles of enhanced recovery protocols are based on the knowledge that stress-induced physiologic responses can adversely impact healing and circulation.[22] The decision to proceed with cosmetic or reconstructive surgery is most often, but not always, elective. During the preoperative phase of preparation for any type of cosmetic or reconstructive surgery, providers should incorporate discussions regarding a patient's expectations of outcomes and explore the motivation driving the decision for surgery. In general, poor outcomes are associated with a history of mood disorders, pursuit of multiple cosmetic procedures, a diagnosis of body dysmorphic disorders, and unrealistic expectations for aesthetic outcomes.[21]

CHAPTER HIGHLIGHTS

- Cosmetic and reconstructive surgery is more common among Caucasian females ranging in age from 40–54 years.
- Breast augmentation is the most common breast surgery performed in America.
- The removal of skin lesions is the most common reconstructive surgery performed.
- Body contouring refers to surgical procedures that enhance the shape of different areas of the body, such as liposuction, body lifts, tummy tucks, and buttock augmentations.
- Gender confirmation surgery is a fast-growing surgical approach for gender transitioning.
- Chest procedures, or "top surgeries," are more common amongst transgender patients than "bottom surgeries."

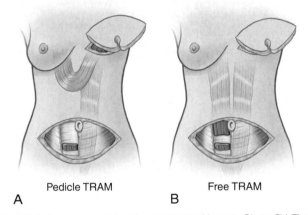

Pedicle TRAM   Free TRAM
A   B

Fig. 34.6 The augmented and reconstructed breast. Ghate SV. The augmented and reconstructed breast. Figure 18.14 in: Joe BN, Lee AY, eds. *Breast Imaging.* 4th ed. Elsevier; 2023.

BOX 34.3 Nursing Assessment of Flaps

Normothermia
Hypotension
Hypovolemia
Capillary refill
Color
Temperature
Swelling
Drainage
Promote comfort
Minimize nausea

Data from: Clifford TL. Plastic and Reconstruction. In: Schick L, Windle PE, eds. *PeriAnesthesia Nursing Core Curriculum: Preprocedure, Phase I and Phase II PACU Nursing.* 4th Ed. Elsevier; 2021.

CASE STUDY

Martha is a 22-year-old Caucasian whose gender assignment at birth was male. Throughout Martha's childhood she expressed a keen interest in wearing girls' clothing. Her parents believed that Martha was going to outgrow her obsession with female interests. As a result of ready access to the Internet, Martha spent time researching ways to change her appearance to match how she felt. Her parents were highly resistant but agreed to explore therapy to better understand the gender experience their "little boy" was having. By the age of eleven, Martha began to beg her parents for hormone therapy to grow breasts and appear as feminine on the outside as she felt on the inside. Finally, at the age of 22, Martha presents to your day surgery center for the first of a series of procedures known as gender confirmation surgery. The patient is scheduled for top surgery today, which is documented in the history and physical examination as a bilateral breast augmentation using saline implants.

As the preoperative nurse, how should you address the patient? Should it be according to the gender assignment at birth or according to the patient's chosen pronouns? Transparency is always the best approach to addressing patients. The preoperative nurse should never assume how a patient would like to be addressed. Rather, the nurse should always ask, "How would you prefer to be addressed?"

Martha expresses concern for pain and comfort management. What are the best options for treating discomfort in patients having chest cosmetic surgery? What nonpharmacologic interventions can help ease discomfort?

Are there any psychosocial implications for this patient of which the postoperative nurse should be aware? Are the parents present? Have they come to accept the changes their child has chosen? What support system does Martha have to help cope with the challenges she may face as she continues this journey?

REFERENCES

1. Asimakopoulou E, Zavrides H, Askitis T. Plastic surgery on body image, body satisfaction and self-esteem. *Acta Chir Plast*. 2020;61 (1-4):3-9.
2. Sarwer DB. Body image, cosmetic surgery, and minimally invasive treatments. *Body Image*. 2019;31: 302-308. Available at: https://doi. org/10.1016/j.bodyim.2019.01.009.
3. American Society of Plastic Surgeons (ASPS). *Plastic Surgery Statistics Report*. ASPS; 2019. Available at: https://www.plasticsurgery. org/documents/News/Statistics/2019/plastic-surgery-statistics-full-report-2019.pdf.
4. American Society of Plastic Surgeons (ASPS). *Breast Augmentation, Augmentation Mammaplasty*. ASPS; 2021. Available at: https://www. plasticsurgery.org/cosmetic-procedures/breast-augmentation/ implants.
5. Hilton L. Which fat reduction technique is right for your patient? *Dermatology Times*. 2016, February;44. Available at: https://web. b.ebscohost.com/ehost/pdfviewer/pdfviewer?vid=6&sid=05 acf7ee-ae8c-4e3f-9bab-13611ae220f4%40sessionmgr102.
6. The American Board of Cosmetic Surgery (ABCS). *Liposuction Guide*. 2021. Available at: https://www.americanboardcosmetic-surgery.org/procedure-learning-center/body/liposuction-guide/.
7. Kaoutzanis C, Gupta V, Winocour J, et al. Cosmetic liposuction: preoperative risk factors, major complication rates, and safety of combined procedures. *Aesthet Surg J*. 2017;37(6):680-694. Available at: https://doi.org/10.1093/asj/sjw243.
8. Bhattacharjee K, Misra, DK, Deori N. Updates on upper eyelid blepharoplasty. *Indian J Opthamol*. 2017;65(7):551-558. Available at: https://doi.org/10.4103/ijo.ijo_540_17.
9. American Society of Plastic Surgeons. *What is Labiaplasty and What Does it Involve?* ASPS; February 2020. Available at: https://www.plasticsurgery. org/news/blog/what-is-a-labiaplasty-and-what-does-it-involve.
10. Centers for Disease Control and Prevention (CDC). *Facts About Anotia/Microtia*. CDC; October 2020. Available at: https://www. cdc.gov/ncbddd/birthdefects/anotia-microtia.html.
11. Seladi-Schulman J. *All about Otoplasty (Cosmetic Ear Surgery)*. Healthline; February 2020. Available at: https://www.healthline. com/health/otoplasty.
12. Jones OT, Ranmuthu CKI, Hall PN, Funston G, Walter FM. Recognising skin cancer in primary care. *Adv Ther*. 2019;37:603-616. Available at: https://doi.org/10.1007/s12325-019-01130-1.
13. Etzkorn JR, Alam M. What is Mohs surgery? *JAMA Dermatol*. 2020;156(6):716. Available at: https://doi.org/10.1001/jamadermatol. 2020.0039.
14. Zito PM, Jawad BA, Mazzoni T. *Z Plasty*. StatPearls. 2020, November 11. Available at: https://www.ncbi.nlm.nih.gov/books/NBK507775/.
15. deLemos DM. *Skin Laceration Repair with Sutures*. UpToDate. 2021, January 4. Available at: https://www.uptodate.com/contents/skin-laceration-repair-with-sutures.
16. Centers for Disease Control and Prevention. *Facts About Cleft Lip and Cleft Palate*. 2020, December 28. Available at: https://www. cdc.gov/ncbddd/birthdefects/cleftlip.html.
17. Nolan IT, Kuhner CJ, Dy GW. Demographic and temporal trends in transgender identities and gender conforming surgery. *Transl Androl Urol*. 2019;8(3):1840190. Available at: https://doi.org/10. 21037/tau.2019.04.09
18. American Society of PeriAnesthesia Nurses. Position statement 16: a position statement on gender diversity. In: *2021-2022 Perianesthesia Standards, Practice Recommendations and Interpretive Statements*. ASPAN;2020:171-173.
19. The Aesthetic Society. *Breast reduction*. 2021. Available at: https:// www.smartbeautyguide.com/procedures/breast/breast-reduction/#label-sbg-procedure-about.
20. American Cancer Society. *Breast Reconstruction Using Your Own Tissues (Flap Procedures)*. 2019. Available at: https://www.cancer.org/ cancer/breast-cancer/reconstruction-surgery/breast-reconstruction-options/breast-reconstruction-using-your-own-tissues-flap-procedures.html.
21. Clifford TL. Plastic and Reconstruction. In: Schick L, Windle PE, eds. *PeriAnesthesia Nursing Core Curriculum: Preprocedure, Phase I and Phase II PACU Nursing*. 4th ed. Elsevier; 2021:770-794.
22. Crosson JA. Enhanced recovery after surgery—the importance of the perianesthesia nurse on program success. *J Perianesth Nurs*. 2018;33(4):366-374. Available at: https://doi.org/10.1016/j. jopan.2016.09.010.

35   Special Procedures in the Ambulatory Setting

Amy Berardinelli, DNP, RN, NE-BC, CPAN, FASPAN

LEARNING OBJECTIVES

A review of the content of this chapter will help the reader to:

1. Describe the impact of outpatient special procedures on surgical outcomes.
2. Describe and define cardiovascular, endoscopic, interventional radiology, and wound procedures in the outpatient ambulatory surgery setting.
3. Describe nursing continuing education related to special procedures in the ambulatory setting.
4. Identify nursing implications for special procedures in an ambulatory surgery center.

OVERVIEW

Ambulatory surgery centers (ASCs) are one example of a modernized healthcare facility. To care for patients safely, effectively, and efficiently across the country, healthcare organizations are challenged with lowering costs and improving care. The most overarching way to meet these goals is with outpatient services. The shift to outpatient procedures in ASCs involves several stakeholders, who must ensure that licensed independent practitioners (LIPs), nurses, and unlicensed assistive personnel are skilled and proficient in medical advances, regulatory changes, and patient management methods in this setting. Decreased operating room minutes due to shorter, less complicated procedures, as well as a decreased patient recovery time after surgery and procedures, has led to cost reductions for the health care organization and the patient.

The special procedures performed in an ASC discussed in this chapter include cardiovascular, endoscopic, interventional radiologic, and wound healing enhancement procedures; however, the procedures vary depending on state laws, regulatory bodies, and facility-specific policies and procedures.

FACTS AND FIGURES

The movement of nonurgent procedures to ACSs has allowed for improvements in hospital utilization by decreasing the patient length of stay and reducing resource needs. Data from 2014 show that 17.2 million hospital visits for ambulatory or inpatient procedures took place and involved invasive therapeutic surgeries. At that time, 57.8% of the surgeries occurred in a hospital-owned ASC, while the remaining 42.2% were in an inpatient facility. Private insurance was the primary payer for 48.2% of the ASC visits (Table 35.1).[1]

SPECIAL PROCEDURES PERFORMED IN AMBULATORY SURGICAL CENTERS

Therapeutic and diagnostic procedures, as well as minimally invasive surgeries, performed in ASCs offer expedient admission and discharge experiences. An ASC nurse is prepared and skilled in admitting patients and helping patients to recover so that the turnover is rapid in these facilities. Due to the increase in the variety of procedures and surgeries performed at ASCs, as well as technologic advancements, ASC nurses are required to have a broad array of knowledge and remain current in evidence-based practices.

Anesthesiologists and anesthesia "front liners" work closely and collaboratively with the ASC nurses, as do the surgeons and proceduralists. The small size of the facility, swift throughput of patients, and expert knowledge required demand a cohesive and highly skilled team of practitioners. Planning, protocols, policies, and continued education are necessities for all team members to ensure that safe, effective, and efficient care is consistently delivered. The goal is for all patients to be safely discharged to go home without a hospital stay.

Cardiovascular Procedures

Cardiovascular procedures, like many other special procedures, are moving from hospitals to ambulatory settings, and this is resulting in reduced costs for the patient, the provider, and the payer. Several advancements in outpatient technologies have driven this shift. Smaller, less expensive equipment has led to minimal incision sizes, a reduced risk of bleeding, earlier ambulation, and a short recovery time. Because patient risks and complications following a procedure have decreased, patients can be safely discharged to go home the same day as surgery. Patient satisfaction and reduced overall costs are direct results.[2]

Vein Ligation, Stripping, and Ablation

The most commonly treated vascular disease is varicose veins, which has an adult morbidity rate of 25% to 40%.[3] The three most common outpatient procedures for treating varicose veins are ligation, stripping, and ablation. Ligation and stripping remain the most popular choices, due to the cost and the success, especially when veins are severely distorted. Vein ligation involves tying off the vein through a small incision in the skin. Vein stripping, most performed on the superficial saphenous vein, involves removal of the vein by use of a guidewire.

Although ablation is the preferred method for treating varicose veins, its disadvantages include its expense (often only partially covered by medical insurance) and its ineffectiveness for severely distorted veins. Vein ablations seal off diseased veins, such as the long saphenous vein in the thigh

TABLE 35.1 Invasive Therapeutic Surgeries, Listed by Body System, Performed in Community Hospitals in the United States by Setting (Ambulatory Versus Inpatient) in 2014

Procedures Listed by CCS Number plus Description	Surgeries, N[a]		Surgeries, N per 100,000 Population[b]		Surgeries Performed in Ambulatory Setting, %
	AS	Inpatient	AS	Inpatient	
OPERATIONS ON THE NERVOUS SYSTEM					
3: Laminectomy, excision intervertebral disc	219,900	438,300	69.3	138.2	33.4
6: Decompression peripheral nerve	322,500	16,300	101.7	5.1	95.2
9: Other OR therapeutic nervous system procedures	81,800	191,100	25.8	60.3	30.0
OPERATIONS ON THE ENDOCRINE SYSTEM					
10: Thyroidectomy, partial or complete	101,600	29,700	32.0	9.4	77.4
12: Other therapeutic endocrine procedures	39,400	38,500	12.4	12.1	50.6
OPERATIONS ON THE EYE					
13: Corneal transplant	30,100	300	9.5	0.1	99.0
15: Lens and cataract procedures	1,419,100	1,000	447.4	0.3	99.9
16: Repair of retinal tear, detachment	109,600	1,000	34.5	0.3	99.1
21: Other extraocular muscle and orbit therapeutic procedures	70,500	6,200	22.2	1.9	91.9
OPERATIONS ON THE EAR					
22: Tympanoplasty	26,500	700	8.3	0.2	97.4
23: Myringotomy	298,600	8,300	94.1	2.6	97.3
24: Mastoidectomy	17,100	2,500	5.4	0.8	87.2
26: Other therapeutic ear procedures	29,800	15,600	9.4	4.9	65.6
OPERATIONS ON THE NOSE, MOUTH, AND PHARYNX					
28: Plastic procedures on nose	164,900	14,600	52.0	4.6	91.9
30: Tonsillectomy and/or adenoidectomy	356,100	16,800	112.3	5.3	95.5
33: Other OR therapeutic procedures on nose, mouth, and pharynx (OR procedures of mouth, nose, and throat, excluding tonsils and teeth)	175,100	76,400	55.2	24.1	69.6
OPERATIONS ON THE RESPIRATORY SYSTEM					
42: Other OR therapeutic procedures on respiratory system and mediastinum	39,100	104,300	12.3	32.9	27.3
OPERATIONS ON THE CARDIOVASCULAR SYSTEM					
48: Insertion, revision, replacement, removal of cardiac pacemaker or cardioverter-defibrillator	286,400	245,600	90.3	77.4	53.8
53: Varicose vein stripping, lower limb	29,700	500	9.4	0.1	98.3
57: Creation, revision, and removal of arteriovenous fistula or vessel-to-vessel cannula for dialysis	150,400	38,400	48.4	12.1	80.0
61: Other OR procedures on vessels other than head and neck (vascular stents and OR procedures, other than head or neck)	206,200	1,000,500	65.0	315.4	17.1
63: Other non-OR therapeutic cardiovascular procedures	33,700	689,600	10.6	217.4	4.7
OPERATIONS ON THE HEMIC AND LYMPHATIC SYSTEM					
67: Other therapeutic procedures, hemic and lymphatic system (lymph node biopsies and excisions, bone marrow procedures)	152,200	301,100	48.0	94.9	33.6
OPERATIONS ON THE DIGESTIVE SYSTEM					
78: Colorectal resection	7,500	302,500	2.4	95.4	2.4
80: Appendectomy	208,800	238,800	65.8	75.3	46.6
84: Cholecystectomy and common duct exploration	577,400	372,600	182.0	117.5	60.8
85: Inguinal and femoral hernia repair	435,900	38,300	137.4	12.1	91.9
86: Other hernia repair (repair of diaphragmatic, incisional, and umbilical hernia)	376,400	239,000	118.7	75.3	61.2

Continued

TABLE 35.1 Invasive Therapeutic Surgeries, Listed by Body System, Performed in Community Hospitals in the United States by Setting (Ambulatory Versus Inpatient) in 2014—cont'd

Procedures Listed by CCS Number plus Description	Surgeries, N[a]		Surgeries, N per 100,000 Population[b]		Surgeries Performed in Ambulatory Setting, %
	AS	Inpatient	AS	Inpatient	
87: Laparoscopy (GI only)	114,900	57,700	36.2	18.2	66.6
94: Other OR upper GI therapeutic procedures	7,700	159,100	2.4	50.2	4.6
96: Other OR lower GI therapeutic procedures	53,200	266,500	16.8	84.0	16.6
99: Other OR gastrointestinal therapeutic procedures	34,400	230,300	10.8	72.6	13.0
244: Gastric bypass and volume reduction[c]	31,400	0	9.9	0.0	100.0
OPERATIONS ON THE URINARY SYSTEM					
100: Endoscopy and endoscopic biopsy of the urinary tract	16,400	161,100	5.2	50.8	9.2
101: Transurethral excision, drainage, or removal of urinary obstruction	4,600	104,300	1.4	32.9	4.2
106: Genitourinary incontinence procedures	88,800	24,100	28.0	7.6	78.7
109: Procedures on the urethra	23,900	28,800	7.5	9.1	45.4
112: Other OR therapeutic procedures of urinary tract	28,100	87,100	8.8	27.4	24.4
OPERATIONS ON THE MALE GENITAL SYSTEM					
113: Transurethral resection of prostate (TURP)	56,400	29,100	17.8	9.2	66.0
114: Open prostatectomy	3,400	61,600	1.1	19.4	5.2
118: Other OR therapeutic procedures, male genital (testicular, prostate, and penile OR procedures)	187,300	22,100	59.1	7.0	89.4
OPERATIONS ON THE FEMALE GENITAL SYSTEM					
119: Oophorectomy, unilateral and bilateral	99,800	182,400	31.5	57.5	35.4
121: Ligation or occlusion of fallopian tubes	103,600	254,500	32.7	80.2	28.9
124: Hysterectomy, abdominal and vaginal	276,100	237,500	87.0	74.9	53.8
125: Other excision of cervix and uterus	16,000	38,100	5.1	12.0	29.6
129: Repair of cystocele and rectocele, obliteration of vaginal vault	68,300	30,000	21.5	9.5	69.5
132: Other OR therapeutic procedures, female organs (vaginal, vulvar, and female pelvic OR procedures)	187,600	74,500	59.1	23.5	71.6
OPERATIONS ON THE MUSCULOSKELETAL SYSTEM					
142: Partial excision bone	251,500	358,900	79.3	113.2	41.2
143: Bunionectomy or repair of toe deformities	185,800	2,900	58.6	0.9	98.5
144: Treatment, facial fracture, or dislocation	53,400	27,200	16.8	8.6	66.3
145: Treatment, fracture or dislocation of radius and ulna	117,800	60,100	37.2	19.0	66.2
147: Treatment, fracture, or dislocation of lower extremity (other than hip or femur)	142,000	196,600	44.8	62.0	41.9
148: Other fracture and dislocation procedure	109,300	167,600	34.5	52.9	39.5
149: Arthroscopy	98,700	9,600	31.1	3.0	91.1
150: Division of joint capsule, ligament, or cartilage	69,200	14,300	21.8	4.5	82.9
151: Excision of semilunar cartilage of knee	513,600	6,900	161.9	2.2	98.7
152: Arthroplasty knee	37,300	753,000	11.8	237.4	4.7
153: Hip replacement, total and partial	21,200	523,100	6.7	164.9	3.9
154: Arthroplasty other than hip or knee	49,900	104,500	15.7	33.0	32.3
157: Amputation of lower extremity	34,500	146,600	10.9	46.2	19.1
158: Spinal fusion	38,000	463,800	12.0	146.2	7.6
160: Other therapeutic procedures on muscles and tendons (muscle, tendon, and soft tissue OR procedures)	755,500	295,300	238.2	93.1	71.9
161: Other OR therapeutic procedures on bone (nonfracture, nonarthroplasty OR procedures on the bone)	279,800	139,800	88.2	44.1	66.7
162: Other OR therapeutic procedures on joints (incision or fusion of joint, destruction of joint lesion)	608,700	147,800	191.9	46.6	80.5

TABLE 35.1 Invasive Therapeutic Surgeries, Listed by Body System, Performed in Community Hospitals in the United States by Setting (Ambulatory Versus Inpatient) in 2014—cont'd

Procedures Listed by CCS Number plus Description	Surgeries, N[a]		Surgeries, N per 100,000 Population[b]		Surgeries Performed in Ambulatory Setting, %
	AS	Inpatient	AS	Inpatient	
164: Other OR therapeutic procedures on musculoskeletal system	36,700	45,700	11.6	14.4	44.5
OPERATIONS ON THE INTEGUMENTARY (SKIN) SYSTEM					
166: Lumpectomy, quadrantectomy of breast	296,500	8,000	93.5	2.5	97.4
167: Mastectomy	61,200	42,600	19.3	13.4	59.0
174: Other non-OR therapeutic procedures on skin and breast	17,600	223,400	5.5	70.4	7.3
175: Other OR therapeutic procedures on skin and breast (OR procedures of skin and breast, including plastic procedures on breast)	325,500	88,100	102.6	27.8	78.7

AS, ambulatory surgery; CCS, Clinical Classifications Software; OR, operating room; GI, gastrointestinal

Notes: Only invasive therapeutic surgeries that are performed and reliably reported in the hospital-based ambulatory surgery setting were included. Procedures are based on the Clinical Classifications Software (CCS) and the CCS for Services and Procedures. Statistics are based on the "narrow" definition of the HCUP Surgery Flag software.

[a] The number of discharges was rounded to the nearest 100.

[b] Based on population estimates from the U.S. Census Bureau.

[c] The gastric bypass and volume reduction CCS category (244) does not exist in the ICD-9-CM categorization. Inpatient gastric bypass and volume reductions are included in alternative categories, such as CCS 94, Other upper GI therapeutic procedures.

Agency for Healthcare Research and Quality (AHRQ), Center for Delivery, Organization, and Markets, Healthcare Cost and Utilization Project (HCUP), National Inpatient Sample (NIS) and nationwide ambulatory surgery analytic file created from the State Ambulatory Surgery and Services Databases (SASD), weighted for national estimates, 2014.

or the short saphenous vein behind the knee, by using electrical current or laser energy to burn and close the veins. Ligation and stripping may be performed under general, monitored anesthesia care or regional anesthesia. Vein ablation is often performed using local anesthesia only, and this makes it a shorter procedure with a quicker recovery time than ligation or stripping.

The newest technique for occluding varicose veins uses a medical-grade glue applied directly into the vein to seal it off. The treatment takes approximately 15 minutes, is done in the physician's office, and requires either local anesthesia or no anesthesia.[4]

Following the procedure, the ASC nurse follows the *nursing implications* of assessing the bandaging, typically an ace wrap, to ensure that the wrap is not too tight, and that proper circulation is present. The affected leg should be elevated and assessed for bleeding. Bleeding that seeps through the ace wrap requires immediate attention, and the LIP should be notified and assess the condition.

> - The medical record must also include pretreatment photographs of the varicose veins for which claims for sclerotherapy are submitted to Medicare. These photographs must be made available to the carrier upon a request for review
> - These are items that the ASC registered nurse may be asked to retrieve from the patient's chart; however, they are the responsibility of the LIP

LCD - Varicose Veins of the Lower Extremity, Treatment of (L33575) (cms.gov)

Transvascular Endomyocardial Biopsy

In 1962, Sakakibara and Konno published an article introducing the transvascular endomyocardial biopsy as a diagnostic procedure that could determine the best treatment plan for cardiac muscle diseases.[5] Since then, advances in medicine and technology, as well as the skills of practitioners, have enabled the use of this technique for the diagnosis of many cardiac conditions.

Evidence-Based Practice: Nursing implications for varicose vein ligation, stripping, and ablation

According to the Centers for Medicare and Medicaid Services, for a patient to receive treatment for varicose veins of the lower extremities, the patient's medical record must document the following:

- History and physical findings supporting a diagnosis of symptomatic varicose veins
- Failure of an adequate trial of conservative treatment
- Exclusion of other causes of edema, ulceration, and pain in the limbs
- Performance of appropriate tests to confirm the presence and location of incompetent perforating veins
- Location and number of varicosities and level of incompetence of the vein and the veins involved
- Necessity of utilizing ultrasound guidance

Evidence-Based Practice: Nursing implications for transvascular endomyocardial biopsy

Post procedurally, the ASC nurse may apply pressure to the incision sites for approximately 10 minutes to prevent hematoma formation. Pressure dressings may be applied to the femoral vein or arterial access sites. Because a sudden and life-threatening complication may occur, cardiovascular resuscitative medication, equipment, and supplies need to be immediately accessible to perform a pericardiocentesis.

The *indications* for transvascular endomyocardial biopsy are heart failure of unknown etiology, heart transplant rejection, cardiac sarcoidosis, hypersensitivity myocarditis, suspected anthracycline cardiomyopathy, heart failure with a restrictive pattern, cardiac tumors, and arrhythmogenic right ventricular cardiomyopathy.

Cardiac Catheterization for Diagnostic and Therapeutic Purposes

A cardiac catheterization is among the most commonly performed modern medical procedures and serves as a diagnostic and therapeutic tool. Patients are often referred for a cardiac catheterization if an electrocardiogram (ECG) or stress test indicates there may be a cardiac condition that requires further diagnostics. Cardiac catheterization procedures include right heart catheterization, left heart catheterization, and coronary angiography with or without intracoronary interventions. The most common use is for the diagnosis of coronary artery disease.[6]

> **Evidence-Based Practice: Nursing implications for cardiac catheterization**
> Because cardiac catheterization involves the insertion of intracardiac or intracoronary instrumentation, cardiac arrhythmias, although relatively low in incidence, are often unavoidable. ASC nurses caring for this patient population are required to identify and be prepared to intervene for the types of arrhythmias and associated risk factors utilizing best practices to reduce risks and improve patient safety. Following the procedure, the nurse may apply manual pressure, a pressure dressing, or a sandbag to the incision site to prevent a hematoma, as well as monitor for hypotension and arrythmias. ASCs may have varying postprocedural policies and guidelines related to the length of time the patient must remain flat or at a 30-degree head elevation until ambulation is allowed.

The *indications* for cardiac catheterization are coronary artery disease, measuring hemodynamics in the right side and left side of the heart, evaluating left ventricular function, evaluating treating cardiac arrhythmias, evaluating and treating valvular heart disease, and assessing pericardial and myocardial diseases.

Electrophysiologic Studies

Electrophysiologic studies are like cardiac catheterizations. The purpose of the studies is to assess a patient's cardiac electrical system or activity. Electrode catheters are placed in the heart's chambers to assess a patient's cardiac electrical system or activity. Cardiac activity is either analyzed in real time or reviewed offline. Cardiac recordings are used to determine activation sequences during arrhythmias. This process is referred to as "mapping."

Electrophysiologic studies determine the mechanisms, physical characteristics, and effects of pharmacologic therapy for arrhythmias, such as bradyarrhythmia, supraventricular tachycardias, and ventricular tachycardia. These determinations assist in confirming whether the arrythmia is best treated pharmacologically, with device implantation, or by ablation.

The *nursing implications* for electrophysiologic studies are like those for cardiac catheterization.

The *indications* for electrophysiologic studies are sinus node dysfunction, atrioventricular conduction malfunction, syncope of unknown origin, wide-complex QRS tachycardia, and ventricular tachycardia.

Pacemaker Generator Change

Pacemakers are devices implanted subcutaneously in the infraclavicular region to regulate heart rhythms for treatment of conditions and symptoms such as bradycardia, syncope, heart failure, and hypertrophic cardiomyopathy. A pacemaker generator gradually becomes depleted over time. The average

generator life is 6–10 years. In the elective replacement indication phase, the pacemaker automatically reprograms itself to extend the generator life. If the generator is not replaced during the elective replacement indication phase, the pacemaker progresses to the end-of-life phase and eventually stops working. Patients experience a varying degree of symptoms and clinical events, such as chest pain, dyspnea, dizziness, fainting or loss of consciousness, palpitations, muscle twitches in the chest or abdomen, frequent hiccups, and heart rate changes.[7]

> **Evidence-Based Practice: Nursing implications for pacemaker generator change**
> **Following the** procedure, the ASC nurse monitors and assesses the pacemaker function, observes for bleeding at the incision sites, and watches for symptoms related to the patient's heart rate, such as dizziness, palpitations, and syncope. Important postprocedural patient teaching includes refraining from wearing tight-fitting clothing, raising the upper extremities above the head, and lifting until the incision is healed. Patients with a pacemaker or an implantable cardioverter-defibrillator must be extremely cautious about avoiding high-voltage, radiation, and magnetic fields. Wearing an identification necklace or bracelet, as well as alerting all healthcare providers, is highly encouraged.

Implantable Cardioverter-Defibrillator

An implantable cardioverter-defibrillator (ICD) is like a pacemaker; the one main difference is that wires are embedded in the heart muscle to deliver an electric shock when an abnormal or life-threatening heart rhythm is detected (Figure 35.1). The shock resets the heart's electrical current, thus correcting the rhythm. Technologic advances in ICDs are launched every few years to improve patient safety and outcomes, as well as reduce costs. Device interrogation can be performed remotely via blue-tooth technology, allowing in-home services.[8]

The *nursing implications* mimic those of patients with pacemaker generator changes. Additionally, the ASC nurse educates the patient on what it feels like if the device delivers a shock, as well as who to notify if this occurs.

The *indications* for implanting an ICD are heart failure, reduced ejection fraction, ventricular tachyarrhythmias, and prevention of sudden cardiac death.

Cardioversion

Cardioversions are performed in ASCs to convert non–life-threatening cardiac dysrhythmias such as atrial flutter, hemodynamically stable fibrillation, and tachyarrhythmias to a sinus rhythm. External cardioversion is performed under sedation or short-acting anesthesia. A 12-lead ECG is needed to determine the baseline cardiac rhythm, as well as be displayed for the appropriate sequence of shock delivery. Electrodes are placed in the anteroposterior or base-apex location to synchronize to the peak of the QRS. Under no circumstances should the shock be delivered on the T wave. Once a satisfactory synchronization is obtained, sedation or anesthesia is initiated and a shock is delivered.[9]

> **Evidence-Based Practice: Nursing implications for cardiac adverse events**
> It is important for the ASC nurse to understand adverse events and monitor the patient for their occurrence, as well as know how to respond to the events. The patient may develop

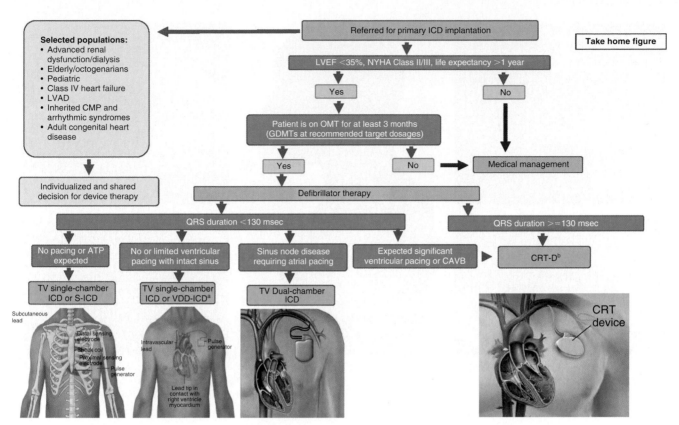

Take home figure

Selected populations:
- Advanced renal dysfunction/dialysis
- Elderly/octogenarians
- Pediatric
- Class IV heart failure
- LVAD
- Inherited CMP and arrhythmic syndromes
- Adult congenital heart disease

Referred for primary ICD implantation

LVEF <35%, NYHA Class II/III, life expectancy >1 year

Yes / No

Patient is on OMT for at least 3 months (GDMTs at recommended target dosages)

Yes / No

Individualized and shared decision for device therapy

Medical management

Defibrillator therapy

QRS duration <130 msec / QRS duration >=130 msec

No pacing or ATP expected | No or limited ventricular pacing with intact sinus | Sinus node disease requiring atrial pacing | Expected significant ventricular pacing or CAVB | CRT-D[b]

TV single-chamber ICD or S-ICD | TV single-chamber ICD or VDD-ICD[a] | TV Dual-chamber ICD

Subcutaneous lead / Distal sensing electrode / Shock coil / Proximal sensing electrode / Pulse generator

Intravascular lead / Pulse generator / Lead tip in contact with right ventricle myocardium

CRT device

Fig. 35.1 Ilan Goldenberg, David T Huang, Jens Cosedis Nielsen, The role of implantable cardioverter-defibrillators and sudden cardiac death prevention: indications, device selection, and outcome, *European Heart Journal*, Volume 41, Issue 21, 1 June 2020, Pages 2003–201.

atrioventricular nodal dysrhythmias, ventricular dysrhythmias, cardiac arrest, hypotension, pulmonary edema, embolism due to cardiac clot disruption, and superficial skin burns. Abnormal cardiac rhythms usually develop within minutes of the cardioversion. Clot dislodgement may lead to a stroke or a pulmonary embolism. Minor skin burns may develop where the external electrodes are placed.

Transesophageal Echocardiography

A transesophageal echocardiogram (TEE) uses echocardiographic sound waves to assess the size and shape of the heart, as well as to visualize how well the heart valves are functioning (Figure 35.2). A TEE can determine areas of damage from previous heart attacks, as well as identify areas of poor blood flow. Once IV sedation is given and a topical anesthetic is applied to inhibit the gag reflex, an ultrasound probe with a transducer is inserted in the esophagus.[10]

The *indications* for TEE are heart valve disease, pericardial effusion, congenital heart disease, left ventricular dysfunction, and endocarditis.

Evidence-Based Practice: Nursing implications for transesophageal echocardiography
Following the procedure, patients are monitored for swallowing due to the topical anesthetic applied. Because the transducer was inserted in the esophagus, a mild sore throat is common. On rare occasions, the transducer can damage the inside of the esophagus, causing bleeding or a tear.

Intravascular Ultrasound

Intravascular ultrasound (IVUS) is a diagnostic procedure used to view the inside of a coronary artery. The catheter-based ultrasound provides a visual image of the inside of the lumen and the atheroma to identify areas of stenosis, plaque distribution and composition, and arterial dissection.

The *indications* for IVUS are coronary artery disease and the assessment of vessel lesions before and after angioplasty, atherectomy, or stenting.

The *nursing implications* for IVUS are mainly monitoring for complications.

Complications after the procedure are rare; however, the ASC nurse needs to understand, identify, and address occlusions, embolisms, myocardial infarcts, angina, and coronary dissection.

Insertion of Central Vascular Access Devices

The Infusion Nurses Society (INS) is a national nursing organization devoted to ensuring that evidence-based practice and optimal care management of central vascular access devices (CVADs) are delivered to all organizations. The INS charges each ASC with developing policies and procedures to align CVAD care with standards of practice. ASCs collect quality outcome data associated with CVADs to drive practices, as well as determine educational and competency needs for the nurses (Table 35.1).[11,12]

A CVAD has been successfully inserted when an x-ray indicates that the catheter tip terminates in the superior vena cava above the right atrium. Insertion sites may vary and include the jugular vein, subclavian vein, and upper extremity veins.

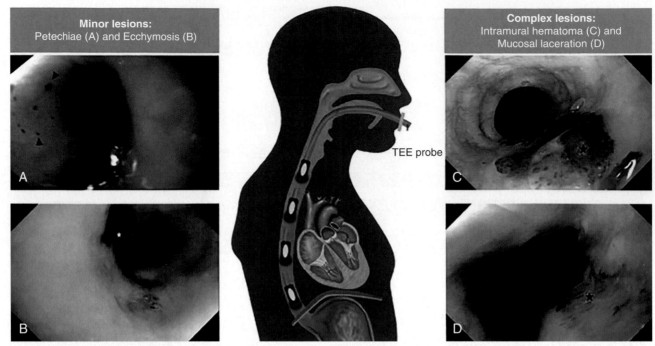

Fig. 35.2 Transesophageal Echocardiography. Types of lesions associated with TEE manipulation during structural cardiac interventions. Freitas-Ferraz AB, Bernier M, Vaillancourt R, et al. Safety of transesophageal echocardiography to guide structural cardiac interventions. *J Am Coll Cardiol.* 2020;75(25):3164–3173. doi: 10.1016/j.jacc.2020.04.069. PMID: 32586591.

The *indications* for inserting a CVAD are therapy that is contraindicated for peripheral IV infusion, long-term medication infusion, and venous monitoring and blood sampling.

> **Evidence-Based Practice: Nursing implications for central vascular access device insertion**
> Central vascular access device insertion at ASC facilities continues to be a prevalent procedure. However, a bloodstream infection, which is preventable, remains a source of patient harm, with a significant negative impact on patients and healthcare costs. Catheter-related bloodstream infections have become less common with the use of single-lumen, antimicrobial-impregnated catheters with a shortened dwelling time of 1–3 weeks.

Arteriovenous Fistula

An arteriovenous fistula is created to connect an artery with a vein. This connection is referred to as an anastomosis. An anastomosis allows blood to bypass the surrounding capillaries, thus diminishing their blood supply. A wider and stronger, surgically created anastomosis aims for increased blood flow and for the insertion of a large-bore needle for hemodialysis. There are both surgically created and nonsurgically percutaneously created arteriovenous fistulas.

The *indication* for creating an arteriovenous fistula is renal failure requiring chronic hemodialysis.

> **Evidence-Based Practice: Nursing implications for arteriovenous fistula**
> Important patient education after creation of an arteriovenous fistula includes ensuring the patient communicates that blood pressure readings, venous blood draws, and IV insertions cannot be performed in the extremity with the arteriovenous fistula.

Wearing a medical identification band on the affected limb is recommended. ASC nurses assess for a bruit, which is audible by stethoscope, and a thrill, which is palpable. Both the bruit and thrill are effects of the vibration caused by arterial blood integrating with deoxygenated blood. The ASC nurse explains to and teaches the patient how to assess the arteriovenous fistula by use of a stethoscope and by palpation with the fingers, as well as how to identify complications. Complications following the creation of an arteriovenous fistula include swelling in the extremity, decreased blood pressure, low flow due to obstruction, thrombosis, hand ischemia, pseudoaneurysm, and infection.

Temporal Artery Biopsy

Temporal artery biopsies are performed to remove a section of the temporal artery for testing and diagnosis. Commonly, these biopsies are completed under local anesthesia. The most common reason for performing the biopsy is to diagnose giant cell arteritis, which is an inflammatory condition of the arteries. The patient may experience headaches, blindness, double vision, aneurysm, or stroke. Advances in technology have led to the use of ultrasound to detect the signs and symptoms of inflamed arteries, and this has reduced the need for biopsy procedures.

The *nursing implications* for temporal artery biopsy involve monitoring the patient for facial nerve damage and stroke.

Gastrointestinal Endoscopy

Gastrointestinal (GI) endoscopy procedures are the primary invasive methods of diagnosis and therapy for GI conditions such as cancer, achalasia, GI bleeds, colitis, and anemia.[13] The digestive system is composed of the GI tract, which is a hollow organs, and the liver, pancreas, and gallbladder, which are solid organs. The tract is a series of organs joined together; they are the mouth, esophagus, stomach, small intestine, large intestine, and anus (Figure 35.3).

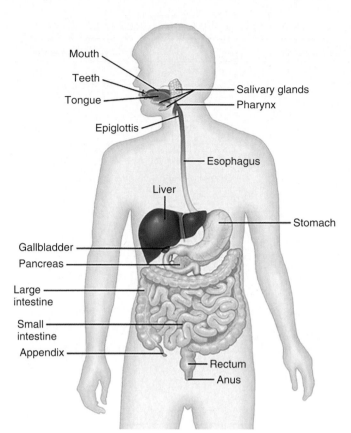

Mouth
Teeth
Tongue
Salivary glands
Pharynx
Epiglottis
Esophagus
Liver
Stomach
Gallbladder
Pancreas
Large intestine
Small intestine
Appendix
Rectum
Anus

Fig. 35.3 Digestive System. Diagram of human digestive tract. https://cdn.britannica.com/39/8039-050-B124FC20/human-digestive-system-front.jpg

The ASC nurse's role in GI endoscopy procedures may include preprocedural, intraprocedural, and postprocedural care. This necessitates a vast amount of knowledge and skill, as the intraprocedural nurse may be administering conscious sedation or technically assisting the proceduralist.

GI procedures are commonly scheduled through an open-access process. This allows for physicians other than GI physicians to directly refer patients to the ASC for a GI procedure. Open access is a cost-effective and time-efficient scheduling practice that negates the need for a GI consultation prior to receiving the procedure. Despite the popularity of open-access scheduling, inferior outcomes continue. Monitoring and evaluation persist to improve the preprocedural obstacles, such as discontinuing anticoagulation and antiplatelet therapy, ordering prophylactic antibiotic drug therapy, conducting an anesthesia consult for possible anesthesia-assisted sedation, and poor bowel preparation. ASC nurses play a key role in preprocedural screening and preparation, as well as intraprocedural care and aftercare. The American Society for Gastrointestinal Endoscopy (ASGE) is dedicated to "advancing digestive care through education, advocacy and promotion of excellence and innovation in endoscopy."[14] The ASGE journal is titled *Gastrointestinal Endoscopy*.

Preprocedural Care

Preprocedural preparation for a GI endoscopy commences in the physician's office when the procedure or treatment is prescribed and scheduled. Education related to the preparation, procedure, and postprocedural care for the patient is delivered to the patient and family member to allow for questions and answers. The gastroenterologist prescribes the preparation based on the individual patient, the procedure, and the patient's medical insurance. The most current guidelines for available bowel preparation products and strategies are available on the ASGE website.[14] Because endoscopic procedures are performed under sedation or anesthesia, the patient may require preadmission testing. The patient is instructed to arrive on the day of procedure accompanied by a responsible individual who will be providing care to the patient after the procedure. The preprocedural education is crucial, as poor patient preparation may lead to delays or cancellations, as well as aggravations for the patient, responsible individual, and ASC caregivers (Tables 35.2 and 35.3).

The patient and responsible individual may be advised to arrive on the day of the procedure 1–2 hours earlier than the scheduled procedure time. During this time, the nurse completes a general health history, paying close attention to GI, respiratory, cardiac, and endocrine system concerns. A physical examination of the patient's abdomen is completed, with a focus on firmness, tenderness, or distention. The patient's height, weight, and vital signs are obtained. A thorough review of recent laboratory and diagnostic tests is completed. Any abnormal results are communicated to the proceduralist for review. The ASC nurse also reviews the patient's medication history and verifies the medications currently prescribed and the most recent dosage taken. Because bleeding is an invasive procedure risk, a careful review of anticoagulation and antiplatelet therapy is necessary. The ASGE has official guidelines on the management of anticoagulation and antiplatelet agents, including recommendations related to whether the medication is held or continued. The recommendations are based on the urgency of the procedure, risk of thromboembolism, and risk of bleeding.[14] Verification that the patient is compliant with the NPO instructions, as well as the successful completion of the prescribed bowel preparation, is extremely important. If the patient could not comply with either of these instructions, the nurse notifies the proceduralist immediately.

ASCs have varied policies and procedures related to patient valuables and clothing, advance directives, and informed consents. The nurse discusses the patient's advance directive status and ensures that the informed consent for the appropriate procedure is completed and signed, as well as provides education to the patient about the risks and benefits of the procedure and what to expect during and after the procedure. This is also the time for the patient and the companion to ask questions. Some facilities may require that all jewelry and all clothing be removed prior to the procedure. Others may require removal for only certain areas of the body. These regulations are specific to the facility and the state in which it is located. The necessity for removal of a patient's dentures or partial dentures, contact lenses, glasses, and hearing aids is based on the type of procedure and facility policies.

Once the preprocedural intake is complete, the nurse or anesthesia provider places an IV catheter. Most GI procedures call for a small-bore IV catheter, either 24 or 22 gauge. The facility policies and LIP orders determine the site of the IV and the IV fluid and rate, as well as IV antibiotic prophylaxis if indicated. GI endoscopies are no longer deemed high-risk procedures; therefore, neither the ASGE nor the American Heart Association recommend the use of antibiotics for endocarditis prophylaxis any longer.[14] At this time, the ASC nurse educates the patient about the GI suite experience. Explanation of the equipment, lighting, sounds, team members, and processes is extremely important for helping to reduce patient anxieties.

Intraprocedural Care

During GI procedures, the ASC nurse may function as either the sedation nurse or technical nurse. Preparation of the GI

TABLE 35.2 Central Venous Access Devices

CVAD Duration	Terminology	Previous Terminology	Types	Abbreviation
Short term (days to weeks if tunnelled)	Centrally Inserted Central Catheter	CVC Central line	Non-tunnelled CICC/standard	CICC
			Tunnelled CICC	t-CICC
	Femorally Inserted Central Catheter	Femoral line	Non-tunnelled FICC/standard	FICC
			Tunnelled FICC	t-FICC
	Apheresis Catheter	Vas-Cath	Non-tunnelled apheresis catheter	A-CICC
			Tunnelled apheresis catheter	t-A-CICC
Intermediate term (potentially weeks, months, or longer)	Peripherally Inserted Central Catheter	PICC	Non-tunnelled PICC	PICC
			Tunnelled PICC	t-PICC
Long term (potentially months to years)	Tunnelled Cuffed Centrally Inserted Central Catheter	Hickman Broviac		tc-CICC
	Totally Implantable Venous Access Device	Port-a-cath Infusaport		TIVAD or portacath
	Tunnelled Cuffed Apheresis Catheters	Permacath Permcath		tc-A-CICC

The **catheter tip** location for CVADs with the greatest safety profile in adult and pediatric patients is at the cavoatrial junction.[1] The lower third of the superior vena cava or the upper right atrium is also acceptable.[1,6]

New CVAD terminology is emerging in the literature and research to standardize CVAD names and definitions globally.

Central venous access devices. Types of CVADs. Available at: https://www.eviq.org.au/clinical-resources/central-venous-access-devices-cvads/112-central-venous-access-devices

TABLE 35.3 Specialized Endoscopy Procedures

Procedure	Definition	Indication	Nursing Implications
Esophagogastro-duodenoscopy (EGD)	Esophagogastroduodenoscopy (EGD), also known as upper endoscopy or gastroscopy, is a diagnostic endoscopic procedure that examines the esophagus, stomach, and duodenum with an endoscope	Abdominal pain Dysphagia Prolonged nausea and vomiting Gastroesophageal reflux disease (GERD) Unexplained weight loss Anemia Hematochezia	Immediately following the procedure, the patient may experience bloating or nausea, as well as a sore throat that may persist for 1–2 days. Due to the local anesthetic applied to the throat, it is important to evaluate the patient's ability to swallow before eating or drinking. Bleeding from the mouth following the procedure may indicate a tear or perforation of the esophagus or stomach, which needs immediate medical evaluation. Important postprocedural patient teaching of the following signs and symptoms that require medical attention: 1. Fever 2. Chest pain 3. Shortness of breath 4. Bloody, black-colored stool 5. Dysphagia 6. Severe or persistent vomiting 7. Hematemesis
Esophageal dilatation	Esophageal dilatation is a therapeutic endoscopic procedure that enlarges or stretches the lumen of the esophagus.	Esophageal scarring from GERD Cancer of the esophagus Esophageal scarring from radiation treatment Esophageal motility disorders	Immediately following the procedure, the patient may experience a sore throat that may persist for one–2 days. Due to the local anesthetic applied to the throat, it is important to evaluate the patient's ability to swallow before eating or drinking. Bleeding from the mouth following the procedure may indicate a tear or perforation of the esophagus, which needs immediate medical evaluation. Important postprocedural patient teaching of the following signs and symptoms that require medical attention: 1. Fever 2. Chest pain 3. Shortness of breath 4. Bloody, black-colored stool 5. Dysphagia 6. Severe or persistent vomiting 7. Hematemesis

TABLE 35.3 Specialized Endoscopy Procedures—cont'd

Procedure	Definition	Indication	Nursing Implications
Sclerotherapy	Sclerotherapy is a procedure to treat and prevent hemorrhaging esophageal varices. An esophagoscope is used to examine and visualize the varices, which are then injected with a hypertonic saline to shrink the vessel. Sclerotherapy has been almost 100% replaced with EVL due to the increased safety and improved patient outcomes.[1]	Manage acute variceal bleeding	Preprocedural awareness: Bacteremia has been reported in up to 50% of patients undergoing sclerotherapy. It is recommended that patients with cirrhosis, those who are immunocompromised, and those with mechanical prosthetic devices, a history of endocarditis, vascular grafts, surgical systemic-pulmonary shunts, or ascites should receive antibiotic prophylaxis before sclerotherapy.[1]
Endoscopic variceal ligation (EVL)	Endoscopic variceal ligation, or endoscopic band ligation, is a procedure that uses elastic bands to treat enlarged esophageal veins, or varices.	Manage acute variceal bleeding	Immediately following the procedure, the patient may experience a sore throat that may persist for one–2 days. Due to the local anesthetic applied to the throat, it is important to evaluate the patient's ability to swallow before eating or drinking. Bleeding from the mouth following the procedure may indicate a tear or perforation of the esophagus, which needs immediate medical evaluation. Important postprocedural patient teaching of the following signs and symptoms that require medical attention: 1. Fever 2. Chest pain 3. Shortness of breath 4. Bloody, black-colored stool 5. Dysphagia 6. Severe or persistent vomiting 7. Hematemesis
Colonoscopy	A colonoscopy is an endoscopic procedure using a thin, flexible colonoscope to examine and visualize the rectum and colon, usually as far as the cecum. It is possible to examine as far as the terminal ileum.	Ulcers Inflammation Hemorrhoids Diverticula Strictures Hematochezia Abdominal pain Diarrhea Change in bowel habits Screen for colon polyps and colon cancer	Following the procedure, the ASC nurse will: Observe the patient for signs of bowel perforation, such as severe abdominal pain, nausea, vomiting, fever, and chills Provide patient privacy and inform patients that they may expel copious amounts of flatus Monitor for rectal bleeding. If a polyp was removed, minimal rectal bleeding is expected for up to 2 days immediately. *Postprocedural patient teaching is the same as for the procedures above. Patients may experience cramping and bloating for several hours following the procedure.
Sigmoidoscopy	Sigmoidoscopy is a less invasive examination than colonoscopy. The exam is of the large intestine from the rectum to the sigmoid colon. There are two types of sigmoidoscopies: Flexible sigmoidoscopy, which uses a flexible endoscope Rigid sigmoidoscopy, which uses a rigid device	Ulcers InflammationHemorrhoids Diverticula Strictures Hematochezia Abdominal pain Diarrhea Change in bowel habits Screen for colon polyps and colon cancer	Same as for colonoscopy
Endoscopic retrograde cholangiopancreatography (ERCP)	Endoscopic retrograde cholangiopancreatography is a diagnostic procedure performed to treat biliary and pancreatic ductal systems issues. It combines the use of fluoroscopy and endoscopy.	Obstructive jaundice Pancreatic ductal system disease Diagnose pancreatic cancer Pancreatitis of unknown cause Manometry for sphincter of Oddi Nasobiliary drainage Biliary stenting for strictures and leakage Drainage for pancreatic pseudocysts	Possible postprocedural complications for the ASC nurse to be aware of: Sepsis Acute pancreatitis Hemorrhage Perforation Signs and symptoms to educate the patient on that need immediate medical evaluation: Fever Rigor Abdominal pain or distention

Adapted from: O'Brien D. Gastrointestinal. Pages 517–536 in: Schick L, Windle PE. *Perianesthesia Nursing Core Curriculum: Preprocedure, Phase I and Phase II PACU Nursing.* 4th ed. Elsevier; 2021.

TABLE 35.4 Other Gastrointestinal Procedures

Procedure	Definition	Indication	Nursing Implications
Liver biopsy	Tissue samples are removed from the liver for microscopic examination of damage or disease. There are three basic types of liver biopsies: Percutaneous (also known as fine-needle biopsy [FNB]); involves insertion of a thin needle through the abdomen and into the liver Transjugular; involves the creation of a small incision over the jugular vein to allow a flexible tube to be passed into the liver to obtain the biopsy; patients with bleeding disorders are candidates for this type of biopsy Laparoscopic; a surgical approach using puncture sites using tube-like instruments that collect the sample through a small incision in the abdomen	Examine tissue under a microscope for signs and symptoms of disease or damage. Digestive system issues Persistent abdominal pain Right upper quadrant abdominal mass Laboratory tests pointing to the liver as an area of concern	Possible postprocedural complications for the ASC nurse to be aware of: Pain at the biopsy site Excessive bleeding that may require a transfusion or surgical intervention Infection due to bacteria entering the abdominal cavity or bloodstream Accidental organ injury from the needle placement
Abdominal paracentesis	Also called an abdominal tap; a procedure that removes ascites (buildup of fluid) from the abdomen; abdominal paracentesis is a simple bedside or clinic procedure in which a needle is inserted into the peritoneal cavity and ascitic fluid is removed	New-onset ascites: fluid evaluation helps to determine etiology, differentiate transudate versus exudate, detect the presence of cancerous cells, or address other considerations Suspected spontaneous or secondary bacterial peritonitis Refractory ascites.	Possible postprocedural complications for the ASC nurse to be aware of: Ascitic fluid leakage Hemorrhage Infection Perforation

Adapted from: Dooley A, Grossman VA. Interventional Radiology and Special Procedures. In: Schick L, Windle PE *PeriAnesthesia Nursing Core Curriculum: Preprocedure, Phase I and Phase II PACU Nursing.* 4th Edition. Elsevier, 2021. P 833-842.

suite, including the equipment, medications, and team members, is determined by ASC policies, local practice, state regulations, and the Society of Gastroenterology Nurses and Associates (SGNA).[15] A monitor showing the noninvasive blood pressure, pulse oximetry, capnography, and cardiac information is available and in clear sight of all team members. After the time-out is completed to ensure the patient is accurately identified, the procedure is verified, and the consent is complete, the nurse further explains the procedure and reassures the patient. For upper endoscopies, topical anesthesia may be sprayed in the back of the patient's throat. This is best tolerated in a seated position to prevent the lidocaine solution from traveling into the patient's lungs. Both upper and lower GI procedures are performed with the patient in the left lateral position.

Moderate or procedural sedation facilitates a safe, comfortable, and efficient endoscopic examination. Both the sedation nurse and the proceduralist are responsible for monitoring the sedated patient. Some facilities may employ anesthesia providers to administer anesthesia and sedation. It is, however, more cost-effective to employ nurses with sedation skills.

There is currently no standard sedation regimen. Proceduralist and facility policy determine the choice of sedation used. Propofol continues to be the most frequently used drug for sedation; however, facility and state regulations are dependent on the medical professional licensed to administer propofol for sedation. Propofol is preferred because it is short-acting and safe for most patient populations.[16] Capnography is widely used when administering propofol to detect hypoventilation sooner than it would be detected by desaturation identified by pulse oximetry or direct observation. A second choice after propofol is a drug from the class of benzodiazepines. Midazolam is the benzodiazepine of choice due to its short duration of action and sound pharmacokinetic effects.

Documentation is always a nursing responsibility when one is caring for patients. Real-time documentation is preferred. Many procedural suites have vital sign auto population records, which decrease the nurse's workload. The nurse documents the patient's status throughout the procedure, including the level of pain and any complications, to depict a clear picture of events. This is also the time when biopsy specimens are verified for appropriate documentation, labeling, and anatomic retrieval location prior to being sent off to the laboratory.

If a patient transitions from moderate/procedural sedation to deep sedation, a reversal agent may be administered, such as naloxone for narcotic reversal or flumazenil for benzodiazepine reversal. Resuscitation equipment, supplemental oxygen, and IV therapy are also readily available. Most states and facilities require sedation nurses and proceduralists to be trained in advanced cardiovascular life support.

When functioning as a technical nurse, the nurse assists the proceduralist during the procedure. This may include obtaining biopsies with a biopsy snare, manipulating the patient's abdomen for improved visualization and being responsible for the operation of equipment throughout the procedure. Some facilities employ GI technicians to assist the proceduralists. Both nurses and GI technicians are educated and competent in high-level disinfection. Regulations and processes are consistently updated by the ASGE and the FDA to provide the safest environment for patients and employees. Germicides and endoscopy scope reprocessors are used to clean and disinfect endoscopic equipment to prevent the spread of germs and disease.

Postprocedural Care

The postprocedural period extends from the completion of the procedure to the time of patient discharge to go home. The postprocedural nurse is responsible for patient monitoring and postprocedural education. Postprocedural monitoring is dependent upon the facility's discharge criteria policy and the guidelines from the SGNA and American Society of PeriAnesthesia Nurses. Typical vital sign monitoring includes the blood pressure, oxygen saturation, and level of consciousness, and they are assessed every 15 minutes until the patient meets the discharge criteria or the criteria established by the anesthesia department. Patients are encouraged to pass flatus, as air and water are infused via the endoscope during the procedure to assist in colon visualization.

Major postprocedural complications for nurses to be aware include adverse reactions to medications, viscous or vessel perforation, and hemorrhage. These complications may occur during, immediately after, or hours after the procedure. Signs of perforation and hemorrhage include severe or increasing pain, increased temperature, abdominal distention, subcutaneous emphysema, shortness of breath, hypotension, diaphoresis, and bleeding. If the patient received a reversal agent during or after the procedure, facility policies will dictate postprocedural length of stay prior to going home. The nurses will educate the patient and responsible individual to ensure they understand the complications, signs, and symptoms that require immediate attention, as well as what to do should these occur.

The importance of safety after sedation and anesthesia is emphasized, such as abstaining from driving a car and using machinery, drinking alcohol, taking sedatives, or sleeping pills, and signing legal documents. Most facilities encourage the responsible individual to remain with the patient for 24 hours following the procedure. Follow-up appointments are usually not necessary. The LIP notifies the patient once biopsy results are known. A follow-up phone call may be offered to track patient satisfaction and ensure the safety of the patient's postprocedural status.

Interventional Radiology Procedures

Patient convenience, insurance reimbursement, and business opportunities have led to profit organizations being owned and managed by interventional radiologists and radiology groups or managed jointly with a hospital system. These centers are referred to as interventional radiology ambulatory surgery centers (irASCs). An interventional radiologic procedure is defined as an interventional surgical procedure performed by an interventionist surgeon. There are over 40 interventional radiologic procedures currently performed at irASCs. An irASC nurse cares for patients receiving minimally invasive image-guided procedures to diagnose and treat diseases in nearly every organ system. The 12 most common irASC procedures are:

1. Percutaneous vertebral augmentation
2. Biliary stent placement
3. Kidney drain placement
4. Ablation of liver tumor
5. Ablation of renal tumor
6. Transcatheter intravascular stent placement
7. Inserted tunneled intraperitoneal percutaneous catheter
8. Nephrostomy
9. Vascular embolization
10. Removal of intravascular foreign body
11. Percutaneous cervicothoracic injection
12. Biliary endoscopy through skin[17]

The irASC nurse functions like a GI nurse. The nurse may be trained to provide care in the preprocedural, intraprocedural, and postprocedural areas. The intraprocedural nurse is trained to assist the LIP technically, as well as to administer sedation. The patient population ranges from those receiving diagnostic procedures and who are in optimal health to those with extremely high acuity needing life-saving measures. An irASC nurse is a highly specialized, highly trained nurse. The need for these nurses is growing fast as ambulatory facilities become increasingly competitive.

Procedures to Enhance the Healing of Wound due to Trauma or Surgical Interventions

Wound healing is a surgical and medical specialty. Wound treatments include cleaning and dressing the wound. The process of wound healing is dependent on how the body restores and replaces the damaged tissue. There are several types of wounds, such as lacerations, hidradenitis suppurativa and pilonidal sinus wounds, wounds from explosions and gunshots, surgical site infections, and burns. The stage of wound healing, wound class, and technique of wound closure determine the course of tissue restoration. The World Health Organization classifies wound healing as having four stages.

Stage 1: Vascular response
Stage 2: Inflammatory response
Stage 3: Proliferative/granulation phase
Stage 4: Remodeling/maturation phase.
The wound classifications are[18]:

1. Clean wound: Uncontaminated wound without transgression into the respiratory, GI, or genitourinary tract. Examples of clean wounds are hernia surgeries and mastectomies, which require a primary closure.
2. Clean-contaminated wound: Wound that enters the GI, genitourinary, or respiratory tract but for which there is no gross contamination or spillage. Examples are cholecystectomy and elective gastric surgeries. The wound usually has primary closure.
3. Contaminated wound: Wound with gross spillage because of puncturing the GI, genitourinary, or respiratory tract. Lavaging the area with saline and antibiotics is necessary to remove all gross contaminants. Closure is dependent on the ability to thoroughly clean the body cavity.
4. Dirty wound: Infected wound with necrotic tissue or an already perforated wound with known organisms. Debridement is necessary, and primary closure is not recommended.

The techniques of wound closure are:

1. Closure by primary intention: Multiple layers of suture are used to approximate the wound edges. The final layer of closure may be wound adhesive or skin tape.
2. Closure by secondary intention: Deeper tissue layers may be closed, leaving the skin layers open.[18]

An ASC nurse is knowledgeable about the stages of wound healing, as well as highly skilled in wound management. Education for the patient and the caretaker is essential. Knowledge of the appropriate cleaning and irrigating treatments for the wound type, the application of topical ointments, and the appropriate dressing choices and techniques are obtained and kept current by ASC wound nurses. Wound management is vital to the patient's path to recovery.

Tissue viability nursing has been a specialty since the 1980s. Along with surgical wound management, the tissue viability nurse also cares for situations in which the soft tissue and skin break down, as in pressure injuries and chronic ulcerations. These nurses are vital team players, as they are often the wound experts teaching the LIPs. Tissue viability nurses may place vacuum-assisted closure devices in the operating room and then continue to manage the devices in the home setting. A foam dressing is applied to the wound using an airtight seal to create negative pressure that pulls exudate from the wound into a canister. The purpose is to keep the wound moist but not wet while promoting healing.

There are several factors that determine the success of wound healing. The World Health Organization credits the following indirect and direct factors as influences on the success of wound healing; age, nutritional status, co-morbidities, type of organ or tissue, severity of injury, wound contamination, time lapse between injury and treatment, local factors related to surgical technique, hemostasis, wound debridement, and timing of closure.

CHAPTER HIGHLIGHTS

- Hospital-based surgical cases are transitioning to ASCs to reduce costs, increase efficiency, and improve patient satisfaction.
- ASC nurses are highly skilled in caring for a vast population of surgical patients and surgical specialties; their skills require consistent and up-to-date education and depend on evidence-based practice.
- Cardiovascular procedures are advancing rapidly, and more of them are being performed in outpatient settings. The ASC nurse should be educated in identifying and treating the signs and symptoms of bleeding, cardiac arrythmias, stroke, and myocardial infarct.
- Gastrointestinal ASC nurses are highly skilled so that they can practice in preprocedural, intraprocedural, and postprocedural areas.
- Interventional radiologic procedures require nursing skills like those of gastrointestinal ASC nurses. Nurses are involved interprocedurally, and their responsibilities include sedation and technical skills.
- Surgical wound healing relies heavily on ASC nurses and their skills and knowledge, as the nurses are educators for the patients and LIPs.

CASE STUDY

The ASC registered nurse made a phone call on the day following a procedure to a 75-year-old man who had presented for a 3-year follow-up colonoscopy for post-stage 2 colon cancer the previous day.

On the day of the procedure, the patient's vital signs and status were as follows:

- Level of consciousness: Alert and oriented to person, place, and time
- Pain: 0/10
- Vital signs: Blood pressure 120/75 mm Hg, heart rate 77 bpm, Respiratory rate 18 breaths per minute, pulse oximetry 98%, temperature 36.9°C
- Abdomen: soft, nondistended
- American Society of Anesthesiologists patient classification: II due to body mass index of 32 and history of deep vein thrombosis
- Colon preparation: successful
- Medications taken day of procedure: none
- Current medications: simvastatin, omeprazole, hydrochlorothiazide, rivaroxaban (stopped 3 days prior to procedure)

Intraprocedural Notes

- Three colon polyps were removed, measuring 3, 4, and 3.5 mm; they were considered diminutive in size
- Zero complications
- Received 25 µg of fentanyl and 3 mg of midazolam intravenously
- Vital signs stable throughout

Postprocedural Notes

The patient remained in the recovery area for 40 minutes. He aroused easily and offered zero reports of pain. He was easily passing flatus and his vital signs were stable. His wife was present during this time. The patient and wife stated they understood the postprocedural instructions.

Follow-up Phone Call

The day after the procedure a member of the nursing staff made a routine follow-up phone call. The patient complained of severe abdominal cramping, nausea, and intermittent vomiting. The perianesthesia nurse asked the patient if he was able to take his temperature. The result was 38.9°C. When the patient was asked if he had had a bowel movement since his colonoscopy, he replied, "Yes; a small amount of stool with a small streak of blood this morning."

Questions

1. What questions are important to ask related to the patient's medications?
2. If the patient is asked to palpate his abdomen, what result do you anticipate hearing?
3. With the information collected, what diagnosis do you anticipate?
4. What are the appropriate next steps?

REFERENCES

1. Steiner CA, Karaca Z, Moore BJ, Imshaug MC, Pickens G. Surgeries in hospital-based ambulatory surgery and hospital inpatient settings, 2014. In: *Healthcare Cost and Utilization Project (HCUP) Statistical Briefs*. Agency for Healthcare Research and Quality (US); Updated July 2020.
2. Anderson M. *The Benefits of Shifting Cardiovascular Procedures to Outpatient Settings*. Becker's ASC Review. Becker's Healthcare; June 2020. Available at: www.beckersasc.com/cardiology/the-benefits-of-shifting-cardiovascular-procedures-to-outpatient-settings.html?tmpl=component.
3. Chen C, Cai Y, Long X, et al. Age is not a barrier to good outcomes following ambulatory high ligation and stripping for varicose veins: a prospective cohort study. *Medicine (Baltimore)*. 2019;98(49):e18085. Available at: https://doi.org/10.1097/MD.0000000000018085.
4. Jayasilan J, Dak Keung BL. The 'Super Glue': Successful use of VenaSeal Closure System for the treatment of varicose vein in Sabah. *Borneo J Med Sci (BJMS)*, 2021;4:15. Available at: https://jurcon.ums.edu.my/ojums/index.php/bjms/article/view/2945/1940.
5. Sakakibara S, Konno S. Endomyocardial biopsy. *Jap Heart J*. 1962; 3(6):537-543. Available at: https://doi.org/10.1536/ihj.3.537.
6. Benjamin EJ, Muntner P, Alonso A, et al. Heart disease and stroke statistics—2019 update: a report from the American Heart Association. *Circulation*. 2019;139(10):e56-e528. Available at: https://doi.org/10.1161/cir.0000000000000659.
7. Liu J, Wen L, Yao S, Zheng P, Zhao S, Yang J. Adverse clinical events caused by pacemaker battery depletion: two case reports. *BMC Cardiovasc Disord*. 2020;20(1):344. Available at: https://doi.org/10.1186/s12872-020-01622-x.
8. Gierula J, Paton MF, Witte KK. Advances in cardiac resynchronization and implantable cardioverter/defibrillator therapy: medtronic cobalt and crome. *Future Cardiol*. 2021;17(4):609-618. Available at: https://doi.org/10.2217/fca-2020-0117.
9. Tracy CM, Akhtar M, DiMarco JP, et al. American College of Cardiology/American Heart Association clinical competence statement on invasive electrophysiology studies, catheter ablation, and cardioversion: a report of the American College of Cardiology/American Heart Association/American College of Physicians–American Society of Internal Medicine task force on clinical competence. *Circulation*. 2000;102(18):2309-2320. Available at: https://doi.org/10.1161/01.cir.102.18.2309.
10. Freitas-Ferraz AB, Bernier M, Vaillancourt R, et al. Safety of transesophageal echocardiography to guide structural cardiac interventions. *J Am Coll Cardiol*. 2020;75(25):3164-3173. Available at: https://doi.org/10.1016/j.jacc.2020.04.069.
11. Meyer BM, Berndt D, Biscossi M, et al. Vascular access device care and management: a comprehensive organizational approach. *J Infus Nurs*. 2020;43(5):246-254. Available at: https://doi.org/10.1097/nan.0000000000000385.
12. Takashima M, Ray-Barruel G, Ullman A, Keogh S, Rickard CM. Randomized controlled trials in central vascular access devices: a scoping review. *PLoS One*. 2017;12(3):e0174164. Available at: https://doi.org/10.1371/journal.pone.0174164.
13. Chandraekhara V, Elmunzer BJ, Khashab MA, Muthusamy VR, eds. *Clinical Gastrointestinal Endoscopy*. 3rd ed. Elsevier; 2018.
14. American Society of Gastrointestinal Endoscopy. Available at: https://www.asge.org.

15. Society of Gastroenterology Nurses and Associates. *Standard Setting Resources*. Available at: https://www.sgna.org/Practice-Resources/Position-Statements-Standards.

16. Dossa F, Megetto O, Yakubu M, Zhang DDQ, Baxter NN. Sedation practices for routine gastrointestinal endoscopy: a systematic review of recommendations. *BMC Gastroenterol*. 2021;21(1):22. Available at: https://doi.org/10.1186/s12876-020-01561-z.

17. Weiss MF, Kronawitter C. *Is There an Interventional Radiology ASC (irASC) in Your Future? Radiology Business*. 2018. Available at: https://www.radiologybusiness.com/topics/healthcare-policy/there-interventional-radiology-asc-irasc-your-future.

18. Mekhail P, Chaturvedi S, Chaturvedi S. Surgical management of wounds. In: Alexandrescu VA, ed. *Wound Healing-New Insights into Ancient Challenges*. IntechOpen; 2016:343-359.

Index